AF443488

Inflammatory Bowel Diseases: Pathophysiology as Basis of Treatment

Inflammatory Bowel Diseases: Pathophysiology as Basis of Treatment

EDITED BY

J. Schölmerich
Medizinische Klinik und Poliklinik I
Universität Regensburg
Franz-Josef-Strauss-Allee 11
W-8400 Regensburg
Germany

H. Goebell
Klinikum Essen
Medizinische Klinik
Hufelandstr. 55
W-4300 Essen 1
Germany

W. Kruis
Innere Abteilung
Evang. Krankenhaus Kalk
Buchforststr. 2
W-5000 Köln 91
Germany

W. Hohenberger
Chirurgische Klinik und Poliklinik
Universität Regensburg
Franz-Josef-Strauss-Allee 11
W-8400 Regensburg
Germany

V. Gross
Medizinische Klinik und Poliklinik I
Universität Regensburg
Franz-Josef-Strauss-Allee 11
W-8400 Regensburg
Germany

*Proceedings of the 67th Falk Symposium held in Regensburg, Germany,
June 25–27, 1992*

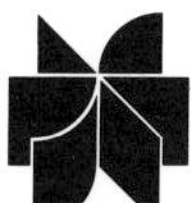

KLUWER ACADEMIC PUBLISHERS
DORDRECHT / BOSTON / LONDON

Distributors

---

for the United States and Canada: Kluwer Academic Publishers, PO Box 358, Accord Station, Hingham, MA 02018-0358, USA
for all other countries: Kluwer Academic Publishers Group, Distribution Center, PO Box 322, 3300 AH Dordrecht, The Netherlands

A catalogue record for this book is available from the British Library

ISBN 0-7923-8996-4

Contents

CONTENTS

CONTENTS

CONTENTS

CONTENTS

xii

Preface

Inflammatory bowel diseases are still a challenging problem in today's gastroenterology. Although their aetiology is still not understood, steady progress has been made during the last years in the understanding of their pathogenesis. This progress has been possible due to the application of innovative molecular biological and cell biological methods. These have improved our knowledge of both the immunology of the gut and the basic mechanisms of inflammatory reactions. There has especially been an explosion of information concerning pro- and anti-inflammatory mediators, the characterization of inflammatory cell types and their functions and molecules mediating cell interactions. Since the main issue of IBD research should be to provide a basis for treatment, many clinicians may ask for the relevance of the findings of basic research. The major aim of a meeting on inflammatory bowel diseases held in Regensburg, 25–27 June 1992, was therefore to close the gap between the new findings in pathophysiology and treatment in order to better understand our current therapeutic concepts and to develop new strategies for the future.

This volume comprises the proceedings of the meeting on 'Inflammatory Bowel Diseases – Pathophysiology as Basis of Treatment'. It contains the lectures given in 15 sessions which covered the fields of aetiology, pathophysiology, extraintestinal manifestations, diagnosis, and treatment. The editors would like to thank all the authors for their contributions which reflect the state of the art in the different fields. To extend the scope the abstracts of posters presented at the meeting are also included in this book.

We are greatly indebted to Dr Herbert Falk and the Falk Foundation, Freiburg for their generous support. We would also like to thank Mr Phil Johnstone from Kluwer Academic Publishers for his cooperation in preparing this volume.

The Editors
September 1992

List of Principal Authors

H. ALLGAYER
Medizinische Klinik I
Städtisches Klinikum
Moltkestr. 14
W-7500 Karlsruhe 1
Germany

K. E. BARRETT
University of California
San Diego Medical Center, 8414
225 Dickinson Street
University of California
San Diego
CA 92103-8414
USA

I. BJARNASON
Department of Clinical Biochemistry
King's College School of Medicine
and Dentistry
King's College London
Bessemer Road
London SE5 9PJ
UK

H. J. BUHR
Chirurgische Klinik der
Universität Heidelberg
Im Neuenheimer Feld 110
W-6900 Heidelberg
Germany

W. F. DOE
Division of Medical Sciences
John Curtis School of Medical Research
Australian National University
POBox 334
Canberra City
AT 2601
Australia

D. A. DROSSMAN
The University of North Carolina
School of Medicine
Chapel Hill
NC 27599-7080
USA

K. W. ECKER
Abteilung Allgemeine Chirurgie
Universitätskliniken im Landeskrankenhaus
Homburg
W-6650 Homburg/Saar
Germany

G. EKELUND
University of Lund
Department of Surgery
Malmö General Hospital
S-21401 Malmö
Sweden

V. E. EYSSELEIN
Harbor-ULCA Medical Center
Division of Gastroenterology
1000 West Carson Street
Torrance
CA 90509
USA

R. G. FARMER
9126 Town Gate Lane
Bethesda
MD 20817-4111
USA

V. W. FAZIO
Department of Colorectal Surgery
Cleveland Clinic Foundation
9500 Euclid Avenue
Cleveland
OH 44195-5014
USA

C. FIOCCHI
Cleveland Clinic Foundation
Research Institute
9500 Euclid Avenue
Cleveland
OH 44195-5014
USA

W. FISCHBACH
Medizinische Poliklinik der Universität
Klinikstr. 8
W-8700 Würzburg
Germany

W. E. FLEIG
Medizinische Klinik I mit Poliklinik
der Universität Erlangen
Krankenhausstr. 12
W-8520 Erlangen
Germany

H. FROMM
Division of Gastroenterology
The George Washington University
Medical Center
2150 Pennsylvania Avenue NW
Washington
DC 20037
USA

H. GOEBELL
Klinikum Essen
Medizinische Klinik
Hufelandstr. 55
W-4300 Essen I
Germany

D. N. GRANGER
Louisiana State University Medical Center
Department of Physiology and Biophysics
PO Box 33932
Shreveport, LA 71130-3932
USA

V. GROSS
Medizinische Klinik und Poliklinik I
Universität Regensburg
Franz-Josef-Strauss Allee 11
W-8400 Regensburg
Germany

F. HARTMANN
Medizinische Klinik
St. Marienkrankenhaus
Richard-Wagner-Str. 4
W-6000 Frankfurt/Main 1
Germany

H. J. F. HODGSON
Department of Medicine
Royal Postgraduate Medical School
Hammersmith Hospital
Du Cane Road
London W12 0NN
UK

W. HOHENBERGER
Chirurgische Klinik und Poliklinik
Universität Regensburg
Franz-Josef-Strauss-Allee 11
W-8400 Regensburg
Germany

S. P. JAMES
Division of Gastroenterology
University of Maryland Hospital
Room N3W62, 22 South Greene Street
Baltimore
MD 21201-1595
USA

B. V. KIRKIN
Institute of Proctology
Department of Therapeutics
Salim Adil. 2
Moscow 123448
Russia

R. A. KOZAREK
Department of Medicine
The Mason Clinic
1100 Ninth Avenue
PO Box 900
Seattle
WA 98111-0900
USA

W. KRUIS
Innere Abteilung, Evang. Krankenhaus Kalk
Buchforststr. 2
W-5000 Köln 91
Germany

P. LAYER
Abteilung für Gastroenterologie
Medizinische Klinik der Universität Essen
Hufelandstr. 55
W-4300 Essen 1
Germany

B. LEMBCKE
Medizinische Universitätsklinik
Theodor-Stern-Kai 7
W-6500 Frankfurt/Main 70
Germany

LIST OF PRINCIPAL AUTHORS

J. E. LENNARD-JONES
St. Mark's Hospital
City Road
London
EC1V 2PS
UK

H. LOCHS
Universitätsklinik für Innere Medizin IV
Gastroenterologie und Hepatologie
Währinger Gürtel 18-20
A-1090 Wien
Austria

M. LOTZ
Department of Medicine (S-045)
University of San California, San Diego
La Jolla
CA 92093-0663
USA

Y. R. MAHIDA
Massachusetts General Hospital
Harvard Medical School
Gastrointestinal Unit
Boston
MA 02114
USA

H. W. MÖLLMANN
Universitätsklinikum Bergmannsheil
Medizinische Poliklinik
Gilsinger Str. 14
W-4630 Bochum
Germany

C. J. J. MULDER
Gastroenterology Dept. of Medicine
Rijnstate Hospital IGZ
PO Box 9555
NL-6800 TA Arnhem
The Netherlands

A. RAEDLER
I. Medizinische Universitätsklinik
Eppendorf
Martinistr. 52
W-2000 Hamburg 20
Germany

W. E. W. ROEDIGER
University of Adelaide
Department of Surgery
The Queen Elizabeth Hospital
Woodville Rd
Woodville
SA 5011
Australia

I. H. ROSENBERG
Human Nutrition – Research Center
Tufts University
711 Washington Street
Boston
MA 02111
USA

J. I. ROTTER
Division of Medical Genetics
Cedars-Sinai Medical Center
UCLA School of Medicine
8700 Beverley Blvd., SSB 3
Los Angeles
CA 90048
USA

H. SANDBERG-GERTZEN
Department of Medicine
Gastroenterology Unit
Örebro Medical Center
S-70185 Örebro
Sweden

R. B. SARTOR
Division of Digestive Diseases
Campus Box 7080
Room 326, Burnett-Womack Bldg.
University of North Carolina
School of Medicine
Chapel Hill
NC 27599-7080
USA

J. SCHÖLMERICH
Medizinische Klinik und Poliklinik I
Universität Regensburg
Franz-Josef-Strauss-Allee 11
W-8400 Regensburg
Germany

A. STALLMACH
Medizinische Klinik
FU Berlin
Klinikum Steglitz
Hindenburgdamm 30
W-1000 Berlin 45
Germany

M. STARLINGER
Chirurgische Klinik und Poliklinik
der Universität Tübingen
Hoppe-Seyler-Strasse 3
W-7400 Tübingen
Germany

W. STOLZ
Klinik und Poliklinik für Dermatologie
Klinikum der Universität Regensburg
Franz-Josef-Strauss Allee 11
W-8400 Regensburg
Germany

L. R. SUTHERLAND
Division of Gastroenterology
Health Sciences Center, University
3330 Hospital Drive NW
Calgary
Alberta T2N 4N1
Canada

S. R. TARGAN
Cedars-Sinai Medical Center
IBD Center, Suite D4063
8700 Beverly Blvd
Los Angeles
CA 90048
USA

W. R. THAYER, Jr
Division of Gastroenterology
Rhode Island Hospital
Brown University
APC Room 421
593 Eddy Street
Providence
RI 02903
USA

A. TOBIN
Gastroenterology/Hepatology Section
Fred Hutchinson Cancer Research Center
Columbia Street
Seattle
WA 98104-2092
USA

W. J. TREMAINE
Division of Gastroenterology
Mayo Clinic
200 First Street, SW
Rochester
MN 55905
USA

B. F. WARREN
Department of Pathology and Microbiology
Bristol Royal Infirmary
Marlborough Street
Bristol BS2 8HW
UK

M. ZEITZ
Abteilung Innere Medizin
Klinikum Steglitz der FU Berlin
Hindenburgdamm 30
W-1000 Berlin 45
Germany

Section I
Aetiology

1
Animal models

B. F. WARREN and P. E. WATKINS

INTRODUCTION

The causes of ulcerative colitis and Crohn's disease remain unknown. There is a need to study mechanisms of inflammation in the gut, their specific responses to treatment and their possible causes. These studies would be most usefully performed in a reproducible model system. Good animal models of disease should be similar in behaviour and appearance to the human disease, should develop similar complications, and should probably be spontaneously occurring. Their responses to treatment should be similar, and the model should preferably be readily available. Animal models of inflammatory bowel disease described so far fall into two broad categories: induced and spontaneously occurring. Both types of model need careful characterization and comparison with the human diseases before they may be considered valid models for investigation. This chapter describes some examples of induced and spontaneously occurring models and summarizes the Bristol work on the cotton-top tamarin model.

INDUCED MODELS

Many models of intestinal inflammation have been induced in an attempt to study the mechanisms of inflammatory bowel disease. Chiodini et al.[1] described a model in infant goats fed on a mycobacterium isolated from a case of human Crohn's disease and which developed segmental granulomatous bowel disease. *In situ* hybridization has permitted the isolation of this bacterium and its identification as *Mycobacterium linda*. This model has led to renewed interest in the search for mycobacteria in cases of Crohn's disease.

The carrageenan-induced model of colonic inflammation in the guinea pig described by Marcus and Watt[2] remains one of the most useful induced models. The induction of granulomatous, usually patchy colitis with carrageenan

3

depends on the use of degraded carrageenan[3] in a colon with normal flora (this will not develop in a germ-free colon[4]). This reproducible model, which shows some overlap between Crohn's disease and ulcerative colitis, has been reported to develop carcinoma[5]. More recently a model of granulomatous ileitis has been developed by injecting live BCG directly into the ileum of guinea pigs[6].

Recent interest in ischaemia as a cause of Crohn's disease, by Wakefield and colleagues[7], has led to the search for a suitable ischaemia-induced model of Crohn's disease by occlusion of the mesenteric vasculature in the ferret with glass spherules[8]. The changes induced in this model provide an excellent picture of intestinal ischaemia and are valuable evidence that pseudomembranous colitis-like changes[9] are really due to ischaemia.

Models of ulcerative colitis have been induced by perfusing the colons, mainly of rodents, with all manner of irritant chemicals[10]. Many of these models do not resemble ulcerative colitis; however, they do have a place in the investigation of mechanisms of inflammation. They may be particularly useful for studying neutrophil movement and its chemotactic factors, and mucin depletion, but their terminology needs care. It is more appropriate to consider these models as models of colonic inflammation; not inflammatory bowel disease.

These substances include acetic acid[11], and formalin with and without prior sensitization[12]. The Arthus reaction will produce a colitis in this way in rabbits[13], but a more realistic model may be produced by the Auer modifcation of this reaction[14]. In this case inflammation is produced at the site of a previous mild inflammation induced by the rectal instillation of formalin, by parenteral administration of egg albumin to an immunized albino hybrid rabbit[12]. This model has been used to study the effects of anti-inflammatory drugs[15]. The colitis becomes chronic if the rabbit is previously sensitized to enterobacterial common antigen. In other words, once the immune defences are weakened, colitis may be maintained by allergic reaction to intraluminal antigens. Indeed some workers have thought it likely that colitis may be caused by a humoral response to colonic bacteria[10]. However, generation of colon autoantibodies by *E. coli* does not always result in colitis[10].

Colitis has also been induced in both rabbits and guinea pigs by sensitization with dinitrochlorobenzene[16]. This substance forms hapten/protein complexes which are recognized as foreign by the host T lymphocytes.

More recently the role of cytokines in the production of colonic inflammation has been studied by infusing recombinant human IL-1β into rabbit colon, to produce a colitis and strengthen the place of IL-1 in production of colitis.

SPONTANEOUSLY OCCURRING MODELS

Spontaneously occurring models of inflammatory bowel disease may be less readily available and reproducible than induced models, but they may bear closer resemblance to the human disease in several ways. Spontaneously occurring granulomatous bowel disorders in the animal world which resemble Crohn's disease have usually been found to be related to infection. Johne's disease in cattle is due to mycobacterial infection, and bears some resemblance to Crohn's disease[17].

Granulomatous terminal ileitis in the Syrian hamster really bears closer resemblance to *Yersinia* infection than Crohn's disease as was originally thought. The causative organism here is a rod-shaped bacillus[18].

Horses sometimes develop a spontaneous granulomatous enteritis for which no infectious cause has been found but, like the pig, which also develops ileitis due to *Campylobacter*, there would be preventive handling difficulties in using it as a model of human disease[10].

Many spontaneously occurring models of colitis have been described including swine dysentery and equine colitis which have known bacterial causes[19]. Boxer dogs develop a usually granulomatous total colitis[10], whereas other dogs may develop a lymphocytic plasmacytic colitis. Cats have been recently observed to develop a steroid-responsive colitis, making infection an unlikely cause[20]. Spontaneous mouse models differ from human ulcerative colitis in a variety of ways, and have been found to be due to bacteria in most cases. Japanese waltzing mice suffer from a predominantly right-sided colitis caused by *Bacillus pyliformis*[10], whereas Swiss Webster mice develop a distal colitis due to *Citrobacter freundii*, which ends in rectal prolapse and death[10]. Transgenic rats with HLA B27 develop a spontaneous colitis which may allow further studies of the relationship between HLA and ulcerative colitis[21].

Spontaneous colitis in primates offers most hope as a model. Lowland gorilla colitis is not particularly useful as a model since endoscopy presents distinct handling difficulties and, histologically, this condition has more features resembling low-grade chronic ischaemia than ulcerative colitis. Many New World monkeys develop a colitis which bears very close resemblance to human ulcerative colitis – clinically, endoscopically, histologically and in its response to treatment[22]. This is particularly true of the cotton-top tamarin, which also develops the complications seen in human ulcerative colitis[23,24]. The cotton-top tamarin's suitability as a model has been under discussion for some time. One of the problems has been that organisms (*Campylobacter*) have been isolated from some cases and not others. Some animals have responded to 5-ASA compounds whereas others have not. Our work in the Bristol colony has helped to clarify this situation. From our clinical, bacteriological, endoscopic, histological and treatment studies, the cotton-top seems to develop not one type, but five types, of colitis. One is an infective colitis due to *Campylobacter jejuni*, another is a rare infection due to *Klebsiella pneumoniae*, a third resembles human pseudomembranous colitis, and the majority are like human inflammatory bowel disease, a very small fraction of which bear closer similarity to Crohn's disease than ulcerative colitis. Cotton-top tamarins with *Campylobacter* colitis have extremely offensive stools, a high peripheral blood white cell count, a total or patchy colitis endoscopically and histological appearances of classical infective colitis[25]. Here there is superficial, predominantly acute inflammation with formation of neutrophil collections in the lamina propria and eccentric crypt abscesses which are also superficial. This condition responds well to oral erythromycin. Failure to recognize it results in the rapid demise of the animal.

Klebsiella pneumoniae colitis is very rare, and is the only colitis in the cotton-top which does not have a direct human counterpart. The histological appearance is of gross mucosal oedema, in which many organisms may be seen.

Pseudomembranous colitis follows antibiotic therapy and is an endoscopically patchy colitis with a histological appearance of intercrypt erosions with volcano-like eruptions of neutrophils and fibrin on the surface. This again is often fatal. We no longer see this in our colony now that antibiotics are no longer the first-line therapy for cotton-top tamarin colitis.

We have only seen four cases which resemble Crohn's disease more closely than ulcerative colitis. Here the endoscopic inflammation and the histological inflammation were patchy, and in two cases mucosal microgranulomas were seen. They responded to the same treatment as the majority of cases of cotton-top tamarin colitis which resemble ulcerative colitis. This disease in some animals is more or less continuous but, in most, follows a pattern of relapse and remission. The majority of cases of cotton-top tamarin colitis resemble human ulcerative colitis.

Histologically, there is a diffuse mixed inflammatory cell infiltrate limited to the mucosa. This is associated with crypt distortion and branching and mucin depletion. When the disease is active, crypt abscesses form, just as in the human disease. Staining for mucin with high iron diamine/alcian blue[26] shows a change from normal colonic-type sulphomucin to small bowel type sialomucin with the development of colitis, as seen in humans[27]. We have treated this condition successfully with 5-aminosalicylic acid in the form of olsalazine. If the colitis is mild this is the only treatment needed. However, if the colitis is more severe (judged endoscopically), treatment with prednisolone and olsalazine is instituted, providing the stool culture is negative. The complications of cotton-top tamarin colitis make it a unique model of human disease. We have known for some time that cotton-top tamarins develop colon cancer as a sequel to ulcerative colitis. Like the carcinomas complicating human ulcerative colitis, these tumours are right-sided, flat and multiple. The only two differences are that these tumours are invariably mucinous and that they have not yet been shown to metastasize to the liver. More recently, liver disease has been recognized in cotton-tops with ulcerative colitis[24]. This liver disease includes periportal chronic inflammation and a histological appearance which resembles human sclerosing cholangitis. The only disadvantage of the cotton-top model is its rarity.

CONCLUSIONS

Induced models of colitis may be useful to study specific features of colonic inflammation, but cannot be used to reliably study the pathogenesis of human inflammatory bowel disease. They should be considered as good models of 'intestinal inflammation' rather than inflammatory bowel disease. Spontaneously occurring models of colitis need careful characterization before they can be useful in the study of aetiology or pathogenesis.

The cotton-top tamarin has an important place as a model of ulcerative colitis once it is realized that it suffers from more than one form of colitis, the majority of which resemble human ulcerative colitis. We believe it is from this model that many of the answers concerning the pathogenesis of ulcerative colitis, the development of its complications, and meaningful studies of its therapy will be made.

ACKNOWLEDGEMENTS

We are extremely grateful for the continued help and support of Professors I. A. Silver and J. W. B. Bradfield, Drs G. R. Pearson and N. Clapp, Mr A. Terlecki and Mr K. Makwakwa. We also acknowledge the generous support of the National Association for Colitis and Crohn's Disease, and Professor R. E. Pounder who kindly supplied our endoscope. We are also grateful to Pharmacia who continue to supply olsalazine powder to us.

References

1. Chiodini RJ, Van Kruiningen HJ, Thayer WR, Merkal RS, Coutu JA. Possible role of mycobacteria in inflammatory bowel disease. I. An unclassified mycobacterium species isolated from patients with Crohn's disease. Dig Dis Sci. 1984;29:1073–9.
2. Marcus R, Watt J. Experimental ulceration of the colon produced by non-algal sulphated products. Gut. 1971;12:868–75.
3. Marcus R, Watt J. Colonic ulceration in young rats fed degraded carrageenan. Lancet. 1971;2:765–6.
4. Onderdonk AB, Hermos JA, Dzink JL, Bartlett JG. Protective effect of metronidazole in experimental ulcerative colitis. Gastroenterology. 1978;74:521–6.
5. Wakabayashi K, Inagaki T, Fujimoto Y, Fukuka Y. Induction by degraded carrageenan of colorectal tumours in rats. Cancer Lett. 1978;4:171–6.
6. Mitchell IC, Turk JL. An experimental model of granulomatous bowel disease. Gut. 1989;30:1371–8.
7. Wakefield AJ, Sawyerr AM, Dhillon AP, Pittilo RM, Rowles PM, Lewis AA, Pounder RE. Pathogenesis of Crohn's disease: multifocal gastrointestinal infarction. Lancet. 1989;2:1057–62.
8. Hudson M, Piasecki C, Sankey EA, Sim R, Wakefield AJ, More LJ, Sawyerr AM, Dhillon AP, Pounder RE. A ferret model of acute multifocal gastrointestinal infarction. Gastroenterology. 1992;102:1591–6.
9. Price AB, Davies DR. Pseudomembranous colitis. J Clin Pathol. 1977;30:1–12.
10. Rhodes JM. Animal models. In: Allan RN, Keighley MRB, Alexander-Williams J, Hawkins C, editors. Inflammatory bowel diseases. London: Churchill Livingstone; 1990:181–6.
11. MacPherson B, Pfeiffer CJ. Experimental colitis. Digestion. 1976;14:424–52.
12. Hodgson HJF, Potter BJ, Skinner J, Jewell DP. Immune complex mediated colitis in rabbits. Gut. 1978;19:225–32.
13. Kirsner JB. Experimental colitis with particular reference to hypersensitivity reactions in the colon. Gastroenterology. 1961;40:307–12.
14. Kraft SC, Fitch FW, Kirsner JB. Histologic and immunohistochemical features of the Auer colitis in rabbits. Am J Pathol. 1963;18:913–27.
15. Rhodes JM, McLaughlin JE, Brown DJC, Nuttall LA, Jewell DP. Inhibition of leucocyte motility and prevention of immune complex experimental colitis by hydroxychloroquine. Gut. 1982;23:181–7.
16. Bicks RO, Rosenberg EW. A chronic delayed hypersensitivity reaction in the guinea pig colon. Gastroenterology. 1964;46:543–9.
17. Dalziel TK. Chronic intestinal enteritis. Br Med J. 1913;2:1068–70.

18. Johnson EA, Jacoby RO. Transmissible ileal hyperplasia of hamster. II. Ultrastucture. Am J Pathol. 1978;91:451–68.
19. Onderdonk AB. Experimental models for ulcerative colitis. Dig Dis Sci. 1985;30:405–55.
20. Ghermai AK. Chronic inflammatory bowel disease in cats. Tiermarztl-Prax. 1989;17:195–9.
21. Hammer RE, Maika SD, Richardson JA, Tang JP, Taurog JD. Spontaneous inflammatory disease in transgenic rats expressing HLA B27 and human beta 2m: an animal model of HLA association human disorders. Cell. 1990;63:1099–112.
22. Clapp N, Henke M, Lushbaugh CC, Humason GL, Gangaware BL. Effect of various biological factors on spontaneous marmoset and tamarin colitis. A retrospective histological study. Dig Dis Sci. 1988;33:1013–19.
23. Kirkwood JK, Pearson GR, Epstein MA. Adenocarcinoma of the large bowel and colitis in cotton top tamarins. J Comp Pathol. 1986;96:507–15.
24. Warren BF, Henke M, Clapp N. Extraintestinal manifestations. In: Clapp N, editor. Cotton top tamarin colitis. Boca Raton: CRC Press; 1992: in press.
25. Day DW, Mandal BK, Morson BC. The rectal biopsy appearances in *Salmonella* colitis. Histopathology. 1978;2:117–31.
26. Spicer SS. Diamine methods for differentiating mucosubstances histochemically. J Histochem Cytochem. 1964;13:211–33.
27. Makwakwa K, Warren BF, Watkins PE. Mucins in cotton cop tamarin colitis. J Pathol. 1992;168:144A.

2

Delineating the major aetiological risk factors for IBD: the genetic susceptibilities

J. I. ROTTER and H. YANG

IMPORTANCE OF THE GENETIC BASIS OF IBD

The inflammatory bowel diseases (IBD) are fundamentally genetic diseases with complex non-Mendelian patterns of inheritance. The support for this proposition will occupy the majority of this paper. But before we turn to this evidence it is important to note two important implications of such a conclusion. First, since the various forms of IBD are due to specific genetic susceptibilities, we must identify those genes and understand how they act, since it is at that fundamental step that the disease process is presumably initiated. This is essential if we are ever to develop methods of disease prevention or fundamentally different therapies. Second, the individual genetic susceptibility will vary tremendously in the population, and thus we will need genetic methods to identify those who are susceptible, for prevention strategies. The power of such a genetic approach can be seen in the advances over the last several years in two other diseases as examples – cystic fibrosis, and insulin-dependent (type 1) diabetes. In cystic fibrosis the gene was localized, cloned, and the mutations identified[1,2]. This has led to new methods of carrier screening and prenatal diagnosis, and the imminent prospects of new therapies including replacing the defective gene. In insulin-dependent diabetes the locations of at least some of the responsible genes have been identified, and we can now identify at-risk individuals years before disease onset, as well as identifying early preclinical stages in the disease process[3,4]. This has led to clinical trials of actual disease prevention. Nothing less should be our goal for aetiological studies in IBD.

GENETIC SUSCEPTIBILITIES ARE THE MAJOR AETIOLOGICAL RISK FACTORS

One can state without exaggeration that the most firmly established and quantitatively largest risk factor for the various forms of IBD is a positive family history[5]. That this familial aggregation has a genetic basis is demonstrated by at least five lines of evidence[5]: one is the increased occurrence of disease in family members widely separated in time and space; the second is the increasing number of recognized genetic syndromes that include a form of IBD among their manifestations; the third is the very recent recognition by workers at the Jackson Laboratories of a genetically determined spontaneous mouse model of colitis[6]; the fourth is the lack of increased frequency in spouses; and the fifth is the increased concordance (both members affected) among monozygotic as opposed to dizygotic twin pairs in which one member has IBD.

It should be emphasized that much more needs to be learned from these family and related genetic epidemiological studies. Thus, for example, the first age-adjusted empirical risks, which are those most appropriate for genetic counselling and genetic modelling, were reported only in 1989[7]. While many more of these and analogous studies need to be done, continued progress is occurring in this area. Three recent studies are particularly noteworthy.

1. Extending the reported observations of ethnic differences in IBD frequencies[8], we in Los Angeles have observed a significantly different familial empirical risk for IBD between Jews and non-Jews[9,10]. In the first-degree relatives of non-Jewish probands the life-time risks for IBD were 5.2% when probands had Crohn's disease (CD) and 1.6% when probands had ulcerative colitis (UC). These were consistently and significantly lower than the corresponding risks for relatives of Jewish patients, 7.8% and 4.5% for CD and UC probands respectively. These data begin to provide the requisite basis for genetic counselling for these disorders.
2. In a study from Baltimore, familiality was also recently observed in clinical characteristics of Crohn's, including location of the inflammation, transmural aggressiveness, and age of onset[11].
3. From New York there has been one intriguing study (as opposed to anecdotal case reports) of the risks to offspring for IBD when both parents themselves have IBD[12]. The results suggested that the risk was substantially greater than that of twice the empirical risk to offspring of couples when one parent has IBD, and was starting to approach the monozygotic twin risks.

Complementary approaches are also becoming productive. An increasing number of genetic syndromes that feature IBD are being recognized[5], and equally significantly, mechanisms are being investigated. The most intriguing observation in this area is that regarding glycogen storage disease type Ib (GSD-Ib). GSD-Ib is an inherited metabolic disorder caused by a defect in the glucose 6-phosphate transport system. This glycogenosis is distinguished clinically from classic GSD-Ia by a predisposition to pyogenic infections caused by neutropenia and neutrophil dysfunction[13,14]. Chronic IBD has been reported in association with GSD-Ib[15,16]. In addition, it has now been reported that long-term treatment with colony-stimulating factors (GM-CSF and G-CSF) can normalize the neutrophil count and bring healing of oral mucosal lesions and IBD in GSD-Ib[17]. These observations suggest the pathogenetic importance of the neutrophil in Crohn's disease. The pathophysiology of IBD in this disorder is therefore a model worthy of further exploration.

A most important resource for genetic studies is the recognition or development of genetically determined animal models of IBD, especially in the mouse. Thus workers at the Jackson Laboratories are to be congratulated for describing recently a heritable form of colitis in the C3H/HeJ strain of mice[6]. These mice suffer from diarrhoea and secondary perianal ulceration. Despite extensive efforts in the past 10 years no pathogens have been isolated from such mice. Pathological analysis has found a colitis with foci of neutrophilic infiltration and crypt abscesses, ulceration, regenerative hyperplasia and submucosal scarring, resembling in many ways human IBD. Once this new animal model is stabilized and expanded it should become a valuable resource for genetic and immunological studies of IBD.

What have these approaches thus far told us about IBD, or UC and CD? First the data regarding empirical risks to family members have allowed rejection of the simple additive polygenic model for IBD as a whole, or either CD or UC[18,19]. Basically what these formal genetic analyses have concluded is that the risk to relatives is too great to be explained by that mode of inheritance. However, the data regarding the different empirical risks for relatives of Jewish and non-Jewish IBD probands, alluded to above, also allow rejection of single Mendelian models for IBD, and for UC and CD individually. The logic is as follows: if the susceptibility to any form of IBD was a simple Mendelian trait (and this includes the factor of reduced penetrance), then one could still observe different frequencies of disease in different ethnic groups due to differences in the frequencies of the underlying disease susceptibilities. However, once one ascertained a family with the disease, the risks would be the same in both ethnic groups. Thus for example, Tay-Sachs disease, an autosomal recessive disorder due to hexosaminidase B deficiency, has a frequency of 1 in 360 000 in US non-Jews, and 1 in 3600 in US Jews. Yet once an affected infant is born in a family the risk is 1 in 4 regardless of ethnic group, that being the risk for an autosomal recessive. Another conclusion comes from the distribution of 'mixed families'. It appeared that, among the multiply affected IBD families, the proportion of families with both UC- and CD-affected individuals was greater in the non-Jewish families than that in the Jewish families (with the greater empirical risks in Jews, the converse would have been expected). These different relative distributions in the type of multiply affected families are consistent with the genetic heterogeneity model for IBD. The inference is that there are different proportions of the various heterogeneous forms of IBD among Jewish and non-Jewish populations. This population heterogeneity has implications for both association and linkage studies. Finally, if the data of Bennett et al.[12] are confirmed regarding the high risk to offspring of two affected parents, this suggests that the actual number of genes predisposing to IBD is limited in number. This is another encouraging observation regarding the potential for success in the search for major genes that predispose to these diseases.

IDENTIFYING THE SUSCEPTIBILITY GENES

Basically, there are two approaches to identifying susceptibility genes. One is to proceed from the disease phenotype and work down towards the genotype (the subclinical marker approach). The second is to work from the genes up (the gene marker approach).

Subclinical markers are parameters used to detect the abnormal genotype in the absence of the full phenotype; e.g. abnormal glucose tolerance and islet cell antibodies in diabetes or serum cholesterol in coronary artery disease. Such a subclinical abnormality may either indicate the genetic abnormality predisposing to a disease, or identify those in whom an earlier phase of disease process is occurring that may or may not eventuate in clinical disease[20]. A number of subclinical markers have been suggested in IBD (Table 1). Recent advances have occurred with three of these.

Colonic glycoprotein composition was recently evaluated in a set of monozygotic twins with IBD[21]. The content of one chromatographically defined component of colonic mucin, designated HCM species IV, was reduced in both patients with ulcerative colitis and their apparently healthy twins, compared with controls. Composition of the mucins in Crohn's disease patients and their affected twins was not significantly different from that in controls. These observations suggest that altered profiles of mucin glycoprotein may be present before the onset of UC, and therefore may be genetically defined. Again, the methodology must be standardized, because some investigators are having difficulties demonstrating the principal finding of abnormal mucin distribution in the UC patients themselves[22].

There have been several new permeability studies in Crohn's disease patients and their family members in the past 2 years[24-27]. On first inspection the results appear inconsistent. It seems that a number of related factors may affect the results of an intestinal permeability study. These may include the type of probes, the method of administration of the probe, e.g. fasting/non-fasting, with meals/without meals, day urine collection/overnight urine collection, length of urine collection, and use of aspirin as a challenge. It is

Table 1 Subclinical genetic markers for IBD

Subclinical marker	Form of IBD	Reference
C3 dysfunction	CD	Elmgreen et al., 1985[29]
Anaerobic faecal flora	CD	van de Merwe et al., 1988[31]
Autoantibodies to epithelial cell-associated antigens	IBD	Fiocchi et al., 1989[30]
Colonic mucins	UC	Tysk et al., 1991[21]
Intestinal permeability	CD	Hollander et al., 1986[23] (and others; see text)
Antineutrophil cytoplasmic antibodies	UC	Shanahan et al., 1992[36]

important to conduct studies to identify a sensitive and reproducible protocol for the permeability testing that reliably separates Crohn's patients (or a subgroup of CD) and controls. The possibility of abnormal permeability in relatives remains an attractive hypothesis[28], either as a genetic abnormality or as a marker of early inflammation. But this field needs additional studies and methodological standardization. Possibly the most interesting approach was presented at the recent American Gastroenterology Association by Pironi et al.[27]. In their study, both healthy relatives of CD patients and healthy controls were given the lactulose/mannitol (L/M) test before and after the administration of aspirin. These investigators concluded that the relatives of CD patients were more sensitive to NSAIDs than healthy controls, i.e. the mean percentage increase of above-baseline L/M values observed after aspirin was greater in relatives than that in controls. Thus, these results suggest that an enhanced small bowel mucosa sensitivity to factors increasing permeability can play a primary role in the pathogenesis of the disease. Clearly this whole area needs additional work.

A distinct subset of anti-neutrophil cytoplasmic antibodies (ANCAs) was recently discovered to be highly specific for ulcerative colitis ($\sim 70\%$ of UC patients are ANCA-positive) compared with other forms of colitis, which included Crohn's (only 6%)[32–35]. To date the presence of ANCAs appears independent of the disease extent and disease activity[32]. ANCAs were also found in UC patients who were 5 years post-colectomy. We have now also observed that the clinically healthy relatives of UC patients have an increased frequency of positive ANCAs (16%) compared with environmental controls (3%)[36]. These cumulative observations – specificity, constancy, and increased prevalence in unaffected relatives – suggest that ANCAs are not simply an epiphenomenon related to active colonic inflammation. The presence of ANCAs in UC may reflect a fundamental disturbance of immune regulation. In this family study it was also shown that the distribution of positivity for ANCA is familial, i.e. that the presence or absence of ANCA was associated within families. This concordant familial distribution strongly indicates heterogeneity within UC. This heterogeneity within UC indicated by ANCAs has been demonstrated to have a genetic basis by use of the HLA class II genes, as discussed below[37]. At the present time, by the combination of family and gene marker studies, ANCAs are the most established subclinical marker for any form of IBD.

As discussed above, the other major approach for gene identification is to examine specific candidate genes, now usually by molecular methods. While there had been some progress in that area[5], definitive HLA class II associations have now been identified. A recent association study between the HLA class II genes and IBD from Los Angeles established that HLA-DR2 was associated with UC in American Caucasian populations[38,39]. It was also suggested that the DR1/DQw5 haplotype was associated with CD. The latter results were confirmed by an independent group in a separate US population[40]. These observations are very important because it now means that we have, for the first time, clearly identified genetic regions for at least one form of UC and one form of CD. These results also indicate that the susceptibility contributed by the HLA class II genes is quite different for the two disorders.

Furthermore, with a combination of HLA class II genes and the UC subclinical marker – anti-neutrophil cytoplasmic antibodies, it was also demonstrated that there is genetic heterogeneity within UC, i.e. ANCA-positive UC was associated with DR2 and ANCA-negative UC was not[37].

The cumulative data now support the concept that IBD is a genetically heterogeneous group of disorders that share the common clinical endpoint of chronic inflammation of the gastrointestinal tract (Table 2). This is true not only for IBD, but for UC and CD individually, i.e. it is likely that there is more than one form of UC and more than one form of CD. The 'mixed' disorder (UC and CD occurring in the same family or individual) could be one of these forms or a further disorder. We will only understand the pathway from genetic susceptibility as we dissect out each of the component disorders from the group of entities we term IBD.

STRATEGIES FOR FUTURE GENETIC STUDIES

This is clearly an exciting time for aetiological genetic research in IBD, as we are just beginning to lift the veil on the mysteries of these genetic susceptibilities to the various forms of these diseases. In that regard there are several strategies that should occupy the gastroenterologist, pathophysiologist, epidemiologist, and geneticist interested in IBD.

1. There are a number of candidate genes that should be investigated in both case–control association and family linkage studies. These include most powerfully the HLA region, but also include the T-cell receptors[41]; complement genes, mucin genes[42], and possibly genes in the inflammatory pathway such as cytokines or adhesion molecules[43].
2. Further studies of the proposed subclinical markers should be conducted and new ones explored.
3. The pathophysiology of the genetic syndromes with IBD should be defined.
4. We should utilize the well-described conservation in the location of genes between the various chromosomal regions of humans and those of the mouse. Thus finding the location of genes or gene regions in the mouse will lead to testing of the analogous gene regions (candidate loci) in humans. Hence gene mapping studies of the rodent models should proceed vigorously, to identify specific regions that lead to IBD in those animals. Those regions then become 'candidates' (or candidate loci) to test for in humans. In this way we may identify genes or gene regions that we otherwise would have never considered in humans.
5. It is not out of the question that as the human gene map is saturated, that this systematic technology of gene mapping the entire genome will become feasible for IBD. It is also an eventual corollary of the animal model work proposed above, but this will absolutely require the existence of a sufficient number of families (in the hundreds).
6. Provide the resources for this gene mapping. To accommodate all these multiple mapping needs we at Cedars–Sinai, with the aid of the Crohn's and Colitis Foundation of America, have established at Cedars–Sinai Medical Center, an international, comprehensive IBD cell-line bank.

Table 2 Current evidence for genetic heterogeneity in IBD (overview)

Category	Genetic syndromes	Clinical differences	Family studies	Polymorphic markers	Subclinical markers
In general	Turner's Hermansky-Pudlak Immunodeficiency Glycogen storage				
Between UC and CD		Disease location Histopathology Associated diseases – PSC, AS		DR2 with UC DR1/DQ5 with CD C3F with CD	
			Aggregation CD > UC Twin concordance CD > UC No mixed MZ twins		C3 with CD ANCA with UC Permeability Mucins
Within UC				DR2 with ANCA + UC	Familial heterogeneity ANCA
CD			Familial concordance in site and transmural aggressiveness	C3F with small bowel	C3

Building on a long-term effort at Cedars–Sinai this CCFA IBD cell-line bank has made great progress in the past 2 years with the combined effort of a consortium of four major IBD clinical centres nationwide (in New York, Chicago, Boston, and Los Angeles). Currently, more than 1000 cell-lines from IBD probands, their family members, and ethnically matched controls have been established. Its eventual growth is planned to well over 2000 individuals. The IBD cell-line bank has been utilized by a number of established scientists investigating the genetics of IBD. The goal is to provide material to dozens and hopefully eventually hundreds of investigators worldwide, to accelerate our mutual goal of mapping and then identifying the genes for IBD.

7. With the identification now of specific subclinical markers and several confirmed genetic markers, longitudinal studies are needed to understand the significance of these markers and the natural history of the disease. The studies may include periodic testing for anti-neutrophil antibodies, intestinal tissue biopsy, etc., in the healthy relatives of the IBD patients. It must be emphasized that these studies are the next logical step in understanding these diseases. However, they are both expensive and long-term. It is precisely these types of studies that have led to the current understanding of the preclinical history of juvenile insulin-dependent diabetes, and is leading to interventions aimed at prevention for that disorder[3,4]. To prevent IBD we must do the same: we must come to understand the pathway from genetic susceptibility to clinical disease.

Acknowledgements

The authors wish to express their appreciation for the research support for this work, which has been supported in part by the National Institutes of Health (DK44482), the Crohn's and Colitis Foundation of America, the Stuart Foundations, and the Cedars–Sinai Board of Governors' Chair in Medical Genetics. We also wish to acknowledge the constant managerial assistance of Ms Deb Dutridge, and the help of our many collaborators and colleagues.

References

1. Rommens JM, Iannuzzi MC, Kerem B-S, Drumm ML, Melmer G, Dean M, Rozmahel R, Cole JL, Kennedy D, Hidaka N, Zsiga M, Buchwald M, Riordan JR, Tsui L-C, Collins FS. Identification of the cystic fibrosis gene: Chromosome walking and jumping. Science. 1989;245:1059–65.
2. Collins FS. Cystic fibrosis: molecular biology and therapeutic implications. Science. 1992;256:774–9.
3. Palmer JP, McCulloch DK. Prediction and prevention of IDDM – 1991. Diabetes. 1991;40:943–7.
4. Vadheim CM, Rotter JI. Genetics of diabetes mellitus. In: Alberti KGMM, DeFronzo RA, Keen H, Zimmet P, editors: International textbook of diabetes mellitus. Chichester: John Wiley & Sons; 1992:31–98.

5. Yang H, Shohat T, Rotter JI. The genetics of inflammatory bowel disease. In: MacDermott RP, Stenson WF, editors. Inflammatory bowel disease. Elsevier, New York; 1992:17–51.
6. Birkenmeier EH, Sundberg JP, Elson CO. A heritable form of colitis in mice. Gastroenterology. 1992;102:A596.
7. Roth M-P, Petersen GM, McElree C, Vadheim CM, Panish JF, Rotter JI. Familial recurrence risk estimates of inflammatory bowel disease in Ashkenazi Jews. Gastroenterology. 1989;96:1016–20.
8. Rotter JI, Yang H, Shohat T. Genetic complexities of inflammatory bowel disease and its distribution among the Jewish people. In: Bonne-Tamir B, Adam A, editors. Genetic diversity among Jews: diseases and markers at the DNA level. New York: Oxford University Press; 1992:395–411.
9. Yang H, McElree C, Roth M-P, Shanahan F, Targan SR, Rotter JI. Familial empiric risks for inflammatory bowel disease: differences between Jews and non-Jews. Gastroenterology. 1992;102:A31.
10. Yang H, McElree C, Roth M-P, Shanahan F, Targan SR, Rotter JI. Familial empiric risks for inflammatory bowel disease: differences between Jews and non-Jews. Gut. 1992; in press.
11. Tokayer AZ, Reydel B, Bayless TM. Possible role of heredity in site and transmural aggressiveness of Crohn's disease. Gastroenterology. 1992;102:A705.
12. Bennett RA, Rubin PH, Present DH. Frequency of inflammatory bowel disease in offspring of couples both presenting with inflammatory bowel disease. Gastroenterology. 1991;100:1638–43.
13. Greene HL. Glycogen storage disease. Semin Liver Dis. 1982;2:291–301.
14. Ambruso DR, McCabe ERB, Anderson D, Beaudet A, Ballas LM, Brandt IK, Brown B, Coleman R, Dunger DB, Falletta JM, Friedman HS, Haymond MW, Keating JP, Kinney TR, Leonard JV, Mahoney DH, Matalon R, Roe TF, Simmons P, Slonim AE. Infectious and bleeding complications in glycogenesis Ib. Am J Dis Child. 1985;139:691–7.
15. Roe TF, Thomas DW, Gilsanz V, Isaccs H, Atkinson JB. Inflammatory bowel disease in glycogen storage disease Ib. J Pediatr. 1986;109:55–9.
16. Couper R, Kapelushnik J, Griffiths AM. Neutrophil dysfunction in glycogen storage disease Ib: association with Crohn's-like colitis. Gastroenterology. 1991;100:549–54.
17. Roe TF, Coates TD, Thomas DW, Miller JH, Gilsanz V. Brief report: treatment of chronic inflammatory bowel disease in glycogen storage disease-Ib with colony-stimulating factors. N Engl J Med. 1992;326:1666–9.
18. Kuster W, Pascoe L, Purrmann J, Funk S, Majewski F. The genetics of Crohn disease: Complex segregation analysis of a family study with 265 patients with Crohn disease and 5,387 relatives. Am J Med Genet. 1989;32:105–8.
19. Monsen U, Iselius L, Johansson C, Hellers G. Evidence for a major additive gene in ulcerative colitis. Clin Genet. 1989;36:411–14.
20. King RA, Rotter JI, Motulsky AG, editors. The genetic basis of common diseases. New York: Oxford University Press, 1992; in press.
21. Tysk C, Riedesel H, Lindberg E, Panzini B, Podolsky D, Jarnerot G. Colonic glycoproteins in monozygotic twins with inflammatory bowel disease. Gastroenterology. 1991;100:419–23.
22. Raouf A, Parker N, Iddon D, Ryder S, Langdon-Brown B, Milton JD, Walker R, Rhodes JM. Ion exchange chromatography of purified colonic mucus glycoproteins in inflammatory bowel disease: absence of a selective subclass defect. Gut. 1991;32:1139–45.
23. Hollander D, Vadheim CM, Brettholz E, Petersen GM, Delahunty T, Rotter JI. Increased intestinal permeability in Crohn's patients and their relatives: a possible etiological factor? Ann Intern Med. 1986;105:883–5.
24. Teahon K, Smethurst P, Levi AJ, Menzies IS, Bjarnason I. Intestinal permeability in patients with Crohn's disease and their first degree relatives. Gut. 1992;33:320–3.
25. Ruttenberg D, Young GO, Wright JP, Isaacs S. PEG-400 excretion in patients with Crohn's disease, their first-degree relatives, and healthy volunteers. Dig Dis Sci. 1992;37:705–8.
26. May GR, Sutherland LR, Meddings JB. Lactulose/mannitol permeability is increased in relatives of patients with Crohn's disease. Gastroenterology. 1992;102:A934.
27. Pironi L, Miglioli M, Ruggeri E, Dallasta MA, Ornigotti L, Valpiani D, Barbara L. Effect of non-steroidal anti-inflammatory drugs (NSAID) on intestinal permeability in first degree relatives of patients with Crohn's disease. Gastroenterology. 1992;102:A679.
28. Hollander D. The intestinal permeability barrier. Scand J Gastroenterol. 1992;27:721–6.

29. Elmgreen J, Both H, Binder V. Familial occurrence of complement dysfunction in Crohn's disease: Correlation with intestinal symptoms and hypercatabolism of complement. Gut. 1985;26:151–7.
30. Fiocchi C, Roche JK, Michener WM. High prevalence of antibodies to intestinal epithelial antigens in patients with inflammatory bowel disease and their relatives. Ann Intern Med. 1989;110:786–94.
31. van de Merwe JP, Schroder AM, Wensinck F, Hazenberg MP. The obligate anaerobic faecal flora of patients with Crohn's disease and their first-degree relatives. Scand J Gastroenterol. 1988;23:1125–31.
32. Saxon A, Shanahan F, Landers C, Ganz T, Targan S. A distinct subset of antineutrophil cytoplasmic antibodies is associated with inflammatory bowel disease. J Allergy Clin Immunol. 1990;86:202–10.
33. Duerr RH, Targan SR, Landers CJ, Sutherland LR, Shanahan F. Antineutrophil cytoplasmic antibodies in ulcerative colitis. Comparison with other colitides/diarrheal illnesses. Gastroenterology. 1991;100:1590–6.
34. Cambridge G, Rampton DS, Stevens TRJ, McCarthy DA, Kamm M, Leaker B. Anti-neutrophil antibodies in inflammatory bowel disease: prevalence and diagnostic role. Gut. 1992;33:668–74.
35. Seibold F, Weber P, Klein R, Berg PA, Wiedmann KH. Clinical significance of antibodies against neutrophils in patients with inflammatory bowel disease and primary sclerosing cholangitis. Gut. 1992;33:657–62.
36. Shanahan F, Duerr RH, Rotter JI, Yang H, Sutherland LR, McElree C, Landers CJ, Targan SR. Neutrophil autoantibodies in ulcerative colitis: familial aggregation and genetic heterogeneity. Gastroenterology. 1992;103:456–61.
37. Yang H, Rotter JI, Toyoda H, Wang S-W, McElree C, Lander CJ, Shanahan F, Targan SR. Ulcerative colitis: A genetic heterogeneous group defined with genetic (DR2) and subclinical markers (anti-neutrophil cytoplasmic antibodies). Gastroenterology. 1992;102:A716.
38. Rotter JI, Wang S-J, Yang H, McElree C, Pressman S, Redford A, Magalong D, Tyan D, Shanahan F, Targan S, Toyoda H. Genetic heterogeneity between ulcerative colitis (UC) and Crohn's disease (CD) identified by molecular HLA class II association. Gastroenterology. 1992b;102:A688.
39. Toyoda H, Wang S-J, Yang H, Redford A, Magalong D, Tyan D, McElree C, Pressman S, Shanahan F, Targan S, Rotter JR. Distinct association of HLA class II genes with inflammatory bowel disease. Gastroenterology. 1992; in press.
40. Neigut D, Proujansky R, Trucco M, Dorman JS, Kocoshis S, Carpenter AB, Ball EJ. Association of an HLA-DQB-1 genotype with Crohn's disease in children. Gastroenterology. 1992;102:A671.
41. Nickerson DA, Whitehurst C, Boysen C, Charmley P, Kaiser R, Hood L. Identification of clusters of biallelic polymorphic sequence-tagged sites (pSTSs) that generate highly informative and automatable markers for genetic linkage mapping. Genomics. 1992;12:377–87.
42. Toribara NW, Gum JR, Culhane PJ, Lagace RE, Hicks JW, Petersen GM, Kim YS. MUC-2 human small intestinal mucin gene structure. Repeated arrays and polymorphism. J Clin Invest. 1991;88:1005–13.
43. Springer TA. Adhesion receptors of the immune system. Nature. 1990;346:425–34.

3
The role of psychosocial factors

D. A. DROSSMAN

INTRODUCTION

The relationship of psychosocial factors with inflammatory bowel disease (IBD) can be an area of confusion and misunderstanding. This chapter will present a framework to understand how psychological and social factors relate to IBD, and will make recommendations for future research.

A CONCEPTUAL MODEL

The traditional understanding of illness and disease* in Western civilization has been the *biomedical model*. This proposes that any illness can be reduced to a single aetiology (reductionism). So, finding and treating this aetiology is sufficient to explain the illness and ultimately lead to cure. Furthermore, illness is dichotomized either to an 'organic' disorder having objectively defined pathophysiology, or a 'functional' disorder, with no specifically identifiable pathophysiology (dualism). This categorization also presumes that organic and functional (i.e. psychological) illness are separate.

While presumed to be clinically useful, there are inconsistencies. First, over 80% of medical illnesses seen in primary care have no structural aetiology, and they are not necessarily psychologically based. Second, for some patients with IBD or other chronic illness, psychosocial factors may take a pre-eminent role. Finally, this model does not encompass the complex medical and psychosocial interactions between the patient, the family, the health-care system, and society.

*For the purpose of this discussion, *disease* is defined as abnormalities in the structure and function of organs and tissues, and *illness* as the experience of ill-health or bodily dysfunction. Illness is a broader concept that is determined by disease activity and its psychosocial influences.

The *systems* or *biopsychosocial* model[1] presumes that an illness is the product of subsystems interacting at multiple levels. As shown in Fig. 1, biological and behavioural factors cannot be separated, because they simultaneously define the illness, which in turn reciprocates with its precedents. So increased disease activity has varying effects on individuals, depending on the status of the other subsystems. A stressful life event, such as the death of a close family member, could affect the severity of symptoms, the patient's psychological status, or any other subsystem in the figure. It will also have differing clinical effects depending on whether pre-existing psychiatric disturbance or a poor social support network exists. Conversely, refractory disease is itself a stressful event, and this may adversely affect the patient's coping ability or psychological status, leading, for example, to clinical depression. Taken from this mutually interacting framework, treatment of the disease, particularly if it is chronic, is not sufficient to ameliorate the illness: attention must also be paid to the intervening psychosocial factors.

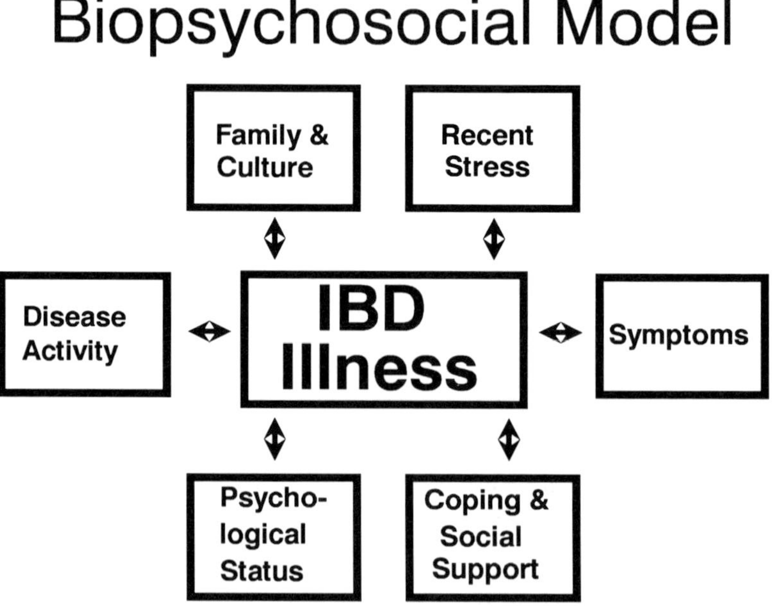

Fig. 1 Systems (biopsychosocial) model of illness for IBD. The illness is shown to result from and, in turn, influence, multiple interacting biological and psychosocial subsystems

THE ROLE OF PSYCHOSOCIAL FACTORS IN IBD

The data relating psychosocial factors to IBD have been conflicting because of methodological difficulties, and the tendencies of some to view the findings from a biomedical perspective. What follows is a summary of these data in consideration of the quality of the studies and from a more comprehensive systems model of illness:

There is a close physiological relationship between brain and gut function.

For centuries it has been recognized that emotional distress can produce changes in bowel function and produce abdominal discomfort, and this is supported by epidemiological and physiological research. Intestinal motor activity can also affect pain perception, mood and other mental functions[2]. It is likely that many of the symptoms which patients with IBD experience may relate to functional changes in motility and pain sensation independent of disease activity.

The biological 'hard-wiring' for these clinical observations is the richly innervated nerve plexes and neuroendocrine associations of the enteric nervous system, and its spinal and autonomic connections to the central nervous system. So, environmental or mental information have, by their neural connections, the capability to affect gastrointestinal (GI) motility and visceral perception, and vice-versa. Further modulation of this brain–gut system occurs via their neurotransmitters, VIP, TRH, 5-HT, CCK, substance P, and the enkephalins, which have integrative activities on GI function and human behaviour depending on their location[2].

Animal research supports an association betweeen stress and changes in mucosal morphology due to activation of disease, but the data in humans are limited.

Physical restraint, prolonged swimming or premature weaning produces acute gastric erosions, called 'stress ulcers' in rats. Chronic GI lesions, including colitis, have been reported in Rhesus monkeys who are restrained in chairs[3]. The cotton-topped tamarin develops colitis and colon carcinoma in captivity. Interestingly, these animals live in an unusual social unit in jungles, with one breeding female, several non-breeding females, and one to three reproductively active males who care for the offspring. Possibly the routine of capturing these animals and caging them in male–female pairs is a disruptive enough social stress to influence the development of these diseases[4]. No other environmental factor such as infection, diet or radiation has been found to explain why these diseases occur in captivity.

The complexity of psychosocial factors in humans makes it difficult to determine its effects on gut morphology, but clinical studies support a relationship. Psychiatric reports beginning 50 years ago have linked experiences of loss with the onset of exacerbation of IBD[3], and these data are consistent with epidemiological studies in other medical fields.

Psychosocial effects on illness and disease may be mediated by immune function.

As stated by Dr Robert Ader, a noted investigator in the field of psycho-immunology: 'The proposition that changes in immune function may mediate the effects of psychosocial factors and stress on susceptibility to, and/or the precipitation or progression of some disease processes is now a tenable hypothesis.' Investigators have found that naturally and experimentally induced stressors can produce alterations in *in vitro* immune function, and this is associated with an increased frequency of acute disease[5]. Given the immune abnormalities in IBD, psychoimmunological research should be considered for the future. Although current studies indicate that the immune effects are too small to have primary effects in causing disease, they may have a permissive role in the timing of disease activation in the predisposed individual.

There is no scientific evidence for a specific IBD personality.

The theory of a specific IBD personality came from psychiatric studies beginning almost 50 years ago[6]. It was proposed that ulcerative colitis, duodenal ulcer, and several non-GI diseases developed from a biological susceptibility *and* specific personality features. With both present, exposure to the proper environmental stress would activate a personality-related conflict, leading to disease activation. For example, the ulcerative colitis personality was characterized by dependence on a dominating parent. Disruption of this relationship by a move from home, or a death, would be particularly distressing, and this event would activate the dependency conflict and lead to the clinical expression of the colitis[6]. While these studies were the first to associate personality disturbance with IBS, better-designed recent studies indicate that this theory is too simplistic.

Psychological disturbance in IBD correlates with the severity of the disease.

Several studies now show an association between IBD and psychiatric morbidity such as depression and anxiety, and patients with Crohn's disease have a greater frequency of psychiatric disturbance, when compared to UC or other medical patients[7,8]. However, most of these studies did not control for the severity of the disease. In a non-clinical sample of 997 members having IBD who belonged to the Crohn's and Colitis Foundation of America (CCFA)[9], we found that those with Crohn's disease do have greater psychological distress and poorer psychological functioning than those with UC. But when we controlled for disease severity, the differences were no longer significant. Further comparisons between IBD members with active disease (CDAI > 182) and inactive disease, confirmed the relationship between psychological disturbance and increased disease activity.

Coping and social support 'buffer' the effects of stress on illness.

Social support and effective coping tend to lower stress levels and improve daily function with illness. We found that CCFA members dealt with disease-related stress predominantly through problem-based coping strategies: seeking social support, self-control, problem-solving and positive reappraisal[9]. They were less likely to use less adaptive emotional strategies: avoiding stressful situations, blaming themselves, or using denial. We also found that these coping patterns are adaptive in minimizing psychological distress and psychosocial dysfunction.

Psychosocial Factors and Outcome

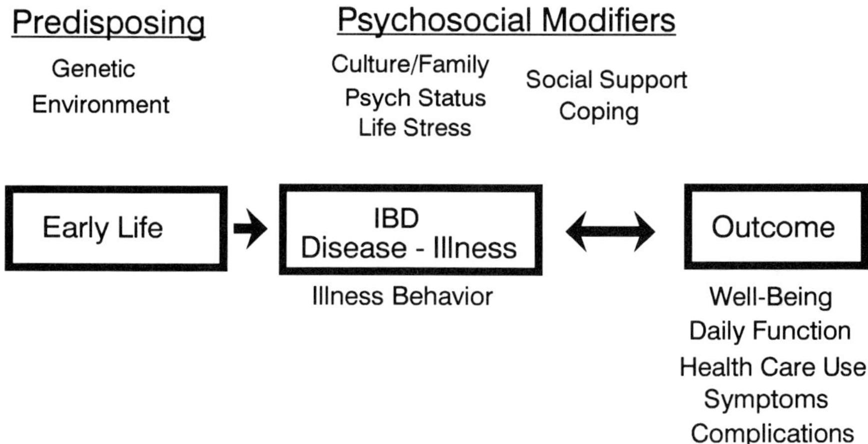

Fig. 2 Psychosocial factors and health outcome in IBD. Relationship of predisposing factors and psychosocial modifiers on disease susceptibility, IBD, and its outcome

Psychosocial factors play an important role in affecting clinical outcome.

As shown in Fig. 2, genetic and environmental factors early in life determine susceptibility to disease. Then psychosocial modifiers will determine when and how the disease is experienced, the person's illness behaviour (see below) and, ultimately, the clinical outcome. In studying the effects of over 20 disease-related and psychosocial variables, in predicting health care utilization[9], six items significantly predicted the frequency of physician visits: three medical factors (greater weight loss, higher steroid dose, female gender), and three psychosocial measures (psychological distress, general well-being and physical dysfunction). In fact, symptom severity did not significantly predict this outcome. In comparison, the frequency of hospitalizations and operations was determined primarily by medical factors.

Based on these observations we recently developed, for research and clinical practice, ulcerative colitis and Crohn's health status scales that incorporate symptoms and psychosocial predictors of health outcome[10]. The scales shown in Table 1 are standardized so that higher scores predict more frequent health-care use, greater psychological distress and poorer physical and psychosocial function. The items are simple to elicit from patients and the resultant score performs better than the Crohn's Disease Activity Index[11] in determining health status. Prospective validation is needed to confirm their role in assessing prognosis and treatment response.

Table 1 Work tables for computing the UC and CD Health Status Scales[10]

Variable*	Possible range		Variable weight	Score
	Minimum	*Maximum*		
Ulcerative colitis				
Perceived well-being	0	4	× 8.8	=
Years of education	0	20	× −1.9	=
Diarrhoea	0	3	× 0.9	=
Loss of bowel control	0	3	× 0.9	=
Frequent trips to the bathroom	0	3	× 0.9	=
No. of bowel movements/week (recoded)	0	3	× 0.9	=
No. of watery stools/day (recoded)	0	3	× 0.9	=
Daily steroid dose (mg)	0	80	× −0.3	=
Dependence on medication for pain	0	3	× 4.4	=
Add a constant:				43
Sum the products to get the final Health Status Score				?
Crohn's disease				
Perceived well-being	0	4	× 8.3	=
Diarrhoea	0	3	× 1.5	=
Frequent trips to the bathroom	0	3	× 1.5	=
No. of bowel movements/week (recoded)	0	3	× 1.5	=
No. of watery stools/day (recoded)	0	3	× 1.5	=
Abdominal pain	0	3	× 2.9	=
Nausea/vomiting	0	3	× 2.9	=
Joint pain/swelling	0	3	× 2.9	=
Eye disease	0	3	× 4.0	=
Dependence on medication for pain	0	3	× 3.6	=
Sum the products to get the final Health Status Score				?

*Scoring system for perceived well-being: 1 = well, 2 = slightly under par, 3 = poor, 4 = very poor, 5 = terrible; for others (unless otherwise indicated) 0 = none, 1 = mild, 2 = moderate, 3 = severe.

THE IMPACT OF IBD

Psychological effects

With chronic disease the major impact is often psychosocial. This relates to working through the personal meaning of the illness, fears of social unacceptability, impaired function at work and at home, and the possibility of untimely death. Those with IBD must specifically learn to: (1) cope with chronic or recurrent symptoms of pain, nausea, diarrhoea, or incontinence; (2) deal with fears of possible surgery, cancer, or the unknown; (3) adjust to the physical and psychological effects of perineal disease, an ostomy, or short bowel syndrome; (4) adjust to possible financial hardship or inability to work or function socially. The longer an illness is present, and the more severe it is, the more adjustments are required. It is therefore not surprising that patients with IBD experience greater impairment in psychosocial (e.g. work, sleep and rest, recreation and social interaction, emotional state), than physical function[12]. How the patient adapts, and the physician's assistance in achieving adaptation, can be crucial to the patients' psychological well-being and the clinical course.

Disease-related concerns

Having IBD understandably leads to worries and concerns, and this may affect satisfaction with care, adjustment to the illness and even the planning of treatment. For example, one of my patients initially rejected our recommendation for a needed colectomy. After further inquiry she disclosed a hidden fear that the surgery would affect her ability to have children. With proper education she agreed to the surgery[13].

We recently developed a standardized question list to evaluate 25 disease-specific concerns for patients with IBD. Table 2 displays these worries and concerns, and their mean severity, on a 0 to 100 scale for members of the CCFA[13]. The most intense concerns related to the uncertain future of their disease, the effects of medication, energy level, surgery (and having an

Table 2 IBD concerns: numerical ranking and comparison of UC and CD scores†

| | All (n = 991) | | UC (n = 320) | | CD (n = 671) | | |
	Mean	(SD)	Mean	(Rank)	Mean	(Rank)	p
Uncertain nature of my disease	58.6	(31.2)	54.3	(4)	60.6	(1)	0.0038
Effects of medication	56.3	(34.3)	54.7	(3)	57.0	(3)	0.3256
Energy level	55.4	(33.7)	48.9	(6)	58.5	(2)	0.0000*
Having surgery	52.9	(33.1)	50.8	(5)	54.0	(4)	0.1471
Having an ostomy bag	52.1	(36.9)	55.6	(1)	50.5	(5)	0.0430
Being a burden on others	47.8	(33.0)	42.6	(8)	50.3	(6)	0.0005*
Loss of bowel control	46.1	(34.1)	47.7	(7)	45.3	(8)	0.2916
Developing cancer	45.4	(33.1)	55.5	(2)	40.6	(12)	0.0000*
Ability to achieve full potential	43.8	(33.3)	38.6	(9)	46.2	(7)	0.0008*
Producing unpleasant odours	41.7	(34.6)	37.4	(12)	43.9	(9)	0.0062
Feelings about my body	40.4	(32.7)	38.1	(10)	41.5	(11)	0.1220
Pain or suffering	39.5	(28.5)	34.3	(14)	42.0	(10)	0.0001*
Feeling out of control	38.0	(32.6)	37.7	(11)	38.2	(13)	0.8295
Attractiveness	35.8	(32.0)	32.1	(16)	37.6	(14)	0.0126
Having access to quality medical care	34.5	(35.2)	33.2	(15)	35.1	(15)	0.4334
Dying early	33.5	(30.5)	36.9	(13)	31.8	(20)	0.0176
Intimacy	32.2	(32.6)	31.2	(17)	32.6	(17)	0.5302
Loss of sexual drive	31.6	(32.9)	30.5	(18)	32.1	(19)	0.4836
Feeling alone	31.0	(31.5)	28.3	(19)	32.3	(18)	0.0654
Financial difficulties	30.3	(30.2)	25.5	(21)	32.8	(16)	0.0002*
Ability to perform sexually	27.6	(31.0)	26.2	(20)	28.3	(22)	0.3294
Passing the disease to others	27.1	(33.3)	22.5	(23)	29.4	(21)	0.0016*
Feeling 'dirty' or 'smelly'	26.1	(30.3)	24.6	(22)	26.8	(23)	0.2786
Being treated as different	21.6	(27.2)	19.7	(24)	22.5	(24)	0.1341
Ability to have children	18.1	(28.9)	18.7	(25)	18.0	(25)	0.7294
Sum score	38.7	(20.4)	37.0		39.6		0.0676

*Significant difference ($p < 0.002$), adjusting for multiple comparisons[8].
†Scores range from 0 = 'not at all', to 100 = 'a great deal'.

ostomy bag), being a burden on others, loss of bowel control, and developing cancer. There were clinically consistent disease-related differences: those with Crohn's disease were more concerned with their energy level, being a burden on others, achieving their full potential, experiencing pain or suffering, financial costs, and passing on the disease to others. Those with ulcerative colitis were more concerned with developing cancer. Further analysis showed that the severity of the concerns correlated with the patient's psychological well-being and daily function. Therefore, it is possible that identifying and addressing some of these concerns through education or counselling will improve the patient's health status.

Physical and social eﬀects

Despite having a chronic illness, several studies now show that most patients with IBD maintain good physical and social functioning. Using a standardized measure of daily functional status, the Sickness Impact Profile, we evaluated several dimensions of physical and social function in 150 patients with IBD (63 UC, 87 CD)[12]. Dysfunction, when present, was greatest for sleep and rest, work, recreation, and general mobility, and was greater for CD than UC. Generally, these patients were able to perform usual home management, eating, ambulation and body care. Sexual dysfunction may be no different from that of the general population; it is reported in 30% of women with IBD, compared to 83% with irritable bowel[14]. There is no increased risk of infertility or pregnancy loss in patients with IBD, but there is a higher rate of pre-term births compared to healthy subjects[15].

FACTORS THAT MODIFY THE IMPACT OF IBD

There are individual differences with regard to the way in which symptoms are perceived, evaluated and responded to (illness behaviours[16]). For example, a patient with Crohn's disease having abdominal pain may not go to the physician if he or she has previously experienced the symptoms without consequence, is worried about losing time from work, grew up in a family where attention to illness was minimized, or believes that complaining is a 'weakness'. Another patient with the same disease activity and symptoms may frequently seek medical assistance if he/she perceives symptoms as potentially dangerous, is seeking disability, is dependent on physicians for health management, or comes from a family where greater attention was paid to illness.

Abnormal illness behaviour

Occasionally, and particularly at the medical centre or in a referral practice, patients may display illness behaviour that is inconsistent with clinical expectations. 'Abnormal' illness behaviour[17] is defined as the patient who: (a) is disabled disproportionate to the observed disease, (b) places responsibility for health care with the physician, (c) feels entitled to be cared for by others, and (d) tends to avoid health-promoting roles ('sick role') such as through exemption from work or family obligations. While seen in a very small proportion of patients with IBD, abnormal illness behaviours can lead to major effects on the family and health-care system.

Social and cultural beliefs

In Western cultures, women with minor complaints are more likely to see physicians, perhaps because males have traditionally been encouraged to be more stoic. Ethnic differences can also be found. In one study, first- and second-generation Jews and Italians were reported to be more dramatic in their response to pain, whereas the Irish tended to deny their symptoms, and the 'Old American' Protestant remained more stoic. Attitudes about pain relief also differed. While Italians were satisfied with relief of pain, the Jewish patients needed to understand the meaning of the pain and its future consequences to be satisfied[18].

Psychiatric diagnosis

Concurrent (co-morbid) psychiatric diagnosis or other psychological disturbances modify the illness experience and its response to treatment. Diagnoses commonly seen in medical patients mostly include depression, anxiety and somatization disorder. Their treatment with psychotherapy or psychopharmacological agents can improve the clinical outcome.

IMPLICATIONS FOR RESEARCH

As this chapter has summarized, the data support the contention that psychosocial factors do modulate the clinical expression of IBD. However, research has lagged behind clinical and epidemiological reports, and multidisciplinary studies using better methodology are needed to address some important issues:

To elaborate the mechanisms for the observed relationships between psychosocial factors, symptoms and disease activity.

Further studies are needed to understand brain–gut 'hard-wiring', and their neurotransmitters as they may affect pain, bowel dysfunction and emotional distress. In addition, studies are needed to evaluate the possible role for psychological factors in modulating *in vivo* immune function and disease activity.

To further investigate health-related quality of life in IBD.

The assessment of health-related quality of life is a means to quantitate, through standardized questionnaires, the subjective experience of illness. It encompasses several domains including general well-being, patient satisfaction, worries and concerns and physical and psychosocial function[19]. For IBD, more studies are needed to improve our ability to guage the effectiveness of surgical interventions[20] and the efficacy of medication[21].

To develop more comprehensive health status measures for research.

From the preceding discussion it is evident that current measures of disease activity are not sufficient to encompass the IBD illness experience (Fig. 1)[21]. The recent development of UC and CD health status scales is a start, since they incorporate medical and psychological variables in their standardization[10]. However, prospective studies are needed to validate their value as predictors of adverse health outcome.

To develop effective behavioural interventions.

Very few studies have studied the effects of behavioural or psychopharmacological treatments in IBD. This may be due to prior emphasis on research designed primarily to control disease activity. Yet for chronic diseases, studies are also needed to determine how patients can best adjust to their illness, possibly through improved coping strategies, family support, stress reduction, or psychopharmacological methods. Effective behavioural interventions will play an important ancillary role in the care of some of these patients.

CONCLUSION

Psychosocial factors are not aetiological for IBD in a direct sense, but they affect the clinical expression of the disease (and vice-versa). These effects may involve symptoms, illness behaviour, the clinical outcome (e.g. health-care use, daily function, health-related quality of life), and possibly disease activity. The biological factors mediating these associations appear to be related to the CNS–ENS neural axis, and possibly through psychoneuroimmunological mechanisms. While there is insufficient evidence to implicate specific IBD personalities, psychosocial disturbance is associated with more severe disease, and 'buffering' factors such as coping and social support may help to ameliorate the illness experience. The clinician's attention to his patient's psychosocial state is likely to lead to an improved clinical outcome.

References

1. Engel GL. The need for a new medical model: a challenge for biomedicine. Science. 1977;196:129–36.
2. Drossman DA. Psychosocial considerations in gastroenterology. In: Sleisenger MH, Fordtran JS, Cello JP, Feldman M, editors. Gastrointestinal disease: pathophysiology, diagnosis, management, 5th edn. Philadelphia: WB Saunders; 1993: in press.
3. Drossman DA. Psychosocial aspects of ulcerative colitis and Crohn's disease. In: Kirsner JB, Shorter RG, editors. Inflammatory bowel disease, 3rd edn. Philadelphia: Lea & Febiger; 1988:209–26.
4. Drossman DA. Is the cotton-topped tamarin a model for behavioral research? Dig Dis Sci. 1985;30:24S–27S.

5. Kiecolt-Glaser JK, Glaser R. Psychosocial moderators of immune function. Ann Behav Med. 1989;9:16–20.
6. Alexander F. Psychosomatic medicine: its principles and applications. New York: WW Norton; 1950.
7. Helzer JE. A controlled study of the association between ulcerative colitis and psychiatric diagnoses. Dig Dis Sci. 1982;27:513–18.
8. Helzer JE. A study of the association between Crohn's disease and psychiatric illness. Gastroenterology. 1984;86:324–30.
9. Drossman DA, Leserman J, Mitchell CM, Li Z, Zagami EA, Patrick DL. Health status and health care use in persons with inflammatory bowel disease: A national sample. Dig Dis Sci. 1991;36:1746–55.
10. Drossman DA, Li Z, Leserman J, Patrick DL. Ulcerative colitis and Crohn's disease health status scales for research and clinical practice. J Clin Gastroenterol. 1992;15:104–12.
11. Best WR, Becktel JM, Singleton JW, Kern F Jr. Development of a Crohn's disease activity index. National Cooperative Crohn's disease study. Gastroenterology. 1976;70:439–44.
12. Drossman DA, Patrick DL, Mitchell CM, Zagami EW, Appelbaum MI. Health related quality of life in inflammatory bowel disease: Functional status and patient worries and concerns. Dig Dis Sci. 1989;34:1379–86.
13. Drossman DA, Leserman J, Li Z, Mitchell CM, Zagami EA, Patrick DL. The rating form of IBD patient concerns: A new measure of health status. Psychosom Med. 1991;53:701–12.
14. Guthrie E, Creed FH. Severe sexual dysfunctioning in women with IBS: comparison with IBD and duodenal ulceration. Br Med J. 1987;295:577.
15. Baird DD, Narendranathan M, Sandler RS. Increased risk of pre-term birth for women with inflammatory bowel disease. Gastroenterology. 1990;99:987–94.
16. Mechanic D. The concept of illness behavior: culture, situation and personal predisposition. Psychol Med. 1986;16:1–7.
17. Pilowsky I. Abnormal illness behavior (dysnosognosia). Psychother Psychosom. 1986;46:76–84.
18. Zborowski M. Cultural response to pain. J Soc Issues. 1952;8:16.
19. Deyo RA. The quality of life, research, and care. Ann Intern Med. 1991;114:695–6.
20. McLeod RS, Churchill DN, Lock AM, Vanderburgh S, Cohen Z. Quality of life of patients with ulcerative colitis preoperatively and postoperatively. Gastroenterology. 1991;101:1307–13.
21. Garrett JW, Drossman DA. Health status in inflammatory bowel disease: Biological and behavioral considerations. Gastroenterology. 1990;99:90–6.

4

Consequences of aetiological hypotheses for the treatment of inflammatory bowel disease

H. LOCHS

The ideal situation for the treatment of any disease is that its aetiology is known and an effective aetiological treatment is available. Neither one of these two prerequisites is fulfilled for the therapy of inflammatory bowel disease (IBD). Consequently treatment strategies have been developed along other lines. On the one hand the mechanism of efficient therapies has been investigated to support pathophysiological hypotheses and help develop new treatment strategies; on the other hand some therapeutic strategies have been developed from pathophysiological hypotheses and have been used to prove or falsify these hypotheses.

In the following I will try to analyse this interaction between aetiological hypotheses and therapeutic strategies with some examples.

In general aetiological hypotheses can be divided into two groups:

1. IBD is initiated by a causative agent with either normal or abnormal reactions of the organism; or
2. abnormal reactions cause the disease without any special agents from the environment[1].

THERAPEUTIC STRATEGIES BASED ON THE HYPOTHESIS THAT CAUSATIVE AGENTS INITIATE IBD (Table 1)

Epidemiological studies suggested that food components might be responsible for the development of IBD. Several studies showed that patients with Crohn's

"

Table 1 Suspected causative agents for IBD and possible therapeutic consequences

Agent	Treatment	Effect
Sugar	Diet	0
Carbohydrates	Diet	?
Different food components	Exclusion diet	Limited
Bacteria	Antibiotics	Not established
Bacterial products (peptides, etc.)	?	Not studied

disease consume more sugar than healthy controls even before the onset of their disease[2]. It was therefore logical to try diets with reduced sugar content in Crohn's disease. Several studies have been performed to investigate the effect of such diets on the maintenance of remission in patients with quiescent Crohn's disease[3,4]. In the studies published to date no advantage of such a diet could be demonstrated. In the largest study, by Ritchie et al.[4], patients were treated either with a diet low in sugar and high in unrefined carbohydrates or with their usual diet. During 2 years no difference in the course of the two groups was found. The latest study investigating the effect of carbohydrates on Crohn's disease is only published as an abstract[5]. In this study not only was the sugar content of the diet reduced, but patients were advised to eat a diet containing less than 80 g of carbohydrates per day. Not all patients randomized to the diet group were compliant with this carbohydrate-reduced diet. The preliminary results indicate that this diet reduced the number of recurrences; however, before drawing conclusions the final publication of this study has to be awaited.

In summary, the studies on dietary treatment of Crohn's disease have been based on an aetiological hypothesis. However, by failing to show therapeutic effects they do not support this hypothesis. On the other hand they cannot invalidate the hypothesis that sugar may play an initiating role, since the reduction of sugar in the diet after the disease has begun might not necessarily eliminate the disease.

Another hypothesis is that individually different food components might cause relapses in Crohn's disease. Based on this hypothesis exclusion diets have been tried. For such diets each patient has to identify those food components which cause symptoms. By eliminating those foods a reduction in the number of relapses could be demonstrated[6]. However, similar results could not be obtained by other groups, which might lead to the conclusion that such an exclusion diet is helpful only for a subgroup of patients.

The use of parenteral nutrition as treatment for the active phase of Crohn's disease was based on the hypothesis of 'bowel rest'. This hypothesis was developed from the general assumption that food components, or the presence of the faecal stream in the gut, maintain inflammatory activity and induce relapses[7]. New studies on the effect of diversion stomata seem to support this hypothesis[8]. Total parenteral nutrition does induce bowel rest and is beneficial in active Crohn's disease. However, it could be shown that enteral nutrition is as effective as parenteral nutrition, indicating that bowel rest might not be the mechanism of action of nutritional treatment. It was assumed that enteral nutrition with elemental diets does in fact induce partial bowel rest, and might therefore be more effective than enteral nutrition with polymeric diets. Several studies have compared elemental and polymeric diets as treatment of the active phase of Crohn's disease. These studies yield different results, leading to no clear conclusion as to whether elemental or polymeric diets are superior. By comparing the published data on the efficacy of parenteral nutrition, enteral nutrition with elemental diets and enteral nutrition with polymeric diets, no significant difference between these three forms of treatment can be found (Table 2).

Table 2 Nutritional therapy in acute CD – effect of parenteral vs. enteral nutrition

	Patients (*n*)	Time (days)	Remission (%)		
			TPN	Elemental	Polymeric
Lochs et al., 1984[9]	25/25	28	73	60	
Greenberg et al., 1988[10]	17/15/19	21	71	60	58
Malchow et al., 1990[11]	51	42		41	
Giaffer et al., 1990[12]	16/14	28		75	36
Raouf et al., 1991[13]	13/11	21		70	73
Cravo et al., 1991[14]	24/15/42	?	75	73	83
Park et al., 1991[15]	7/7	28		29	71
Lochs et al., 1991[16]	55	42		60	
$\Sigma \bar{x}$	66/197/93		73 ± 1	59 ± 6	64 ± 8

TPN = Total parenteral nutrition.

In this regard nutritional therapy based on an aetiological hypothesis proved this hypothesis wrong, despite being effective as a therapeutic strategy.

Besides food components infectious agents have always been suspected as the cause of IBD. Based on this hypothesis several antibiotics have been tried in IBD. However, this kind of treatment is not generally considered to be effective. This does not, however, invalidate the initial hypothesis since it easily could be the case that (a) the infectious agent cannot be eliminated by the drugs used, and (b) infections are only an initiating event and do not contribute to the continuation of the disease.

THERAPEUTIC STRATEGIES BASED ON THE HYPOTHESIS THAT ABNORMAL REACTIONS CAUSE THE DISEASE

Studies have shown pathological cellular immune reactions in patients with IBD (Table 3). Many of the established medical therapies, e.g. corticosteroids or azathioprine, are based on this hypothesis. The most specific therapy to influence cellular immune reactions is probably the use of CD4 antibodies. This treatment – though still experimental – is based on the observation that the number of CD4-positive cells is elevated in patients with Crohn's disease. It could be shown that injection of CD4 antibodies not only reduces the number of CD4-positive cells, but also reduces disease activity in these patients[17]. This appears to indicate that a specific intervention in cellular

Table 3 Abnormal reactions as cause of IBD and possible therapeutic consequences

Reaction	Treatment	Effect
Immune reactions	Corticosteroid	+
	Azathioprine	+
	Methotrexate	?
	CD4 antibodies	+
Increased permeability	Misoprostol	Not investigated
	Corticosteroids	+
	Enteral nutrition	+

immune reactions does result in the predicted effect on the disease. Corticosteroids also influence immune reactions and are the most effective treatment in both Crohn's disease and ulcerative colitis. However, as will be discussed later, corticosteroids do have several other effects, and it is not clear if the immunosuppressive effect of corticosteroids is responsible for the effect on clinical activity of IBD.

Another abnormal reaction in patients with IBD is increased intestinal permeability[18]. It is not clear whether this increase in intestinal permeability is an initiating factor or if it occurs in early phases of IBD. However, the hypothesis was put forward that normalization of intestinal permeability might decrease inflammatory activity. In a study we could show that corticosteroids do normalize intestinal permeability, and this normalization is accompanied by a reduction in disease activity. In fact, all those patients who reacted with a decrease of the Crohn's disease activity index to corticosteroid therapy also showed a reduction of their increased intestinal permeability[19]. A completely different therapy – enteral nutrition – also reduces increased intestinal permeability in patients with active Crohn's disease. Again a good correlation between the effect of enteral nutrition on disease activity and intestinal permeability could be shown[18]. This might indicate that both treatments – corticosteroids as well as enteral nutrition – work via a different mechanism than initially assumed.

Over many years research has focused on altered mediators as aetiology for inflammatory bowel disease (Table 4). On the one hand studies showed

Table 4 Altered mediators as cause of IBD and possible therapeutic consequences

Mediator	Treatment	Effect
Cytokines	Corticosteroids	+
	5-ASA	+
	IL-1 receptor antagonists	?
	Interferon	?
Leukotrienes	SASP	+
Thromboxanes	5-ASA/4-ASA	+
	Omega-3 fatty acids	?
	5-Lipoxygenase inhibitors	?

elevated concentrations of several cytokines in peripheral blood[20] as well as in lamina propria cells in patients with IBD; on the other hand it is known that production of leukotrienes and thomboxanes is abnormal in IBD. The fact that corticosteroids do reduce IL-1 and IL-6 concentrations in peripheral blood might indicate that this is the mechanism of action of corticosteroids in the treatment of IBD. However, other substances, such as interferon which also reduce IL-6 concentration, do not have favourable effects on disease activity in patients with IBD.

Sulphasalazine and 5-ASA interfere with the leukotriene production which was considered to be the mechanism of action of these drugs in IBD. Several drugs which have similar but more specific effects on leukotriene production have been tested in IBD, but do not give comparable clinical results. Omega 3-fatty acids, for example, cause similar changes in the production of leukotrienes as sulphasalazine but have much lower clinical efficiency[21]. Recently lipoxygenase inhibitors have been tested in ulcerative colitis and appeared to be less effective than 5-ASA, which might indicate that the clinical effect of 5-ASA is multifactorial. This view is supported by the finding that 5-ASA has several other effects besides influencing leukotriene production. It does, for example, also reduce IL-1 concentrations[22].

From the above-mentioned examples it becomes clear that: (a) some therapeutic strategies were developed from aetiological hypotheses. Only a part of these therapies is clinically efficient. In some cases it could be shown that the mechanism of action of treatments is different from the initial hypothesis which led to the introduction of the treatment. (b) Some therapies which are clinically effective led to the formulation of an aetiological hypothesis and consequently to the testing of other substances with the same mechanism. Many of these substances were not effective.

In summary it can be concluded that the aetiology of IBD is multifactorial, and hypotheses about single aetiological factors might not lead to efficient therapies.

References

1. Podolsky DK. Inflammatory bowel disease. N Engl J Med. 1991;325:928–37.
2. Lorenz-Meyer H, Brandes JW. Gibt es eine diätetische Behandlung des Morbus Crohn in der Remission? Dtsch Med Wochenschr. 1988;108:595–7.
3. Brandes JW, Lorenz-Meyer H. Zuckerfreie Diät: Eine neue Perspektive zur Behandlung des Morbus Crohn. Eine randomisierte kontrollierte Studie. Z Gastroenterol. 1981;19:1–2.
4. Ritchie JK, Wadsworth J, Lennard-Jones JE *et al*. Controlled multicentre therapeutic trial of an unrefined carbohydrate, fibre rich diet in Crohn's disease. Br Med J. 1987;295:517–20.
5. Lorenz-Meyer H, Purrmann J, Scheurlen C *et al*. Crohnstudie V; Ergebnisse der Studie zur Erhaltung der Remission bei Morbus Crohn mit 0-3-FS bzw. einer kohlenhydratarmen Kost. Z Gastroenterol. 1992;9:654.
6. Jones VA, Workman E, Freeman AH *et al*. Crohn's disease: maintenance of remission by diet. Lancet. 1985;2:177–80.
7. Harper PH, Lee ECG, Kettlewell MGW *et al*. Role of the faecal stream in the maintenance of Crohn's colitis. Gut. 1988;26:279–84.
8. Rutgeerts P, Goboes K, Peeters M *et al*. Effect of faecal stream diversion on recurrence of Crohn's disease in the neoterminal ileum. Lancet. 1991;338:771–4.

9. Lochs H, Egger-Schödl M, Pötzi R *et al*. Enterale Ernährung – eine Alternative zur parenteralen Ernährung in der Behandlung des Morbus Crohn? Leber-Magen-Darm. 1984;14:64–7.
10. Greenberg GR, Fleming CR, Jeejeebhoy KN *et al*. Controlled trial of bowel rest and nutritional support in the management of Crohn's disease. Gut. 1988;29:1309–15.
11. Malchow H, Steinhardt HJ, Lorenz-Meyer H *et al*. Feasibility and effectiveness of a defined formula diet regimen in treating active Crohn's disease: European Cooperative Crohn's Disease Study III. Scand J Gastroenterol. 1990;25:235–44.
12. Giaffer MH, North G, Holdsworth CD. Controlled trial of polymeric versus elemental diet in treatment of active Crohn's disease. Lancet. 1990;335:816–19.
13. Raouf AH, Hildrey V, Daniel J *et al*. Enteral feeding as sole treatment for Crohn's disease: controlled trial of whole protein v amino-acid based feed and a case study of dietary challenge. Gut. 1991;32:702–7.
14. Cravo M, Camilo ME, Correia JP. Nutritional support in Crohn's disease: which route? Am J Gastroenterol. 1991;86:317–21.
15. Park RHR, Galloway A, Danesh BJZ *et al*. Double-blind controlled trial of elemental and polymeric diets as primary therapy in active Crohn's disease. Eur J Gastroenterol Hepatol. 1991;3:483–90.
16. Lochs H, Steinhardt HJ, Klaus-Wentz B *et al*. Comparison of enteral nutrition and drug treatment in active Crohn's disease. Results of the European Cooperative Crohn's disease study IV. Gastroenterology. 1991;101:881–8.
17. Emmrich J, Seyfarth M, Fleig WE *et al*. Treatment of inflammatory bowel disease with anti-CD4 monoclonal antibody. Lancet. 1991;338:570–1.
18. Sanderson IR, Boulton P, Menzies I *et al*. Improvement of abnormal lactulose/rhamnose permeability in active Crohn's disease of the small bowel by an elemental diet. Gut. 1987;28:1073–6.
19. Wyatt J, Vogelsang H, Lochs H. Effect of corticosteroids on intestinal permeability in patients with active Crohn's disease. Gastroenterology. 1992;102:A947.
20. Gross V, Andus T, Caesar I *et al*. Evidence for continuous stimulation of interleukin-6 production in Crohn's disease. Gastroenterology. 1992;102:514–19.
21. Stenson WF, Cort D, Rodgers J *et al*. Dietary supplementation with fish oil in ulcerative colitis. Ann Intern Med. 1992;116:609–14.
22. Mahida YR, Lamming CED, Gallagher A *et al*. 5-Aminosalicylic acid is a potent inhibitor of interleukin 1β production in organ culture of colonic biopsy specimens from patients with inflammatory bowel disease. Gut. 1991;32:50–4.

Section II
Pathophysiology — Immunology

5

The mucosal immune system: structure and function

A. TOBIN

INTRODUCTION

Recent decades have wrought enormous changes in the study of the immune system. The field of immunology has expanded to embrace many other disciplines such as biochemistry, molecular biology and genetics. The pace of new discovery continues to gain speed as ever more powerful and sophisticated research tools become available.

Despite our increasingly detailed knowledge of cellular processes within the immune system, the cause or causes of inflammatory bowel disease remain conjectural. Ulcerative colitis and Crohn's disease form the ends of a spectrum of chronic inflammatory disorders of the intestine in which no infectious agent has been implicated. The inability to establish an infectious basis for these diseases led many investigators to postulate that an endogenous immune defect triggers and maintains chronic inflammation and tissue damage. Indirect evidence that immune mechanisms may be important in inflammatory bowel disease is provided by several clinical observations. The natural history of recurrent relapse and remission, the frequent involvement of joints, skin, liver and eyes, and the tendency for inflammatory bowel disease sufferers to have an increased incidence of organ-specific autoimmune disorders[1] point to an immune pathogenesis, while the response to immunosuppressive doses of corticosteroids is often dramatic in acute but not in chronic disease[2].

It remains unknown whether inflammatory bowel disease reflects a primary immunoregulatory defect, an ineffectual attempt to clear an as yet unidentified agent or a secondary failure to shut off an appropriate inflammatory response. Nevertheless, it is clear that the ongoing tissue inflammation and injury is mediated to a large degree by the host immune response. While earlier hopes of discovering a curable cause remain unfulfilled, our improved understanding of the escalation from immune response to inflammation holds the promise of being able to selectively intervene to block the inflammatory process without exposing the host to the risks of generalized immunosuppression.

Early workers, studying readily accessible peripheral blood cells, described a variety of abnormalities of the systemic immune system in inflammatory bowel disease. Disappointingly, most have turned out to be non-specific sequelae of chronic disease, malnutrition and immunosuppression, rather than specific markers of the disease itself. The availability of techniques to isolate and purify mucosal cell populations has led to a shift in emphasis from the secondary events of the systemic circulation to the primary site of disease, the intestine itself, and the complex interrelationships and regulatory circuits of the mucosal immune system.

This chapter will begin by focusing on selected aspects of mucosal immunity before going on to consider the alterations present in the immune system in inflammatory bowel disease.

MUCOSAL IMMUNE SYSTEM – ORGANIZATION

The mucosal immune system monitors the largest interface in the body and mounts appropriate immune responses to luminal antigens. The digestive function of the gastrointestinal tract has dictated the evolution of several attributes of the mucosal immune system. While remaining unresponsive to the myriad harmless antigens present in gut commensals and foods, it must recognize and vigorously respond to mucosal pathogens without generating inflammatory responses which would impair the assimilation of nutrients; it must limit the entry of exogenous antigen to the internal milieu, and it must regulate the response of the systemic immune system to common environmental agents that would otherwise overwhelm the system with response to trivial antigen.

The enormity of this task is reflected in the size of the intestinal immune system. Composed of lymphoid and non-lymphoid cells arranged around the gut lumen, the gut associated lymphoid tissue (GALT) accounts for one-half to one-third of the lymphoid cell population of the body. Thus, in addition to its nutritive function, the gut accommodates the largest lymphoid organ in the body, which occupies a quarter of its volume.

Arranged in afferent and efferent limbs which link the mucosa to the systemic circulation and other non-intestinal mucosal tissues, the GALT can be considered to contain three distinct compartments. The organized lymphoid structures such as the Peyer's patches, tonsils and appendix contain generative or 'afferent' areas where sampled luminal antigen and mitogens initiate cell activation and differentiation. 'Efferent' or receiving areas include the lamina propria and the intra-epithelial compartment, where antigens interact with cells to induce terminal differentiation leading to antibody production or cytotoxic reactions. Whereas the lamina propria is populated by a heterogeneous collection of cells including T cells, B cells, macrophages, mast cells and other non-lymphoid cells, the majority of the intraepithelial lymphocytes bear mature T cell markers. The strategic location of these cells, in close proximity to the lumen, strongly suggests that they play a key role in local immune homeostasis.

Each of these three locations function as discrete compartments, harbouring cell subpopulations whose collective function is specific for that micro-environment and whose constituent cell types are stable but not static. The Peyer's patches serve as major sites of luminal antigen sampling. Constant immune surveillance of the intestinal contents takes place via their specialized overlying dome epithelium. Here, reduced mucus and secretory immunoglobulin A facilitate active uptake by the microfold-containing cells of both viable particulate and soluble antigen[3]. This is transported to the underlying macrophages and dendritic cells, which process them and present them to adjacent T cells within the patch. Interleukin-2, among other signals secreted by the activated T cell, in turn stimulates the clonal expansion of T and B lymphoblasts, which continues as they migrate from the follicle through the mesenteric lymph nodes, thoracic duct and circulation before homing to the lamina propria and intestinal epithelium. In this way the organized lymphoid follicles serve as the major sites of activation and programming of Ig-A producing B cells and mucosally directed effector T cells; the reactions which take place within the follicle give rise to the differentiated cells which eventually home to and populate the other compartments within the mucosa.

The maintenance of such compartmentalization of cell type and function depends upon the massive and highly regulated circulation of lymphocytes. Constant cell traffic links these microenvironments to each other and to the systemic circulation; an estimated 10^{10} cells migrate between the intestinal lymph and peripheral circulation each day, sufficient to replace the blood content of lymphocytes 10–20 times per day. The majority of these cells are lymphocytes that had emigrated from the blood several hours earlier, and return to initiate another cycle; they are joined by immunoblasts, memory cells and terminally differentiated effector cells. Such an enormous throughput enhances the likelihood of an antigen sequestered in a lymphoid follicle encountering one of the typically rare lymphocytes which can respond to it, and facilitates the dissemination of responding effector cells to locations remote from their initial site of antigen presentation.

LYMPHOCYTE MIGRATION

How lymphocytes home to and lodge in various tissues is a major area of research with profound implications for inflammatory bowel disease, where the normal cellular composition of the mucosa is disturbed and there is an influx of acute inflammatory cells. The entry of blood-borne lymphocytes into lymphoid follicles is by means of adhesion to the specialized cuboidal endothelium of the high endothelial venule (HEV)[4]. Current research indicates that the interaction between lymphocytes and the HEV is extraordinarily specific, involving binding of specific 'homing receptors' or addressins on the lymphocytes with complementary ligands on the HEV. This bond depends on cell subset, maturity, prior antigenic stimulation and level of activation, as well as the anatomical location of the HEV. There is evidence that macrophages and other cells, by means of their secreted products, may act to induce adhesive ligands on HEV. *In vitro*, exposure of cultured umbilical vein endothelium to IL-1, IFN-γ and TNF augments its ability to bind lymphocytes.

CELL-MEDIATED IMMUNITY

A large and confusing literature exists on the subject of the state of activation and immunomodulatory function of intestinal lymphocytes. It is becoming clear that substantial inter-species differences exist, making extrapolation from animal studies unreliable. Awareness is also growing that marked regional variation exists within the intestine, and that studies of small bowel isolates may not reflect activity in the colon. This complex area has been the subject of many excellent reviews, and will be addressed elsewhere in this book. Accordingly, it will not be dealt with in detail here.

Several different lines of evidence indicate that the lamina propria represents a site of enhanced cell activation. Studies of morphological and phenotypical markers of activation accord with functional studies demonstrating enhanced spontaneous proliferation and uptake of tritiated thymidine. Although the proportions of CD4 and CD8 T cells in lamina propria and organized lymphoid structures are similar to those in the circulation[5,6], significant differences exist in their immunoregulatory function. Intestinal CD4 cells provide more help for immunoglobulin synthesis than peripheral blood CD4 cells. Unlike peripheral blood CD4 cells, incubation with anti-leu-8 antibody does not induce suppressor function, reflecting lower levels of leu-8 antigen expression[7]. Mucosal CD4, leu-8 + cells appear similar to peripheral blood in exhibiting low levels of suppression for IgM synthesis in the absence of concanavalin A.

In contrast with the predominance of helper function in the lamina propria, CD4 cells within the lymphoid follicles have been shown to preferentially induce suppressor cells, and can themselves suppress immunoglobulin synthesis. Depending on experimental conditions, intestinal CD8 cells can exhibit either helper or suppressor function[8]. Recent studies suggest that lamina propria lymphocytes are more resistant than peripheral blood lymphocytes to down-regulation by compounds generated during inflammation, such as prostaglandin E2. In a series of experiments where cells were stimulated via the CD2 or CD3 pathways in the presence of PGE_2, LPL were found to be more sensitive to down-regulation when activated via the CD3 pathway, and less so when pre-activated by incubation with phytohaemagglutinin, suggesting that susceptibility to down-regulation is influenced by mechanism and level of activation[9].

Investigation of cytotoxicity has been a major area of interest. The proportion of natural killer (NK) cells expressing leu-7 antigen within the mucosa is considerably lower than in the circulation, and most studies conclude that mucosal levels of NK function are low, although this may be due to failure to recognize phenotypic variants or to utilize the appropriate targets in functional assays. Inducible cytotoxicity has been widely demonstrated;

LAK cells may readily be induced by incubation of lamina propria cells with Il-2 and are active against a wide range of targets. There are varying reports of the level of other forms of killing, including antibody-dependent cellular cytotoxicity and mitogen-induced cytotoxicity, again due to differences in cell isolation and assay techniques.

The importance of the role played by non-lymphoid cells such as macrophages is increasingly being recognized. These heterogeneous cells, of which over 90% express class II molecules, carry out a wide range of functions including antigen presentation, microbicidal and tumoricidal activity, phagocytosis and enzyme and cytokine secretion. Morphologically, there are marked regional variations within the gut, whose functional significance is not known. Cellular aggregates incorporating macrophages have been among the earliest alterations found in the bowel in Crohn's disease, fuelling intense study of this cell type's pluripotent function in inflammatory bowel disease.

The demonstration of the heavy innervation of lymphoid tissue, and in particular of the proximity of nerve endings to mucosal mast cells, has stimulated study of the bidirectional communication between the neuroendocrine and immune systems. Neural cells have receptors for lymphokines such as IL-1, which influences the central nervous system. Under certain circumstances lymphocytes can secrete not only interleukins and other cytokines, but endorphin-like neuropeptides and ACTH, and possess receptors for a wide range of neuropeptides. Although in its infancy, the study of this additional level of function of the mucosal immune system may translate into potential for new therapeutic strategies.

HUMORAL IMMUNITY – SECRETORY IgA

One of the hallmarks of the mucosal immune system is its preferential utilization of immunoglobulin A (IgA) in response to antigenic stimuli. In contrast to circulating monomeric IgA of bone marrow origin, most IgA secreted at mucosal surfaces is produced by plasma cells within the lamina propria in the form of a dimer of IgA linked by a J (joining) chain. Additional stability to withstand the harsh intraluminal environment is conferred by binding to secretory component, which functions as a unique 'sacrificial receptor' to transport the complex across the epithelial cell to the intestinal lumen. Most circulating IgA is in the form of IgA_1, which is particularly susceptible to proteases produced by many bacteria as virulence factors; in the intestine the proportion of the more resistant IgA_2 rises steadily in luminal secretions from the small bowel to the rectum[10], reflecting the higher proportion of IgA_2 producing cells in the distal colon and rectum[11]. This preponderance may be partly antigen-driven, as lipopolysaccharide from Gram-negative bacteria is known to primarily elicit an IgA_2 response[12].

Several properties of secretory IgA (sIgA) make it particularly suitable for the task of disarming and eliminating potential pathogens in a non-inflammatory way. Inefficient at killing microorganisms, it does not bind complement and is a poor opsonin. Secretory IgA appears to be an infrequent and relatively ineffectual mediator of antibody-dependent cellular cytotoxicity[13]. Despite its lack of participation in inflammatory reactions, sIgA secreted into the gut lumen can bind to invasive bacteria, preventing their adhesion to gut epithelium[14]. It also appears to prevent enteric viral colonization and infection[15], and can block absorption of proteins across the gut epithelium[16]. Much has been made of the role of sIgA in 'immune exclusion', that is, inhibition of uptake of non-viable antigen at mucosal surfaces. This scavenging function is not confined to the mucosa – circulating IgA-bound antigen binds to transmembrane secretory component on hepatocytes in the rat[17] and other species, and is excreted into bile. A similar mechanism involving ductal epithelial cells has been described in humans[18].

ISOTYPE REGULATION

Over 90% of the B cells and plasma cells in the normal lamina propria express IgA. The mechanisms governing this isotype predominance are undoubtedly complex, and include regulation by T cells and their secreted lymphokines in at least two stages. T cells that induce immature IgM-bearing cells to switch to IgA have been isolated from murine Peyer's patches[19]. Once switched, other T cell factors induce further proliferation and maturation.

In 1986 two subgroups of T helper clones in mice were defined on the basis of their differing patterns of lymphokine secretion[20,21]. In conjunction with *in vitro* work with recombinant cytokines, evidence has accumulated that the Th2-specific cytokines IL-4, 5 and 6 preferentially provide help for B cell growth and differentiation and exert a major influence on the isotype and amount of antibody produced to a given antigen. Although in humans the distinction between T helper clones is not as distinct, these findings are of great relevance to the disordered pattern of immunoglobulin secretion found in inflammatory bowel disease. The replacement of IgA by IgG_1 in ulcerative colitis and IgG_2 in Crohn's disease may reflect altered ratios of secreted lymphokines in the mucosa. Recent reports of increased levels of IL-1, IL-6[22,23] and IL-8[24,25] in the circulation and mucosa of patients with Crohn's disease, and an imbalance between secretion of IL-1 and IL-1 receptor antagonist[26,27] lend weight to this view. Better understanding of this complex area depends on elucidation of the factors driving differential induction of T helper subsets, which may be influenced by the type of antigen-presenting cell involved, or the antigen itself.

ANTIGEN HANDLING – ABSORPTION, PROCESSING AND PRESENTATION

The traditional view of mucosal immunity has tended to focus on humoral defences while neglecting the role of cellular regulation of immunity. The normal human intestine abounds in cell types other than those necessary for B cell responses, reminding us that cellular immune reactions in the digestive tract are also of major importance, and that humoral defences constitute only part of the array of host mechanisms active at mucosal surfaces. Although agglutination of pathogens followed by peristaltic clearance reduces the antigenic load at the mucosal surface, large amounts of antigen gain access to the immunocompetent cells lying beneath the intestinal epithelium. Most are harmless, frequently encountered antigens to which a state of unresponsiveness or tolerance must be maintained. Several studies have demonstrated that fed antigen tends to elicit specific suppressor T cells which directly, and by means of soluble factors, induce systemic unresponsiveness, with or without the production of local specific IgA. This phenomenon, known as oral tolerance, is a major homeostatic mechanism which prevents the host being overwhelmed by response to trivial antigen. The conditions which dictate the outcome of interaction with antigen are incompletely understood. Physical properties of the antigen – such as size and type of antigen, whether cellular, particulate or soluble – appear important, as is the maturity and prior exposure of the host. The site of initial interaction between antigen and intestinal immune system may be critical, determining subsequent handling and the type of cells to which it is presented. There are three potential sites where antigen crosses the epithelium. As described earlier, most attention has been directed to the active transport mechanisms of the specialized microfold containing cells overlying lymphoid aggregates.

Antigen may also pass between epithelial cells, though this paracellular mechanism probably only operates where the intercellular tight junctions are disrupted by inflammation. This route presumably assumes considerable importance in inflammatory bowel disease, where there is chronic loss of mucosal integrity.

Another possible route of entry is through the epithelial cell itself. This last portal of entry is potentially of major importance, as a novel role for enterocytes as antigen-presenting cells has been proposed. The role of antigen-presenting cells is currently an area of great interest. Hitherto, the formation of the trimolecular complex composed of the T cell receptor binding antigen coexpressed with class II determinants on the surface of an antigen-presenting cell, has been viewed as the pivotal event in the generation of specific immunity. There is a growing appreciation that the uptake, processing and presentation of antigen by different cell types may profoundly influence the rate and type of response generated. Several groups have reported that epithelial cells are able to present antigen to T cell[28] *in vitro*, but they differ in several respects from conventional antigen-presenting cells. Current evidence indicates that they have a far more limited ability to process bound antigen, and may simply bind peptides which have been degraded by luminal proteases. Epithelial cells also lack the macrophages' capacity to elaborate cytokines such as IL-1 and IL-6, which amplify T cell responses by inducing expression of IL-2 receptors. These limitations suggest that epithelial cells may present antigen only to specific T cell clones, a hypothesis borne out by the finding that, in contrast to conventional antigen-presenting cells which elicit a $CD4^+$ helper response, normal epithelial cells preferentially activate suppressor cells[29]. This potentially important mechanism for maintaining non-reactivity to antigen absorbed across the epithelium has been reported to be disturbed in inflammatory bowel disease[30]. In inflammatory bowel disease, epithelial cell/T cell cultures fail to elicit suppression, instead activating T helper cells, which in turn secrete cytokines such as IFN-γ, further promoting inflammation by inducing local macrophage activation and epithelial class II expression.

Attention is now focusing on other cell types as potential antigen-presenters. Recently, evidence was presented that M cells possess acidic lysosomal compartments containing structures on which MHC class II determinants are expressed – characteristics necessary for antigen processing and presentation[31].

While the *in vivo* significance of these new findings is not yet known, they afford tantalizing glimpses of the complexity of mucosal immunoregulation, and of a potentially crucial defect in inflammatory bowel disease.

IMMUNOPATHOLOGY IN INFLAMMATORY BOWEL DISEASE

In inflammatory bowel disease the defences of the mucosal barrier and secretory IgA are breached, and the highly antigenic contents of the gut lumen come into direct contact with the immunocompetent cells of the mucosa. Inevitably multiple immune reactions take place; the difficulty lies in distinguishing between those which are epiphenomena and those which mediate the disease. Examination of early lesions may afford clues about triggering events and initial responses unobscured by secondary changes due to chronicity or treatment. Such early lesions have been documented in Crohn's disease; even in patients with clinically inactive or distant disease, biopsy of endoscopically normal rectal mucosa yields microgranulomas in up to 18% of cases[32]. Using a magnifying endoscope and dye staining distorted areas of epithelium overlying small collections of lymphocytes and prominent macrophages have been detected[33]. Microgranulomas and granulomas were present in 70% of these areas, compared with 30% in adjacent normal tissue. Further study of these microscopic lesions confirmed that they exhibited similar changes to those seen in severely diseased surgical specimens[34]: an absolute increase in T cells but with preservation of the normal CD4/CD8 ratio, expression of HLA-D by colonic epithelium, and the presence of distinct subpopulations of macrophages which are rare in uninflamed areas. Some of these are positive for RDF9, a marker also expressed by epithelioid cells present in granulomas, and 3G8, which recognizes a receptor for IgG, whose function is unknown but may mediate clearance of immune complexes[35].

The presence of these lesions distant from overtly involved bowel suggests that the whole intestine may be abnormal in Crohn's disease, while the fact that these microscopic lesions contain the same cellular infiltrate and granuloma formation as mature lesions indicated that these may be primary events. The superficial nature of the inflammatory infiltrate and granulomas in association with a functional impairment of the epithelium (the inability to take up dye) may represent an epithelial reaction to a luminal stimulus. On the other hand, earlier studies where cellular infiltrates were present in the absence of any evidence of epithelial change were interpreted to mean that inflammatory foci within the mucosa damaged the epithelium as a secondary event[36].

No such preclinical lesions have been identified in ulcerative colitis, perhaps in part because of the comparative inaccessibility of normal bowel in a disease that begins distally and extends proximally. Interestingly, although the increase in macrophage numbers in the mucosa in ulcerative colitis is often less marked than in Crohn's disease, aggregates of RDF$^+$ and 3G8$^+$ macrophages have also been reported in ulcerative colitis[37].

Mature inflammatory lesions in both ulcerative colitis and Crohn's disease have been the subject of intense study. Drawing on immunohistochemical studies of intact tissue, cell extraction techniques, and more recently monoclonal antibody staining of cell surface markers, an attempt can be made to piece together a composite picture of events within the mucosa.

Several factors contribute to the weakening of the mucosal barrier in inflammatory bowel disease. It has long been recognized that goblet cell numbers and mucus production are reduced in ulcerative colitis. Abnormal glycosylation of mucus has been reported; in ulcerative colitis monoclonal antibodies to mucin glycoproteins recognize an antigen not expressed in normal or diseased controls[38]. This antigen, which appears independent of inflammation, may mark a biochemical abnormality in which normal mucosal constituents are exposed to pathogenic responses. Circulating antibodies reacting with goblet cells and glycocalix have been reported in ulcerative colitis[39,40], while large amounts of tissue-bound IgG specific to ulcerative colitis recognize a 40 kDa protein constituent of normal mucosa[41]. Abnormal mucus may be more susceptible to bacterial degradation, and may be further denatured by reactive oxygen species produced by phagocytes attracted into the mucosa in IBS.

Although the number of IgA-bearing cells in the lamina propria is doubled, overall IgA production is reduced[42]. The normal secretory pattern of c. 70% dimeric IgA, of which c. 40% is IgA$_2$, is replaced by production of mainly monomeric IgA$_1$[42], which is more susceptible to enzymatic degradation within the lumen.

The combination of abnormal IgA and mucus production increases the epithelium's vulnerability to bacterial attack, and allows the diffusion of bacterial products, such as N-formyl-methionyl-leucyl-phenylalanine (FMLP) and endotoxin, into the lamina propria where they may attract and activate phagocytic cells, initiating an inflammatory response. Animal experiments have demonstrated that FMLP activation of migrating neutrophils increases mucosal permeability due to capillary damage and inflammation[43].

Within the lamina propria the numbers of mononuclear cells increase 2–4-fold. Lymphoid follicles increase in number and size, and may contain multiple germinal centres. Although T-cell subsets within inflammatory bowel disease lesions appear similar to control intestinal tissue[5], increased surface expression of a variety of markers attests to enhanced cell activation[44–46]. There are dramatic alterations in immunoglobulin isotype and subclass profile, though the relative contribution of extravasated peripheral blood cells and altered local production is not known. The normal marked preponderance of locally produced IgA gives way to a 30-fold increase in

IgG-bearing cells; IgM-bearing cells are also increased[47,48]. In ulcerative colitis most of the IgG is of the IgG_1 subclass, with some IgG_3, while in Crohn's disease IgG_2 is the major subclass produced[49,50]. Antibody isotype and subclass response are in part determined by the nature of the antigen; proteins preferentially elicit an IgG_1 response, while carbohydrates have been shown to primarily evoke IgG_2. This is one piece of evidence that the mucosal stimulus may be different in ulcerative colitis and Crohn's disease. Interestingly, elevations of IgG_1 have also been reported in autoimmune diseases such as rheumatoid arthritis and systemic lupus erythematosus, as well as glomerulonephritis and ulcerative colitis.

Functionally, the replacement of scavenging IgA with the more biologically active IgG has major implications for local immunity. IgG can activate complement, induce cell-mediated cytotoxicity and initiate phagocytosis. IgG_1 and IgG_3 are more efficient complement pathway activators and opsonins than IgG_2; their increased production in ulcerative colitis might suggest a more important role for complement activation in local tissue injury than in Crohn's disease. Increased turnover of C3 has been reported in inflammatory bowel disease, implying activation of the classical pathway by immune complexes, while recent studies using a monoclonal antibody to the terminal complement complex demonstrated complement deposition in submucosal vessels to the same extent in both diseases[51].

Macrophages are increased in both ulcerative colitis and Crohn's disease; cells thought to act as scavengers increase in number and staining intensity, particularly in the deeper layers of the mucosa and submucosa, while two subtypes appear which are rare in normal intestine and infectious colitis[37].

Despite their designation as chronic inflammatory diseases, both ulcerative colitis and Crohn's disease are characterized by the presence of acute inflammatory cells such as neutrophils and monocytes attracted from the circulation. There is convincing evidence that neutrophil- and monocyte-mediated damage is a major contributor to mucosal injury. Products of granulocyte arachidonate metabolism such as prostaglandin E_2, leukotriene B_4 (LTB_4) and platelet-activating factor are increased in ulcerative colitis mucosa, and their levels correlate with disease activity and degree of mucosal inflammation. The damaged mucosa contains several potential chemotactic agents in addition to LTB_4. Bacterial cell wall products such as FMLP, lipopolysaccharide (LPS) and the product of complement activation, C5a, may also play a role. A study which examined the chemoattractant properties of fractionated colonic mucosa found that LTB_4, of which neutrophils are the major source, accounted for most of the chemotactic activity in inflammatory bowel disease mucosa[52]. Recent work suggests that other potent neutrophil chemoattractants and activators may also be increased; increased messenger RNA for IL-1β, IL-6 and IL-8 has been reported in cultures of inflammatory bowel disease mucosa[53].

Monocytes attracted from the circulation to the mucosa ingest antigen, become activated and secrete IL-1. Evidence has accumulated which suggests that the production of IL-1 and other monocyte–macrophage products is abnormal. Spontaneous[54] and LPS-stimulated[55] production of IL-1 by peripheral blood monocytes is increased in Crohn's disease, while their increased prostaglandin E_2 production has been thought to mediate excessive suppression of T cell proliferative responses in both ulcerative colitis and Crohn's disease. Similar abnormalities have been described at mucosal level; intestinal lamina propria mononuclear cells in both Crohn's disease and ulcerative colitis have been reported to produce increased amounts of granulocyte colony-stimulating factor and IL-1[44], both major mediators of granulocyte proliferation, chemotaxis and activation. Not only are absolute levels of IL-1 increased; it appears that there is also discordant production of its physiological antagonist, IL-1 receptor antagonist, which competitively binds IL-1 surface receptors. Recent reports suggest that the ratio of IL-1 to IL-1 receptor antagonist is abnormally low in ulcerative colitis and Crohn's disease[26,27], which may result in an impaired ability to down-regulate, favouring the perpetuation of inflammation.

CLINICAL IMPLICATIONS FOR TREATMENT

For many years the best we could offer our patients with inflammatory bowel disease was a range of empirically derived therapies, whose beneficial effects were unpredictable and whose side-effects were numerous. The clinical impression that inflammatory bowel disease was a heterogeneous disorder, with varying disease patterns and responses to theapy, was not paralleled by any available means to discriminate among them.

The avalanche of new information emerging on immune function in health and disease has not only added greatly to our understanding of the abnormalities at mucosal level, but holds the promise of being able to identify different patterns of disease, permitting a more rational approach to therapy. Information on immunoregulatory networks is beginning to translate into exciting new avenues of therapy for immune-mediated disease. The genes for most of the known cytokines and their receptors can be cloned and expressed using recombinant DNA technology, allowing the molecules of the immune system to be harnessed as therapeutic agents. Monoclonal antibodies directed against specific subsets of T cells and their receptors should enable their modulation in a highly circumscribed fashion. Clinical trials using anti-CD4 monoclonal antibodies have already shown promising results in the treatment of inflammatory bowel disease[56]. The use of soluble receptors such as IL-1 receptor will allow the selective down-regulation of the inflammatory process. Knowledge of the mechanisms regulating secretion of naturally occurring competitive inhibitors, such as IL-1 receptor antagonist, may permit their manipulation.

The diversity and versatility of the secretory products of the mucosal immune system will doubtless confound many attempts to specifically influence one small part of it. Implementation of these new modalities of treatment will not occur overnight. The translation of new advances at the molecular and cellular level to the clinical level is accompanied by an exponential increase in complexity. Nevertheless, early evidence of therapeutic success in experimental models of immune disease confirms the value of a more specific immunotherapy. Tailoring the treatment of the patient with inflammatory bowel disease should reduce risks and side-effects while permitting fundamental alteration of the natural history of the disease.

References

1. Greenstein AJ, Janowity HD, Sacher DB. The extra-intestinal complications of Crohn's disease and ulcerative colitis: a study of 700 patients. Medicine. 1982;55:401.
2. Truelove SC, Witts LJ. Cortisone and corticotrophin in ulcerative colitis. Br Med J. 1959;1:387.
3. Wolf JL, Bye WA. The membranous epithelial (M) cell and the mucosal immune system. Ann Ren Med. 1984;35:95.
4. Stamper HB, Woodruff JJ. Lymphocyte homing into lymph nodes: *in vitro* demonstration of the selective affinity of recirculating lymphocytes for high endothelial venules. J Exp Med. 1975;144:828–931.
5. Selby WS, Janossy G, Bofull M, Jewell DP. Intestinal lymphocyte subpopulations in inflammatory bowel disease: analysis by immunohistological and cell isolation techniques. Gut. 1984;25:32.
6. James SP, Fiocchi C, Graeff AS, Strober W. Phenotypic analysis of lamina propria lymphocytes: predominance of helper-inducer and cytolytic T cell phenotypes and deficiency of suppressor-induced phenotypes in Crohn's disease and control patients. Gastroenterology. 1986;21:1483.
7. Kanoff ME, Strober W, Fiocchi C *et al.* CD4 positive Leu-8 negative helper-inducer T cells predominate in the human intestinal lamina propria. J Immunol. 1988;141:3029–36.
8. Lee A, Sugerman H, Elson CO. Regulatory activity of the human CD8$^+$ cell subset: a comparison of CD8$^+$ cells from the intestinal lamina propria and blood. Eur J Immunol. 1988;18:21–7.
9. Deem RL, Nel A, Targan SR. Relative refractoriness of lamina propria vs peripheral blood T-cell cytokine production to down-regulation by prostaglandin E2. Digestive Diseases Week 1992, abstract no. 955.
10. Delacroix DL, Dive C, Rambaud JC, Vaerman JP. IgA subclasses in various secretions and in serum. Immunology. 1982;47:383.
11. Andre C, Andre F, Faigier MC. Distribution of IgA1 and IgA2 plasma cells in various normal human tissues and in the jejunum of plasma IgA deficient patients. Clin Exp Immunol. 1978;33:327.
12. Mestecky J, Russell MW. IgA subclasses. Monogr. Allergy. 1986;19:277.
13. Kagnoff MF, Campbell S. Antibody dependent cell mediated cytotoxicity: comparative ability of murine Peyer's patches and spleen cells to lyse lipopolysaccharide coated and uncoated erythrocytes. Gastroenterology. 1976;70:341.
14. Williams RC, Gibbons RJ. Inhibition of bacterial adherence by secretory immunoglobulin A: a mechanism of antigen disposal. Science. 1972;177:697.
15. Ogra PL, Karzon DT. Distribution of poliovirus antibody in serum, nasopharynx and alimentary tract following segmental immunization of bowel alimentary tract with poliovaccine. J Immunol. 1969;102:1423.
16. Andre C, Lambert R, Bazin H, Heremans JF. Interference of oral immunisation with the intestinal absorption of heterologous albumin. Eur J Immunol. 1974;4:701.
17. Sztul ES, Howell KE, Palade GE. Intracellular and transcellular transport of secretory component and albumin in rat hepatocytes. J Cell Biol. 1983;97:1582.
18. Nagura H, Smith PD, Natane PK, Brown WR. IgA in human bile and liver. J Immunol. 1981;126:587.
19. Kawanishi H, Ozato K, Shober W. Mechanisms regulating IgA class-specific immunoglobulin production in murine gut-associated lymphoid postswitch SIgA bearing Peyer's patch B cells. J Exp Med. 1983;158:649.
20. Mossmann TR, Cherwinski HM, Bond MW *et al.* Two types of murine helper T cell clones. I. Definition according to profiles of lymphokine activities and secreted proteins. J Immunol. 1986;136:2348.
21. Cherwinski HM, Schumacher JH, Brown KD *et al.* Two types of mouse helper T cell clones. III. Further differences in lymphokine synthesis between Th1 and Th2 clones revealed by

DNA hybridization, functionally monospecific bioassays and monoclonal antibodies. J Exp Med. 1987;166:1229.

22. Gross V, Andus T, Caesar I, Roth M, Scholmerich J. Evidence for continuous stimulation of interleukin-6 production in Crohn's disease. Gastroenterology. 1992;102:514–19.

23. Raedler A, Steffen M, Reinecker C, Witthoft T, Schreiber S *et al*. Lamina propria mononuclear cells in patients with inflammatory bowel disease secrete enhanced levels of IL-1β, TNF-α and IL-6. Digestive Diseases Week 1992, abstract no. 1204.

24. Fu RD, Izutani R, Muraki T, Sartor RB, MacDermott RP. Increased secretion of interleukin-8 from peripheral monocytes in patients with Crohn's disease. Digestive Diseases Week 1992, abstract no. 1325.

25. Izutani R, Loh EY, Rombeau JL *et al*. Enhanced expression of interleukin-8 mRNA and increased IL-8 production by colonic mucosa in inflammatory bowel disease. Digestive Diseases Week 1992, abstract no. 2044.

26. Cominelli F, Fiocchi C, Eisenberg SP *et al*. Imbalance of IL-1 and IL-1 receptor antagonist synthesis in the intestinal mucosa of Crohn's disease and ulcerative colitis patients: a novel pathogenetic mechanism. Digestive Diseases Week 1992, abstract no. 1202.

27. Isaacs KL, Sartor RB, Haskill JS. Relative expression of IL-1 and IL-1 receptor antagonist in inflammatory bowel disease. Digestive Diseases Week 1992, abstract no. 1203.

28. Mayer I, Schlien R. Evidence for function of Ia molecules on gut epithelial cells in man. J Exp Med. 1987;166:1471–83.

29. Mayer L, Siden E, Becker S, Eisenhardt D. Antigen handling in the intestine mediated by normal enterocytes. In: MacDonald TT, Challacombe SJ, Bland PW, Stokes CR, Heatly RV, Mowat AMcI, editors. Advances in mucosal immunology. Dordrecht: Kluwer; 1990:23–28.

30. Mayer I. Eisenhardt D. Lack of induction of suppressor T cells by intestinal epithelial cells from patients with inflammatory bowel disease. J Clin Invest. 1990;86:1255–60.

31. Allan CH, Mendrick DL, Trier JS. M cells contain acidic compartments and express Class II MHC determinants. Digestive Diseases Week 1992, abstract no. 1213.

32. Korelitz BL, Somers SC. Rectal biopsy in patients with Crohn's disease. Normal mucosa on sigmoidoscopic examination. J Am Med Assoc. 1977;237:274.

33. Makiyama K, Bennett MK, Jewell DP. Endoscopic appearances of the rectal mucosa of patients with Crohn's disease visualized with a magnifying colonoscope. Gut. 1984;25:337.

34. Gionchetti P, Mahida R, Patel S, Jewell DP. Macrophage and lymphocyte subpopulations in magnifying endoscopic lesions of Crohn's disease. Clin Exp Immunol. 1988;72:373.

35. Clarkson SD, Kimberley RP, Valinsky SE *et al*. Blockage of clearance of immune complexes by an anti-Fc Gamma receptor monoclonal antibody. J Exp Med. 1986;164:474.

36. Schmitz-Moorman P, Becker H. Histologic studies on the formal pathogenesis of the epithelial cell granuloma in Crohn's disease. In: Pena AS, Weterman IT, Booth CC, Strober W, editors. Recent advances in Crohn's disease. The Hague: Martinus Nijhoff; 1981:76.

37. Mahida YR. Patel S, Gionchetti P, Vaux D, Jewell DP. Macrophage subpopulations in lamina propria of normal and inflamed colon and terminal ileum. Gut. 1989;30:826.

38. Podolsky DK, Fournier DA. Alterations in mucosal content of colonic glycoconjugates in inflammatory bowel disease defined by monoclonal antibodies. Gastroenterology. 1988;95:379.

39. Broberger O, Perlmann P. Demonstration of an epithelial antigen in colon by means of fluorescent antibodies from children with ulcerative colitis. J Exp Med. 1962;115:13.

40. Wright R, Truelove SC. Auto-immune reactions in ulcerative colitis. Gut. 1966;7:32.

41. Takahashi F, Das KM. Isolation and characterisation of a colonic autoantigen specifically recognised by colon tissue bound IgG from idiopathic ulcerative colitis. J Clin Invest. 1985;76:311.

42. MacDermott RP, Nash GS, Bertovich MJ *et al*. Altered patterns of secretion of monomeric IgA and IgA sub-class I by intestinal mononuclear cells in inflammatory bowel disease. Gastroenterology. 1986;91:379.

43. Von Ritter C, Be R, Granger D. Neutrophilic proteases: mediators of F Met-Leu-Phe induced ileitis in rats. Gastroenterology. 1989;97:605.

44. Pullman WE, Elsbury S, Kobayashi M *et al*. Enhanced mucosal cytokine production in inflammatory bowel disease. Gastroenterology. 1992;102:529–37.

45. Pallone F, Fais S, Squarcia O *et al*. Activation of peripheral blood and intestinal lamina

propria lymphocytes in Crohn's disease. *In vivo* state of activation and *in vitro* response to stimulation as defined by the expression of early activation antigens. Gut. 1987;28:745–53.
46. Fiocchi C, Gattisto JR, Garmer RG. Studies on isolated gut mucosal lymphocytes in inflammatory bowel disease. Detection of activated T cells and enhanced proliferative response to *Staphylococcus aureus* and lipopolysaccharides. Dig Dis Sci. 1981;36:728–36.
47. Brandtzaeg P, Baklien P, Fausa O *et al.* Immunohistochemical characterisation of local immunoglobulin formation in ulcerative colitis. Gastroenterology. 1974;66:1123.
48. Baklien K, Brandtzaeg P. Comparative mapping of the local distribution of immunoglobulin containing cells in ulcerative colitis and Crohn's disease of the colon. Clin Exp Immunol. 1975;22:197.
49. Kett K, Rognum TO, Brandtzaeg P. Mucosal subclass distribution of IgG producing cells is different in ulcerative colitis and Crohn's disease of the colon. Gastroenterology. 1987;93:919.
50. Scott MG, Nahn MH, Macke K *et al.* Spontaneous secretion of IgG subclasses by intestinal mononuclear cells: differences between ulcerative colitis, Crohn's disease and controls. Clin Exp Immunol. 1986;66:209.
51. Halstenen TS, Mollnes TE, Fausa O, Brandtzaeg P. Deposits of terminal complement complex (TCC) in muscularis mucosal and submucosal vessels in ulcerative colitis and Crohn's disease of the colon. Gut. 1989;30:361.
52. MacDermott RP, Stenson IVF. The role of the immune system in inflammatory bowel disease. Immunol Allergy Clin N Am. 1988;8:521.
53. Izutani R, Loh EY, Rombeau JL *et al.* Enhanced expression of interleukin-8 mRNA and increased IL-8 production by colonic mucosa in inflammatory bowel disease. Digestive Diseases Week 1992, abstract no. 2044.
54. Satsangi J, Wolstencroft RA, Cason J *et al.* Interleukin-1 in Crohn's disease. Clin Exp Immunol. 1987;67:594.
55. Suzuki Y, Tobin A, Quinn D, Whelan A, O'Morain C. Interleukin-1 in Crohn's disease. Eur J Gastroenterol Hepatol. 1991;3:45–9.
56. Deusch K, Reiter C, Mauthe B, Riethmuller G, Classen M. Chimeric monoclonal anti-CD4 antibody therapy proves effective for treating inflammatory bowel disease. Digestive Diseases Week 1992, abstract no. 1981.

6

Phenotypic and functional characteristics of intestinal lamina propria T lymphocytes

M. ZEITZ, D. C. SCHMIDT, R. ULLRICH, H. L. SCHIEFERDECKER and T. SCHNEIDER

INTRODUCTION

The intestinal mucosa is in close contact with a large number of foreign antigens and mitogenic substances in the gut lumen. To protect the host against invasion of potential pathogens or an inappropriate immune response to the enormous number of antigens, a highly specialized immune system in the intestinal mucosa has developed, the so-called gut-associated lymphoid system (GALT)[1-3]. Disturbances in this local immune compartment may lead to characteristic diseases of the intestine and/or disease manifestations in other organs[4]. Examples of diseases in which the major primary event is thought to be located in the gut-associated immune system are the idiopathic inflammatory bowel diseases (Crohn's disease and ulcerative colitis), coeliac disease, the primary gastrointestinal B and T cell lymphomas (MALTomas), and primary IgA deficiency. In other diseases disturbances in the local immune system of the intestine are responsible for major clinical symptoms, e.g. the gastrointestinal manifestations of HIV infection.

In inflammatory bowel disease a chronic relapsing inflammation leads to severe destruction of the mucosa and to multiple extraintestinal manifestations. The characteristics of the clinical course, and the histological appearance of the mucosa in IBD, are indicative of an endogenous immunological defect, which is most likely located in the local immune system of the intestinal mucosa[5,6]. Recent studies have shown that intestinal lymphocytes undergo a specific differentiation process adapted to their specific tasks in the mucosal immunological compartment, and that this differentiation process is disturbed in inflammatory bowel disease. This review will primarily focus on studies on T lymphocytes in the human intestinal lamina propria. Data will be presented which indicate that T cell function in the lamina propria is disturbed in idiopathic inflammatory bowel disease.

HUMAN INTESTINAL LAMINA PROPRIA T CELLS UNDER NORMAL CONDITIONS

'Memory' phenotype of lamina propria T cells

In studies using both immunohistology of frozen tissue sections and flow cytometry of isolated cells it has been shown that more than 95% of human intestinal lamina propria T cells bear the α/β isotype of the antigen-specific T cell receptor[7,8], CD4- and CD8-positive T cells are present in the lamina propria in a similar proportion compared to the peripheral blood (Table 1)[9–11]. Thus, regarding the major T cell subpopulations, there are no clear differences between peripheral blood T cells and lamina propria T cells.

It is supposed that lymphocytes in the intestinal mucosa encounter antigen in the afferent limb of the gut-associated lymphoid tissue comprising the organized lymphoid tissue of the mucosa, the Peyer's patches of the small intestine and the lymphoid follicles of the colon and rectum. Lymphocytes then leave the mucosa, enter the circulation via the thoracic duct, and finally migrate back to the efferent limb of the mucosal immune system, comprising lymphocytes diffusely spread in the lamina propria and lymphocytes in the intraepithelial compartment above the basement membrane. Since lamina propria lymphocytes and intraepithelial lymphocytes have developed into effector cells after antigen contact, these cells might represent memory cells[12,13].

Monoclonal antibodies against certain T cell surface antigens are used to distinguish between T cells which had no prior contact to specific antigens

Table 1 Comparison of T cell phenotype and function under normal conditions and in Crohn's disease. Characteristic disturbances in T cell differentiation in inflammatory bowel disease might occur and contibute to disease pathogenesis

	Normal	*Crohn's disease*
T cell subsets (CD4/CD8 ratio)	Similar to peripheral blood	Similar to normal intestinal tissue
T cell activation	Increased compared to the peripheral blood	Increased compared to normal intestinal tissue
T cell function	No proliferation after antigenic stimulation	Proliferation after antigenic stimulation
Consequences for mucosal integrity	Mucosal structure regulated by lamina propria T cell activation	Destruction of intestinal epithelial cells by factors from activated T cells, overshooting immune response

(naive T cells) and T cells which were already stimulated by antigen (memory T cells). Naive and memory T cells can be distinguished by their high or low expression of different antigen specificities of the CD45 cell surface glycoprotein complex[14,15]. The transition from naive to memory T cell function is accompanied by a shift from the 205/220 kDa determinant (CD45RA recognized by 2H4) to the 180 kDa form (CD45R0 recognized by UCHL1) of the CD45 cell surface glycoprotein complex[16,17]. Additional markers have been described which are coexpressed with the CD45 glycoprotein complex after the transition from naive to memory T cells[14]. Naive T cells can be characterized as CD45RA-high, CD58 (LFA-3)-low, CD2-low, CD11A/CD18 (LFA-1)-low, CD45R0-low, and CD29-low; memory T cells are the reciprocal subset.

In flow cytometric studies it was shown that only 10% of lamina propria lymphocytes express CD45RA in comparison to 33% CD45RA-positive cells in the peripheral blood[11]. Staining of isolated human lamina propria lymphocytes with monoclonal antibody UCHL-1 revealed that about 90% of this lymphocyte population is CD45R0-positive[11]. This phenotype resembles that of memory T cells. However, expression of another marker of memory T cells, CD29 (β_1 chain of integrins) is not increased in the lamina propria compared to the peripheral blood. The phenotype of lamina propria lymphocytes therefore only partially corresponds with that of memory T cells. These phenotypic studies are a first indication that T cells in the intestinal lamina propria represent a specialized memory T cell subset.

Another finding indicating maturational differences between circulating and intestinal T cells is a low expression of L-selectin (Leu-8) on human and non-human primate lamina propria T cells[10,11,18]. L-selectin is now used to define a subset of memory T cells[19], and it has been shown that L-selectin is the human equivalent of the Mel-14 protein, the mouse homing receptor for peripheral lymph nodes[20]. This finding might explain the lack of L-selectin expression in the intestinal lamina propria.

T cell receptor triggered function of lamina propria lymphocytes

Memory T cells differ from naive T cells not only in their phenotype but also in their response to antigens, and in the profile of cytokines secreted: memory T cells are capable of mounting a high proliferative response to recall antigen while naive cells have a low proliferative response to triggering the T cell receptor[14]. Limited data are available on the T cell receptor triggered function of lamina propria lymphocytes. This question was addressed in a study in which non-human primates were immunized by rectal intramucosal injection of *Chlamydia trachomatis* followed by isolation of lymphocytes from various origins and testing for their responsiveness to stimulation with specific antigen *in vitro*[21]. As already suggested by their only partially overlapping phenotype, clear differences between the *in vitro*-defined memory T cells and lamina propria lymphocytes were found: lymphocytes isolated from the intestinal lamina propria, the site of immunization, had no proliferative response to recall stimulation by *Chlamydia trachomatis* antigens *in vitro*, whereas peripheral blood lymphocytes, lymphocytes from the spleen, and mesenteric lymph node lymphocytes proliferated after antigenic stimulation. Similarly, rectal immunization with other protein antigens such as BCG or tetanus toxoid did not result in detectable proliferative responses of isolated lamina propria T cells to these antigens. However, lamina propria T lymphocytes did respond to recall antigen in providing helper function for immunoglobulin synthesis by spleen B cells after antigenic stimulation with *Chlamydia trachomatis* antigens *in vitro*[21]. Thus, lamina propria T cells do not proliferate after stimulation with recall antigen, but manifest a T cell effector function, i.e. helper activity, in response to antigen. Recent studies have also shown that the pattern of lymphokines produced by lamina propria T cells and the responsiveness to certain lymphokines differ from those of other lymphocyte populations[22,23].

Another indication of a different responsiveness of the antigen-specific T cell receptor is also given in recent studies which showed a decreased responsiveness of lamina propria T cells to stimulation with immobilized antibodies to CD3 and an undisturbed responsiveness to mitogenic anti-CD2 monoclonal antibodies[24]. In related studies an impairment of calcium mobilization and phosphatidylinositol response through the T cell receptor/CD3 complex was shown, and it has been speculated that the T cell receptor activation pathway may be down-regulated in the lamina propria[25]. However, the finding of an antigen-induced helper function of lamina propria T cells clearly demonstrates responsiveness through the antigen-specific T cell receptor, and indicates an altered pathway in signal transduction in lamina propria T cells compared to other T cell populations.

Activation of lamina propria T cells

Activation of T cells is followed by a rapid expression of the IL-2 receptor on the cell surface, and this event is critical in T cell function[26]. Northern blot analyses revealed that mRNA for CD25 (α-chain of the IL-2 receptor) is clearly detectable in freshly isolated lymphocytes from the intestinal lamina propria of non-human primates, whereas in other lymphocyte populations from the spleen, mesenteric lymph nodes, or the peripheral blood CD25 mRNA was found only after activation *in vitro*[27]. Correspondingly, using flow cytometry it was shown that 15% (range 6–29%) of freshly isolated intestinal lamina propria lymphocytes were CD25-positive, but less than 3% of the other lymphocyte populations expressed CD25. A high proliferative response of lamina propria lymphocytes to low doses of IL-2 indicates that the IL-2 receptors are functional. In addition, lamina propria lymphocytes express MHC class II antigens[27] and other T cell activation markers[28], and it was demonstrated that these cells are able to synthesize large amounts of IL-2[27]. In humans these findings have been confirmed by the immunohistological and cytofluorometric detection of CD25 on lamina propria lymphocytes[11,29].

The finding that the mucosal T cell-associated antigen recognized by HML-1 is an activation antigen further supports the concept of an increased activation of lamina propria T cells[11].

INTESTINAL LAMINA PROPRIA T CELLS IN INFLAMMATORY BOWEL DISEASE

Disturbed differentiation of lamina propria T cells in inflammatory bowel disease

Earlier studies did not reveal major differences in the relative proportions of the T cell subpopulations CD4 or CD8 in the mucosa of patients with inflammatory bowel disease compared to controls[10]. Preliminary immunohistological studies from our laboratory indicate that L-selectin expression is increased in the inflamed intestinal mucosa in Crohn's disease, but not in uninvolved areas or in ulcerative colitis when compared to control tissue. As discussed above, normal lamina propria T cells very rarely express L-selectin, the peripheral lymph node homing receptor. In addition, the number of T cells expressing CD29, another marker used for the definition of memory T cells, seems to be lower in the intestinal lamina propria of patients with inflammatory bowel disease (own unpublished results). These phenotypic data are a first indication that T cell differentiation might be disturbed in inflammatory bowel disease.

Proliferating (i.e. Ki67-positive) lamina propria cells are absent in normal intestinal tissue as shown by immunohistology; however, Ki67-positive cells are frequently found in the inflamed mucosa of patients with inflammatory bowel disease[30,31] (also unpublished results). This finding is supported by recent functional studies by Pirzer and co-workers which showed that the responsiveness to antigenic stimulation differs fundamentally between lamina propria T cells from inflamed intestinal tissue compared to intestinal T cells from uninflamed areas: isolated lamina propria mononuclear cells from inflamed and unaffected intestine from patients with Crohn's disease as well as circulating T cells were stimulated with an array of recall antigens *in vitro*, and proliferative responses were compared. As expected, T cells from normal mucosa were unresponsive with regard to proliferation but T cells from inflamed mucosa responded with proliferation comparable to circulating T cells[32]. These findings indicate that the differentiation process of lamina propria T cells is disturbed in Crohn's disease which may lead to uncontrolled proliferation and expansion of T cells in the gut wall (Table 1).

Intestinal epithelial cells express MHC class II antigens and are able to present antigens to T cells. It has been shown that antigen presentation by intestinal epithelial cells leads to a preferential stimulation of CD8-positive cells with suppressor function under normal conditions[33]. However, intestinal epithelial cells from patients with IBD stimulate CD4-positive cells with helper function under identical *in vitro* conditions[34]. This induction of helper mechanisms might contribute to an overshooting immune response in the GALT in inflammatory bowel disease.

Increased activation of lamina propria T cells in inflammatory bowel disease

In studies investigating the state of activation of lamina propria mononuclear cells in patients with inflammatory bowel disease large intestinal biopsies from patients with Crohn's disease and ulcerative colitis were stained with monoclonal antibodies recognizing the α-chain of the IL-2 receptor (CD25). Inflamed areas as determined by endoscopic criteria were compared to uninvolved areas in patients with IBD and normal controls. The number of mononuclear cells expressing CD25 was increased in involved areas in Crohn's disease compared to uninvolved areas or control tissue[30,31] (also unpublished results). Macroscopically uninvolved mucosa from IBD patients did not differ from control tissue. In ulcerative colitis the proportion of CD25-positive mononuclear cells was only slightly increased and not significantly different from control biopsies. Since the number of macrophages identified as CD68-positive cells was not different in IBD compared to controls the increase in CD25-positive cells is most likely due to T cells[30]. In addition to an increased CD25 expression in inflamed intestinal tissue in Crohn's disease it has recently been demonstrated that mRNA levels for IL-2 are also elevated in inflammatory lesions of patients with Crohn's disease, but not in the colonic mucosa in patients with ulcerative colitis[35]. These findings demonstrate an increased state of T cell activation in intestinal inflammatory lesions in patients with Crohn's disease (see Table 1).

Another finding documenting increased activation of T cells in Crohn's disease is the demonstration of higher concentrations of circulating soluble IL-2 receptors in the serum of patients with active Crohn's disease compared with controls[36,37], (also own unpublished results). However, we found similarly low numbers of circulating CD25-positive T cells in patients with IBD and controls[30]. Thus, the increased concentrations of soluble IL-2 receptors in patients with active Crohn's disease probably reflect mucosal T cell activation.

Consequences of T cell activation for intestinal epithelial cell proliferation and function

Increased mucosal T cell activation is found not only in inflamed areas of patients with Crohn's disease but also in intestinal diseases accompanied by hyperregenerative villus atrophy, such as coeliac disease or certain infections of the intestine[30,38]. Activation of mucosal T cells of fetal intestinal tissue *in vitro* is followed by crypt hyperplasia and partial villus atrophy, the changes being blocked by cyclosporin A co-incubation[39]. These experimental and clinical findings indicate that activated T cells interact with intestinal epithelial cells and influence viability and proliferation of these cells.

In recent investigations it has been shown that soluble factors of activated T cells inhibit proliferation and decrease viability of the human colon cancer-derived intestinal epithelial cell line HT29[40-42]. The epithelial cell line HT29 differentiates under certain *in vitro* conditions and gains some characteristics of mature enterocytes. If this cell line is incubated with supernatants of anti-CD3-stimulated T cells a decrease in viability occurs as measured by the MTT test or by propidium iodide staining. Applying cell cycle analysis by propidium iodide staining of fixed and permeabilized cells, together with surface staining for MHC class II expression (HLA-DR), we showed that proliferation is inhibited and HLA-DR expression is increased by soluble T cell factors[40] (also own unpublished results). The effects of the T cell supernatant can at least partially be mimicked by incubating HT29 cells with a combination of interferon-γ and tumour necrosis factor-α[40]. These findings show that T cell-derived factors profoundly influence proliferation and viability of an intestinal epithelial cell line. The increased expression of MHC class II antigens induced by T cell factors may indicate a differentiation event of the epithelial cell, and probably has effects on its antigen-presenting capability.

CONCLUSIONS

The intestinal lamina propria contains T cells which have a distinctive phenotype and which are activated. Functionally these T cells can be characterized as differentiated effector lymphocytes which respond to triggering the antigen-specific T cell receptor by secreting helper factors for B cells. Lamina propria T cells thus represent a subset of memory T cells with a unique maturational state adapted to the specific tasks in the intestinal mucosa. An antigen-specific response of intestinal lamina propria T cells in the form of a down-regulation of proliferation and an increase in the secretion of regulatory factors would prevent potentially harmful clonal expansion of T cells in the mucosa, and at the same time allow protective immune responses, e.g. immunoglobulin secretion.

An increased activation and a disturbed differentiation process of lamina propria T cells in Crohn's disease might lead to a different responsiveness of the T cell receptor with an inappropriate expansion of mononuclear cells in the intestinal mucosa (Table 1). Such altered T cells might also secrete a different pattern of lymphokines. In addition, an imbalance between helper and suppressor mechanisms in the intestinal mucosa could result in a sustained and overshooting inflammatory and immune reaction against antigens normally occurring in the intestinal lumen. The increased activation of intestinal T cells in inflammatory bowel disease may also have important consequences for intestinal epithelial cell viability, proliferation, and function. However, further studies on T cell differentiation and function at the mucosal level in inflammatory bowel disease are clearly needed to characterize the defects in mucosal immunoregulation and their role in the pathogenesis of IBD.

ACKNOWLEDGEMENTS

The studies of T cell function in the intestinal lamina propria under normal conditions and in inflammatory bowel disease were supported by the Deutsche Forschungsgemeinschaft (Ze 188/3-1, Ze 188/4-1, and Ze 188/4-2).

References

1. Pabst R. The anatomical basis for the immune function of the gut. Anat Embryol. 1987;176:135–44.
2. Strober W, Jacobs D. Cellular differentiation, migration, and function in the mucosal immune system. In: Gallin JI, Fauci AS, editors. Advances in host defense mechanisms, Vol. 4. New York: Raven Press; 1985:1–30.
3. Zeitz M, James SP, Strober W. Die Funktion des gastrointestinalen Immunosystems in der Abwehr enteropathogener Bakterien. Z. Gastroenterol. 1986;24:43–52.
4. Zeitz M. Störungen des darmassoziierten Immunosystems. In: Goebell H, editor. Innere Medizin der Gegenwart – Gastroenterologie, Band 11. München, Wien, Baltimore: Urban & Schwarzenberg; 1992:590–606.
5. Strober W, James SP. The immunologic basis of inflammatory bowel disease. J Clin Immunol. 1986;6:415–32.
6. Zeitz M. Immunoregulatory abnormalities in inflammatory bowel disease. Eur J Gastroenterol Hepatol. 1990;2:246–50.
7. Ullrich R, Schieferdecker HL, Ziegler K, Riecken EO, Zeitz M. Gamma delta T cells in the human intestine express surface markers of activation and are preferentially located in the epithelium. Cell Immunol. 1990;128:619–27.
8. Ullrich R, Schieferdecker HL, Zeitz M. Gamma-delta T cells in the human intestine. Immunol Res. 1991;10:306–9.
9. Selby WS, Janossy G, Bofill M, Jewell DP. Lymphocyte subpopulations in the human small intestine. The findings in normal mucosa and in the mucosa of patients with adult coeliac disease. Clin Exp Immunol. 1983;52:219–28.
10. James SP, Fiocchi C, Graeff AS, Strober W. Phenotypic analysis of Lamina propria lymphocytes. Predominance of helper-inducer and cytolytic T-cell phenotypes in Crohn's disease and control patients. Gastroenterology. 1986;91:1483–9.
11. Schieferdecker HL, Ullrich R, Weiss-Breckwoldt AN, Schwarting R, Stein H, Riecken EO, Zeitz M. The HML-1 antigen of intestinal lymphocytes is an activation antigen. J Immunol. 1990;144:2541–9.
12. James SP, Zeitz M, Kanof ME, Kwan WC. Intestinal lymphocyte populations and mechanisms of cell-mediated immunity. In: Kagnoff MF, editor. Immunology and allergy clinics of North America, vol. 8, number 3: Gut and intestinal immunology. Philadelphia: WB Saunders; 1988:369–91.
13. Zeitz M, Schieferdecker HL, James SP, Riecken EO. Special functional features of T-lymphocyte subpopulations in the effector compartment of the intestinal mucosa and their relation to mucosal transformation. Digestion. 1990;46(Suppl. 2):280–9.
14. Sanders ME, Malegapuru W, Makgoba MW, Shaw S. Human naive and memory T cells: reinterpretation of helper-inducer and suppressor-inducer subsets. Immunol. Today. 1988;9:195–9.
15. Sanders ME, Makgoba MW, Sharrow SO, Stephany D, Springer TA, Young HA, Shaw S. Human memory T lymphocytes express increased levels of three cell adhesion molecules (LFA-3, CD2, and LFA-1) and three other molecules (UCHL-1, CDw29, and Pgp-1) and have enhanced IFN-g production. J Immunol. 1988;140:1401–7.
16. Akbar AN, Terr L, Timms A, Beverley PCL, Janossy G. Loss of CD45R and gain of UCHL1 reactivity is a feature of primed T cells. J Immunol. 1988;140:2171–8.
17. Streuli M, Hall LR, Saga Y, Schlossman SF, Saito H. Differential usage of three exons generate at least five different mRNAs encoding human leucocyte common antigens. J Exp Med. 1987;166:1548–66.
18. James SP, Graeff AS, Zeitz M. Predominance of helper-inducer T cells in mesenteric lymph nodes and intestinal lamina propria of normal nonhuman primates. Cell Immunol. 1987;107:372–83.
19. Tedder TF, Matsuyama T, Rothstein D, Schlossman SF, Morimoto C. Human antigen-specific memory T cells express the homing receptor (LAM-1) necessary for lymphocyte recirculation. Eur J Immunol. 1990;20:1351–7.
20. Camerini D, James SP, Stamenkovic I, Seed B. Leu-8/TQ1 is the human equivalent of the Mel-14 lymph node homing receptor. Nature. 1989;342:78–82.
21. Zeitz M, Quinn TC, Graeff AS, James SP. Mucosal T cells provide helper function but do not proliferate when stimulated by specific antigen in Lymphogranuloma venereum proctitis in nonhuman primates. Gastroenterology. 1988;94:353–66.

22. James SP, Kwan WC, Sneller MC. T cells in inductive and effector compartments of the intestinal immune system of nonhuman primates differ in lymphokine mRNA expression, lymphokine utilization, and regulatory function. J Immunol. 1990;144:1251–6.
23. James SP, Mullin GE, Kanof ME, Zeitz M. Role of lymphokines in immunoregulatory function of mucosal T cells in humans and nonhuman primates. Immunol Res. 1991;10:230–8.
24. Pirzer UC, Schürmann G, Post S, Betzler M, Meuer SC. Differential responsiveness to CD3-Ti vs. CD2-dependent activation of human intestinal T lymphocytes. Eur J Immunol. 1990;20:2339–42.
25. Quiao L, Schürmann G, Betzler M, Meuer SC. Functional properties of human lamina propria T lymphocytes assessed with mitogenic monoclonal antibodies. Immunol Res. 1991;10:218–25.
26. Greene WC, Leonard WJ, Depper JM. Growth of human T lymphocytes: an analysis of interleukin 2 and its cellular receptor. Prog Hematol. 1986;14:283–301.
27. Zeitz M, Greene WC, Peffer NJ, James SP. Lymphocytes isolated from the intestinal lamina propria of normal nonhuman primates have increased expression of genes associated with T cell activation. Gastroenterology. 1988;94:647–55.
28. Peters M, Secrist H, Anders KR, Nash GS, Schloemann S, MacDermott RP. Increased expression of cell surface activation markers by intestinal mononuclear cells. Clin Res. 1986;35:462.
29. Ullrich R, Zeitz M, Heise W, L'age M, Ziegler K, Bergs C, Riecken EO. Mucosal atrophy is associated with loss of activated T cells in the duodenal mucosa of human immunodeficiency virus (HIV)-infected patients. Digestion. 1990;46(Suppl. 2):302–7.
30. Zeitz M, Ullrich R, Schieferdecker HL, Weiss-Breckwoldt AN, James SP, Riecken EO. Characterization of T cell subpopulations in the intestinal lamina propria in inflammatory bowel disease. In Goebell H, Ewe K, Malchow H, Koelbel C, editor. Inflammatory bowel diseases – Progress in basic research and clinical implications. Lancaster: Kluwer; 1991:63–70.
31. Ullrich R, Zeitz M, Schieferdecker H, Brunn C, Riecken EO. Expression von aktivierungs- und proliferationsabhängigen Antigenen in der intestinalen Lamina propria (LP) von Kontrollpersonen und Patienten mit chronisch entzündlichen Darmerkrankungen (CED). Klin Wochenschr. 1989;67(Suppl. XIV):234.
32. Pirzer U, Schönhaar A, Fleischer B, Hermann E, Meyer zum Büschenfelde KH. Reactivity of infiltrating T lymphocytes with microbial antigens in Crohn's disease. Lancet. 1991;338:1238–9.
33. Mayer L, Shlien R. Evidence for function of Ia molecules on gut epithelial cells in man. J Exp Med. 1987;166:1471–83.
34. Mayer L, Eisenhardt D. Lack of induction of suppressor T cells by intestinal epithelial cells from patients with inflammatory bowel disease. J Clin Invest. 1990;86:1255–60.
35. James SP, Mullin GE. Lymphokine production by mucosal T cells in inflammatory bowel disease. In Goebell H, Ewe K, Malchow H, Koelbel C, editors. Inflammatory bowel diseases – Progress in basic research and clinical implications. Lancaster: Kluwer; 1991:71–81.
36. Mueller C, Knoflach P, Zielinski CC. T-cell activation in Crohn's disease. Increased levels of soluble interleukin-2 receptor in serum and in supernatants of stimulated peripheral blood mononuclear cells. Gastroenterology. 1990;98:639–46.
37. Brynskov J, Tvede N. Plasma interleukin-2 and a soluble/shed interleukin-2 receptor in serum of patients with Crohn's disease. Effect of cyclosporin. Gut. 1990;31:795–9.
38. Riecken EO, Stallmach A, Zeitz M, Schgulzke JD, Menge H, Gregor M. Growth and transformation of the small intestinal mucosa – importance of connective tissue, gut associated lymphoid tissue and gastrointestinal regulatory peptides. Gut. 1989;30:1630–40.
39. MacDonald TT, Spencer J. Evidence that activated mucosal T cells play a role in the pathogenesis of enteropathy in human small intestine. J Exp Med. 1988;167:1341–9.
40. Schmidt DC, Schieferdecker HL, Jahn HU, Hirseland H, Riecken EO, Zeitz M. Cytokines released by activated T cells decrease viability and proliferation, and increase MHC II expression of a colonic cancer cell line (HT29). FASEB J. 1992;6:A1993.
41. Deem RL, Shanahan F, Targan SR. Triggered mucosal T Cells release tumour necrosis factor alpha and interferon-gamma which kill human colonic epithelial cells. Clin Exp Immunol. 1991;83:79–84.
42. Lowes JR, Priddle JD, Jewell DP. Production of epithelial cell growth factors by lamina propria mononuclear cells. Gut 1991;33:39–43.

7

Role of inflammatory cell types

C. M. GELBMANN and K. E. BARRETT

INTRODUCTION

The chronic inflammatory bowel diseases of ulcerative colitis and Crohn's disease remain of unknown aetiology despite intense investigation. There have been a large number of studies suggesting a genetic predisposition to these disorders, and more limited work providing evidence of an infectious aetiology (recently reviewed in ref. 1). It is, however, well recognized that activation of immunological effector cells, both specific (such as lymphocytes) and non-specific (inflammatory cells) is likely to contribute to the pathogenesis of these diseases.

Whatever the initial inciting event, inflammatory bowel disease is thought to result from the failure of regulatory mechanisms that normally serve to limit mucosal immune and inflammatory responses. The concept is emerging of an intestinal mucosa that is in a perpetual state of immunological readiness to deal with the massive antigenic load that is presented to the lumen. This normal state of readiness may well resemble a chronic, low-grade 'inflammation' in extraintestinal tissue sites. In inflammatory bowel disease, inappropriate stimulation or perpetuation of this inflammatory response appears to occur, either due to an increase in stimulatory events, or a failure of suppressive events, or both. In the absence of knowledge of the specific primary event for disease initiation, most current approaches to therapy of inflammatory bowel disease focus on interrupting the secondarily amplified inflammatory events. Thus this chapter will discuss specific inflammatory networks that may become established in inflammatory bowel disease, the mediators and cells that comprise these networks, and how the actions of these cells and mediators may contribute to disease pathogenesis and tissue damage. We will also examine in detail the ability of two particular inflammatory cells, the mast cell and the neutrophil, to induce the most prominent symptom of both ulcerative colitis and Crohn's disease; inflammatory diarrhoea. Involvement of the 'specific' arm of the mucosal response (i.e. lymphocytes) in disease pathogenesis is discussed elsewhere in this volume.

'NON-SPECIFIC' IMMUNE EFFECTOR CELLS

Neutrophils

Neutrophils are considered to be the predominant inflammatory cell type in inflammatory bowel disease, particularly in ulcerative colitis where they are frequently encountered in luminal aggregates referred to as crypt abscesses[1]. Further, circulating neutrophils in patients with inflammatory bowel disease display morphological features consistent with an enhanced degree of activation *in vivo*, particularly when cells from patients with active, rather than quiescent, disease were examined[2]. This accumulation and activation of neutrophils is an indicator of disease activity, and also thought to be important in mediating tissue injury in inflammatory bowel disease[3-5].

To date there has been no clear evidence for an intrinsic defect in neutrophil function in inflammatory bowel disease, although this hypothesis has been widely studied in terms of chemotaxis, migration, phagocytic and respiratory activity (reviewed in ref. 4). While these studies have revealed differences in neutrophil function in patients, these could be explained by a general activation of neutrophils that occurs in all inflammatory responses. Nevertheless, since neutrophils appear to be significant determinants of tissue injury in inflammatory bowel disease, knowledge regarding the mechanisms of neutrophil actions and activation, and modulation of this cell type, is likely to be necessary for effective therapy.

Important neutrophil functions include the generation of reactive oxygen metabolites and release of lysosomal granule constituents. These can be observed following stimulation with substances that also cause neutrophil chemotaxis, such as LTB_4 and formyl-methionyl-leucyl-phenylalanine (FMLP)[6,7]. However, in general the initiation of these processes requires significantly higher concentrations of these agents than required to promote migration. This may reflect the presence of high- and low-affinity receptors mediating different cell functions[8-10]. This may also suggest that control mechanisms have evolved to delay the release of neutrophil products until the cells have migrated into the inflammatory focus.

Reactive oxygen products and lysosomal granule constituents are the major leucocyte-derived products likely to be important for leucocyte-induced mucosal damage. Stimulation of neutrophils results in an activation of the membrane-associated NADPH-oxidase system with the subsequent generation of large amounts of superoxide anion ($O_2^{\cdot-}$) and hydrogen peroxide (H_2O_2). Activated neutrophils also secrete myeloperoxidase (MPO) into the extracellular fluid, which catalyzes the generation of hypochlorous acid (HOCl) from H_2O_2 and Cl^- (see ref. 11). Hypochlorous acid is an extremely powerful oxidizing and chlorinating agent with approximately 100–1000-fold greater toxicity than either $O_2^{\cdot-}$ or H_2O_2. HOCl also reacts rapidly with primary amines to form N-chloramines. One such N-chloramine, monochloramine, has been implicated as a mediator of inflammatory diarrhoea[12]. The cytotoxicity associated with HOCl and N-chloramines is a result of sulphydryl oxidation, haemoprotein and cytochrome inactivation, protein and amino acid degradation, and chlorination of DNA bases[13,14].

Primary granules of neutrophils are classical lysosomes and contain microbicidal enzymes (myeloperoxidase, lysozyme), neutral serine proteases such as elastase, acid hydrolases, and cationic proteins. The specific granules contain lysozyme, collagenase, lactoferrin, vitamin B_{12} binding protein, and plasminogen activator. In addition, the membranes of specific granules contain cytochrome b, which is thought to be important for the NADPH oxidase enzyme system. Gelatinase has been found in a third type of granule[15]. The most potent enzymes with respect to tissue damage are probably the serine proteinase, elastase, and the metalloproteinases, collagenase and gelatinase. All three have the ability to destroy extracellular matrix components and thereby disrupt the architecture of the tissue. Extracellular fluid contains very effective protease inhibitors such as α_2-macroglobulin and α_1-antiprotease, which normally serve to protect tissue from damage by these enzymes. However, if these antiproteases are exposed to significant quantities of MPO-generated hypochlorous acid they are inactivated. In addition, hypochlorous acid activates the inactive, latent forms of collagenase and gelatinase[13]. Overall, powerful oxidants such as hypochlorous acid are by nature short-lived, and can therefore have only localized effects on tissue damage. However, their ability to alter the tissue protease/antiprotease balance represents an important indirect mechanism for tissue injury.

Finally, another recent finding that pertains to neutrophil involvement in inflammatory bowel disease is that of serum antineutrophil cytoplasmic antibodies in the majority of patients with ulcerative colitis, but not in patients with Crohn's disease or other colitides. These antineutrophil cytoplasmic antibodies show a characteristic perinuclear immunofluoresence pattern, which is distinct from the diffuse cytoplasmic pattern associated with Wegener's granulomatosis. The pathophysiological importance of these characteristic antibodies in ulcerative colitis is unknown, but their presence might be an expression of altered immune regulation[16-19].

In summary, the attraction and activation of neutrophils into the lamina propria provides a mechanism – involving the interaction of reactive oxidative metabolites, proteinases and antiproteinases – whereby much of the tissue damage observed in inflammatory bowel disease can be achieved. However, while it has been shown that many substances are able to stimulate neutrophils *in vitro*, the actual presence of such stimuli and their interactions and relative importance in inflammatory bowel disease have not been fully elucidated.

Mast cells

Mast cells are a prominent cellular constituent of the intestinal lamina propria, and their numbers are generally thought to be increased in the inflammatory foci of both ulcerative colitis[20] and Crohn's disease[21] (though not all authors have found this, see ref. 22). There is additional evidence that mast cells in the intestine of patients with inflammatory bowel disease are activated, based both on ultrastructural evidence of ongoing degranulation[21], and studies showing an increased spontaneous release of mediators from mast cells either present in[23], or isolated from[24], inflamed tissue. Mast cells contain, or can synthesize upon activation, a large number of mediators of relevance to the pathogenesis of inflammatory bowel disease[25]. These include histamine, adenosine, proteases, leukotrienes and platelet-activating factor. It is also becoming increasingly recognized that mast cells serve as an important tissue source of a number of cytokines[26]. In particular, there is evidence that mast cells are an unusual source of the cytokine TNF-α. While many cells can synthesize this molecule *de novo* following stimulation, mast cells may represent a source of preformed TNF-α that can be rapidly released into tissues once the cell is activated[27].

The classical stimulus for mast cell activation is the combination of antigen with cell-fixed IgE molecules. There are limited data to support the concept that inflammatory bowel disease might result from an allergic reaction of this type, with many conflicting reports regarding the association of these diseases with food allergy or the allergic diathesis[28]. However, mast cells may also be activated via mechanisms other than antigenic stimulation. Notably, mast cells can be stimulated to release mediators by a number of neuropeptides[29], and there are both functional and morphological data for an association of mast cells with the enteric nervous system, and particularly with peptidergic nerve endings[29].

One function of mast cells that has been described in other tissues, but has not been specifically addressed in the setting of the intestine, is their ability to modulate fibroblast proliferation and fibrosis. A number of mast cell products appear to be directly mitogenic for fibroblasts, including histamine and granular proteoglycans[30]. More recently, Caughey and co-workers have described the ability of a purified mast cell protease, tryptase, to both directly stimulate the proliferation of fibroblasts and also to synergistically enhance growth in response to other growth factors[31]. This protease is known to be present in the mast cells of the lamina propria. The ability of mast cells to enhance fibroblast growth may have implications for disease progression, and also may be representative of an amplification mechanism for inflammatory diarrhoea, since part of the secretory effect of certain mast cell mediators on the intestinal epithelium appears to be indirect, and due to the release of prostaglandins from subepithelial fibroblasts[32] (see also below).

Macrophages

Macrophages have long been recognized to be an important constituent of most inflammatory responses[33], and are thought by some to play a central role in initiating the inflammatory response seen in inflammatory bowel disease. They are increased in number in the mucosa of patients with ulcerative colitis and Crohn's disease, and there is also evidence that they display differences in their functional and morphological properties compared with normal macrophages[34,35]. The turnover of peripheral blood monocytes, which are likely to be the main source of intestinal macrophages, is additionally increased[36].

Intestinal macrophages are heterogeneous with a wide spectrum of morphological and phenotypic expressions. The development of various monoclonal antibodies has provided the opportunity to study macrophage subpopulations. The antibody RFD1 labels a unique class II antigen preferentially associated with 'dendritic' cells; RFD7 specifies tissue macrophages with strong acid phosphatase (AP) activity; RFD9 epithelioid cells and tingible body macrophages, and UCHM1, a CD14a MoAb, identifies monocytes. Dendritic cells (RFD1+, RFD7−, AP−) are considered to be specialized for antigen presentation to lymphocytes and are therefore important for the initiation of immune responses. They are morphologically and functionally distinct from scavenger macrophages (RFD1−, RFD7+, AP+), the classical phagocytic tissue macrophage. Epithelioid cells (RFD9+) are only weakly phagocytic and are seen characteristically in association with granulomas. There are further intermediate cell types in this spectrum of macrophage subsets which lie between the cells mentioned in terms of their immunohistochemical and enzyme characteristics. For example, the majority of macrophages in the normal colon are positive for both RFD1 and RFD7, but negative for UCHM1. The proportion of macrophages displaying this normal RFD1+/RFD7+ phenotype was significantly reduced in tissue from inflammatory bowel disease patients, and largely replaced by macrophages which were only RFD7+. However, there is also an increase in RFD1+/RFD7− cells, particularly in ulcerative colitis in association with lymphoid infiltrates. Many of these RFD1−/RFD7+ and RFD1+/RFD7− cells were also positive for UCHM1, the peripheral blood monocyte marker. Also remarkable was the presence of clusters of extrafollicular RFD9+ cells (epithelioid cells), predominantly in Crohn's disease but also in ulcerative colitis. Therefore heterogeneity of morphology and phenotypic expression of macrophage-like cells is much greater in ulcerative colitis and Crohn's disease than in normal colon, particularly in severely inflamed sections[34,37−40].

Leucocyte adhesion molecules play a fundamental role in the interaction of macrophages with lymphocytes. Together with its specific ligand, intercellular adhesion molecule 1 (ICAM-1, CD54), the lymphocyte function-associated antigen 1 (LFA-1, CD11a/CD18) mediates T-cell recognition, antigen presentation, and T-cell activation. In normal colon only a few macrophages express CD11a and ICAM-1 at high densities. In contrast, in ulcerative colitis the percentage of macrophages expressing ICAM-1 was increased 10-fold, and in Crohn's disease 7-fold[41], whereas CD11a expression was only slightly enhanced. These changes in adhesion molecule expression by macrophages in inflammatory bowel disease are specific, in that they are not paralleled by corresponding changes in macrophage complement receptors. This would suggest that the antigen-presenting capabilities of macrophages are up-regulated in inflammatory bowel disease, while adhesion molecules contributing to the function of these cells as 'scavenger' macrophages are unaltered. The mediators responsible for the increase in ICAM-1 expression are unknown, though cytokines such as IL-1, IFN-γ and TNF-α induce this molecule in other systems.

Activation of oxygen uptake and production of toxic oxygen metabolites (the respiratory burst) is one of the main functional responses by which phagocytes mediate antimicrobial and cytotoxic effects. In theory this could be a mechanism whereby macrophages contribute to epithelial disruption in inflammatory bowel disease, particulary since macrophages have been identified clustered around crypts in inflamed tissue. Furthermore, in comparison to macrophages isolated from normal terminal ileal or colonic mucosa, macrophages from the mucosa of ulcerative colitis or Crohn's disease appear to be primed for activation, in that a greater proportion of these cells undergo a respiratory burst when stimulated with phorbol ester (PMA) or zymosan[42].

The levels of various cytokines with potent inflammatory and immuno-regulatory activities are increased in the mucosa of patients with active inflammatory bowel disease[43] (also recently reviewed in refs. 44–47). Many cell types are now known to be able to synthesize various cytokines, but macrophages remain a prominent source. They produce IL-1, IL-6, TNF, IFN, G-CSF, GM-CSF, M-CSF, TGF-β1 and the recently reported macrophage inflammatory protein (MIP) and neutrophil-activating peptide (NAP-I/IL-8) (reviewed in ref. 33), and may be quantitatively the most important source of some of these molecules, particularly IL-1. IL-1 has been extensively studied with regard to its role in inflammatory processes. Macrophages release significantly greater amounts of IL-1β in active inflammatory bowel disease than under normal conditions[48]. In addition to its inflammatory effects, IL-1 appears to prime mesenchymal elements such as subepithelial fibroblasts for enhanced prostaglandin synthesis, with implications for the ability of this cell type to mediate amplified intestinal secretory responses to other inflammatory mediators[49].

IL-6, another inflammatory cytokine largely produced by macrophages and monocytes, is found to be increased in the serum of patients with active inflammatory bowel disease[50,51]. Similarly, tissue levels of both mRNA for IL-6, and IL-6 protein were increased in inflammatory bowel disease[52,53]. In Crohn's disease, synthesis of TNF-α by mononuclear cells was also found to be increased, but T-cells may also contribute significant amounts of this cytokine in the mucosa[54,55]. Increased tissue levels of the potent chemotactic cytokine neutrophil-activating peptide/interleukin-8 (NAP-1/IL-8) were measured in active ulcerative colitis[56]. NAP-1/IL-8 was originally described as a product of mononuclear phagocytes, but is now shown to be expressed by a wide variety of cells after stimulation with IL-1 or TNF-α. However, the fact that monocytes and macrophages also release this cytokine after stimulation with LPS might be important by virtue of the increased permeability for bacterial endotoxins that occurs in inflammatory bowel disease[57].

Finally, the ability of macrophages to synthesize leukotrienes and prostaglandins, particularly under inflammatory conditions, suggests that tissue macrophages could contribute to the orchestration of additional inflammatory cell influx, as proposed for mast cells above. In summary, by virtue of their function as accessory cells in the presentation of antigen to T-cells, their ability to perform phagocytic and cytotoxic functions, and their capacity to secrete a variety of mediators and enzymes, macrophages are likely to play an important role in the pathogenesis of inflammation[33]. However, it remains the case that we know considerably more about macrophage function *in vitro* than *in vivo*. Since the tissue microenvironment has the capability to modulate macrophage function, additional studies are warranted to dissect the precise contribution of this cell type to inflammatory bowel diseases.

Eosinophils

Like mast cells, eosinophils have been shown to be increased in number in inflammatory foci of ulcerative colitis[20] and Crohn's disease[21], and to exhibit morphological features consistent with ongoing degranulation in the latter condition[21]. Similarly, eosinophil cationic protein appears to be actively secreted into the small intestinal lumen in Crohn's disease, even in apparently uninvolved segments[58]. Eosinophils are well recognized to be directly injurious to a wide variety of cell types, including epithelium; this may result from their ability to synthesize reactive oxygen species, as well as their granular content of a number of cytotoxic proteins including major basic protein, eosinophil cationic protein, eosinophil peroxidase and eosinophil-derived neurotoxin. However, somewhat surprisingly perhaps, the eosinophil has not been extensively studied in terms of its ability to cause tissue damage in inflammatory bowel disease (reviewed in ref. 59).

Eosinophil cytotoxicity in some settings has been shown to be moderated by mucins[60]. Thus the observation that epithelial mucin secretion is disregulated both quantitatively and qualitatively in inflammatory bowel disease[61] may have implications regarding the propensity of the epithelium to fall victim to 'innocent bystander' damage by activated eosinophils. This is a hypothesis that would certainly be worthy of testing in the setting of the intestine.

CONTROL OF INFLAMMATORY CELL INFLUX

Chemotactic factors

Neutrophils, eosinophils and monocytes appear to be attracted into the inflamed foci of ulcerative colitis and Crohn's disease by the activity of chemotactic factors. Such agents may be exogenous and derived from the intestinal lumen, such as bacterial f-met peptides, or can be derived from cells resident in the mucosa.

Chemotactic activity in the intestinal mucosa of inflammatory bowel disease patients is markedly increased. Leukotriene B_4 (LTB_4) appears to be the major chemotactic signal and is present in high concentrations in the mucosa[62,63]. LTB_4 is chemotactic for neutrophils in the nanomolar concentration range[64]. This eicosanoid is synthesized by a variety of inflammatory cell types including mast cells, eosinophils and neutrophils themselves, via the 5-lipoxygenase pathway. At least in animal models of intestinal inflammation, much of the neutrophil infiltration and associated tissue damage can be prevented by inhibition of 5-lipoxygenase or antagonism of LTB_4[65,66]. There is also preliminary evidence that intestinal epithelial cells express 5-lipoxygenase and may be able to synthesize small amounts of LTB_4 under certain circumstances[67]. By analogy with other epithelial tissues, such as the airway, neutrophil migration into tissues under the influence of LTB_4 could potentially be amplified by a process that has been referred to as transcellular metabolism. The precursor of LTB_4, LTA_4, is produced in excess by inflammatory cells and a portion can be taken up by other cells and subsequently metabolized via the enzyme LTA_4 hydrolase. LTA_4 hydrolase is known to be present in airway epithelial cells[68], but its existence in intestinal epithelium has yet to be examined.

Because LTB_4 is a predominant arachidonic acid metabolite of stimulated neutrophils themselves, an amplification mechanism for inflammation is implied[69]. Likewise, platelet-activating factor is generated by neutrophils and has chemoattractant properties for this cell type as well as eosinophils, and may thus function as auto- or paracrine amplifier of responses to other stimuli[70]. Evidence for local complement activation in inflammatory bowel disease may also be of relevance, since C5a is, after LTB_4, one of the most potent chemoattractants for neutrophils[71–73].

Another very potent chemotactic substance for neutrophils is the bacterial-derived peptide FMLP[74]. This substance may assume particular importance in the setting of increased intestinal permeability[75,76]. It is also able to enhance mucosal permeability itself[77] and in animal models it has the ability to induce colonic inflammation[78,79]. In Crohn's disease, but not in ulcerative colitis, an increased expression of surface receptors for FMLP on circulating neutrophils was demonstrated. This difference between neutrophils isolated from the two patient populations probably reflects the influence of the different inflammatory milieu rather than an intrinsic difference[80].

LTB_4, platelet-activating factor, C5a and FMLP act via specific receptor binding and their receptors are differentially regulated by cellular activation. This suggests that neutrophil recruitment can result from the concerted and/or sequential action of multiple stimuli[9].

Additional mediators with direct or indirect chemotactic activity whose tissue levels are increased in IBD include IL-8, IL-1 and TNF-α[44–47,81]. IL-8 is produced by macrophages[33] and possibly also by the intestinal epithelium[82]. Levels of this potent cytokine are elevated in the tissues of patients with active ulcerative colitis[56]. The production of this chemotactic factor can be induced by other cytokines, and also by bacterial products such as endotoxin which may have greater access to the lamina propria across a damaged epithelium.

Eosinophil migration is primarily stimulated by mast cell products, including platelet-activating factor, IL-5, and a variety of poorly defined eosinophil chemotactic factors of anaphylaxis which may be small peptides[83,84].

Adhesion molecules

In addition to responding to a chemotactic gradient, inflammatory cells must adhere to the endothelium in inflammatory foci in order to migrate out of the circulation and into the tissues. There has been rapid recent progress in the understanding of the molecular basis of the adhesive interactions that mediate inflammatory cell diapedesis[85]. It is beyond the scope of this chapter to provide a comprehensive review of this area; instead, we will focus on the possible control of inflammatory cell/endothelial interactions by mediators that have been implicated in inflammatory bowel disease (Table 1).

The primary molecules mediating the interactions of inflammatory cells, particularly neutrophils, with the vascular endothelium include two selectins expressed on endothelium, ICAM-1 and GMP-140 (CD62), and heterodimeric β-2 integrins expressed on neutrophils, CD11/CD18. The endothelial cell ligands differ in their kinetics of expression and in the mediators that induce their expression. GMP-140 is rapidly mobilized, presumably from an intracellular store, in response to histamine and thrombin, and is thought to be necessary to initially 'tether' the neutrophil to the endothelial cell[86]. The expression of GMP-140 is additionally thought to be transient in nature. However, of interest, oxidants can also induce expression of GMP-140, and this effect is prolonged in time-course. This might have a bearing on the continued influx of neutrophils into inflammatory foci. More prolonged adhesion is also mediated by the slower expression of molecules such as ICAM-1, thought to be at least one type of counter-receptor for the β-2 integrins on the neutrophil surface. Expression of ICAM-1 and another molecule with apparently similar function, ELAM-1, requires *de novo* protein synthesis, and can be stimulated by IL-1 and TNF-α[85]. The ability of endothelial cells to synthesize a membrane-bound form of platelet-activating factor also appears to contribute to the adhesive interaction by binding to neutrophil receptors for this lipid, activating neutrophil signal transduction pathways that in turn lead to increased $\beta2$-integrin expression[86]. Expression of the CD11/CD18 dimer is also enhanced by factors which are chemotactic for neutrophils, as described above, including IL-8, LTB$_4$ and FMLP.

Similar mechanisms play a role in the migration of monocytes into the lamina propria[85]. However, there are some important differences between the adhesion of neutrophils and monocytes, because there is a high level of binding of unstimulated monocytes to endothelial cells in the absence of activation of the endothelium by cytokines. This may simply reflect the fact that it is difficult to isolate monocytes from peripheral blood without activating them. However, the findings do imply that there may be a novel

Table 1 Regulation of adhesion molecule expression by inflammatory mediators

Adhesion molecule	Class	Mediators inducing expression
ELAM-1, ICAM-1	Selectin	IL-1, TNF-α
GMP-140 (CD62)	Selectin	Histamine, thrombin, oxidants, leukotrienes
CD11/CD18 family	Integrin	IL-8, platelet-activating factor, leukotriene B$_4$, chemotactic factors

endothelial ligand for monocyte adherence that is not utilized by neutrophils[85]. This may also have implications for the different types of inflammatory infiltrates seen at different stages of inflammatory bowel disease, and may provide clues as to the relative cytokine environments existing.

The modulation of adhesive interactions between cells may hold considerable promise as a therapeutic strategy for inflammatory bowel disease. The experimental manoeuvres most commonly employed to inhibit binding, monoclonal antibodies to the various adhesion proteins, are likely to prove impractical for clinical use. However, increased understanding of adhesive interactions may permit the design of related therapies such as soluble adhesion molecules or small chemicals designed to interrupt ligand–receptor binding.

EFFECTS OF INFLAMMATORY CELLS ON EPITHELIAL FUNCTION

Barrier function and epithelial integrity

One mechanism whereby inflammatory responses in the intestinal mucosa could be perpetuated would be an inappropriate decrease in epithelial barrier function such that an increased antigenic load could be delivered to the lamina propria and thus cause ongoing activation of the immune system. An increase in mucosal permeability has long been associated with inflammatory bowel disease, and may even be a primary defect under genetic control, since it reportedly occurs in unaffected relatives of patients[75].

It appears that inflammatory cells have the potential to cause a reduction in barrier integrity via both cytotoxic and non-cytotoxic mechanisms. First, a number of the products of inflammatory cell types, as alluded to above, have the potential to be directly injurious to the intestinal epithelium. In particular these include reactive oxygen species, cationic proteins derived from eosinophils, and proteases from neutrophils and mast cells. Sloughing of the epithelium from the basement membrane would constitute a considerable breakdown in epithelial integrity which would certainly allow the passage of macromolecules into the lamina propria. Second, alterations in epithelial permeability that do not simply result from loss of epithelial cells are also possible. Some cytokines may alter the permeability of epithelial tight junctions without directly killing the cells. An example of this would be IFN-γ, produced by lymphocytes and mast cells, which significantly reduced the resistance of intestinal epithelial cell monolayers grown in tissue culture without altering the viability of the cells[87]. Intriguingly, there is also evidence that sensitization of rats to produce an IgE antibody response, without even a requirement for a secondary antigen challenge, increases tissue permeability[88]. The mediator(s) of this effect has not yet been identified.

There can also be alterations in epithelial permeability caused by transmigration of inflammatory cells across the epithelium into the intestinal lumen. This has been most extensively studied for the case of neutrophil migration by Madara and co-workers. Migration of neutrophils across epithelial monolayers requires an adhesive interaction that depends on the presence of a β2-integrin on the neutrophil surface (CD11b/CD18)[89], and results in a profound decrease in monolayer resistance as the neutrophils migrate through intercellular tight junctions[89,90].

Effects on ion transport

The cardinal symptom of inflammatory bowel disase is diarrhoea. Clinically, diarrhoea results when there is an imbalance between the opposing processes of fluid absorption and secretion. The processes are driven, in turn, by the active absorption and secretion of solutes. One mechanism whereby the balance can be tipped in favour of secretion is by the stimulation of active chloride secretion by the intestinal epithelium. If this occurs without a compensatory rise in absorption (or, indeed, if absorption is simultaneously inhibited) diarrhoea will result. It has long been suspected that a considerable part of inflammatory diarrhoea results from the effects of mediators on chloride secretion. In this section we will review the pathways whereby mediators from two inflammatory cell types, the neutrophil and the mast cell, can influence epithelial ion transport via both direct and indirect mechanisms.

Some of the immune mediators which have been shown to have effects on intestinal secretion are listed in Table 2, together with the cell type most commonly associated with their generation, and their proposed mechanism of action. A casual inspection reveals that many of the substances present in the inflamed mucosa could theoretically be responsible for diarrhoea. Further, many of the listed substances interact synergistically, such that when they act in concert on the epithelium the end-result is a potentiation of the overall secretory effect.

Table 2 Mediators implicated in the pathogenesis of inflammatory diarrhoea

Substance	*Primary source/stimulus*	*Proposed mechanism(s) of action*
Histamine	Mast cells	Increased calcium in epithelium (H_1); effects on nerves (H_2); stimulation of PG production
Adenosine, NDS	Mast cells, neutrophils; ischaemia	Direct effect on epithelium (unknown messenger)
PGs	Many cells	Increased cAMP in epithelium; ? effects on nerves
PAF	Mast cells; neutrophils, ?eosinophils	Activation of nerves; stimulation of PG formation
H_2O_2	Neutrophils; macrophages	Stimulation of PG formation
Monochloramine	Neutrophils	Increased calcium in epithelium
IL-1, IL-3	Macrophages; many immunocytes	Priming of fibroblasts; stimulation of PG formation
IFN-γ	Many immunocytes	Increased paracellular transport
Sulphidopeptide LTs	Mast cells; eosinophils	Decreased active absorption of electrolytes

PG = prostaglandin; NDS = neutrophil-derived secretagogue; PAF = platelet-activating factor; LT = leukotriene

Diarrhoea has long been known to be associated with conditions that involve significant activation of mast cells, such as systemic anaphylaxis, food allergies, and systemic mastocytosis. In a variety of animal models, challenge of sensitized intestinal tissue with an appropriate antigen leads to marked secretion of chloride and water (reviewed in ref. 91). This response can be inhibited by mast cell-stabilizing drugs and, depending on the species, by competitive antagonists of mast cell mediators such as histamine and 5-hydroxytryptamine, and/or inhibitors of prostaglandin synthesis via cyclooxygenase. Mast cell mediators can act directly at the level of the epithelium to provoke secretion, as is thought to be the case for histamine, adenosine, and prostaglandin D_2[92,93]. However, indirect pathways of activation are also likely to be important. For example, a significant portion of the secretory response of intact tissue to antigen challenge, or to the mast cell mediator platelet-activating factor, can be blocked by neurotoxins acting on the enteric nervous system[94,95]. Similarly, as alluded to above, mast cell mediators such as histamine may induce at least part of their secretory effect via the stimulation of prostaglandin generation by subepithelial fibroblasts[32].

There is also evidence that chronic exposure of the epithelium to mast cell products, such as might occur in foci of ongoing inflammation where mast cells appear to be activated continuously[21], can alter the responsiveness of the epithelium such that it becomes more sensitive to the normal neurohumoral 'tone'. Thus the growth of monolayers of intestinal epithelial cells in the presence of mast cell lysates for 1 week selectively increased their ability to secrete chloride when subsequently stimulated with VIP, the muscarinic agonist carbachol, or a bacterial enterotoxin, ST_a[96].

A variety of neutrophil products have also been implicated as inflammatory secretagogues. Activation of neutrophils in intact tissue specimens by the bacterial chemoattractant FMLP leads to chloride secretion which, like that induced by mast cell activation, involves direct mechanisms, enteric nerves, and the generation of prostaglandins. Reactive oxygen species generated by neutrophils have been implicated in the secretory response, since mono-chloramine[12] and hydrogen peroxide[97] can induce secretion in several models. Like the response to histamine, the response to hydrogen peroxide in intact tissue is likely to be amplified by mesenchymal elements such as fibroblasts[32]. There has also been the recent description of a novel secretagogue which shares similarities with adenosine, and this is interesting in that it appears to induce secretion only if supplied to the apical surface of the epithelium[98]. This situation (i.e. release of mediators from neutrophils onto the apical aspect of epithelial cells) is likely to pertain in crypt abscesses, a prominent feature of ulcerative colitis.

In summary, it is easy to link, at least at the level of hypothesis, the ability of various inflammatory cells to secrete and synthesize mediators to the pathogenesis of inflammatory diarrhoea. However, we are far from a complete understanding of this area, because no comprehensive information is available regarding the precise mediator complement, and possible interactions between mediators that exist in the tissues of human subjects with inflammatory bowel disease. We need to know that the concentrations of inflammatory mediators required to produce secretory effects *in vitro* are actually attained in clinical settings, and how the generation of these mediators is controlled. With this information in hand we will be able to undertake a more rational approach to the therapy of inflammatory diarrhoea.

CONCLUSIONS – FUTURE DIRECTIONS

Clearly, the cells that migrate into the lamina propria in inflammatory bowel disease, together with resident inflammatory cell types such as mast cells, and specific immunocytes such as T- and B-cells, have the capability to generate the pathological lesions that are characteristic of these diseases, as well as the symptomatology. The concept is developing of an autoamplifying network of cells, mediators and cytokines that establishes a vicious cycle of inflammation and thus the perpetuation of disease. A simplified view of some of the possible components of this network is presented in Fig. 1. Mediators released from mast cells and macrophages can induce the expression of adhesion molecules on endothelial cells with the resulting infiltration of neutrophils and eosinophils. In turn, the activation of neutrophils in the lamina propria amplifies the inflammation and attracts more inflammatory

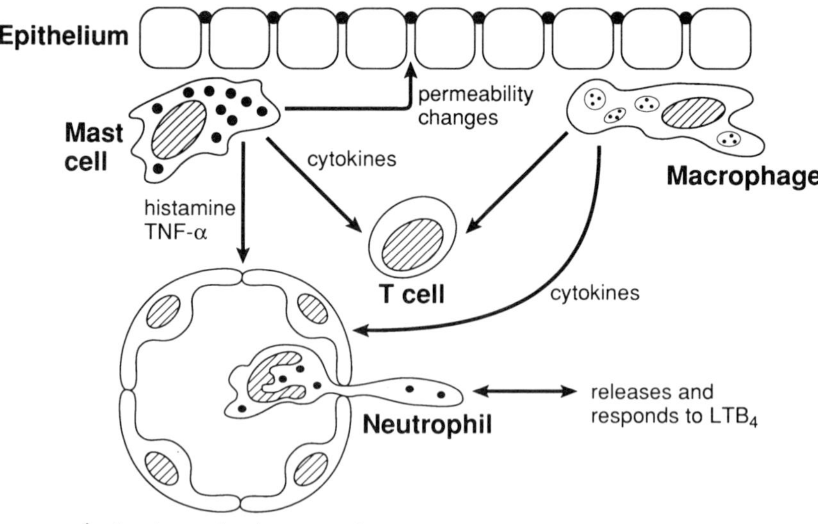

Fig. 1 Examples of some inflammatory networks that may lead to the perpetuation of inflammatory bowel disease. Mast cells and macrophages resident in the lamina propria release cytokines that can activate T cells. These cells also synthesize chemoattractants and induce the expression of various adhesion molecules on the vascular endothelium, resulting in the influx of neutrophils and eosinophils into the inflammatory focus. Once present in the tissue, neutrophils can amplify the response still further by themselves synthesizing chemoattractants. Mast cell mediators have also been associated with acute alterations in epithelial barrier function; this could increase the antigenic load presented to the intestinal immune system and thereby amplify tissue destruction in innocent bystander reactions. For further details, see text

cells into the focus. All the cell types discussed have the capability to interact additionally with mesenchymal elements such as fibroblasts, with the enteric nervous system, and with the intestinal epithelium to induce changes in fluid transport and diarrhoea, deficits in epithelial barrier function, and further amplification of the inflammatory response by the stimulation of prostaglandin, leukotriene, and cytokine synthesis by these non-inflammatory cell types.

Much of the information regarding the involvement of inflammatory cells in inflammatory bowel disease has been extrapolated from *in vitro* models. While these reductionist approaches to an extremely complex system undoubtedly both were necessary, and have yielded much useful information, the challenge now is to understand the actual events that are of importance *in vivo*. This will not be an easy task, with the bewildering and ever-increasing repertoire of all the cell types discussed in terms of their ability to synthesize cytokines, to interact with each other, and to alter the function of non-inflammatory cells. It will only be by understanding what are the relative contributions of different cells and mediators in the clinical setting that we can begin to design targeted therapies. In the meantime, however, it is clear that our emerging knowledge already holds out the promise of more effective drugs for inflammatory bowel disease, such as anti-adhesins, modulators of transcellular metabolism of eicosanoids, and cytokine antagonists.

ACKNOWLEDGEMENTS

We thank Ms Glenda Wheeler for her assistance with manuscript preparation. Studies from the authors' laboratory have been supported by grant numbers AI 24992 and DK 28305 from the National Institutes of Health (USA). Dr Gelbmann is the recipient of a fellowship grant from the Deutsche Forschungsgemeinschaft (Germany).

References

1. Podolsky DK. Inflammatory bowel disease (first of two parts). N Engl J Med. 1991;325:928–37.
2. McCarthy DA, Rampton, DS, Liu Y-C. Peripheral blood neutrophils in inflammatory bowel disease: morphological evidence of *in vivo* activation in active disease. Clin Exp Immunol. 1991;86:489–93.
3. Riddell, RH. Pathology of idiopathic inflammatory bowel disease. In: Kirsner JB, Shorter RG, editors. Inflammatory Bowel Disease, 3rd edn. Philadelphia: Lea & Febiger; 1988:329–50.
4. Elson CO. The immunology of inflammatory bowel disease. In: Kirsner JB, Shorter RG, editors. Inflammatory bowel disease, 3rd edn. Philadelphia: Lea & Febiger, 1988:97–164.
5. Saverymuttu SH, Peters AM, Lavender JP, Chadwick VS, Hodgson HJF. *In vivo* assessment of granulocyte migration to diseased bowel in Crohn's disease. Gut. 1985;26:378–83.
6. Bokoch GM, Reed PW. Effect of various lipoxygenase metabolites of arachidonic acid on degranulation of polymorphonuclear luekocytes. J. Biol Chem. 1981;256:5317–20.
7. Nast CC, LeDuc LE. Chemotactic peptides. Mechanisms, functions and possible role in inflammatory bowel disease. Dig Dis Sci. 1988;33:50S–7S.
8. Goldman DW, Goetzl EJ. Heterogeneity of human polymorphonuclear leukocyte receptors for leukotriene B_4. Identification of a subset of high affinity receptors that transduce the chemotactic response. J Exp Med. 1984;159:1027–41.
9. Pike MC. Chemoattractant receptors as regulators of phagocytic cell function. In: Grinstein

S, Rotstein OD, editors. Current topics in membranes and transport, 1st edn, vol. 35: Mechanisms of leukocyte activation. San Diego: Academic Press; 1990:19–43.

10. Snyderman R, Pike MC. Chemoattractant receptors on phagocytic cells. Ann Rev Immunol. 1984;2:257–81.

11. Klebanoff SJ. Phagocytic cells: products of oxygen metabolism. In: Gallin JI, Goldstein IM, Snyderman R, editors. Inflammation: basic principles and clinical correlates, 1st edn. New York: Raven Press; 1988:391–444.

12. Tamai H, Gaginella TS, Kachur JF, Musch MW, Chang EB. Ca-mediated stimulation of Cl secretion by reactive oxygen metabolites in human colonic T84 cells. J Clin Invest. 1992;89:301–7.

13. Weiss SJ. Tissue destruction by neutrophils. N Engl J. Med. 1989;320:365–76.

14. Grisham MB, Granger DN. Neutrophil-mediated mucosal injury. Role of reactive oxygen metabolites. Dig Dis Sci. 1988;33:6S–15S.

15. Boxer LA, Smolen JE. Neutrophil granule constituents and their release in health and disease. Hematol Oncol Clin N Am. 1988;2:101–34.

16. Rump JA, Scholmerich J, Gross V et al. A new type of perinuclear anti-neutrophil cytoplasmic antibody (p-ANCA) in active ulcerative colitis but not in Crohn's disease. Immunobiology. 1990;181:406–13.

17. Duerr RH, Targan SR, Landers CJ, Sutherland LR, Shanahan F. Anti-neutrophil cytoplasmic antibodies in ulcerative colitis. Comparison with other colitides/diarrheal illnesses. Gastroenterology. 1991;100:1590–6.

18. Saxon A, Shanahan F, Landers C, Ganz T, Targan S. A distinct subset of anti-neutrophil cytoplasmic antibodies is associated with inflammatory bowel disease. J Allergy Clin Immunol. 1990;86:202–10.

19. Falk RJ, Sartor RB, Jones DA, Jeffries BD, Jennette JC. Anti-neutrophil cytoplasmic antibodies (ANCA) in ulcerative colitis. Clin Res. 1990;38:387A.

20. Sarin SK, Malhotra V, Sen Gupta S, Karol A, Guar SK, Anand BS. Significance of eosinophil and mast cell counts in rectal mucosa in ulcerative colitis. A prospective controlled study. Dig Dis Sci. 1978;32:363–7.

21. Dvorak AM, Monahan RA, Osage JE, Dickersin GR. Crohn's disease: Transmission electron microscopic studies. II. Immunologic inflammatory response. Alterations of mast cells, basophils, eosinophils and the microvasculature. Hum Pathol. 1980;11:606–19.

22. Sanderson IR, Leung KBP, Pearce FL, Walker-Smith JA. Lamina propria mast cells in biopsies from children with Crohn's disease. J Clin Pathol. 1986;39:279–83.

23. Knutson L, Ahrenstedt O, Odlind B, Hallgren R. The jejunal secretion of histamine is increased in active Crohn's disease. Gastroenterology. 1990;98:849–54.

24. Fox CC, Lazenby AJ, Moore WC, Yardley JH, Bayless TM, Lichtenstein LM. Enhancement of human intestinal mast cell mediator release in active ulcerative colitis. Gastroenterology. 1990;99:119–24.

25. Barrett KE, Pearce FL. Mast cell heterogeneity. In: Foreman JC, editor. Immunopharmacology of mast cells and basophils. New York: Academic Press; 1993: in press.

26. Gordon JR, Burd PR, Galli SJ. Mast cells as a source of multifunctional cytokines. Immunol Today. 1990;11:458–64.

27. Gordon JR, Galli SJ. Mast cells as a source of both preformed and immunologically inducible TNF-α/cachetin. Nature. 1990;346:274–6.

28. Barrett KE, Metcalfe DD. Mucosal mast cells and IgE. In: Jones AL, Heyworth MF, editors. Immunology of the gastrointestinal tract and liver. New York: Raven Press; 1988:65–92.

29. Bienenstock J, Denburg J, Scicchitano R, Stead R, Perdue M, Stanisz A. Role of neuropeptides, nerves and mast cells in intestinal immunity and physiology. Monogr Allergy. 1988;24:124–33.

30. Jordana M, Befus AD, Newhouse MT, Bienenstock J, Gauldie J. Effect of histamine on proliferation of normal human adult lung fibroblasts. Thorax. 1988;43:552–8.

31. Ruoss SJ, Hartmann T, Caughey GH. Mast cell tryptase is a mitogen for cultured fibroblasts. J Clin Invest. 1991;88:493–9.

32. Berschneider HM, Powell DW. Fibroblasts modulate intestinal secretory responses to inflammatory mediators. J Clin Invest. 1992;89:484–9.

33. Keshav S, Chung L-P, Gordon S. Macrophage products in inflammation. Diagn Microbiol Infect Dis. 1990;13:439–47.

34. Allison MC, Poulter LW. Changes in phenotypically distinct mucosal macrophage populations may be a prerequisite for the development of inflammatory bowel disease. Clin Exp Immunol. 1991;85:504–9.
35. Thyberg T, Graf W, Klingenstrom P. Intestinal fine structure in Crohn's disease. Lysosomal inclusions in epithelial cells and macrophages. Virchows Arch (A). 1981;39:141–52.
36. Meuret G, Bitzi A, Hammer B. Macrophage turnover in Crohn's disease and ulcerative colitis. Gastroenterology. 1978;74:501–3.
37. Allison MC, Cornwall S, Poulter LW, Dhillon AP, Pounder RE. Macrophage heterogeneity in normal colonic mucosa and in inflammatory bowel disease. Gut. 1988;29:1531–8.
38. Mahida YR, Patel S, Gionchetti P, Vaux D, Jewell DP. Macrophage subpopulations in lamina propria of normal and inflamed colon and terminal ileum. Gut. 1989;30:826–34.
39. Seldenrijk CA, Drexhage HA, Meuwissen SGM, Pals ST, Meijer CJLM. Dendritic cells and scavenger macrophages in chronic inflammatory bowel disease. Gut. 1989;30:484–91.
40. Selby WS, Poulter LW, Hobbs S, Jewell DP, Janossy G. Heterogeneity of HLA-DR positive histiocytes in human intestinal lamina propria: a combined histochemical and immunohistological analysis. J Clin Pathol. 1983;36:379–84.
41. Malizia G, Calabrese A, Cottone M et al. Expression of leukocyte adhesion molecules by mucosal mononuclear phagocytes in inflammatory bowel disease. Gastroenterology. 1991;100:150–9.
42. Mahida YR, Wu KC, Jewell DP. Respiratory burst activity of intestinal macrophages in normal and inflammatory bowel disease. Gut. 1989;30:1362–70.
43. Ligumsky M, Simon PL, Karmeli F, Rachmilewitz D. Role of interleukin 1 in inflammatory bowel disease – enhanced production during active disease. Gut. 1990;31:686–9.
44. Sartor RB. Cytokines in inflammatory bowel disease. Progr Inflamm Bowel Dis. 1991;12:5–8.
45. Sartor RB. Pathogenetic and clinical relevance of cytokines in inflammatory bowel disease. Immunol Res. 1991;10:465–71.
46. Fiocchi C. Production of inflammatory cytokines in the intestinal lamina propria. Immunol Res. 1991;10:239–46.
47. Gross V, Andus T, Leser H-G, Roth M, Scholmerich J. Inflammatory mediators in chronic inflammatory bowel diseases. Klin Wochenschr. 1991;69:981–7.
48. Mahida YR, Wu K, Jewell DP. Enhanced production of interleukin 1-beta by mononuclear cells isolated from mucosa with active ulcerative colitis or Crohn's disease. Gut. 1989;30:835–8.
49. Hinterleitner TA, Berschneider HM, Powell DW. Fibroblast-mediated Cl$^-$ secretion by T$_{84}$ cells is amplified by interleukin-1β. Gastroenterology. 1991;100:A690.
50. Gross V, Andus T, Caesar I, Roth M, Scholmerich J. Evidence for continuous stimulation of interleukin-6 production in Crohn's disease. Gastroenterology. 1992;102:514–9.
51. Mahida YR, Kurlak L, Gallagher A, Hawkey CJ. Circulating and tissue interleukin 6 (IL6) levels in inflammatory bowel disease. Gastroenterology. 1990;98:A461.
52. Isaacs K, Sartor RB, Wang A, Haskill JS. Profiles of cytokine activation in inflammatory bowel disease tissue: measurement by cDNA amplification. Gastroenterology. 1990;98:A455.
53. Stevens C, Walz G, Zanker B, Singaram C, Lipman M, Strom TB. Interleukin-6 (IL-6), interleukin-1 beta (IL-1b) and tumor necrosis factor alpha (TNFa) expression in inflammatory bowel disease (IBD). Gastroenterology. 1990;98:A475.
54. Andus T, Targan SR, Deem R, Toyoda H. Measurement of TNF-α mRNA in lamina propria lymphocytes (LPL) isolated from mucosal biopsies of patients with inflammatory bowel diseases by reverse transcriptase quantitative polymerase chain reaction. Gastroenterology. 1992;102:A590.
55. MacDonald TT, Hutchings P, Choy M-Y, Murch S, Cooke A. Tumour necrosis factor-α and interferon-γ production measured at the single cell level in normal and inflamed human intestine. Clin Exp Immunol. 1990;81:301–5.
56. Mahida YR, Ceska M, Effenberger F, Kurlak L, Lindley I, Hawkey CJ. Enhanced synthesis of neutrophil-activating peptide-I/interleukin-8 in active ulcerative colitis. Clin Sci. 1992;82:273–5.
57. Baggiolini M, Walz A, Kunkel SL. Neutrophil-activating peptide-1/interleukin 8, a novel cytokine that activates neutrophils. J Clin Invest. 1989;84:1045–9.
58. Hallgren R, Colombel JF, Dahl R et al. Neutrophil and eosinophil involvement of the small bowel in patients with celiac disease and Crohn's disease: studies on the scretion rate and immunohistochemical localization of granulocyte granule constituents. Am J Med.

1989;86:56–64.
59. Walsh RE, Gaginella TS. The eosinophil in inflammatory bowel disease. Scand J Gastroenterol. 1991;26:1217–24.
60. Hates DE, Silberstein DS, Rodrique SW, Kufe DW. DF3 antigen, a human epithelial cell mucin, inhibits adhesion of eosinophils to antibody coated targets. J Immunol. 1990;145:962–70.
61. Podolsky DK, Isselbacher KJ. Glycoprotein composition of colonic mucosa. Specific alterations in ulcerative colitis. Gastroenterology. 1984;87:991–8.
62. Lobos EA, Sharon P, Stenson WF. Chemotactic activity in inflammatory bowel disease. Role of leukotriene B_4. Dig Dis Sci. 1987;32:1380–8.
63. Sharon P, Stenson WF. Enhanced synthesis of leukotriene B_4 by colonic mucosa in inflammatory bowel disase. Gastroenterology. 1984;86:453–60.
64. Goetzl EJ, Pickett WC. Novel structural determinants of the human neutrophil chemotactic activity of leukotriene. Br J Exp Med. 1981;153:482–7.
65. Fretland DJ, Widomski D, Tsai B-S, et al. Effect of the leukotriene B_4 receptor antagonist SC-41930 on colonic inflammation in rat, guinea pig and rabbit. J Pharmacol Exp Ther. 1990;255:572–6.
66. Wallace JL, MacNaughton WK, Morris GP, Beck PL. Inhibition of leukotriene synthesis markedly accelerates healing in a rat model of inflammatory bowel disease. Gastroenterology. 1989;96:29–36.
67. Cortese JF, Eisinger W, Spannhake EW, Yang VW. The 5-lipoxygenase pathway in cultured human intestinal epithelial cells. Gastroenterology. 1992;102:A206.
68. Bigby TD, Lee DM, Meslier N, Gruenert DC. LTA_4 hydrolase activity of human airway epithelial cells. Biochem Biophys Res Commun. 1989;164:1–7.
69. Borgeat P, Samuelsson B. Transformation of arachidonic acid by rabbit polymorphonuclear leukocytes. J Biol Chem. 1979;254:2643–6.
70. Baggliolini M, Dewald B, Thelen M. Effects of PAF on neutrophils and mononuclear phagocytes. Prog Biochem Pharmacol. 1988;22:90–105.
71. Baklien K, Brandtzaeg P. Immunohistochemical localization of complement in intestinal mucosa. Lancet. 1974;2:1087–8.
72. Halstensen TS, Brandtzaeg P. Local complement activation in inflammatory bowel disease. Immunol Res. 1991;10:485–92.
73. Fernandez H, Henson PM, Otani A, Hugli TE. Chemotactic response to human C3a and C5a anaphylatoxins. I. Evaluation of C3a and C5a leukotaxis in vitro and under stimulated in vivo conditions. J Immunol. 1978;120:109–15.
74. Marasco WA, Phan SH, Krutzsch H, et al. Purification and identification of formyl-methionyl-leucyl-phenylalanine as the major peptide neutrophil chemotactic factor produced by Escherichia coli. J Biol Chem. 1984;259:5430–9.
75. Hollander D, Vadheim CM, Brettholz E, Petersen GM, Delahunty T, Rotter JI. Increased intestinal permeability in patients with Crohn's disease and their relatives. Ann Intern Med. 1986;105:883–5.
76. Ukabam SO, Clamp JR, Cooper BT. Abnormal small intestinal permeability to sugars in patients with Crohn's disease of the terminal ileum and colon. Digestion. 1983;27:70–4.
77. VonRitter C, Sekizuka E, Grisham MB, Granger DN. The chemotactic peptide n-formyl-methionyl-leucyl-phenylalanine increases mucosal permeability in the distal ileum of the rat. Gastroenterology. 1988;95:651–6.
78. LeDuc LE, Nast CC. Chemotactic peptide-induced acute colitis in rabbits. Gastroenterology. 1990;98:929–35.
79. Chester JF, Ross JS, Malt MA, Weitzman SA. Acute colitis produced by chemotactic peptides in rats and mice. Am J Pathol. 1985;121:284–90.
80. Anton PA, Targan SR, Shanahan F. Increased neutrophil receptors for and response to the proinflammatory bacterial peptide formyl-methionyl-leucyl-phenylalanine in Crohn's disease. Gastroenterology. 1989;97:20–8.
81. Larsen CG, Anderson AO, Oppenheim JJ, Matsushima K. Production of interleukin-8 by human dermal fibroblasts and keratinocytes in response to interleukin-1 or tumor necrosis factor. Immunology. 1989;68:31–6.
82. Schurer-Maly CC, Maly FE, Kagnoff MF. T84 colon epithelial cells produce interleukin-8, a neutrophil chemoattractant. Gastroenterology. 1992;102:A692.
83. Wang JM, Rambaldi A, Biondi A, Chen ZG, Sanderson CJ, Mantovani A. Recombinant

human interleukin-5 is a selective eosinophil chemoattractant. Eur J Immunol. 1989;19:701–5.

84. Wardlaw AJ, Moqbel R, Cromwell O, Kay AB. Platelet-activating factor. A potent chemotactic and chemokinetic factor for eosinophils. J Clin Invest. 1986;78:1701–10.

85. Carlos TM, Harlan JM. Membrane proteins involved in phagocyte adherence to endothelium. Immunol Rev. 1990;114:5–28.

86. Lorant DE, Patel KD, McIntyre TM, McEver RP, Prescott SM, Zimmerman GA. Coexpression of GMP-140 and PAF by endothelium stimulated by histamine or thrombin: a juxtacrine system for adhesion and activation of neutrophils. J Cell Biol. 1991;115:223–34.

87. Madara JL, Stafford J. Interferon-γ directly affects barrier function of cultured intestinal epithelial monolayers. J Clin Invest. 1989;83:724–7.

88. Crowe SE, Perdue MH. Jejunal morphology in sensitized rats before and after luminal antigen (Ag) challenge. Gastroenterology. 1992;102:A611.

89. Parkos CA, Delp C, Arnaout MA, Madara JL. Neutrophil migration across a cultured intestinal epithelium. Dependence on a CD11b/CD18 mediated event and enhanced efficiency in physiological direction. J Clin Invest. 1991;88:1605–12.

90. Nash S, Stafford J, Madara JL. Effects of polymorphonuclear leukocyte transmigration on the barrier function of cultured intestinal epithelial monolayers. J Clin Invest. 1987;80:1104–13.

91. Barrett KE. Immune regulation of intestinal ion transport: implications for inflammatory diarrhea. Progr Inflamm Bowel Dis. 1991;12:8–11.

92. Wasserman SI, Barrett KE, Huott PA, Beuerlein G, Kagnoff M, Dharmsathaphorn K. Immune-related intestinal Cl^- secretion. I. Effect of histamine on the T_{84} cell line. Am J Physiol. 1988;254:C53–62.

93. Barrett KE, Cohn JA, Huott PA, Wasserman SI, Dharmsathaphorn K. Immune-related intestinal chloride secretion. II. Effect of adenosine on T_{84} cell line. Am J Physiol. 1990;258:C902–12.

94. Hanglow AC, Bienenstock J, Perdue MH. Effect of platelet activating factor on ion transport in isolated rat jejunum. Am J Physiol. 1989;257:G845–50.

95. Crowe SE, Sestini P, Perdue MH. Allergic reactions of rat jejunal mucosa. Ion transport responses to luminal antigen and inflammatory mediators. Gastroenterology. 1990;99:74–82.

96. Barrett KE. Immune-related intestinal Cl^- secretion. III. Acute and chronic effects of mast cell mediators on chloride secretion by a human colonic epithelial cell line. J Immunol. 1991;147:959–64.

97. Karayalcin SS, Sturbaum CW, Wachsman JT, Cha J-H, Powell DW. Hydrogen peroxide stimulates rat colonic prostaglandin production and alters electrolyte transport. J Clin Invest. 1990;86:60–8.

98. Nash S, Parkos C, Nusrat A, Delp C, Madara JL. *In vitro* model of crypt abscess: a novel neutrophil-derived secretagogue activity. J Clin Invest. 1991;87:1474–7.

8
Crohn's disease: an adjuvant disease?

W. E. W. ROEDIGER

INTRODUCTION

The 'adjuvant response' infers a range of immune responses but in the main implies enhancement of immune reactions that are, under ordinary conditions, weak or hardly measurable. Freund *et al.*[1] in 1937 utilized paraffin oil and killed mycobacteria to enhance the immune response to mycobacteria, a response tested by tuberculin sensitivity or antibody formation to mycobacteria. Subsequently the reaction has been elicited with equal success by employing oils with fragments or chemical derivatives of mycobacteria[2,3]. The semblance of Crohn's disease (CD) to an 'adjuvant disease' lies in the proposal that a lipid, oil or sterol, plus bacterial fragment are essential to produce a strong immune response (Fig. 1) and that subsequent re-exposure to such a combination of antigenic agents occurs in the gastrointestinal tract to cause, by the adjuvant response, mucosal ulcers or necrosis.

An implication of the 'adjuvant response' in CD is that it is specific for the disease and does not occur in ulcerative colitis, where immune reactions are of a different nature. Experimental evidence supports a difference of immune responses in the two diseases. Significantly interleukin-2 (IL-2) receptors on macrophages are more prominent in CD[4], circulating levels of IL-6 are higher in active CD[5,6] and generation of IL-1B is greater in CD[7] than in active ulcerative colitis.

The strong antigenic responses in CD focus attention on two factors needed for the adjuvant response: (a) lipids and (b) bacteria which strongly associate with or depend upon lipids to maintain viability and demonstrate pathogenic expression.

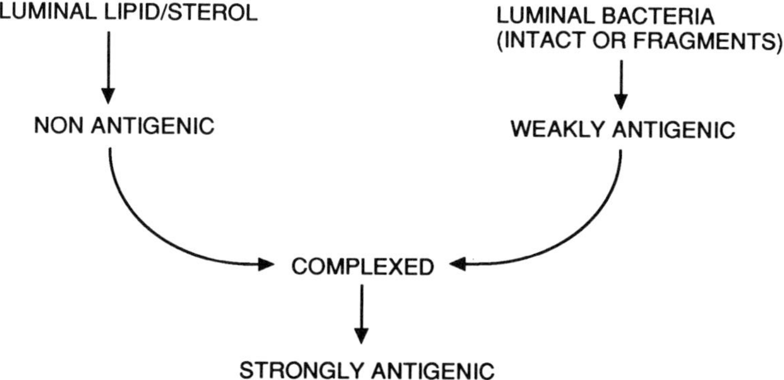

Fig. 1 Combination of lipids with bacteria/bacterial fragments provokes a stronger immune (adjuvant) response than each agent individually

ENTERAL LIPIDS IN CROHN'S DISEASE

Parenteral and enteral nutritional support have been used with success in active CD to redress depleted nutritional levels associated with severe disease. The role of elemental nutrition given enterally as a primary therapeutic means is less clear, but where therapeutic benefit has been reported the mechanism of action remains unexplained. The number of studies now available (Table 1) should have prompted a meta-analysis, but diversity of methods and types of feeds make such an analysis difficult[8]. The opposite ends of therapeutic responses are worthy of comparison. Studies by O'Morain *et al.*[9], Giaffer *et al.*[10], Okada *et al.*[11], Teahon *et al.*[12] and Rigaud *et al.*[13] with elemental diets where the caloric content from fat was less than 1.5%, revealed good clinical responses to enteral feeding. In contrast the elemental diets utilized by Park *et al.*[14] and Lochs *et al.*[15] were less effective than the above studies and not better than steroid therapy as observed in the therapeutically successful diets.

The different therapeutic responses are not easily explainable: the degree of allergenicity of protein hydrolysate or lack of allergenicity of constituent amino acids have been invoked. Notable is the low caloric contribution (<1.5%) made by fats in those diets, which have been shown to produce remarkable reversal of Crohn's inflammation compared to 10% or more in those diets which were less efficacious. This feature has been put to the test by Hiwatashi *et al.* in Japan[16], who concluded that lack of fat in enteral feeds was responsible for the therapeutic effect. Enteral diets low in fat reduce the chemiluminescent response in whole blood[17], suggesting immunological as well as nutritional improvement with these diets in active CD.

Table 1 Controlled trials comparing elemental diets with other treatment options in active Crohn's disease

Date	Ref.	Observation time in weeks	Elemental diet (nos/remission)	Control treatment (nos/remission)	How assessed
1984 randomized	9	4	Vivonex (11), 82%	Prednisolone (10), 80%	Activity index
1990 randomized	10	4	Vivonex (16), 75%	Polymeric diet (14), 35%	Activity index
1990 randomized	11	6	Vivonex equivalent (10), 90%	Prednisolone (10), 20%	X-ray appearance
1990 historical	12	24	Vivonex (52), 80%	Prednisolone (37), 75%	Patient and physician assessment
1991 randomized	13	4	Vivonex (15), 66%	Polymeric diet (15), 73%	Activity index
1991 randomized	14	4	Elemental 028 (7), 29%	Polymeric diet (7), 71%	Clinical score
1991 randomized	15	6	Peptisorb (55), 53%	Prednisolone (52), 79%	Activity index

LIPID–BACTERIAL CONNECTIONS

Long-chain fatty acids or cholesterol are essential for mycoplasma and mycobacteria[18,19] (Fig. 2), organisms which have previously been associated with the pathogenesis of CD.

Mycobacteria

Atypical mycobacteria have been strongly invoked as a cause of CD[20–22]. Mycobacteria require exogenous fatty acids for growth[18] and about one-third of their dry weight is constituted by lipids. In tissues mycobacteria may be found as intact organisms, fragments of organisms, spheroplasts or cords. As mycobacterial genomes (DNA) have both been reported[22,23] and denied to exist in CD[24] the combination of lipid with mycobacteria could either be with fragments of bacteria or with whole bacteria. Antimycobacterial therapy has not been of clinical efficacy in active CD[25] while prednisolone, in experimental infections with atypical mycobacteria, causes deterioration of mycobacterial disease[26]. Antibodies to *M. paratuberculosis* are rare in CD but more frequent in cases with active pulmonary tuberculosis[27]. Clinically the manifestation of proven intestinal tuberculosis[28–30] is usually in the ileocaecal region where 90% of CD cases will eventually have a disease focus. The case for or against mycobacteria as a causative agent of CD has not yet been resolved.

Mycoplasma

Mycoplasma are found widely throughout the plant and animal world in both vertebrates and invertebrates[31], and grow anaerobically in the colon of animals[32]. The genome size of mycoplasma is one-fifth that of *E. coli*[33]; mycoplasma actively pump sodium out of the bacterial body and depend on external energy sources to maintain osmotic integrity. Mycoplasma have

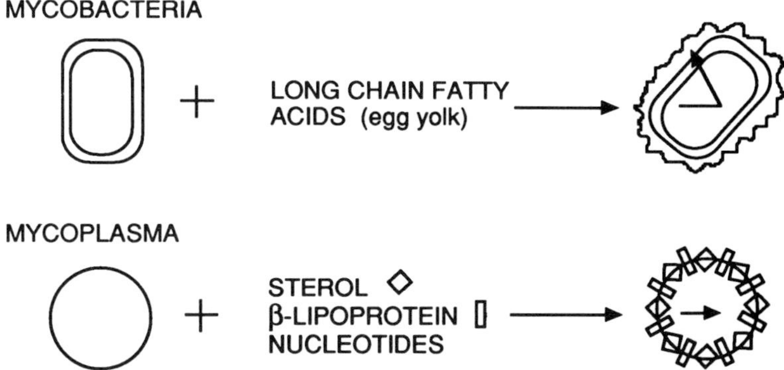

Fig. 2 Lipid requirements for bacteria. Mycobacteria require long-chain fatty acids for capsule formation, and mycoplasma require sterols and β-lipoprotein for membrane stabilization

been referred to as 'cell wall deficient' or 'wall-less', but nevertheless have a limiting membrane which avidly associates with cholesterol and human β-lipoprotein[34] (Fig. 2). Mycoplasma-like organisms have not been observed in Crohn's tissue[35] but noted in tissue culture inoculated with Crohn's tissue[35] where their growth was considered a contaminant[36].

Two indirect techniques have been employed to attempt to identify mycoplasma in CD.

Electron microscopic evidence for mycoplasma

In almost all cases of CD enterocytes show epithelial inclusion bodies (Fig. 3) (see ref. 37 for detailed literature survey). Because mycoplasma only have a limiting membrane they will appear as intracellular organelles (Fig. 4). Osmotic fragility will lead to lysosomal scavenging in which regard lysosomal bodies (lamellar bodies) have been found in almost all cases with CD[37]. The abundance of lamellar bodies has been suggested to be a defect in the normal processing of lipoproteins[38] with which, as mentioned above, mycoplasma may be associated. The appearance of epithelial lamellar bodies is a non-specific tissue response[38] and these bodies undergo transcytosis to the lamina propria[39] or may be extruded into the mucus of epithelial cells. Electron micrographs of CD show no evidence of atypical mycobacteria but bodies that resemble mycoplasma organisms (Fig. 4).

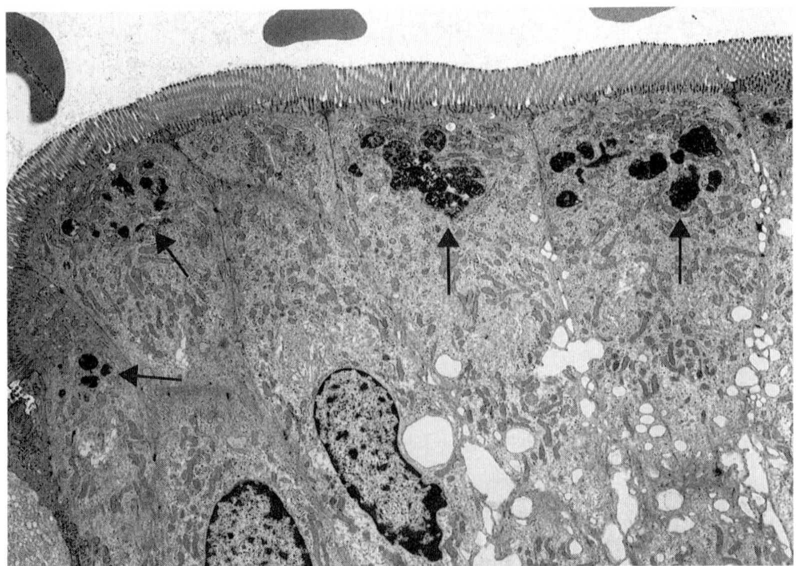

Fig. 3 Ileal enterocytes in active CD show numerous lamellar bodies (arrows) and intracellular vesicles suggestive of cell damage. Original magnification ×5000

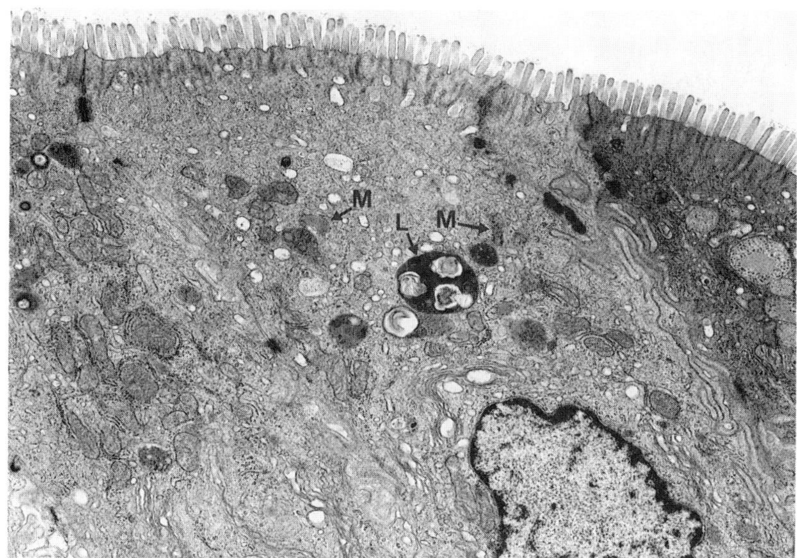

Fig. 4 Ileal enterocyte in active CD with lamellar bodies (L) and (?) mycoplasma (M). Numerous apical vesicles from endocytosis. Original magnification ×12000

Mycoplasma DNA staining in enterocytes

As specific immunofluorescent stains for intestinal mycoplasma are not available a search for mycoplasma DNA with a specific fluorochrome stain (Hoechst 33258)[40] was made in Crohn's tissue obtained within 5 min of operation. Cryostat sections, 5 µm, of fresh ileal mucosal tissue abutting on ulcers from three cases of CD were stained according to the method of Chen[40] with Hoechst 33258, at either 2.5 or 5.0 µg/ml. All three cases studied contained in a number of crypts cytoplasmic granules in enterocytes (Fig. 5a and 5b) which in appearance were similar to mycoplasma infestation of cultured cells observed by Hay *et al.*[41] and Russell *et al.*[42] with the same staining method. The terminal ileum of three control cases obtained from right hemicolectomies for colonic carcinoma showed cellular granulations in one case where an obstructing carcinoma of the ascending colon was present, but not in the other two control cases. The fluorescent stain is specific for mycoplasma DNA and 17 different species or strains have reacted positively[40]. Staining of mitochondrial DNA[43] is also possible, but no cells in the adjacent lamina propria or other enterocytes showed cytoplasmic accentuations (Fig. 5).

Mycoplasma and cell culture

The growth of mycoplasma in tissues from CD[35,36] and other tissues[41,42] is invariably regarded as a sign of 'contamination' of cell cultures. Such a

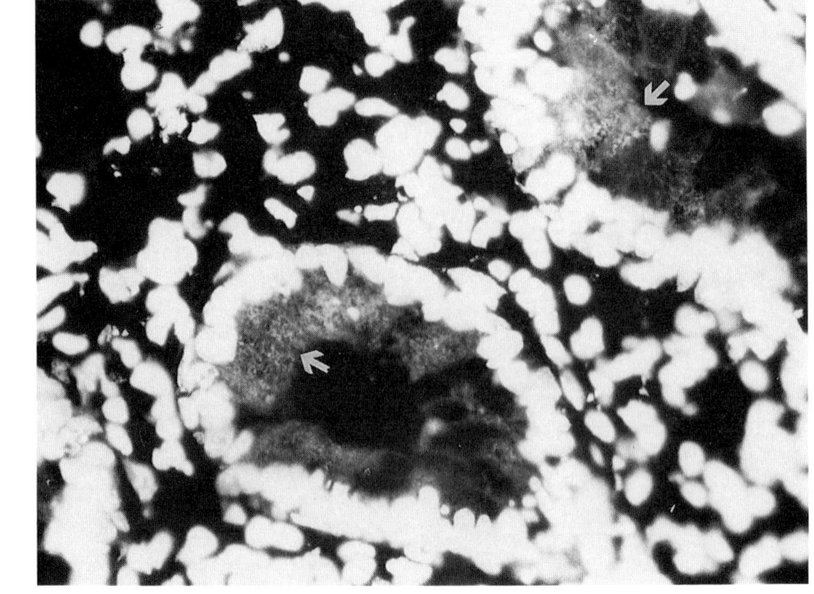

Fig. 5 Cryostat section of ileal mucosa in active CD stained with Hoechst 33258 for DNA. Cytoplasmic granules in enterocytes but not·in inflammatory cells (**a**) Original magnification ×650; (**b**) original magnification ×1000

perceived view would be a disinclination to ascribe a pathogenic role to mycoplasma should they be found in tissue culture systems or other culture systems in CD.

Mycoplasma in the intestinal tract

Mycoplasma are found in the oral cavity as commensals[44]; however, no search for mycoplasma has been undertaken in oral CD. Intestinal mycoplasma are most likely to be pathogenic where bacteria, cholesterol absorption and emulsifying agents are readily found, principally the distal ileum and colon but also at other sites such as the proximal small bowel. Epithelial cells of the intestinal tract contain fatty acid binding protein[45], which may be important for mycoplasma organisms. Mycoplasma organisms have been found in children with diarrhoea[46] and in the animal colon[32], but no studies in the human colon appear to have been carried out. Special conditions in growth media are required for detection of mycoplasma[47,48]. Some lipids within the colon[49] are of bacterial as well as dietary origin and the latter may make a variable contribution to luminal lipids. Lipid encrustation of the colonic mucosa may occur with high lipid intake[50]. Because some lipids are bacterial in origin dietary restriction of lipids for large bowel Crohn's disease may not be as effective as such restriction for disease in the small bowel[9-15].

LIPIDS AND POST-RESECTIONAL RECURRENCE OF CROHN'S DISEASE

The frequent recurrence of CD proximal to an ileocolonic anastomosis[51,52] can to some degree be explained by the new hypothesis. By diminishing the reflux of bacterial contents with a mucosal valve the incidence of recurrent CD can be diminished proximal to bowel anastomosis[53]. After distal small bowel resection in experimental animals the absorption of fat proximal to the anastomosis is significantly increased[54]. Should this occur in humans then increased absorption of fat after ileal resection, together with bacterial reflux, may be an explanation for the frequent recurrence of CD proximal to anastomoses.

A NEW HYPOTHESIS FOR CROHN'S DISEASE AND CLINICAL IMPLICATIONS

The present proposals are outlined in Fig. 1. Non-antigenic luminal lipid may be complexed with weakly antigenic bacteria, the combination of which would exert a strong adjuvant response at the mucosal level. Evidence from electron microscopy and observations with enteral nutrition support such a possibility. At present mycoplasma and cholesterol are a favoured combination. Other organisms such as streptococci[55] and mycobacterial fragments[56], when injected into the bowel wall, also cause inflammatory changes resembling CD. Thus the new proposals may not be unique to a single organism. The regional distribution of tuberculosis in the intestine is dependent upon lipids, and viable mycobacteria appear to gain entry to the intestinal mucosa. The clinical similarities between intestinal tuberculosis, and as now purported, mycoplasma involvement of the intestine, is summarized in Table 2. In a recent survey six out of six patients with inflammatory bowel disease who had respiratory tract infections due to *Mycoplasma pneumoniae* also had gastrointestinal symptoms[57]. No relationship bwetween *Mycoplasma pneumoniae* and CD is known to exist, and presumably other intestinal mycoplasma, as now proposed, must be involved in CD. The implication of the adjuvant response for clinical management is that disease expression would depend upon: (a) luminal bacteria (mycoplasma, mycobacteria, streptococci); (b) luminal lipids; and (c) the antigenic response of an adjuvant reaction (Fig. 6). The variability of clinical expression may be due to differences of interaction at all three levels. Diversion of the luminal stream should and has been shown to produce clinical improvement[58], providing support for the luminal origin of organisms.

Current proposals for CD may be difficult to prove in concordance with proposals based on Koch's postulates for living organisms, but the revised Koch's principles for non-viable organisms or molecular pathology applied to CD might be more pertinent[59]. These principles incorporate precise identification and temporal sequence of the pathological processes linked with reproducibility of the process and subsequent correction of molecular defects by removing causative factors. To conduct fruitful scientific work Pavlov advised gradual development of scientific processes while admitting to a lack of knowledge, but maintaining a passion to pursue new concepts[60]. This should be achievable in investigating the disease process of CD.

Table 2 Correlation of disease processes in lung and gastrointestinal tract involved with tuberculosis or mycoplasma

		Microorganism	
Organ	*Parameter*	*Tuberculosis*	*Mycoplasma*
Lung	Infective	Yes	Yes
	Age	Young	Young
	Nutrition	Poor	Good
	Lipid source	Surfactant	Surfactant
Gastrointestinal tract	Infective	Yes	Yes, proposed for CD
	Age	Young–Middle age	Young
	Nutrition	Poor	Good
	Lipid source	Luminal (LCFA)	Luminal (cholesterol)
	Main site	Ileocolonic	Ileocolonic
	Same organism for both organ sites	Yes	Probably not (? *M. intestinalis*)

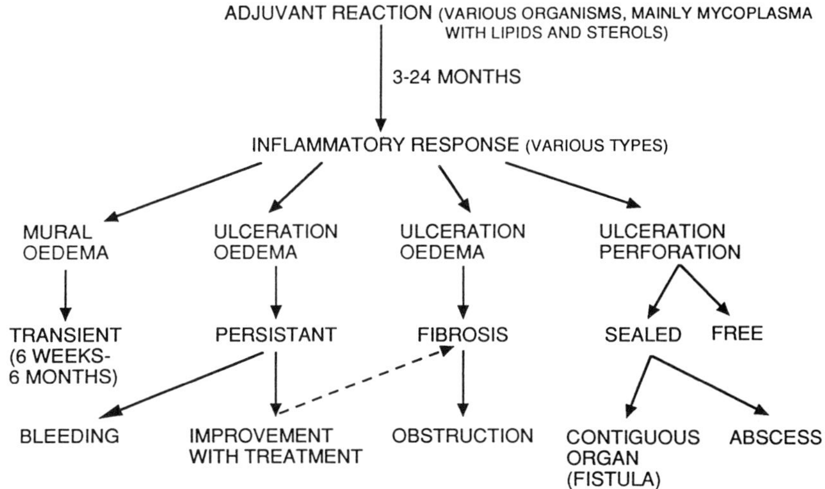

Fig. 6 Clinical manifestations attributable to the adjuvant response

ACKNOWLEDGEMENTS

I am grateful to the Electron Microscope Unit and Histopathology Department of the Queen Elizabeth Hospital for their assistance with tissue processing, and to Mrs E. Mazel for her skilful secretarial help.

References

1. Freund J, Casals J, Hosmer EP. Sensitization and antibody formation after injection of tubercle bacilli and paraffin oil. Proc Soc Exp Biol Med. 1937;37:509–13.
2. Bekierkunst A, Levij IS, Yarkoni E, Vilkas E, Adam A, Lederer E. Granuloma formation induced in mice by chemically defined mycobacterial fractions. J Bacteriol. 1969;100:95–102.
3. Kato K, Yamamoto K-I. Role of adjuvant and immunogenic moieties of M tuberculosis in pathogenicity. In: Bendinelli ML, Friedman H, editors. Mycobacterium tuberculosis. Interactions with the immune system. New York: Raven Press; 1988:39–58.
4. Choy MY, Walker-Smith JA, Williams CB, MacDonald TT. Differential experience of CD25 (interleukin-2 receptor) on lamina propria T cells and macrophages in the intestinal lesions in Crohn's disease and ulcerative colitis. Gut. 1990;31:1365–70.
5. Mahida YR, Kurlac L, Gallagher A, Hawkey CJ. High circulating concentrations of interleukin-6 in active Crohn's disease but not ulcerative colitis. Gut. 1991;32:1531–4.
6. Gross V, Andus T, Caesar I, Roth M, Scholmerich J. Evidence for continuous stimulation of interleukin-6 production in Crohn's disease. Gastroenterology. 1992;102:514–19.
7. Hodgson HJF, Mazlam MZ. Cytokines – are they different in ulcerative colitis and Crohn's disease? In: Goebell H, Ewe K, Malchow H, Koelbel Ch, editors. Inflammatory bowel disease: Progress in basic research and clinical implications. Lancaster: Kluwer; 1991:161–8.
8. Murray GD. Meta-analysis. Br J Surg. 1990;77:243–4.
9. O'Morain C, Segal AW, Levi AJ. Elemental diet as primary treatment of acute Crohn's disease: a controlled trial. Br Med J. 1984;288:1859–62.

10. Giaffer MH, North G, Holdsworth CD. Controlled trial of polymeric versus elemental diet in treatment of active Crohn's disease. Lancet. 1990;335:816–19.
11. Okada M, Yao T, Yamamoto T, Takenaka K, Mamura K, Maeda K, Fujita K. Controlled trial comparing an elemental diet with prednisolone in the treatment of active Crohn's disease. Hepato-gastroenterology. 1990;37:72–80.
12. Teahon K, Bjarnason I, Pearson M, Levi AJ. Ten years' experience with an elemental diet in the management of Crohn's disease. Gut. 1990;31:1133–7.
13. Rigaud D, Cosnes J, LeQuintrec Y, Rene E, Gendre JP, Mignon M. Controlled trial comparing two types of enteral nutrition in treatment of active Crohn's disease: elemental *v* polymeric diet. Gut. 1991;32:1492–7.
14. Park RHR, Galloway A, Danesh BJZ, Russell RI. Double-blind controlled trial of elemental and polymeric diets as primary therapy in active Crohn's disease. Eur J Gastroenterol Hepatol. 1991;3:483–90.
15. Lochs H, Steinhardt HJ, Klaus-Wentz B et al. Comparison of enteral nutrition and drug treatment in active Crohn's disease. Results of the European Co-operative Crohn's disease study IV. Gastroenterology. 1991;101:661–8.
16. Hiwatashi N, Yamazaki H, Suzuki K, Kayaba Y, Toyota T. The therapeutic effect of enteral hyperalimentation for active Crohn's disease (CD) – with special reference to the mechanism, in the development of effects. Proceedings, World Congress Gastroenterology, Sydney: 1990:729.
17. Okabe N, Maeda K, Okado M, Uekt M et al. Effects of nutritional therapy on chemiluminescence in Crohn's disease. Dig Dis Sci. 1991;36:1661.
18. Wheeler PR, Bulmer K, Ratledge C. Enzymes for biosynthesis de novo and elongation of fatty acids in mycobacteria grown in host cells: is mycobacterium leprae competent in fatty acid biosynthesis? J Gen Microbiol. 1990;136:211–17.
19. Razin S, Rottem S, Hasin M, Gershfeld NL. Binding of exogenous proteins and lipids to mycoplasma membranes. Ann NY Acad Sci. 1973;225:28–37.
20. Burnham WR, Lennard-Jones JE, Stanford JL, Bird RG. Mycobacteria as a possible cause of inflammatory bowel disease. Lancet. 1978;2:693–6.
21. Chiodini RJ, Van Kruiningen HJ, Thayer WR, Coutu JA. Spheroplastic phase of mycobacteria isolated from patients with Crohn's disease. J Clin Microbiol. 1986;24:357–63.
22. Sanderson JD, Hermon-Taylor J. Mycobacterial diseases of the gut: some impact from molecular biology. Gut. 1992;33:145–7.
23. Sanderson JD, Moss M, Malik Z, Tizard M, Green EP, Hermon-Taylor J. Polymerase chain reaction detects mycobacterium paratuberculosis in Crohn's disease tissue extracts. Gut. 1991;32:A572 (abstract).
24. Wu SWP, Pao CC, Chan J, Benedict Yen TS. Lack of mycobacterial DNA in Crohn's disease tissue. Lancet. 1991;337:174–5.
25. Jarnerot G, Rolny P, Wickbom G, Alewmayehu G. Antimycobacterial therapy ineffective in Crohn's disease after a year. Lancet. 1989;1:164–5.
26. Follett DM, Czuprynski CJ. Cyclophosphamide and prednisolone exacerbate the severity of intestinal paratuberculosis in mycobacterium paratuberculosis monoassociated mice. Microb Pathogen. 1990;9:407–515.
27. Brunello F, Martini S, Marino L, Astegiand M, Barletti C, Gastaldi P, Verme G, Emanuell IG. Antibodies to *Mycobacterium paratuberculosis* in patients with Crohn's disease. Dig Dis Sci. 1991;36:1741–5.
28. Klimach OE, Ormerod LP. Gastrointestinal tuberculosis: a retrospective review of 109 cases in a district general hospital. Q J Med. 1985;56:569–78.
29. Pettengell KE, Larsen C, Garb M, Mayet FGH, Simjee AE, Pirie D. Gastrointestinal tuberculosis in patients with pulmonary tuberculosis. Q J Med. 1990;74:303–8.
30. Shan S, Thomas V, Mathan M, Chacko A, Chandy G, Ramakrishna BS, Rolston DDK. Colonoscopic study of 50 patients with colonic tuberculosis. Gut. 1992;33:347–51.
31. Razin S. The mycoplasmas. Microbiol Rev. 1978;42:414–70.
32. Petzel JP, Hartman PA. Aromatic amino acid biosynthesis and carbohydrate catabolism in strictly anaerobic mollicutes (*Anaeroplasma* spp). Syst Appl Microbiol. 1990;13:240–7.
33. Neidhardt FC, Ingraham JL, Schaechter M. Physiology of the bacterial cell. A molecular approach. Sunderland, Mass: Sinauer Associates, 1990:14,243.
34. Efrati H, Oschry Y, Eisenberg S, Razin SD. Preferential uptake of lipids by mycoplasma membranes from human plasma low-density lipoproteins. Biochemistry. 1982;21:6477–82.

35. Cave D, Kirsner J *et al.* Infectious agents in inflammatory bowel disease (IBD) A status report. Gastroenterology. 1980;78:1185 (abstract).
36. Kapikian AZ, Barile MF, Wyati RG, Yolken RH, Tully JG, Greenberg HB, Kalica AR, Chanock RM. Mycoplasma contamination in cell culture of Crohn's disease material. Lancet. 1979;2:466–7.
37. Roediger WEW. A new hypothesis for the aetiology of Crohn's disease – evidence from lipid metabolism and intestinal tuberculosis. Postgrad Med J. 1991;67:666–71.
38. Schmitz G, Muller G. Structure and function of lamellar bodies, lipid-protein complexes involved in storage and secretion of cellular lipids. J Lipid Res. 1991;32:1539–70.
39. Mostov KE, Simister NE. Transcytosis. Cell. 1985;43:389–90.
40. Chen TR. *In situ* detection of mycoplasma contamination in cell cultures by fluorescent HOECHST 33258 stain. Exp Cell Res. 1977;104:255–62.
41. Hay RJ, Macy ML, Chen TR. Mycoplasma infection in cultured cells. Nature. 1989;339:487–8.
42. Russell WC, Newman C, Williamson DH. A simple cytochemical technique for demonstration of DNA in cells infected with mycoplasmas and viruses. Nature. 1975;253:461–2.
43. Borst P. Structure and function of mitochrondrial DNA. TIBS. 1977;2:31–4.
44. Evans AS, Brachman PS. Bacterial infections in humans: epidemiology and control, 2nd edn. New York: Plenum; 1989:443.
45. Ockner RK, Manning JA, Poppenhausen RB, Ho WKL. A binding protein for fatty acids in cytosol of intestinal mucosa, liver, myocardium and other tissues. Science. 1972;177:56–8.
46. Poley JR. Chronic nonspecific diarrhea in children: investigation of the surface morphology of small bowel mucosa utilizing the scanning electron microscope. J Pediatr Gastroenterol Nutr. 1983;2:71–94.
47. Davies S, Eggington R. Recovery of *Mycoplasma hominis* from blood culture media. Med Lab Sci. 1991;48:110–13.
48. Jacobs F, Van De Stadt J, Gelin M, Nonhoff C, Gay F, Adler M, Thys J-P. Mycoplasma hominis infection of perihepatic hematomas in a liver transplant recipient. Surgery. 1992;111:98–100.
49. James AT, Webb JPW, Kellock TD. The occurrence of unusual fatty acids in faecal lipids from human beings with normal and abnormal fat absorption. Biochem J. 1961;78:333–9.
50. Binder HJ, Van Noorden S. The distribution of lipid in colonic mucosa. Proc Soc Exp Biol Med. 1969;131:1119–23.
51. Williams JG, Wong WD, Rothenberger DA, Goldberg SM. Recurrence of Crohn's disease after resection. Br J Surg. 1991;78:10–19.
52. Olaison G, Smedh K, Sjodahl R. Natural course of Crohn's disease after ileocolic resection: endoscopically visualized ileal ulcers preceding symptoms. Gut. 1992;33:331–5.
53. Smedh K, Olaison G, Sjodahl R. Ileocolonic nipple valve anastomosis for preventing recurrence of sugically treated Crohn's disease. Dis Colon Rectum. 1990;33:987–90.
54. Thomson ABR. Uptake of lipids into rabbit jejunum and colon following ileal resection. Dig Dis Sci. 1986;31:193–201.
55. Sartor RB, Cromartie WJ, Powell DW, Schwab JH. Granulomatous enterocolitis induced in rats by purified bacterial cell wall fragments. Gastroenterology. 1985;89:587–95.
56. Mitchell IC, Turk JL. An experimental animal model of granulomatous bowel disease. Gut. 1989;30:1371–8.
57. Kangro HO, Chong SKF, Hardiman A, Heath RB, Walker-Smith JA. A prospective study of viral and mycoplasma infections in chronic inflammatory bowel disease. Gastroenterology. 1990;98:549–54.
58. Rutgeerts P, Goboes K, Peeters M *et al.* Effect of faecal stream diversion on recurrence of Crohn's disease in the neoterminal ileum. Lancet. 1991;338:771–4.
59. Hall PA, Lemoine NR. Koch's postulates revisited. J Pathol. 1991;164:283–4.
60. Pavlov IP. Bequest of Pavlov to the academic youth of his country. Science. 1936;83:369.

9
Treatment implications of immunological abnormalities

S. P. JAMES

INTRODUCTION

In order to understand the immunological abnormalities associated with inflammatory bowel disease (IBD) it is first necessary to understand the function of the mucosal immune system in the normal gastrointestinal tract. A large proportion of the total lymphoid cell population of the body is associated with the gastrointestinal tract, and the mucosal immune system carries out many important roles in host defence[1]. The gastrointestinal mucosa contains a large number of B cells and plasma cells that secrete IgA, an immunoglobulin class present in secretions that is thought to protect the host from pathogens. Both the intestinal lamina propria and epithelial layer contain a large number of T cells, and recent studies have demonstrated that these populations of cells have many characteristics that are important for host defence in the intestine. The pathogenesis of the idiopathic IBD, Crohn's disease and ulcerative colitis, is probably multifactorial and is probably different for each of the two diseases. Both the B cell and T cell components of the mucosal immune system are activated in these diseases, and a number of different abnormalities have been defined. However, so far the significance of these abnormalities is uncertain and as yet no entirely unique immunological abnormality has been associated with IBD. Nonetheless, it seems likely that these cells are important in pathogenesis of the disease, and therapies that are known to have effects on lymphoid function have empirically been found to have efficacy in IBD. Many of the treatments that have been used in IBD have relatively non-selective effects on lymphocyte function. However, recent advances suggest that it may be possible to treat IBD with therapies that have much more selective effects on the mucosal immune system. Ultimately, if the nature of the lymphoid cells involved and the inciting antigens can be defined precisely, it may be possible to develop highly selective therapies for IBD.

MUCOSAL IMMUNE SYSTEM

The mucosal immune system consists of lymphoid tissues associated with the lacrimal, salivary, gastrointestinal, respiratory and urogenital tracts and lactating breasts. Quantitatively, the lymphoid tissues associated with these sites, in particular with the gastrointestinal tract, contain the majority of the lymphoid tissue of the body. This fact presumably reflects the continuous activation of local immune mechanisms in response to the numerous potential pathogens and the complex array of antigens normally present at mucosal surfaces. This conclusion is supported by the observation first made many years ago that germ-free animals have a largely atrophic mucosal immune system. There are a number of important features of the gastrointestinal mucosal immune system. The mucosal immune system contains specialized structures, such as the Peyer's patches, where immune responses are thought to be initiated. Secondly, there is a pattern of relatively specific recirculation of lymphoid cells to the mucosa, known as mucosal homing. Thirdly, subsets of lymphoid cells, particularly IgA B cells and memory T cells, predominate at mucosal surfaces. Fourthly, the predominant mucosal immunoglobulin, secretory IgA, is particularly well-adapted to host defence at mucosal surfaces. These elements of the gastrointestinal mucosal immune system function together to generate an immune response which on the one hand protects the host from harmful pathogens, but on the other hand is tolerant of the ubiquitous dietary antigens and normal microbial flora.

T-cells in the Peyer's patches and mesenteric lymph nodes are a mixed population, containing both CD4 and CD8 cells in similar proportions to that in peripheral blood[2]. It is thought that CD4 cells carry out the same critical helper functions in response to antigens displayed on MHC class II antigen-presenting cells as in the peripheral immune system. Similarly, there is evidence in animal models that CD8 cells may differentiate into cytolytic T cells in response to pathogens present in the mucosa.

The functional capabilities of T cells present in the intestinal lamina propria compartment are more specialized and restricted in comparison to T-cells in the peripheral circulation. First, T-cells in the lamina propria bear surface glycoproteins typical of so-called memory lymphocytes, i.e. cells that have undergone differentiation in response to antigen exposure. These include the presence of low molecular weight components of the T200 family of glycoproteins (CD45R0) and absence of the high molecular weight glycoproteins characteristic of naive lymphocytes (CD45RA)[2]. In addition, virtually all of the lymphocytes in the diffuse lamina propria compartment lack the MEL-14/Leu-8 human peripheral lymph node homing receptor, which is found on about 60% of circulating lymphocytes[3]. An increased proportion of lymphocytes, both T and B cells, in the lamina propria have evidence of recent activation, as evidenced by expression of the IL-2 receptor alpha chain (CD25) on about 15% of lamina propria lymphocytes[4]. It has also been shown that although intestinal lamina propria lymphocytes have the capacity to proliferate in response to conventional mitogens, they show minimal or no proliferative responses to conventional protein antigens[5]. This is not due to the absence of antigen-specific T cell receptors on this population, since these lymphocytes have the capacity to mediate typical T cell functions, such as providing helper activity in response to specific antigens. Although the reason for lack of proliferation is unknown, it may be analogous to the functional tolerance that is observed with T cell clones following certain types of activation. T cells in the lamina propria have high capacity to produce lymphokines such as IL-2, IL-4, IL-5 and interferon-γ, consistent with their 'memory' cell phenotype[6]. It is likely that production of these lymphokines accounts in part for the functions of differentiated lymphocytes, including providing help for B cell immunoglobulin production and maturation of cytolytic effector cells. These and other lymphokines may also be important in the growth and differentiation of non-lymphoid cells such as mast cells and eosinophils, both of which are normally present in large numbers in the lamina propria. Similarly, lamina propria T cells have the ability to suppress immunoglobulin production and to mediate CD3-dependent cytolytic function typical of cytolytic effector cells. There is some evidence that T cells in mucosal sites may have a selective ability to enhance IgA production by B cells. This may be in part due to greater production of soluble factors such as IL-5, which appear to have a relatively greater enhancing effect on IgA production than other immunoglobulin isotypes.

Although both CD4 and CD8 cells are present in the mucosa, their distribution in the lamina propria is not uniform. CD4 cells outnumber CD8 cells by a 2–3:1 ratio in the lamina propria; however, nearly all of the T cells present in the intraepithelial cell layer are CD8 cells. The increased cytoplasmic/nuclear ratio and presence of granules has suggested that intraepithelial lymphocytes are cytolytic effector cells, for which there is some evidence in animal models[7]. However, whether lysis of potential target cells is the only role that these cells play is presently uncertain. In healthy individuals, most of the T cells associated with the gastrointestinal tract bear the α,β heterodimer T cell receptor. Only a minority express the γ,δ T cell receptors[8], unlike in rodents, where the latter account for a significant proportion of T cell receptors in the intestinal mucosa. CD8 intraepithelial lymphocytes in particular are enriched in cells expressing γ,δ T cell receptors. The role of $\gamma,\delta+$ T cells in host defence is presently uncertain[9]. There is experimental evidence that $\gamma,\delta+$ T cells make up an important component of T cells responding early in particular types of immune responses. Their proportion is increased in certain disease states such as gluten-sensitive enteropathy; however, their function in these situations is still unknown. In addition to their potential role as cytolytic effector cells, CD8+ T cells may secrete factors that are important in regulating the growth and function of epithelial cells.

It is clear that perturbations of this system occur in many diseases, and may actually underlie the pathogenesis of a number of diseases, including food allergies, autoimmune diseases such as systemic lupus erythematosus, and specific gastrointestinal diseases such as ulcerative colitis and Crohn's disease. In addition, an understanding of the mechanisms of generation of protective and tolerizing immune responses at mucosal surfaces is critical to developing immunological strategies for immunotherapy.

LYMPHOCYTE ABNORMALITIES IN IBD

The idiopathic inflammatory bowel diseases (IBD) ulcerative colitis and Crohn's disease are characterized by intense chronic inflammation in the gastrointestinal mucosa with a significant increase in the presence of activated mucosal T and B cells. The pathogenesis of these diseases is likely to be multifactorial, including environmental factors, host factors including the intestinal microflora, genetic factors and the mucosal immune system itself. Although IBD has been associated with particular MHC class II phenotypes, extensive studies have failed to prove the presence of unique aetiological antigens or pathogens in patients with IBD. Nonetheless, the clinical observations that the use of parenteral nutrition or enteral alimentation is associated with improvement in disease activity, and that oral antibiotics may diminish inflammation in IBD, have suggested that lumenal antigens may be important in the disease.

The immunological search for unique aetiological immune mechanisms has been hampered by the problem that the diseased gastrointestinal mucosa in IBD may provide access to the mucosal immune system of a myriad of commensal lumenal bacterial products that may secondarily lead to marked activation of lymphocytes. Therefore, the search for specific immunological abnormalities in IBD has been difficult. A number of fundamental observations are likely to be important in the pathogenesis of IBD (Table 1). It has been shown that soluble IL-2 receptors are present in the serum of patients with both ulcerative colitis and Crohn's disease, and this is probably a reflection of activation of T cells, B cells and monocytes in the intestinal mucosa, but this abnormality provides no further insight into the mechanism of activation of these cells[10].

With regard to B cell abnormalities, the most prominent abnormalities have been an increase in the presence of activated B cells in the intestine, an increase in the presence of IgG secreting plasma cells in the intestine (that

Table 1 Lymphocyte alterations in IBD

B cells
Increased numbers in diseased tissues
   Increased activation
   Increase in IgG secreting cells in tissues
Autoantibodies

T cells
Increased numbers in diseased tissues
Polyclonal TCR
Lymphocyte activation
   Soluble IL-2R
   Lymphokine gene expression

are normally infrequent) and the presence of autoantibodies in the serum[11]. Recent interest has focused on anti-neutrophil antibodies in patients with ulcerative colitis; however, there is as yet no evidence that these antibodies or other autoantibodies are specific for this disease or play a pathogenic role. Some authors have suggested that unique autoantigens associated with epithelial cells may be the targets of autoreactivity in IBD.

With regard to T cells in IBD, the most obvious abnormality, as mentioned above, is that the number of T cells is increased in the mucosa, and there is a significant proportion of cells that are activated. Previous studies of T cell receptor genes have failed to demonstrate evidence of oligoclonal expansion of T cells in the intestinal mucosa in IBD, but this would not be expected in a non-malignant disease. However, Posnett et al.[12] have provided evidence that T cells associated with the gastrointestinal tract may be selectively activated in IBD, in that the mesenteric lymph nodes of patients with Crohn's disease contain an increased proportion of T cells expressing the TCR-Vβ8 family of T cell receptors. Interestingly, this increase was not found in the intestinal lamina propria, the most prominent site of involvement of this disease, suggesting the possibility that T cells that had been activated in the afferent limb of the mucosal immune system either did not recirculate, or may have been deleted prior to their entry into the lamina propria. Since many of the functional effects of T cells are mediated by release of cytokines, there has been great interest in determining the nature of cytokines produced in IBD that are likely to be important in disease pathogenesis. Recently, it was demonstrated that IL-2 mRNA was increased in the intestinal lamina propria of patients with Crohn's disease, but not ulcerative colitis, suggesting that the pattern of cytokine activation may be different in these two diseases[13]. The complete pattern of cytokine production by T cells in the intestine in IBD is yet to be defined, but it is very likely that the nature of the secreted cytokines will be very useful in defining the nature of the inflammatory process and hopefully provide some clues to pathogenesis and new avenues of treatment.

IMPLICATIONS FOR TREATMENT

With the above information as background, it is obvious at the present time that the precise role of the lymphoid system in the pathogenesis of IBD is uncertain. Nonetheless, it has clearly been found from empirical studies that treatments that alter the mucosal immune system may be beneficial in IBD, and furthermore, several new areas of investigation suggest that further advances in modifying the activity of the immune system may be possible. General approaches to immunomodulation in disease include drugs with relatively non-specific immunosuppressive effects, approaches that have more selective effects on the immune system, and approaches that are highly selective and may be disease-specific (Table 2).

The adrenocorticosteroids have been studied and used extensively in the treatment of IBD, but at this point we do not have a complete understanding of their mechanism of benefit, again because the pathogenesis of IBD is

Table 2   General approaches to immunomodulation in IBD

Nonspecific
Immunosuppressive drugs
  Prednisone, azathioprine, 6-mercaptopurine, methotrexate

Selective
Drugs that inhibit cell function
  Cyclosporin, FK506
Cell depletion
  Lymphapharesis
  Monoclonal antibodies: anti-CD4, anti-IL-2R
  IL-2-toxin conjugate
Cytokine antagonists
  IL-1 receptor antagonist
Soluble cytokine receptors

Potentially specific
Remove antigen
  Modify intestinal flora
Oral tolerance

---

incompletely understood. It is likely that much of the beneficial effect of corticosteroids is due to their anti-inflammatory effects. In addition, the corticosteroids are potent inhibitors of macrophage activation. It is possible that one of the more important long-term effects of corticosteroids in IBD is that they inhibit macrophage activation and lymphokine production, thus secondarily inhibiting activation of T and B lymphocytes and their secreted products. Other non-specific immunomodulatory agents that have benefit in IBD include drugs which have potent immunosuppressive activity, azathioprine, 6-mercaptopurine and methotrexate. Azathioprine and 6-MP are purine analogues that interfere with DNA and RNA synthesis, and it is presumed that their long-term effect in IBD is to interfere with the replication of long-lived lymphoid cell populations that are important in disease pathogenesis. However, there is no proof as yet that this is the case. Methotrexate is a folic acid analogue that interferes with DNA and RNA synthesis, and has many effects on cell function. This drug also has been shown in open trials to have efficacy in the treatment of IBD, and as for corticosteroids the mechanism of action of this drug probably occurs at multiple levels.

More recently there has been interest in trying to use drugs to treat IBD that have more selective effects on the immune system. The best-studied agent is cyclosporin. This cyclic undecapeptide is a potent immunosuppressive drug that is the mainstay of organ transplantation and has been used extensively in attempts to treat autoimmune diseases. The mechanism of action of this drug has been worked out in great detail. Cyclosporin binds a specific cytoplasmic protein called cyclophilin, and the cyclosporin–cyclophilin complex then inhibits a cytoplasmic phosphatase called calcineurin. Inhibition of the activity of this enzyme inhibits the activation of a cytoplasmic factor called NF-AT, which is required for activation of gene transcription in the nucleus. The immediate effect of this drug is that it inhibits gene transcription in activated lymphocytes, and in particular inhibits lymphokine production. The selectivity of this drug is probably based on the fact that levels of calcineurin are rate-limiting in T cell activation. These effects of cyclosporin probably explain the beneficial effects that have been observed in the treatment of IBD[14], and correlate well with the observation mentioned above that IL-2 mRNA levels are increased in lesions of patients with active Crohn's disease. However, it is still uncertain whether cyclosporin will achieve long-term success in the treatment of IBD, in part due to its significant toxicity. Therefore, the search for other approaches to immunosuppression continues.

A completely different approach to immunosuppression in IBD has been therapeutic lymphapharesis. In open trials this approach has been reported to achieve success in some patients[15]. However, this treatment has never been subjected to randomized trials. Furthermore, it is expensive and inconvenient for patients, and therefore has not gained popularity. Nonetheless, this approach to treatment points to the possibility that lymphocyte depletion has potential for treating IBD if better methods can be developed to achieve this. The development of monoclonal antibody technology has in fact brought this type of approach to the level of therapeutic trials. As a background observation, it has been known for a number of years that patients with well-established IBD may achieve remission of their disease when they acquire HIV infection, with its subsequent CD4 T cell immunodeficiency[16]. This observation, coupled with the knowledge that CD4 T cells play a central role in initiating and maintaining many types of immune responses, led to the possibility that depletion of circulating lymphocytes with monoclonal antibodies that react with CD4 could be therapeutically beneficial in patients with IBD. Small studies have been carried out suggesting possible benefit of murine monoclonal anti-CD4 in IBD[17]; however, murine antibodies have the major disadvantage that they cannot be administered repeatedly because of immune reactions against the foreign murine protein. With the advent of molecular engineering, it is now possible to create chimeric monoclonal antibodies that have the variable region of murine anti-CD4 and constant regions of human IgG. These synthetic antibodies can be administered repeatedly and will deplete CD4 cells from the circulation. Two different groups of investigators have reported preliminary observations suggesting that CD4 T cell depletion with chimeric monoclonal antibodies may be beneficial in the treatment of IBD[18,19]. Furthermore, other types of monoclonal antibodies might be of use in IBD[20]. In particular, approaches that are directed at activated T cells, by using anti-IL-2 receptor monoclonal antibodies, might merit exploration. An alternative approach would be to use the ligand for the receptor coupled to the toxin, as has been carried out for IL-2-toxin conjugates. Yet another approach that has been used in experimental models of autoimmunity is to deplete specific subpopulations of T cells defined by their T cell receptor families. As a prelude to such an approach we have carried out preliminary studies to determine whether any specific families of TCR-Vβ families are overexpressed in the intestine in patients with IBD, but the results to date have not shown evidence that one specific family of T cells is highly expressed.

There are many other approaches to immunomodulation that could be explored in the future in IBD. An area of great interest has been to try to block the effects of lymphoid cells at the level of their secreted products, using either receptor antagonists (such as IL-1 receptor antagonist) or multivalent synthetic receptors that complex and block the effects of cytokines (such as soluble TNF-receptor). A completely different approach is to try to harness the inherent capacity of the mucosal immune system to generate negative or tolerogenic signals to fed antigens. The mechanisms by which antigen feeding leads to inhibition of subsequent systemic immune responses to the antigen are probably multiple, and may involve deletion or inactivation of particular cell populations and the generation of circulating suppressor T cells. In animal models of autoimmunity it has now been clearly demonstrated that it is possible to decrease the activity of autoimmune disease by feeding of the relevant disease-inducing antigen. Whether this approach will be possible in IBD is as yet uncertain. Further progress along these lines will require a better understanding of the antigens which are responsible for lymphocyte activation in the disease, to determine whether this approach is practical. Furthermore, it is possible that the fundamental defect in IBD in fact involves a selective inability to generate the necessary tolerogenic signals to the disease-provoking antigens, thus making it impossible to use this approach.

References

1. Strober W, James SP. The mucosal immune system. In: Stites DP, Terr A, editors. Basic and clinical immunology. Norwalk: Appleton & Lange; 1991:175–86.
2. James SP. Mucosal T cell function. Gastroenterol Clin N Am. 1991;20:597–612.
3. Berg M, Murakawa Y, Camerini D, James SP. Lamina propria lymphocytes are derived from circulating cells that lack the Leu-8 lymph node homing receptor. Gastroenterology. 1991;101:90–99.
4. Zeitz M, Green WC, Peffer NJ, James SP. Lymphocytes isolated from the intestinal lamina propria of normal non-human primates have increased expression of genes associated with T cell activation. Gastroenterology. 1988;94:647–55.
5. Zeitz M, Quinn TC, Graeff AS, James SP. Mucosal T cells provide helper function but do not proliferate when stimulated by specific antigen in Lymphogranuloma venereum proctitis in non-human primates. Gastroenterology. 1988;94:353–66.
6. James SP, Kwan WC, Sneller MC. T cells in inductive and effector compartments of the intestinal mucosal immune system of nonhuman primates differ in lymphokine mRNA expression, lymphokine utilization, and regulatory function. J Immunol. 1990;144:1251–6.
7. Klein JR, Kagnoff MF. Spontaneous in vitro evolution of lytic specificity of cytotoxic T lymphocyte clones isolated from murine intestinal epithelium. J Immunol. 1987;138:58–62.
8. Porcelli S, Brenner MB, Band H. Biology of the human gd T cell receptor. Immunol Rev. 1991;120:137–83.
9. Kiyono H, Fujihashi K, Taguchi T, Aicher WK, McGhee JR. Regulatory functions for murine intraepithelial lymphocytes in mucosal responses. Immunological Res. 1991;10:324–30.
10. Matsuura T, West GA, Klein JS, Ferraris L, Fiocchi C. Soluble interleukin-2 and CD8 and CD4 receptors in inflammatory bowel disease. Gastroenterology 1992;102:2006–14.
11. Schreiber S, Raedler A, Stenson W, MacDermott RP. The role of the mucosal immune system in inflammatory bowel disease. Gastro Clin N Am. 1992;21:451–502.
12. Posnett DN, Schmelkin I, Burton DA, August A, McGrath H, Mayer LF. T cell antigen receptor V gene usage. Increased in V beta 8+ T cells in Crohn's disease. J Clin Invest. 1990;85:1770–6.
13. Mullin GE, Lazenby AJ, Harris ML, Bayless TM, James SP. Increased interleukin-2 messenger RNA in the intestinal mucosal lesions of Crohn's disease but not ulcerative colitis. Gastroenterology. 1992;102:1620–7.

14. Brynskov J, Freund L, Rasmussen SN *et al.* A placebo controlled, double-blind, randomized trial of cyclosporine therapy in active chronic Crohn's disease. N Eng J Med. 1989;321:845–50.
15. Bicks RO, Groshart KD. Editorial: the current status of T-lymphocyte apheresis (TLA) treatment of Crohn's disease. J Clin Gastroenterol. 1989;11:136–8.
16. James SP. Remission of Crohn's disease following human immunodeficiency virus infection. Gastroenterology. 1988;95:1667–9.
17. Emmrich J *et al.* Treatment of IBD with anti-CD4 monoclonal antibody. Lancet. 1991;388:571.
18. Stronkhorst A, Yong SL, Radema S, ten Berge I, Das PK, Tytgat GN, van Deventer SJH. Phase 1 multiple-dose pilot study of chimeric monoclonal M-T412 (anti CD4) antibodies in Crohn's disease. Preliminary data. Gastroenterology. 1992;102:A702.
19. Deusch K, Reiter C, Mauthe B, Riethmüller G, Classen M. Chimeric monoclonal anti-CD4 antibody therapy proves effective for treating inflammatory bowel disease. Gastroenterology. 1992;102:A615.
20. Sriram S. Immunotherapy of autoimmune disease with anti-T cell antibodies. In: Cruse JM, Lewis RE Jr, editors. Therapy of autoimmune diseases. Concepts in Immunopathology. Karger: Basel; 1989:7:162–72.

Section III
Pathophysiology — Cytokines and Mediators

10

The cytokine network

M. LOTZ

INTRODUCTION

In the mature organism, cytokines are physiological mediators of host defence responses to injury such as trauma or infection. In these responses, cytokine synthesis is triggered directly or indirectly by microbial antigens, activation products of humoral inflammatory systems or degraded extracellular matrix components. In homeostasis most cytokines are not produced and cytokine receptors are not expressed, or only at low levels. This feature of inducibility is consistent with the role of cytokines as mediators of host defence responses. Upon generation of one or a small number of cytokines, interactions between cytokines and their receptors on different cell types lead to a sequence of events that is referred to as cytokine cascade. These interactions define the particular biological functions of a specific cytokine since the effects of one cytokine can be mediated or modulated by other cytokines that are present simultaneously or sequentially. Most cytokines are capable of enhancing their own synthesis, which is referred to as autoinduction or stimulate the expression of other cytokines.

A particular cell proliferative or secretory response can be induced by more than one cytokine. This may in part be related to the induction of secondary cytokines, or represent redundancy in that a given cellular response is independently regulated by more than one cytokine. When distinct cytokines induce qualitatively similar responses in the same cell type this is generally mediated through different cell surface receptors. Only few cytokines share common receptors and these cytokines are in general structurally related. This discussion will highlight interactions of peptide regulatory factors in the regulation of cytokine expression and in the modulation of their biological activities.

REGULATION OF CYTOKINE EXPRESSION

Most cytokine genes are not transcribed during homeostasis. In response to injury such as infection or trauma, stimuli are generated that trigger the induction of cytokine gene transcription. Such inciting stimuli can be microbial antigens, fragments of degraded extracellular matrix or products resulting from the activation of humoral mediator systems such as the complement components C3a and C5a. These agents bind to specific cell surface receptors and activate intracellular second messenger systems. This results in the activation of DNA binding proteins which recognize specific regions in the promoters of cytokine genes. Multiple binding motifs which are determined by specific sequences of approximately eight to 14 nucleotides have been identified in cytokine promoters. Motifs that are found in several cytokine genes include the binding sites for the transcription factors AP-1, NF-kB, NF-IL-6, CREB or SP-1. Protein binding to several of these sites is required for high levels of cytokine gene expression. Figure 1 illustrates some of the events involved with the induction of cytokine gene expression using IL-6 as a model. Binding of a cytokine inducer to its cell surface receptor results in the activation of intracellular signals and activation of protein kinases or phosphatases which regulate the activity of DNA binding proteins. Analysis of the activation of the IL-6 gene showed that the levels of the activated forms of the transcription factors AP-1 and NF-IL-6 do not correlate with the absence or presence of IL-6 mRNA. These factors are constitutive and may be required for maximal levels of IL-6 gene transcription, but they do not appear to be the critical regulators. In contrast, the DNA binding protein NF-kB is not present in unstimulated cells and its levels correlate with the induction of IL-6 transcription[1,2]. NF-kB is a transcription factor that is composed of two subunits which are inactive when bound to the cytoplasmic inhibitor IkB[3]. Phosphorylation of this inhibitor by protein kinase C or protein tyrosine kinase releases NF-kB, which then translocates to the nucleus and binds to the specific motif in promoter of IL-6 or other genes. In addition to the protein-kinase-mediated activation

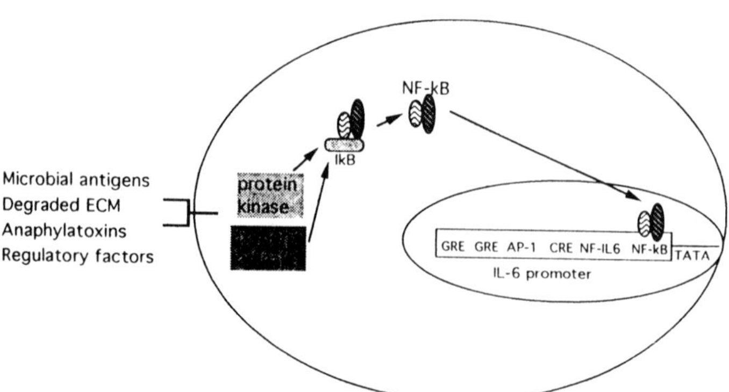

Fig. 1 Regulation of cytokine gene expression

of NF-kB a new mechanism that depends on oxygen radicals has recently been identified[4].

Upon activation of the essential transcription factors or inhibition of negative transcriptional regulators, cytokine mRNA production is initiated. At this level, cytokine expression can be influenced by the rate and duration of transcription. In the case of IL-1 expression in human monocytes, LPS primarily increases the rate of transcription while preincubation of the cells results in increased mRNA levels via longer duration of transcription and increased mRNA stability[5]. Many cytokines share an ATTTA sequence in their 3' end which is responsible for rapid mRNA degradation[6].

The presence of cytokine mRNA does not necessarily result in the production of protein, and regulation at the translational level is important in the expression of several cytokines. Examples for this include IL-1, TNF-α and CSF-1 whose mRNA can be induced by monocyte adherence, but protein is only produced upon further stimulation of the cells with LPS[7,8].

Some cytokines are secreted upon complete intracellular processing; others are stored in large quantities intracellularly, and additional stimuli are required to trigger secretion. When secreted from the cell most cytokines are biologically active. However, others such as TGF-βs are secreted in a biologically inactive or latent form and require further extracellular processing to be biologically active[9].

Cytokines can be distinguished with respect to their cellular sources. Some cytokines such as IL-2 or IFN-γ are produced by a limited number of cell types, while others such as IL-6, TGF-β, IL-8 or monocyte chemoattractant protein-1 (MCP-1) are expressed in most tissues.

Cytokines interact in the regulation of their expression. These interactions occur at the transcriptional or post-transcriptional level, and can present in the form of autoinduction, stimulation of another cytokine, as well as inhibition of cytokine expression. Cytokines which can induce their own expression include IL-1[10], IL-2, IL-6, LIF and TGF-β. Autoinduction represents a potent mechanism for the amplification of the signal generated by the primary stimulus that induces host defence responses. IL-1, TNF and LIF induce each other's expression and that of a series of other cytokines including IL-2, IL-6, IL-8, MCP-1 and colony-stimulating factors (CSF).

Inhibition of cytokine expression represents an important regulatory mechanism by which differentiation of cellular responses and potentially detrimental cytokine activities are controlled. TGF-β, IL-4 and IL-10 are the best-characterized inhibitors of cytokine production. TGF-β can inhibit IL-1 or LPS-induced TNF or IL-6 synthesis in monocytes[11,12] while stimulatory or bifunctional effects of TGF-β on cytokine synthesis in other cell types have been observed. IL-4 is a potent inhibitor of monocyte activation and interferes with the production of IL-1, TNF, IL-6[13] and IL-8[14] in response to different stimuli. IL-4 can reduce, although not completely inhibit, the production of IL-10 in monocytes[15]. IL-10 is a cytokine that has been discovered on the basis of its ability to inhibit IFN-γ production by T lymphocytes[16]. It is also a potent monocyte deactivator, produced in relatively large quantities by monocytes, and inhibits synthesis of several cytokines by monocytes in an autoregulatory role[15].

IL-10 is able to inhibit its own synthesis in monocytes in a negative feedback mechanism. Through the inhibition of cytokine synthesis and monocyte activation IL-10 is capable of inhibiting antigen-driven T cell responses and of down-regulating inflammatory responses.

CYTOKINE RECEPTORS

Once a cytokine is secreted from a cell and biologically active it can bind to a specific receptor on cell membranes, to a carrier protein, soluble receptors or associate with extracellular matrix components (Fig. 2). Functionally most important are cell surface receptors which can activate intracellular messenger systems. The tissue distribution of cytokine receptors defines the spectrum of biological activities of cytokines. Cytokine receptors are not expressed or present at low levels on resting cells. Receptor density at the cell surface can be increased by the same agents that trigger cytokine production, or by cytokines themselves. A cytokine can up-regulate the expression of the autologous or of a heterologous receptor. IL-1 contributes to the up-regulation of IL-2 receptors. TGF-β has been shown in some cell types to inhibit the expression of IL-1 receptors and this may represent one mechanism by which it interferes with the biological effects of IL-1. The IL-6 binding component of the IL-6 receptor is induced by TGF-β in cartilage cells[17].

Cytokine binding and signal transduction can be functions of the same receptor protein or represent separate functions of receptor subunits. Association of subunits can also modulate affinity for the cytokines. Cloning of the genes encoding cytokine receptors has resulted in the identification of different receptor families that are defined on the basis of common structures[18]. The type 1 cytokine receptor family which shares the c-terminal amino acid sequence Trp-Ser-X-Trp-Ser (W-S-X-W-S) includes the receptors for IL-2, IL-3, IL-4, IL-5, IL-6, IL-7, GM-CSF, G-CSF, erythropoietin, Leukaemia inhibitory factor (LIF), oncostatin M (OSM) and ciliary neurotropic factor (CNTF). Receptors with short intracellular domains appear to require association with signal transducing membrane proteins. This has recently

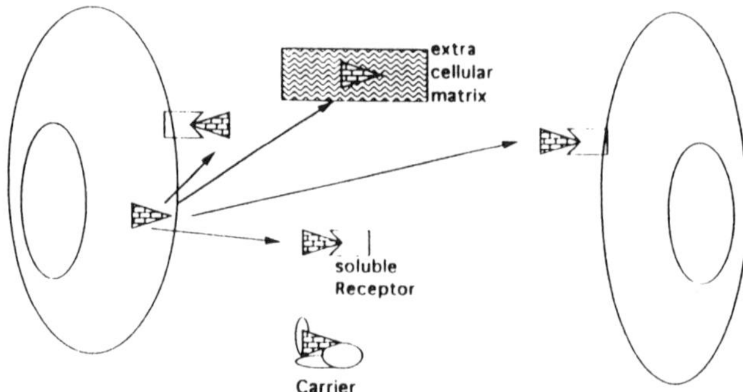

Fig. 2 Cytokine binding structures

been demonstrated for several members of this receptor family. The IL-6, LIF, OSM and CNTF receptors are composed of two subunits where one chain is responsible for ligand binding and defines ligand specificity. All of these different ligand binding chains associate with the same signal transducing molecule, gp130[27,28]. The two IL-1 receptors represent a distinct family of cytokine receptors and are characterized by extracellular immunoglobulin-like domains. Two receptors for TNF have been cloned and their extracellular regions contain cysteine-rich motifs which are the common feature of the nerve growth factor/tumour necrosis factor receptor family. Most receptors are specific for one ligand. This applies in particular to cytokines which are structurally unique. Cytokines that share a high degree of homology such as IL-1α and IL-1β, TNF-α and TNF-β, the different forms of IFN-α and/or the different isoforms of TGF-β utilize the same receptors.

In addition to membrane-associated cytokine receptors, soluble forms have been described for the IL-2R, the TNFR, IL-6R, IFN-γR, IL-4R and the IL-7R. Soluble IL-2R and TNFR are generated by cleavage of the membrane-associated protein. The soluble IL-4R and IL-7R are products of differentially spliced mRNAs[19,20]. Soluble receptors are generated in response to cell activation and measurements of IL-2R in body fluids were found in some studies to correlate with disease activity in conditions that are associated with activated immunological or inflammatory responses[21]. Soluble TNF receptors bind TNF and block its biological activity[29,30] while inhibition of IL-2 activity by soluble IL-2R requires higher receptor concentrations. The biological function of soluble cytokine receptors may be to modulate cytokine activity. Soluble forms of cytokine receptors that do or do not exist physiologically are being tested for therapeutic efficacy in experimental models of disease and in some clinical trials.

Further binding cytokine binding structures are carrier proteins. α_2-Macroglobulin has been shown to bind IL-1, IL-6 and TGF-β. When bound to this carrier, IL-1 appears to be inactive while IL-6 maintains its biological activity. TGF-β also binds to a proteoglycan, termed betaglycan, which exists in soluble and membrane associated forms. The membrane-bound proteoglycan does not induce intracellular signals upon TGF-β binding. Cytokines can bind to extracellular matrix and this has been documented for the family of heparin-binding growth factors and the family of chemotactic cytokines that includes IL-8 and MCP-1. Secreted and matrix-associated forms of leukaemia inhibitory factor have been described[22]. Alternative usage of the first exon in the LIF gene is responsible for the production of the different forms of this cytokine. Matrix association of cytokines may generate a reservoir of cytokines that can rapidly be mobilized in response to tissue injury.

Upon cytokine binding to specific cell surface receptors intracellular signals are activated, and this elicits secretory or proliferative responses and differentiation in target cells. Interactions within the cytokine network are critical at this level. Depending on the number and types of cytokines that act on the same target cell they can additively or synergistically enhance their effects or act as antagonists. The quality of the interactions depends on the types of second messengers that are generated. Information on this level of cytokine interactions is limited, and the signals generated in response to binding of one ligand to its receptor are now being characterized. The following section summarizes findings on signal transduction pathways involved with differential regulation of gene expression by cytokines. Distinct functional programmes can be induced in human articular chondrocytes by IL-1β and TGF-β. IL-1 induces catabolic events including the expression of matrix metalloproteinases (MMP) while TGF-β stimulates chondrocyte proliferation and synthesis of extracellular matrix proteins. In some of these responses IL-1 and TGF-β antagonize each other's effects. Based on studies with promoter constructs, the transcription factor complex binding to the AP-1 motif had previously been suggested to be important in the induction of the MMPs collagenase and stromelysin. In human articular chondrocytes AP-1 activity was detectable under conditions where MMPs are not expressed, or present at low levels. More importantly, AP-1 was not increased by IL-1 which strongly up-regulated MMP mRNAs. In contrast, TGF-β increased AP-1 activity but not MMP expression. MMP promoters contain binding sites for NF-kB and some of the IL-1 effects are mediated by this factor. NF-kB activity was weak or absent in resting chondrocytes and increased very strongly in response to IL-1. TGF-β did not increase NF-kB activity and did not inhibit the IL-1 effect in co-stimulation experiments. This suggested that, in intact chondrocytes, the activation of endogenous MMP promoters is primarily regulated by NF-kB.

We had previously shown that pre-proenkephalin, a cyclic AMP-induced gene, is induced by TGF-β and inhibited by IL-1[23], suggesting that transcription factor activity binding to the cyclic AMP response element (CREB) may be involved in differential and antagonistic effects of IL-1 and TGF-β. It was increased by TGF-β and strongly suppressed by IL-1.

These results indicate that activation of NF-kB but not AP-1 may be the trigger for the expression of MMPs by IL-1. The levels of NF-kB and CREB are differentially regulated by IL-1 and TGF-β, and can mediate the opposing effects of these two cytokines in the regulation of gene expression in chondrocytes.

CYTOKINE INTERACTIONS DURING DISTINCT PHASES OF HOST DEFENCE RESPONSES TO INJURY

Much of the diversity of cytokine activities and interactions has been established on the basis of *in-vitro* systems (Table 1). These are often removed from highly complex networks of cells and mediator systems *in vivo* to the minimal number of components to allow demonstration of one or a limited number of interactions *in vitro*. In attempting to integrate these interactions into a functionally meaningful process, distinct phases of host defence responses to injury can be proposed and particular cytokines associated with them (Fig. 3). In the description of these phases we will discuss redundancy, additive, synergistic and antagonistic interactions of cytokines in the regulation of cell function.

The early phase, immediately following injury, is triggered by microbial

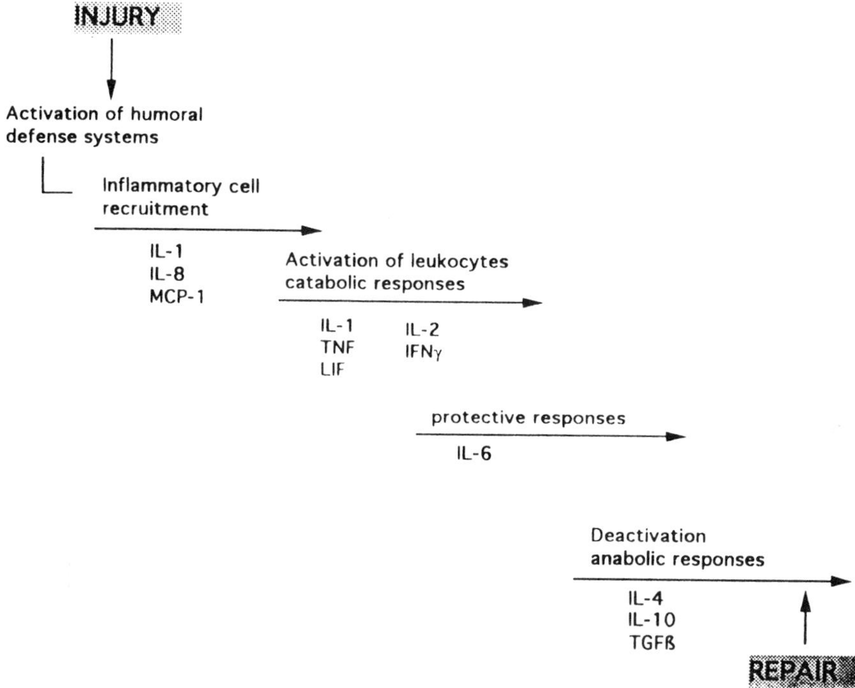

Fig. 3 Function of cytokines in different phases during host defence responses to injury

antigens, extracellular matrix antigens or activation products of preformed components of humoral defence systems. It consists of cell recruitment and the induction of those cytokines which contribute to activation of proinflammatory, immunostimulatory and catabolic responses.

This first group of cytokines is composed of IL-1, TNF, LIF, OSM and a set of chemotactic factors whose primary function is to promote recruitment of inflammatory cells. Chemotactic factors are relatively cell-specific[31]. IL-8 is the principal neutrophil chemoattractant, MCP-1 is selective for monocytes, IL-1 attracts lymphocytes. Monocytes and neutrophils migrate in response to TGF-β. The chemotactic factors, in particular IL-1, IL-8 and MCP-1, are induced directly by the inciting agent and by the cytokines in this first group. These cytokines have a broad spectrum of target cells. At the site of injury they act on stromal and parenchymal cells, as well as on recruited leucocytes. Their effects on mesenchymal cells are characterized by catabolic responses. Most important is the induction of metalloproteinases which degrade extracellular matrix. In the context of the repair response to injury this serves to remove damaged connective tissue. Effects on monocytes include the stimulation of cytokine and protease production and lymphocytes respond with increased proliferation and differentiation. These cytokines also participate in the systemic adaptation to injury and act on the CNS, liver and the bone marrow. This is manifested by the induction of fever, the hepatic

Table 1 Cytokine activities in host defence response

	IL-1	TNF	IL-6	LIF	IL-2	IFN-γ	IL-8	MCP-1	IL-4	IL-10	TGF-β
Immune responses											
Monocyte activation	+	+	+	+	+	+	−	−	+	+	−
T cell growth/differentiation	+	+	+	+	+	+	0	0	+	−	−
B cell growth/differentiation	+	+	+	?	+	+	0	0	+	+	−
Inflammation											
PGE$_2$ synthesis	+	+	0	+	0	0	0	0	0	−	±
Induction of integrins	+	+	0	?	0	0	0	0	0	?	±
Chemotaxis	+	+	0	?	0	0	+	+	+	?	+
Connective tissue metabolism											
Cell proliferation	+	+	+	?	0		0	0	0	0	+
Proteases	+	+	−	+	0		−	−	0	0	−
Protease inhibitors	(+)	(+)	+	?	0		0	0	0	0	+
Bone resorption	+	+	+	+	0		0	0	?	?	−
ECM	−	−	0	?	0		0	0	0	0	+
Systemic adaptation in host defence											
Fever	+	+	+	?	0		0	0	0	0	0
Anorexia	+	+	0	+	0	0	?	?	?	?	?
Hepatic acute phase	+	+	+	+	−	+	0	0	0	0	+
Haematopoiesis	+	+	+	?	+	0	0	0	0	0	−

+, Stimulation; −, inhibition; 0, no effect; ?, not known

110

acute phase response and the stimulation of increased formation of white blood cells and platelets.

IL-6 is induced by all of the cytokines in the first group. However, IL-6 induces cellular responses that distinguish it from the former cytokines and it may induce protective responses against the proinflammatory and catabolic effects in the first group of cytokines. IL-6 does not stimulate the production of proteases but is a potent inducer of protease inhibitors. Several of the hepatic acute-phase proteins are protease inhibitors and IL-6 is the major inducer of the hepatic acute-phase response. In monocytes and connective tissue cells it increases the production of the tissue inhibitor of metallo-proteinases[26]. IL-6 is the principal differentiation factor for B cells and promotes the production of immunoglobulins.

In this intermediate phase of host defence responses, effector mechanisms have been generated and defend against and eliminate the agent responsible for injury. Depending on the nature of the inciting stimulus it is cleared primarily via effector mechanisms generated by inflammatory cells or by immunological responses, and distinguished by distinct time kinetics and duration.

The third phase begins with successful clearance of the inciting stimulus and tissue or cells damaged by it. Inflammatory and immunological responses are deactivated or down-regulated. Cytokine interactions that are operative in this phase have not yet been as well characterized as those that mediate the activation phase. This phase, however, is as critical to the successful completion of the host defence response to injury. It is associated with the initiation of active anti-inflammatory and anabolic factors and cellular functions primarily characterized by cell proliferation and the formation of new and tissue specific extracellular matrix. Cytokines such as IL-4, IL-10 and TGF-β are potent deactivators of proinflammatory and catabolic responses, and TGF-β is an important stimulus for the formation of new connective tissue.

This scenario is tentative and based on the predominant biological activities of the different cytokines. The spectrum of bioactivities of some cytokines is too broad to allow assignment to only one phase, while for some the complete spectrum of activities has not been characterized. Distinct phases as proposed here may occur in host defence responses to an injury that is successfully cleared. Similar activation and deactivation events are operative in different disease states and contribute to pathology. In many diseases uncontrolled activation of the cytokine network is a central pathogenetic factor. The natural course of chronic inflammatory diseases which is characterized by fluctuating levels of disease activity is the result of the balance between cytokines that activate versus those that deactivate immune and inflammatory responses. In these disease states both are simultaneously activated and their balance is a manifestation of the multiple factors that are responsible for aetiology and pathogenesis. A series of approaches to therapeutically modulate this balance is now being tested. Modulation of cytokine activity can be achieved by the administration of antagonistic cytokines, natural inhibitors such as the IL-1 receptor antagonist, antibodies to cytokines or their receptors and soluble forms of cytokine receptors.

References

1. Zhang B, Geng Y, Lotz M. Signal transduction pathways involved with differential gene expression by IL-1 and TGFβ in human articular chondrocytes. Arthritis Rheum. 1992 (abstract) (in press).
2. Zhang B, Gross V, Geng Y, Lotz M. Induction of IL-6 and NF-kB by IL-1 are protein kinase C independent and dependent on oxygen radicals. Arthritis Rheum. 1992 (abstract) (in press).
3. Baeuerle P. The inducible transcription factor NF-kB: regulation by distinct protein subunits. Biochim Biophys Acta. 1991;1072:63–80.
4. Schreck R, Baeuerle PA. A role for oxygen radicals as second messengers. Trends Cell Biol. 1991;1:39.
5. Arend WP, Gordon DF, Wood W, Janson RW, Joslin FG, Jameel S. IL-1β production in human monocytes is regulated at multiple levels. J Immunol. 1989;143:118–26.
6. Caput D, Beutler B, Hartog K, Thayer R, Brown-Shimer S, Cerami A. Identification of a common nucleotide sequence in the 3′-untranslated region of mRNA molecules specifying inflammatory mediators. Proc Natl Acad Sci USA. 1986;83:1670.
7. Haskill S, Johnson C, Eierman D, Becker S, Warren K. Adherence induces selective mRNA expression of monocyte mediators and protooncogenes. J Immunol. 1988;140:1690.
8. Schindler R, Clark BD, Dinarello CA. Dissociation between interleukin-1β mRNA and protein synthesis in human peripheral blood mononuclear cells. J Biol Chem. 1990;265:10232–7.
9. Miyazono K, Yuki K, Takaku F, Wernstedt C, Kanzaki T, Olofsson A, Hellman U, Heldin CH. Latent forms of TGFβ: Structure and Biology. Ann NY Acad Sci. 1990;593:51–8.
10. Warner SJK, Auger KR, Libby P. Human interleukin-1 induces interleukin-1 gene expression in human vascular smooth muscle cells. J Exp Med. 1987;165:1316.
11. Chantry D, Turner M, Abnet E, Feldman M. Modulation of cytokine production by transforming growth factor-β. J Immunol. 1990;142:4295–300.
12. Musso T, Espinosa-Delgado I, Pulkki K, Gusella GL, Longo DL, Vaserio L. Transforming growth factor β downregulates interleukin-1 (IL-1)-induced IL-6 production by human monocytes. Blood. 1990;76:2466–9.
13. te Velde AA, Huijbens RJF, Heije K, de Vries J, Figdoe CG. Interleukin-4 (IL-4) inhibits secretion of IL-1β, tumor necrosis factor a and IL-6 by human monocytes. Blood. 1990;76:1392–7.
14. Standiford TJ, Strieter RM, Chensue SW, Westwick J, Kasahara K, Kunkel SL. IL-4 inhibits the expression of IL-8 from stimulated human monocytes. J Immunol. 1990;145:1435–9.
15. de Waal Malefyt R, Abrams J, Bennett B, Figdor CG, de Vries JE. Interleukin-10 (IL-10) inhibits cytokine synthesis by human monocytes: an autoregulatory role of IL-10 produced by monocytes. J Exp Med. 1991;174:1209–20.
16. Howard M, O'Garra A. Biological properties of interleukin-10. Immunol Today. 1992;13:198–200.
17. Guerne PA, Lotz M. Regulation of Swarm rat chondrosarcoma cell proliferation: synergy between interleukin-6 (IL-6) and transforming growth factor-β (TGFβ). J Cell Physiol. 1991;149:117–24.
18. Miyajima A, Kitamura T, Harada N, Yokota T, Arai K. Cytokine receptors and signal transduction. Ann Rev Immunol. 1992;10:295–331.
19. Mosley B, Beckmann MP, March CJ, Idzerda RL, Gimpel SD, VandenBos T, Friend D, Alpert A, Anderson D, Jackson J, Wignall JM, Smith C, Ballis B, Sims JE, Urdal D, Widmer MB, Cosman D, Park LS. The murine interleukin-4 receptor: molecular cloning and characterization of secreted and membrane bound forms. Cell. 1989;59:335–48.
20. Goodwin RG, Friend D, Ziegler SF, Jerzy R, Falk BA, Gimpel S, Cosman D, Dower SK, Namen AE, Park LS. Cell. 1990;60:941–51.
21. Rubin LA. The soluble IL-2 receptor in rheumatic disease. Arthritis Rheum. 1990;33:1145–8.
22. Rathjen PD, Toh S, Willis A, Heath JK, Smith AG. Differentiation inhibiting activity is produced in matrix-associated and diffusible forms that are generated by alternate promoter usage. Cell. 1990;62:1105–14.
23. Villiger P, Lotz M. Expression of preproenkephalin by human articular chondrocytes is linked to cell proliferation. EMBO J. 1992;11:135–43.

24. Villiger PM, Geng Y, Lotz M. Induction of cytokine expression by leukemia inhibitory factor. J Clin Invest. 1992; (in press).
25. Villiger PM, Terkeltaub R, Lotz M. Monocyte chemoattractant protein-1 (MCP-1) expression in human articular cartilage: Induction by peptide regulatory factors and differential effects of dexamethasone and retinoic acid. J Clin Invest. 1992;90:488–96.
26. Lotz M, Guerne PA. Interleukin-6 induces the synthesis of tissue inhibitor of metalloproteinases-1/erythroid potentiating activity (TIMP-1/EPA). J Biol Chem. 1991;266:2017.
27. Gearing DP, Thut GJ, VandeBos T, Gimpel SD, Delaney PB, King J, Price V, Cosman D, Beckmann MP. Leukemia inhibitory factor receptor is structurally related to the IL-6 signal transducer, gp130. EMBO J. 1991;10:2839.
28. Gearing DP, Comeau MR, Friend DJ, Gimpel SD, Thut CJ, McGourty J, Brasher KK, King JA, Gillis S, Mosley B, Ziegler SF, Cosman D. The IL-6 signal transducer, gp130: an oncostatin M receptor and affinity converter for the LIF receptor. Science. 1992;255:1434.
29. Nophar Y, Kemper O, Brackebusch C, Engelmann H, Zwang R, Aderka D, Holtman H, Wallach D. Soluble forms of tumor necrosis factor receptors (TNF-Rs). The cDNA for the type 1 TNF-R, cloned using amino acid sequence data of its soluble form, encodes both the cell surface and a soluble form of the receptor. EMBO J. 1990;10:3269–78.
30. Seckinger P, Zhang JH, Hauptmann B, Dayer JM. Characterization of a tumor necrosis factor α (TNF-α) inhibitor: evidence of immunological cross-reactivity with the TNF receptor. Proc Natl Acad Sci USA. 1990;87:5188–92.
31. Oppenheim JJ, Zachariae COC, Mukaida N, Matsushima K. Properties of the novel proinflammatory supergene 'intecrine' cytokine family. Ann Rev Immunol. 1991;9:617–48.

11

Proinflammatory cytokines and mediators

M. Z. MAZLAM and H. J. F. HODGSON

INTRODUCTION

In recent years intense research effort has concentrated on the mediators of inflammatory processes. In the context of chronic inflammatory bowel disease – ulcerative colitis and Crohn's disease – the number of publications on the potential mediators of the inflammatory processes within the gastrointestinal mucosa far exceeds those on the underlying cause of the conditions. In part this reflects the frustrating lack of progress in defining the aetiology of the diseases – I judge only a minority of workers in the field believe there is a simple 'cause' like a bacteria which can be eliminated and result in 'cure'. In part, current research in IBD follows basic scientific advances which have made rapid progress in defining inflammatory processes at the molecular level. Finally, there is hope that defining mediators that are critical for the initiation, amplification or expression of the inflammatory process may allow therapy to be improved.

A speculative list of important proinflammatory mediators relevant to gut inflammation in IBD commences in the gut lumen, where bacterial products, including both cell wall polysaccharide, and bacterial peptides such as formyl-met-leu-phe, are present[1]. The peptides are powerfully chemo-attractant, particularly to polymorphonuclear leucocytes, and the lipopolysaccharides are particularly relevant in terms of this chapter as a powerful stimulator of monocyte and macrophage activation.

Within the gut mucosa, a wide variety of humoral inflammatory mediators have been implicated. Immune complex formation – predictable from the presence of locally generated IgG antibody to antigens present in the gut such as anaerobic bacteria – is likely to lead to the activation of complement via the classical pathway[2]. Alternative pathway activation of complement may also follow lipopolysaccharide penetration into diseased mucosa[3]. Evidence for deposition of activated complement within the diseased mucosa in inflammatory bowel disease has recently been enhanced by further immunohistochemical data from Brandtzaeg's group, demonstrating activated early complement components and terminal complement complex deposition[4]. Eicosanoids, in particular leucotrienes and thromboxanes[5], and platelet-activating factor[6], are all demonstrable in enhanced amounts in the mucosa or in gut content dialysates. Polymorphonuclear leucocyte enzymes such as elastase are released into the interstitium of the bowel walls[7].

More recently, attention has turned to cytokines as potential mediators of inflammation in inflammatory bowel disease, playing this role not only within the mucosa, but also responsible for systemic reactions in inflammatory bowel disease. The term cytokine, a low molecular weight glycoprotein released from a variety of cell types, embraces both lymphokines and monokines. These were initially described from their predominant cell of origin, but the more general term cytokine acknowledges their similarities independent of their cell of origin, and the fact that a wide variety of cells can in fact produce these polypeptides. Interleukin was a term originally coined to indicate production from a white cell, and the property of affecting growth or differentiation of other leucocytes. Current nomenclature describes new cytokines by their biological properties, and assigns an interleukin number when the amino acid sequence of the human polypeptide is determined. The original – TNF-α – remains a time-honoured exception.

THE SYSTEMIC ACUTE PHASE RESPONSE

Our interest in the role of cytokines developed from two related aspects of inflammatory bowel disease. The uncertain relationship between ulcerative colitis and Crohn's disease – whether different conditions or part of a continuous disease spectrum – prompts careful examination of those differences which can be defined[8]. The interest in our laboratory on the assessment of the inflammatory activity of these conditions, particularly the use of acute-phase reactants, highlighted one such difference[9].

The acute-phase response describes the dramatic changes in the pattern of certain plasma proteins synthesized by the liver during inflammation. The concentration of the acute-phase reactants, such as fibrinogen, haptoglobin, α_1-acid glycoprotein, and α_2-macroglobulin increases, and that of constitutively expressed proteins such as albumin decreases[10]. In the particular context of the differences between ulcerative colitis and Crohn's disease, the increases in C-reactive protein and serum amyloid A component (SAA) are particularly striking[11].

C-reactive protein has been described as the prototype acute phase reactant. Coded on chromosome 1, it has structural similarities to the P-component of amyloid, both representatives of a small class of proteins named pentraxins from their pentagonal shape[12]. The serum levels of CRP can rise by over 1000-fold within hours of the onset of inflammation, reflecting enhanced synthesis by hepatocytes. Its biological role is not fully understood, but it plays a role as an opsonin, and also complexes with DNA released from lysed cells, perhaps aiding the subsequent degradation of this. It may also modulate the expression of the immune response by interactions with lymphocytes and monocytes[13,14].

C-reactive protein levels are elevated in patients with active inflammatory bowel disease. This is particularly apparent in the context of Crohn's disease, as when patients with similar extent, distribution and activity of colonic inflammation with ulcerative colitis and Crohn's disease are compared, the levels in Crohn's disease are strikingly higher[9]. CRP has been defined as one of the best markers for inflammation in Crohn's disease, the levels correlating with the extent and activity of inflammation, and with other objective parameters such as leucocyte excretion into bowel[15]. Serial CRP elevations have been effectively used in serial studies to assess therapeutic drugs[16].

The stimulus, at the level of the hepatocyte, to the production of CRP has been extensively investigated as one feature of the integrated acute-phase response. Experimental systems using isolated hepatocytes, and *in vivo* systems involving cytokine infusions, have defined the central role of monocyte-derived cytokines as initiators of the switch of hepatocytes to producing acute-phase proteins[17]. The relative strength of individual cytokines as initiators of protein synthesis varies, and different liver cell lines used for experiments differ in their ability to respond. *In vitro*, IL-1 determines a restricted set of acute phase proteins[18], and TNF-α a smaller, partially overlapping set[19]: similarly IL-6 stimulates many but not all, indicating that an integrated acute-phase response requires cooperativity between a number of monocyte-derived cytokines[20]. The precise interpretation of *in vitro* experiments is difficult as most available hepatocytes for study – well-differentiated tumour-derived cell lines – do not all give either similar or representative acute-phase protein release.

We initially posed the question – does the difference in acute-phase protein response seen in Crohn's disease reflect differences in the amount of monocyte-derived cytokines released by monocytes from patients with Crohn's disease? We investigated peripheral blood monocytes, as representatives of the monocyte macrophage lineage, and stimulated a given number of normal, Crohn's disease-derived or ulcerative colitis-derived monocytes, with lipopolysaccharide to release cytokines *in vitro*. By starting from an identical number of cells we avoided the possibility that a greater cytokine response in one disease – as reported *in vivo* – might merely reflect a greater number of cells involved in an inflammatory response, or more extensive areas of gut involved – because the motive behind the experiments was to explore whether there were qualitative rather than merely quantitative differences behind the differences in acute-phase response in ulcerative colitis and Crohn's disease.

The predominant difference that emerged was that monocytes from patients with Crohn's disease had a greater tendency to produce IL-1β than either controls or patients with ulcerative colitis, and the TNF-α response in ulcerative colitis was reduced[21]. Since the design of the experiments was intended to avoid the possibility that this was merely secondary to disease activity, the results implied that this reflected a greater innate tendency to develop IL-1 – and perhaps quite different profiles of a variety of cytokines – between patients with different types of inflammatory bowel disease. The concept is attractive as it may (as discussed below) set the scene for a number of differences between the two conditions. Thus, in the same way as we know possession of the HLA B8[22] haplotype is associated with the tendency to develop liver disease in association with IBD, possibly the cytokine profile an individual is genetically programmed to produce will determine the type of IBD they develop.

AIMS

The further development of this line of argument in the context of the acute-phase response differences between the two forms of idiopathic IBD lead to the specific aims of the experiments reported here:

1. To study a group of patients with UC and CD, measure the CRP levels in serum, and confirm the differences between the two conditions.
2. To culture identical numbers of monocytes from those patients, and harvest monocyte-conditioned media.
3. To quantitate cytokine release into the conditioned media.
4. To assess the effect of the conditioned media in initiating release of CRP from a hepatocyte-derived cell line.
5. To explore the hypothesis that a greater CRP release would occur with Crohn's disease monocytes, reflecting a greater release of one or more monocyte cytokines.

METHODS

Twenty-two patients with CD, 22 with UC and 11 healthy controls were studied. In the Crohn's disease (CD) group 11 patients were quiescent and 11 had active disease (Harvey Bradshaw index mean of 6.2 (0.8 SEM). Nine had ileitis, five ileocolitis, and eight colitis. Eleven patients with ulcerative colitis (UC) were active (Truelove and Witts), seven mildly and four moderately.

Cytokine generation

Peripheral blood mononuclear cells were separated, and monocytes purified by adherence. Monocytes were cultured with or without $10\,\mu g/ml$ of lipopolysaccharide for 24 h, and monocyte-conditioned medium collected and stored at $-70°C$. Cytokines IL-1β and IL-6 were measured by ELISA techniques. The lower detection limit of IL-1β was 20 pg/ml and the IL-6 50 pg/ml. There was no crossreactivity between these antigens, nor with TNF-α and IL-1α. Serum CRP was measured in venous blood by an ELISA.

CRP release

The PLC/PRF/5 (Alexander) cell line was grown in Dulbecco's modified Eagle's medium. A suspension of cells (100 000 cells/ml) was grown in 24-well tissue culture plates to confluence, and a 50/50 mixture of monocyte-conditioned medium and fresh complete medium added for 72 h. After 72 h supernatant was collected for analysis of CRP release by ELISA assay. The lower detection limit of the CRP assay was 0.05 ng/ml.

Statistics

Non-parametric procedures were employed for statistical significance testing. Comparisons between groups were assessed by Kruskal–Wallis and Mann–Whitney U test. Correlation coefficients were by Kendall rank correlation results.

RESULTS

Serum CRP levels

CD serum CRP levels were mean 29.7 mg/l (range 0.5–142.5), CRP in UC mean 6.8 mg/l (0.05–23.18), CRP in inactive CD (5.7 ± 2.6 mg/l) was not significantly different from UC (3.0 ± 1.5 mg/l). Serum CRP in patients with active CD (53.6 ± 16.2) was significantly elevated compared with active UC (10.7 ± 2.3) and normal controls (1.6 ± 0.6 mg/l). The levels in active CD were also significantly higher than those in inactive CD (Fig. 1).

IL-1β generation

A fixed number of monocytes were taken from patients with CD, UC and normal controls. The number of peripheral blood monocytes for CD ($5.3 \pm 0.4 \times 10^5$/ml) was greater compared to UC (4.6 ± 0.35) and normal controls ($3.3 \pm 0.5 \times 10^5$/ml). The difference between CD and normal controls was statistically significant, but not the difference between the two forms of inflammatory bowel disease.

Spontaneous IL-1β release by monocytes in CD (562 ± 2.1 pg/ml) was significantly elevated compared to UC (75 ± 9.1 p/ml, $p < 0.05$) and normal controls (29.7 ± 7.4 pg/ml, $p < 0.05$). Lipopolysaccharide-stimulated IL-1β generation in CD ($16\,573.5 \pm 5879.8$ pg/ml) was also significantly higher than compared with UC (4508 ± 1403 pg/ml, $p < 0.005$) and normal controls (3678 ± 1000 pg/ml, $p < 0.05$).

In patients with inactive CD both spontaneous and LPS-stimulated IL-1β (967.2 ± 545.1 and $11\,791 \pm 4995$) release were significantly more than inactive UC (41.2 ± 21.2 and 3404 ± 1378 pg/ml, $p < 0.05$). In active CD, both spontaneous and LPS-stimulated IL-1β (158.0 ± 66.2 and $21\,355 \pm 10\,755$ respectively) released from monocytes were elevated compared with active UC (108 ± 53.8 and 5606 ± 2476 pg/ml), although this difference did not reach statistical significance.

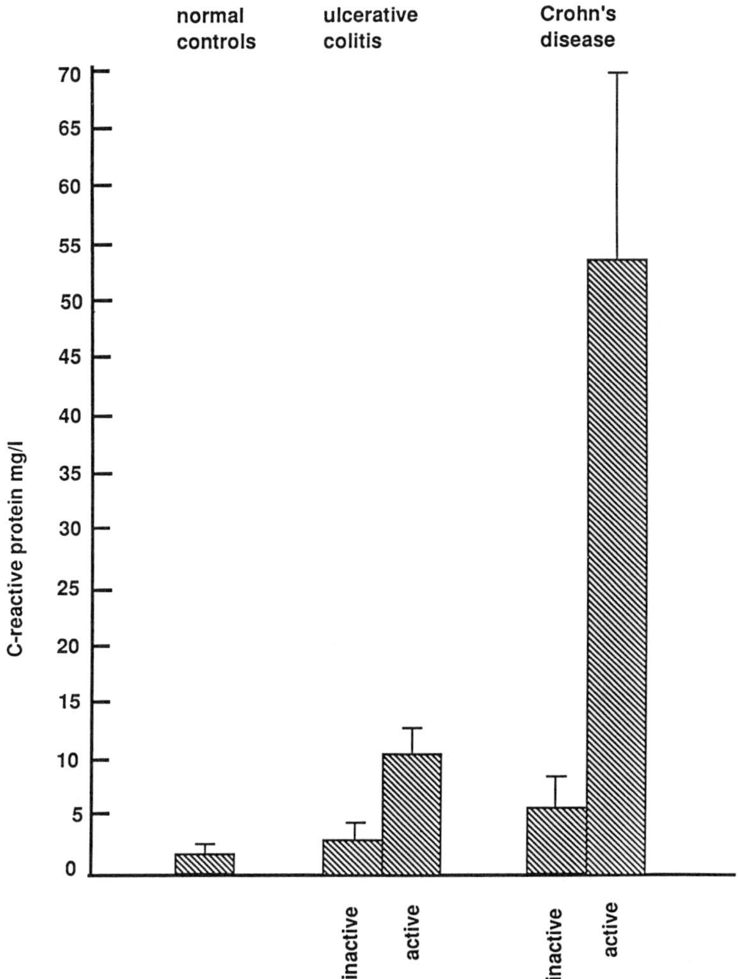

Fig. 1 Serum C-reactive protein (mg/l). Serum CRP is markedly elevated in patients with active Crohn's disease ($n = 11$, $p < 0.02$ Mann–Whitney) compared to active ulcerative colitis ($n = 11$) and normal controls ($n = 11$). In inactive CD ($n = 11$, $p > 0.05$ Mann–Whitney) serum CRP is not significantly different compared to inactive UC ($n = 11$)

IL-6 generation

In contrast to the findings of IL-1β, no difference was found between the capacity of the same number of monocytes from patients with UC and CD to generate IL-6. Both spontaneous and LPS-stimulated IL-6 production from patients with CD (1606 $\pm$ 294.6 and 3244 $\pm$ 363 pg/ml) were similar to UC (1064 $\pm$ 155 and 2456 $\pm$ 250 respectively) and normal controls (1473 $\pm$ 295.9

and 2802 ± 352.1). No further differences emerged on considering active and inactive groups separately.

Cytokine release related to monocyte numbers in whole blood

In a separate exercise, the IL-6 and IL-1β producing capacities of patients with CD and UC were calculated from the production of the cytokines from a given number of monocytes, related to the number of monocytes present in peripheral blood. When spontaneous and LPS-stimulated IL-6 production were related to the total count of monocytes from patients with CD, the IL-6 production was significantly greater compared with UC and normal controls. The figures for spontaneous and LPS-stimulated release were CD 3992 ± 603 and 8540 ± 1276 pg, UC 2372 ± 363.9 and 5479 ± 546, $p < 0.05$, normal controls 2549 ± 579 and 4220 ± 552 pg.

As expected from the higher mean monocyte count found in CD compared with UC, the difference in production of IL-1β between CD and UC became even more marked when this was reflected to the total count of monocytes. The overall figures showed a much higher level in CD (1949 ± 929 pg for spontaneous and 49 151 ± 1971 for LPS-stimulated, compared with UC 134 ± 43 and 8613 ± 2362 pg).

Effect of monocyte-conditioned medium on CRP release

Both unstimulated and LPS-stimulated monocyte-conditioned medium from patients with active Crohn's disease (mean (SEM) 1.73 (0.40) ng/ml and 3.48 (0.87) ng/ml, respectively) caused significantly greater CRP release from Alexander cells than monocyte-conditioned medium from active ulcerative colitis (mean (SEM) 0.67 (0.17) ng/ml; $p < 0.02$ Mann–Whitney and 2.01 (0.38) ng/ml; $p < 0.05$ Mann–Whitney, respectively) and normal controls (mean (SEM) 0.61 (0.09) ng/ml; $p < 0.02$ Mann–Whitney and 1.30 (0.12) ng/ml; $p < 0.002$ Mann–Whitney, respectively) (Fig. 2).

Release of CRP from Alexander cells by unstimulated and LPS-stimulated monocyte-conditioned medium from patients with inactive Crohn's disease (mean (SEM) 0.79 (0.20) ng/ml and 1.50 (0.32) ng/ml, respectively) was not significantly different compared to inactive ulcerative colitis (mean (SEM) 0.68 (0.14) ng/ml and 2.0 (0.19) ng/ml, respectively; $p > 0.05$ Mann–Whitney) and normal controls (mean (SEM) 0.61 (0.09) ng/ml and 1.30 (0.12) ng/ml, respectively; $p > 0.05$ Mann–Whitney).

Correlation of IL-1β and IL-6 release with *in vitro* CRP synthesis

Analysis performed on all IBD patients combined showed statistically significant correlations between *in vitro* CRP synthesis in response to monocyte-conditioned medium, and the IL-1β and IL-6 levels in those media, when the conditioned was obtained in the absence of LPS ($r = 0.74$; $p < 0.001$ Kendall's rank correlation and $r = 0.18$; $p < 0.05$ Kendall's rank correlation, respectively) although not in the presence of LPS ($r = 0.14$; $p > 0.05$ Kendall's

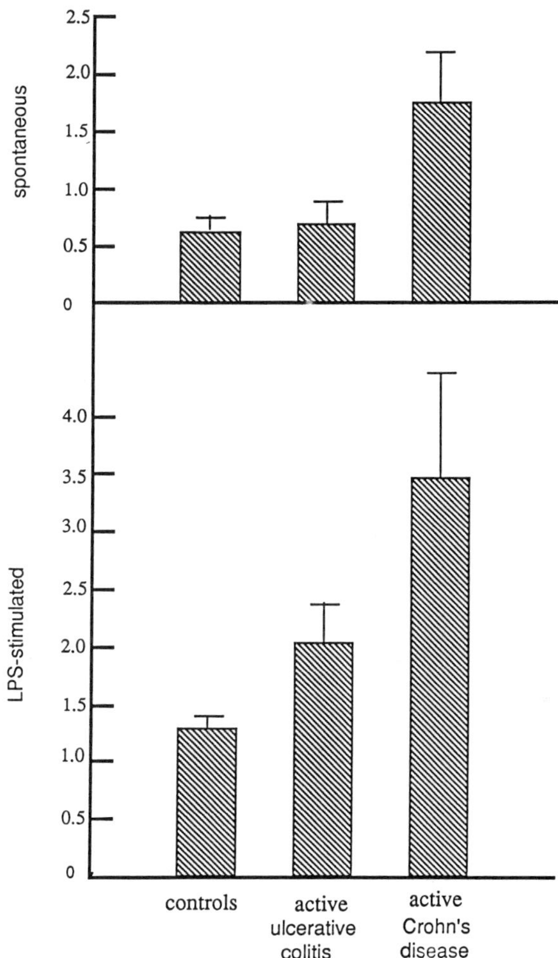

Fig. 2 *In vitro* C-reactive production (ng/ml). Both unstimulated and LPS-stimulated monocyte-conditioned medium (MoCM) from patients with active CD ($n = 11$, $p < 0.02$ Mann–Whitney and $p < 0.05$ Mann–Whitney, respectively) caused greater CRP release from Alexander cells than McCM from active UC ($n = 11$) and normal controls ($n = 11$)

rank correlation and $r = -0.14$; $p > 0.05$ Kendall's rank correlation, respectively).

IL-1β and IL-6 correlations with serum CRP concentration

Table 1 summarizes the correlation coefficients and significance values between IL-1β, and IL-6 and serum C-reactive protein concentrations in

Table 1 Correlations of cytokine generation with serum C-reactive protein in ulcerative colitis and Crohn's disease

	Crohn's disease	*Ulcerative colitis*
Interleukin-1β		
Spontaneous	n.s.	$r = 0.42, p < 0.05$
LPS-stimulated	$r = 0.35, p < 0.05$	n.s.
Interleukin-6		
Spontaneous	$r = -0.32, p < 0.05$	n.s.
LPS-stimulated	$r = -0.26, p < 0.05$	n.s.
Spontaneous (related to total monocyte count)	n.s.	n.s.
LPS-stimulated (related to total monocyte count)	n.s.	n.s.

Crohn's disease and ulcerative colitis. We found statistically significant but weak positive correlations between serum CRP and LPS-stimulated IL-1β production in Crohn's disease. However, we found significant negative though weak correlations between serum CRP, and spontaneous IL-6 and LPS-stimulated IL-6 production in Crohn's disease. In ulcerative colitis neither spontaneous nor LPS-stimulated IL-6 production significantly correlated with serum CRP. When analysis was performed by using the amount of IL-6 release related to the total count of monocytes per 10 ml blood we found no significant correlation between serum CRP, with either spontaneous or LPS-stimulated IL-6 production either in Crohn's disease or in ulcerative colitis.

DISCUSSION

The results from this study may be summarized as follows:

1. The enhanced propensity of monocytes from patients with CD to generate IL-1β, both in response to lipopolysaccharide *in vitro* and emphasized when monocytes are taken from patients with active inflammation, was confirmed.
2. There was no apparent enhanced propensity of monocytes to generate IL-6 in CD, although the larger number of circulating monocytes indicates that there may be a greater overall ability of an individual with active CD to generate IL-6, if this is typical of the monocyte macrophage pool generally.
3. The greater elevation of CRP associated with active CD may be correlated with enhanced propensity to generate interleukins, particularly IL-1.

In further discussion of this, and the potential role of cytokines in IBD, we shall concentrate on two aspects. Firstly we shall place our cytokine results in context with those published by others, and secondly we shall speculate on the potential impact of a different panel of cytokines in the manifestations of IBD, over and above the generation of CRP.

A number of other studies on systemic cytokine production in inflammatory bowel disease have reported that peripheral blood mononuclear cells (PBMC) or monocytes from patients with Crohn's disease produce more IL-1 compared to patients with ulcerative colitis and normal individuals. In a study using the mouse thymocyte stimulation assay, Satsangi *et al.* (1987) measured lymphocyte-activating factor (LAF) activity in supernatants from cultures of peripheral blood mononuclear cells from 16 patients with Crohn's disease, six with ulcerative colitis, and 10 healthy subjects, and reported spontaneous release of LAF in cultures of unstimulated cells from six patients with Crohn's disease and, to a lesser extent, from one with ulcerative colitis and from one healthy control[23]. Suzuki *et al.* reported that peripheral blood monocytes from patients with IBD provoked more IL-1β than controls[24], and Crohn's disease to produce significantly elevated levels compared with ulcerative colitis[25]. Duclos *et al.* demonstrated a significant elevation of IL-1 blood levels in Crohn's disease compared to ulcerative colitis or controls[26,27]. Reports on circulating IL-6 by several workers have demonstrated elevated levels in Crohn's disease compared to ulcerative colitis and controls[28–30]. A number of studies also support the enhanced production of TNF-α in Crohn's disease[21,31,32].

Involvement of cytokines in the inflammatory and immune sequences which may account for the perpetuation of the inflammatory responses in inflammatory bowel disease are readily appreciated, although the prior triggering event is not fully understood. Initially antigenic stimulation leads to monocyte/macrophage activation. Activated monocytes/macrophages release monokines which may stimulate their own production[33,34] and also each other's production in a highly complex manner in monocytes/macrophages and other cell types[35,36]. Such a mechanism of cell–monokine interaction provides for a powerful amplification circuit during the inflammatory response.

IL-1 produced by macrophages acts on multiple target cells. IL-1 induces T cells to produce IL-2, which in turn provides the growth signal for clonal expansion of various helper, suppressor, and cytolytic T cells and augments natural killer cell activity. IL-1 in conjunction with other cytokines IL-4, IL-5 and IL-6 can induce B cell proliferation and antibody production[37]. IL-6, which is a major inducer of B cell terminal differentiation, can enhance IgG, IgA and IgM production in activated B cells[38,39]. Increased IgG secretion can activate the complement system and subsequently cause activation of the kinin system. IL-1 also induces production of platelet-activating factor and the arachidonic acid cascade of inflammatory mediators, resulting in increased production of the products of the cyclooxygenase and lipoxygenase pathways[40]. Activated macrophages also generate cytokines such as TNF-α, IL-6, IL-8[41,42] and TGF-β[43]. These cytokines have complex interrelationships with IL-1 and with each other. Interleukin-8 (IL-8), which is also called neutrophil-activating peptide-1 (NAP-1) could bring about accumulation of neutrophils. Activation of neutrophils induces expression of surface adhesion molecules, release of storage enzymes and production of reactive oxygen metabolites[44]. The end-result is an amplificatory process with further recruitment of acute inflammatory cells and continuing tissue destruction occurring in inflammatory bowel disease.

Cytokines and CRP release in inflammatory bowel disease

In the present study we have examined the role of cytokines in acute-phase protein synthesis in inflammatory bowel disease. We have shown that CRP plasma levels and *in vitro* CRP production in Crohn's disease were significantly elevated compared to ulcerative colitis. Our data accord with the suggestion that more enhanced CRP response in the setting of Crohn's disease may reflect differences in the profile of cytokines produced by macrophages from patients with Crohn's disease. This was suggested by the presence of significant though low correlations between IL-1β and with serum CRP in Crohn's disease in our studies. In Crohn's disease serum CRP was also shown to be significantly correlated with circulating IL-6 level by some workers[29].

Discrepancies between acute-phase proteins and cytokine levels *in vitro* and *in vivo* may arise because of a number of reasons such as the complexities in the types of inflammatory mediators produced by various inflammatory cells, effect of treatment on the state of activation of inflammatory cells, and differences in the half-life between acute-phase proteins and cytokines. Cytokines have short circulatory half-life, in the order of minutes, in contrast to the circulatory half-life of serum proteins, which are in the order of days. These may account for the low or absent correlation between plasma proteins and cytokine production found in these studies.

Nevertheless, since each of IL-1, IL-6 and TNF-α has been implicated to modulate CRP synthesis, the tendency for the acute-phase reactant, CRP, to be markedly elevated in Crohn's disease compared to ulcerative colitis can be explained by the combined stimulatory effects of IL-1, IL-6 and TNF-α on the hepatic synthesis of this protein.

Other implications of differing cytokine profiles in CD and UC

There are other significant clinical differences between ulcerative colitis and Crohn's disease which may also reflect differences in the profile of cytokines between Crohn's disease and ulcerative colitis, and require further investigation.

The tendency to transmural granulomatous inflammation and fibrosis, and resultant gut stenosis, is one of the most striking differences between Crohn's disease and ulcerative colitis. Increased fibrosis reflects enhanced collagen synthesis by fibroblasts, which may be due to production by mononuclear cells of inflammatory mediators that are responsible for initiating and/or perpetuating the fibrotic response.

Several macrophage-derived cytokines are potentially fibrogenic, including IL-1, TNF-α, transforming growth factor-β, platelet-derived growth factor and basic fibroblast growth factor[45]. IL-1 and TNF individually stimulate cell proliferation and collagen production, although findings differ amongst various studies[46-48]. Production of IL-1 in tissues may contribute to local effects such as fibrosis and the influx of inflammatory cells. IL-1 can directly increase the transcription of type I and type III collagen and type IV collagen[49,50]. IL-1 and TNF increase fibroblast proliferation[51]. The tendency for Crohn's disease patients to generate more IL-1 and TNF-α, and other potentially fibrogenic cytokines may thus play a role in the marked fibrosis seen in this condition. It may be that patients who have Crohn's disease manifest this form of inflammation because of the innate tendency to generate a cytokine network that leads to transmural inflammation and marked fibrosis, while patients with ulcerative colitis have a tendency to generate a cytokine network that tends to cause diffuse mucosal inflammation.

Granulomas and cytokines in inflammatory bowel disease

Another feature of Crohn's disease is the typical non-caseating granuloma. Histopathologically, the bulk of a granuloma is composed of cells of the monocyte lineage (macrophages, epithelioid cells, and giant cells) together with lymphocytes and eosinophils. In Crohn's disease the exact stimulus for granuloma formation remains unknown.

The production of IL-1 and TNF within the colonic mucosa in IBD may lead to activation of the microvascular endothelium. Both of these monokines can then stimulate the production of leucocyte adhesion molecules on endothelial cells, and thereby promote the adhesion of neutrophils, monocytes and lymphocytes at sites of inflammation. In view of the predominant participation of macrophages in experimental granulomas *in vivo* and *in vitro*, it is reasonable to assume that chemotactic activity and inflammatory signals of monokines are responsible for the initiation and/or development of granulomas.

Studies on the role of cytokines in the intercellular interactions that lead to formation and maintenance of granulomas have shown that *in vivo* IL-1 may be important in initiation of granuloma in an animal model[52]. Reports in mice using antibodies directed against tumour necrosis factor have shown that this cytokine is important in the development and maintenance of granulomas in response to intravenous injection of bacille Calmette–Guérin[53].

In a study by Shikama *et al.* (1989) *in vitro* granulomas were induced by culturing murine spleen cells in the presence of artificial microparticles. Culture supernatants of dextran-induced granulomas contained high levels of IL-1 activity but not IL-2 or IL-4 activity. IL-1 activity was correlated with granuloma size. Additionally, granulomas were produced by culturing spleen cells in the presence of agarose beads coupled to recombinant IL-1 or recombinant TNF-α[54].

IL-1 and TNF thus appear to be centrally involved in granuloma formation in animal models. Further studies are required to delineate their role in the development and maintenance of granuloma in humans, and the role of these cytokines in contributing to the histological pattern of macrophage infiltration in Crohn's disease.

One final note of speculation. The interrelation between smoking and IBD is intriguing, with epidemiological evidence associating smoking with Crohn's disease and non-smoking with ulcerative colitis. C-reactive protein is reported to be increased in cigarette smokers[55,56]. Smokers also produce higher levels of interleukin-1 than non-smokers. Nagai *et al.* reported that IL-1 activity released from LPS-stimulated bronchoalveolar lavage fluid macrophages was significantly higher in smokers than in non-smokers. LPS-stimulated monocytes in smokers also showed a similar significant increase in IL-1, raising the possibility of a 'flow of stimulating substances' from the lung to systemic circulation[57].

It appears that both smoking and Crohn's disease are individually associated with elevated IL-1 production, suggesting that IL-1 may be a common mechanism of action. The association between smokers and Crohn's disease could be accounted for by smokers also tending to have elevated IL-1 production, hence actively promoting Crohn's disease in a population subgroup genetically predisposed to developed IBD.

In summary: generation of cytokines in patients with CD and UC is likely to mediate and amplify the inflammatory process; the precise spectrum of cytokines generated (whether this reflects differing stimuli, or a genetic predisposition in favour of a certain group of cytokines) may define the histopathological and clinical features which we use to classify idiopathic inflammatory bowel disease.

ACKNOWLEDGEMENT

We acknowledge the generous support of the National Association for Colitis and Crohn's Disease of Great Britain.

References

1. Broom MF, Mellor DM, Chadwick VS. Purification and amino acid sequences of naturally occuring N-formyl methioyl oligopeptides from E. Coli. Experientia. 1989;45:1097–99.
2. Monteiro E, Fossey J, Shiner M, Drasad BS, Allison AC. Antibacterial antibodies in rectal and colonic mucosa in ulcerative colitis. Lancet. 1971;i:249.
3. Fearon DT, Tuddy S, Schur PH, McCabe WR. Activation of the properdin pathway of complement in patients with gram-negative bacteremia. New Engl J Med. 1975;292:937.
4. Halstensen TS, Mollnes TE, Garred P, Fausa O, Brandtzaeg P. Epithelial deposition of immunoglobulin G1 and activated complement (c3b and terminal complex) in ulcerative colitis. Gastroenterology. 1990;98:1264–71.
5. Nielson OH, Ahnfelt-Ronne I, Elmgreen J. Abnormal metabolism of arachadonic acid in chronic inflammatory bowel disease: enhanced release of leukotriene B_4 from activated neutrophils. Gut. 1987;28:181–5.
6. Rosam AC, Wallace JL, Whittle B. Potent ulcerogenic actions of platelet-activating factor on the stomach. Nature. 1986;319:54–6.
7. Adeyemi EO, Neumann S, Chadwick VS, Hodgson HJF, Pepys MB. Circulating human leucocyte elastase in patients with inflammatory bowel disease. Gut. 1985;26:1306–11.
8. Hodgson HJF. Assessment of drug therapy in inflammatory bowel disease. Br J Clin Pharmacol. 1982;14:159–70.
9. Saverymuttu SH, Hodgson HJF, Chadwick VS, Pepys MB. Differing acute phase responses in Crohn's disease and ulcerative colitis. Gut. 1986;27:809–13.
10. Baumann H. Hepatic acute phase reaction in vivo and in vitro. In Vitro Cellular & Developmental Biology. 1989;25:115–26.
11. Chambers RE, Stross P, Barry RE, Whicher JT. Serum amyloid A protein compared with C-reactive protein, alpha 1-antichymotrypsin and alpha 1-acid glycoprotein as a monitor of inflammatory bowel disease. Eur J Clin Invest. 1987;17:460–67.
12. Pepys MB, Baltz BL. Acute phase proteins with special reference C-reactive protein and related proteins (pentraxins) and serum amyloid A protein. Adv Immunol. 1983;34:141–212.
13. Robey FA, Jones KD, Steinberg AD. C-reactive protein mediates the solubilization of nuclear DNA by complement *in vitro*. J Exp Med. 1985;161:1344–56.

14. Robey FA, Ohura K, Futai S, Fujii N, Yajima H, Goldman N, Jones KD, Wahl S. Proteolysis of human C-reactive protein produces peptides with potent immunomodulating activity. J Biol Chem. 1987;262:7053–7.
15. Saverymuttu SH, Chadwick VS, Hodgson HJF. Granulocyte migration in ulcerative colitis. Eur J Clin Invest. 1985b;15:60–3.
16. Hodgson HJF, Mazlam MZ. Review article: assessment of drug therapy in inflammatory bowel disease. Aliment Pharmacol Therap. 1991;5:555–84.
17. Kushner I, Ganapathi M, Schultz D. The acute phase response is mediated by heterogenous mechanisms. Ann NY Acad Sci. 1989;557:19–29.
18. Taylor AW, Ku N-O, Mortensen RF. Both IL-1 and IL-6 induce synthesis of C-reactive protein (CRP) by PLC/PRF/5 hepatoma cell line. Ann NY Acad Sci. 1989;557:532–3.
19. Ganapathi MK, Schultz D, Mackiewicz A, Salmols D, Hu S-I, Brabenec A, Macintyre SS, Kushner I. Heterogenous nature of the acute phase response. Differential regulation of human serum amyloid A, C-reactive protein and other acute phase proteins by cytokines in Hep 3B cells. J Immunol. 1988;141:564–9.
20. Heinrich PC, Castell JV, Andus T. Interleukin-6 and the acute phase response. Biochem J. 1990;265:621–36.
21. Mazlam MZ, Hodgson HJF. Peripheral blood monocyte cytokine production and acute phase response in inflammatory bowel disease. Gut. 1992;33:773–8.
22. Schrumpf E, Fausa O, Forre O, Dobloug JH, Ritland S. HLA antigens and immunoregulatory T-cells in ulcerative colitis associated with hepatobiliary disease. Scand J Gastroenterol. 1982;17:187–91.
23. Satsangi J, Wolstencroft RA, Cason J, Ainley CC, Dumonde DC, Thompson RPH. Interleukine 1 in Crohn's disease. Clin Exp Immunol. 1987;67:594–605.
24. Suzuki K, Murata Y, Niida N, Shiotani K, Munakata M, Moriya N, Satoh M, Ishizuka K, Saitoh H, Munakata A, Yoshida Y. Increased synthesis of interleukin-1β (IL-1β) by monocytes from patients with inflammatory bowel disease. Gastroenterology. 1991;100:A619 (abstract).
25. Suzuki Y, Tobin A, Quinn DG, Whelan CA, O'Morain C. Interleukin 1 production by monocytes in Crohn's disease and ulcerative colitis. British Society for Immunology, Autumn meeting, London. 1989; Po 1.41 (abstract).
26. Duclos B, Reimund JM, Dumont S, Sapin R, Chamouard P, Baumann R, Poindron P, Weill JP. Discrepancy between tumor necrosis factor (TNF) and interleukine 1 (IL1) blood levels and cytotoxic activity of blood monocytes in Crohn's disease (CD). Gastroenterology. 1991b;100:A576 (abstract).
27. Duclos B, Reimund JM, Lehr L, Sapin R, Derlon A, Chamouard P, Baumann R, Weill JP. Interleukin 1 (IL1), 6 (IL6) and tumor necrosis factor (TNF) serum levels in Crohn's disease (CD). Gastroenterology. 1991a;100:A576 (abstract).
28. Gross V, Andus T, Caesar I, Roth M, Schölmerich J. Evidence for continuous stimulation of interleukin-6 production in Crohn's disease. Gastroenterology. 1992;102:514–19.
29. Lobo AJ, Jones SC, Evans SW, Banks R, Rathbone BJ, Axon ATR. Plasma interleukin-6 in inflammatory bowel disease. Gut. 1990;31:A1194 (abstract).
30. Mahida YR, Kurlak L, Hawkey CJ. High circulating concentrations of interleukin-6 (IL-6) in active Crohn's disease but not ulcerative colitis. Gut. 1991;32:1531–4.
31. MacDonald TT, Hutchings P, Choy M-Y, Murch S, Cooke A. Tumour necrosis factor-alpha and interferon-gamma production measured at the single cell level in normal and inflamed human intestine. Clin Exp Immunol. 1990;81:301–5.
32. Mitsuyama K, Toyanaga A, Sasaki E, Ikeda H, Tsurata O, Harada K, Tanikawa K. Interleukin-8 and regulatory cytokines (interleukin-1 and tumor necrosis factor-α) in inflammatory bowel disease. American Gastroenterological Association. 1992:1586 (abstract).
33. Philip R, Epstein LB. Tumor necrosis factor as immunomodulator and mediator of monocyte cytotoxicity induced by itself, gamma-interferon and interleukin-1. Nature. 1986;323:86–9.
34. Van Damme J, Opdenakker G, Simpson RJ, Rubira MR, Cayphas S, Vink A, Billiau A, van Snick J. Identification of the human 26 kD protein, interferon β_2 (IFN-β_2) as a B cell hybridoma/plasmacytoma growth factor induced by interleukin-1 and tumor necrosis factor. J Exp Med. 1987;165:914–19.
35. Warner SJC, Auger KR, Libby P. Interleukin-1 induces interleukin-1. II. Interleukin-1 induces production of interleukin-1 by adult human vascular endothelial cells in vitro.

J Immunol. 1987;139:1911–17.

36. Dinarello CA, Canon JG, Wolff SM, Bernheim HA, Beutler B, Cerami A, Figari IS, Palladino MA, O'Connor JV. Tumor necrosis factor (cachectin) is an endogenous pyrogen and induces production of interleukin 1. J Exp Med. 1986;163:1433–50.

37. Kishimoto T, Hirano T. Molecular regulation of B lymphocyte response. Ann Rev Immunol. 1988;6:485–512.

38. Muraguchi A, Hirano T, Tang B, Matsuda T, Horii Y, Nakajima K, Kishimoto T. The essential role of B cell stimulatory factor 2 (BSF-2/IL-6) for the terminal differentiation of B cells. J Exp Med. 1988;167:332–44.

39. Beagley KW, Eldridge JH, Lee F, Kiyono H, Everson MP, Koopman WJ, Hirano T, Kishimoto T, McGhee JR. Interleukins and IgA synthesis. Human and murine interleukin 6 induce high rate IgA secretion in IgA-committed B cells. J Exp Med. 1989;169:2133–48.

40. Wardle TD, Turnberg LA. Interactions between interleukin 1 and phospholipid derivatives in ulcerative colitis. Gut. 1992; suppl 33, T100 (abstract).

41. Yoshimura T, Matsushima K, Oppenheim JJ, Leonard EJ. Neutrophil chemotactic factor produced by lipopolysaccharide (LPS)-stimulated human blood mononuclear leukocytes: partial characterization and separation from interleukin 1 (IL-1). J Immunol. 1987;139:788–93.

42. Peveri P, Walz A, Dewald B, Baggiolini M. A novel neutrophil-activating factor produced by human mononuclear phagocytes. J Exp Med. 1988;167:1457–1559.

43. Assoian RK, Fleurdelys BE, Stevenson HC, Miller PJ, Madtes DK, Raines EW, Ross R, Sporn MB. Expression and secretion of type β transforming growth factor by activated human macrophages. Proc Natl Acad Sci. 1987;84:6020–24.

44. Baggiolini M, Walz A, Kunkel SL. Neutrophil-activating peptide-1/interleukin 8, a novel cytokine that activates neutrophils. J Clin Invest. 1989;84:1045–9.

45. Piguet PF, Collart MA, Grau GE, Sappino A-P, Vassalli P. Requirement of tumour necrosis factor for development of silica-induced pulmonary fibrosis. Nature. 1990;344:245–7.

46. Kähäri V-M, Heino J, Vuorio E. Interleukin-1 increases collagen production and mRNA levels in cultured skin fibroblasts. Biochim Biophys Acta. 1987;929:142–7.

47. Postlethwaite AE, Raghow R, Stricklin GP, Poppleton H, Seyer JM, Kang AH. Modulation of fibroblast functions by interleukin 1: increased steady-state accumulation of type 1 procollagen messenger RNAs and stimulation of other functions but not chemotaxis by human recombinant interleukin 1α and β. J Cell Biol. 1988;106:311–18.

48. Elias JA, Freundlich B, Kern JA, Rosenbloom J. Cytokine networks in the regulation of inflammation and fibrosis in the lung. Chest. 1990;97:1439–45.

49. Canalis E. Interleukin-1 has independent effects on DNA and collagen synthesis in cultures of rat calvariae. Endocrinology. 1986;118:74–81.

50. Matsushima K, Bano M, Kidwell WR, Oppenheim JJ. Interleukin-1 increases collagen type IV production by murine epithelial cells. J Immunol. 1985;134:904–9.

51. May LT, Helfgott DC, Sehgal PB. Anti-β-interferon antibodies inhibit the increased expression of HLA-B7 mRNA in tumor necrosis factor-treated human fibroblasts: structural studies of the β_2 interferon involved. Proc Natl Acad Sci. 1986;83:8957–61.

52. Kobaysahi K, Allred C, Cohen S, Yoshida T. Role in interleukin 1 in experimental pulmonary granuloma in mice. J Immunol. 1985;134:358–64.

53. Kindler V, Sappino A, Grau GE, Piguet PF, Vassalli P. The inducing role of tumor necrosis factor in the development of bactericidal granuloma during BCG infection. Cell. 1989;56:731–40.

54. Shikama Y, Kobayashi K, Kasahara K, Kaga S, Hashimoto M, Yoneya I, Hosoda S, Soejima K, Ide H, Takahashi T. Granuloma formation by artificial microparticles *in vitro*. Macrophages and monokines play a critical role in granuloma formation. Am J Pathol. 1989;134:1189–99.

55. Heiskell CL, Miller JN, Aldrich HJ, Carpenter CM. Smoking and serologic abnormalities. JAMA. 1962;181:88–91.

56. Palosuo T, Husman T, Koistinen J, Aho K. C-reactive protein in population samples. Acta Med Scand. 1986;220:175–9.

57. Nagai S, Takeuchi M, Watanabe K, Aung H, Izumi T. Smoking and interleukin-1 activity released from human alveolar macrophages in healthy subjects. Chest. 1988;94:694–700.

12

Anti-inflammatory mechanisms: cytokines, cytokine binding proteins, acute-phase response

V. GROSS, T. ANDUS, I. CAESAR and J. SCHÖLMERICH

INTRODUCTION

Cytokines are important mediators which orchestrate inflammatory and immunological host defence reactions. When produced in excess, cytokines cause local or systemic toxic effects. Therefore, mechanisms which counteract the induction and/or the effects of various proinflammatory peptide mediators exist. Since inflammatory bowel diseases (IBD) are characterized by a chronic inflammatory state the analysis of these anti-inflammatory mechanisms is of interest. In the following we will concentrate on four basic anti-inflammatory principles:

1. anti-inflammatory effects of certain cytokines,
2. anti-inflammatory action of acute-phase proteins,
3. inhibition of cytokine activities by soluble cytokine receptors,
4. inhibition of interleukin-1 (IL-1) effects by soluble interleukin-1 receptor antagonist (IL-1ra).

ANTI-INFLAMMATORY EFFECTS OF CYTOKINES

Besides mainly proinflammatory cytokines such as IL-1 and TNF-α[1] other cytokines exert also certain anti-inflammatory effects. IL-4, IL-6, TGF-β and IL-10 belong to this group of cytokines[2].

IL-4, also known as B cell stimulatory factor, is mainly synthesized by activated lymphocytes. It is a stimulatory factor for both B and T cells. Although it positively influences lymphocyte functions, it impairs certain monocyte functions. IL-4 inhibits human macrophage colony formation[3], monocyte-derived H_2O_2 production[4], and the release of the inflammatory mediators TNF, IL-1 and PGE_2[5].

IL-6 is synthesized by various cell types such as monocytes[6-8], fibroblasts[9-12], endothelial cells[12-14], B and T lymphocytes[15] and other cell types upon adequate stimulation. Among its various effects, i.e. B cell maturation, induction of acute-phase protein synthesis, etc. it downregulates certain monocyte functions. Pretreatment of monocytes with IL-6 impairs synthesis of IL-1 and TNF[16,17]. Furthermore, injection of IL-6 stimulates release of corticotropin, ACTH, and cortisol into the blood stream, which are immunosuppressive and anti-inflammatory hormones[18].

TGF-β exerts stimulatory and inhibitory effects on the immune system. It is a chemotactic agent for monocytes[19] and fibroblasts[20] and enhances the expression of Fc-γ III receptors (CD 16) on monocytes[21]. On the other hand, TGF-β is a potent monocyte deactivating agent. It impairs the production of oxygen radicals and the synthesis of other cytokines in response to other stimuli, e.g. endotoxin[22,23]. It furthermore impairs the interferon gamma (IFN-γ)-induced expression of HLA-DR[24]. TGF-β is in addition a potent regulator of lymphocyte proliferation. It inhibits the proliferation of B and T cells, and the generation of cytotoxic T cells and of lymphokine-activated killer cells[25].

IL-10 is produced by T cells[26], B-cells[27], or monocytes activated by LPS[28]. IL-10 inhibits cytokine production by Th 1 cell clones when they are activated under conditions requiring the presence of antigen-presenting cells. Furthermore, IL-10 inhibits cytokine synthesis by Th 1 cells stimulated with the super-antigen *Staphylococcus* enterotoxin B. IL-10 shows its inhibitory effects only when macrophages, but not when B-cells, are used as antigen-presenting cells[29]. IL-10 strongly reduces antigen-specific human T cell proliferation by diminishing the antigen-presenting capacity of monocytes via down-regulation of class II MHC expression[30]. It does not act via an inhibition of antigen processing. In addition, IL-10 also inhibits cytokine production by activated macrophages, e.g. LPS-induced expression of IL-1α, IL-6 or TNF-α[31]. IL-10 thus plays a role not only in the regulation of T cell activation but also in acute inflammatory responses.

The synthesis of IL-6 and TGF-β has been studied in patients with IBD. In the case of IL-4 and IL-10 no published data on their expression in IBD are available.

For IL-6 there is evidence for a continuous stimulation of its production in Crohn's disease[32]. In an unselected population of 70 patients with Crohn's disease (median CDAI 88, range 0–328) and of 23 patients with ulcerative colitis (median Rachmilewitz index 2.5, range 0–11) serum concentrations of biologically active IL-6 were significantly increased in patients with Crohn's disease (6.8 $\pm$ 0.9 U/ml, mean $\pm$ SEM) compared with patients with ulcerative colitis (mean < 4 units/ml) and healthy controls (mean < 4 units/ml); 65.5% of patients with Crohn's disease, 21.7% of patients with ulcerative colitis and 0% of healthy controls had serum IL-6 concentrations $\geqslant 4\,U/ml$ (Fig. 1). There was a tendency towards higher serum IL-6 concentrations in patients with active Crohn's disease than in patients with inactive Crohn's disease. These differences were, however, not statistically significant. Similarly, Mahida et al.[33] found high circulating concentrations of immunologically active IL-6 in active Crohn's disease but not in ulcerative colitis. IL-6 was detected in the plasma of 18 of 21 patients with Crohn's disease (median 47, range < 20–250 pg/ml), but in only two of 20 with ulcerative colitis and two of 16 controls.

Concerning the main source of circulating IL-6 in inflammatory bowel disease both mononuclear cells from peripheral blood[34,35] and intestinal inflammatory cells[36,37] seem to contribute to its increased serum levels.

TGF-β1 production has been analysed in human IBD by in situ hybridization[38]. Virtually all of the hybridized cells were eosinophils. TGF-β produced by intestinal cells in Crohn's disease was 92% active as compared to 68% activated from tissues in ulcerative colitis and 73% activated from control biopsies. These differences might partially explain the greater tendency towards fibrosis in Crohn's disease.

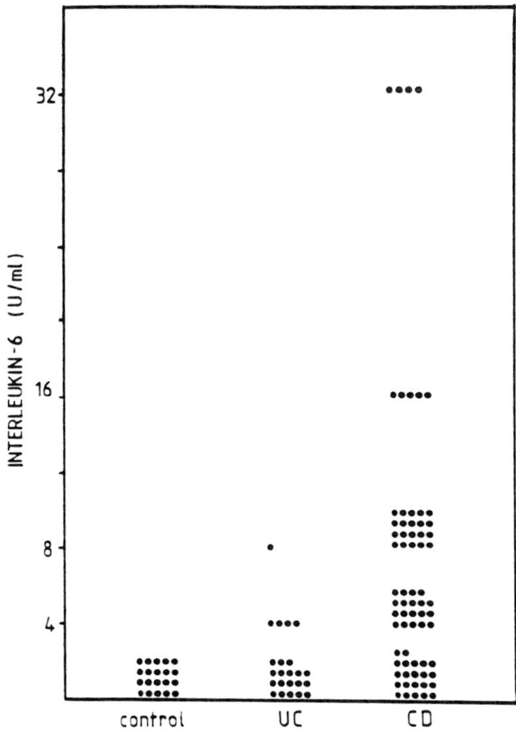

Fig. 1 Serum concentration of IL-6 in patients with IBD and in healthy controls. IL-6 bioactivity was determined in the serum of 70 patients with Crohn's disease, 23 patients with ulcerative colitis and 20 healthy controls by the B9 cell bioactivity assay

ACUTE-PHASE PROTEINS

The increased synthesis of acute-phase proteins forms part of the body's answer to disturbances of its homeostasis. Major functions of acute-phase proteins are to limit and to counteract proinflammatory and tissue-disturbing reactions induced by activated neutrophils and mononuclear cells. The ability of these cells to damage tissues *in vivo* relies mainly on two components: (1) the formation of reactive oxygen metabolites and (2) the release of proteolytic enzymes[39,40]. Released proteinases may lead not only to local tissue destruction but also to an activation of the proteolytic cascades in blood, i.e. the coagulation, the fibrinolytic, the complement and the kallikrein–kinin system. Inhibition of proteinases is a major function of acute-phase proteins such as α_1-antitrypsin, α_1-antichymotrypsin, C1-inhibitor, or α_2-anti-plasmin[41,42]. Caeruloplasmin has the ability to bind reactive oxygen metabolites and thus to reduce tissue destruction. Similarly, α_1-antitrypsin can be oxidized by oxygen radicals. Oxidized α_1-antitrypsin, however, loses its proteinase inhibitory activity[43]. α_1-Acid glycoprotein may interfere with the endothelial adhesion of neutrophils, which is an important step for neutrophil extravasation[44].

Acute-phase proteins are mainly synthesized in the liver[45,46], although secondary sites of synthesis exist, e.g. monocytes or macrophages[47]. During recent years several cytokines have been identified which may up-regulate the synthesis of various acute-phase proteins in the liver (Table 1). Among these are IL-1[48,49], IL-6[50,51], IL-11[52], TNF-α[53,54], IFN-γ[55], leukaemia inhibitory factor[56], oncostatin M[57], EGF[58] and TGF-β[59]. Among these cytokines IL-6, IL-11, leukaemia inhibitory factor and oncostatin M induce the same spectrum of acute-phase proteins. The molecular explanation for this phenomenon is that these cytokines share a similar signal transducing membrane glycoprotein, which forms part of the IL-6 receptor complex[60]. Compared with this group of cytokines IL-1, TNF-α, IFN-γ and TGF-β only induce a limited spectrum of acute-phase proteins.

Although the *in vitro* activities of IL-6, IL-11, leukaemia inhibitory factor and oncostatin M seem to be comparable, no comparative *in vivo* studies during inflammation exist in humans. While there are many reports demonstrating increased serum levels of IL-6 during acute-phase conditions such as major surgery[61,62], severe burns[63], bacterial infections[64,65], or acute pancreatitis[66], which correlate with the induction of acute-phase proteins, e.g. CRP[66], no comparable data are available for IL-11, leukaemia inhibitory factor or oncostatin M.

Table 1 Cytokines inducing acute-phase protein synthesis by hepatocytes

IL-1	INF-γ
IL-6	Leukaemia inhibitory factor
IL-11	Oncostatin M
EGF	Ciliary derived neurotropic factor
TNF-α	TGF-β

In patients with active IBD increased serum concentrations of acute-phase proteins such as α_1-acid glycoprotein, α_1-antitrypsin, α_1-antichymotrypsin, β_2-microglobulin, C-reactive protein, and serum amyloid A have been described[32,67-77]. Acute-phase protein serum levels usually correlate well with clinical activity indices in inflammatory bowel disease[32]. On the other hand, however, there is no significant correlation between acute-phase protein levels and serum concentrations of IL-6 in patients with inflammatory bowel disease[32]. This lack of correlation might have several reasons, e.g. the short circulatory half-life of IL-6 ($t_{1/2}$ *ca.* 5 min)[78] versus the much longer half-life (several days) of most acute-phase proteins. An alternative explanation would be that other cytokines such as IL-11, leukaemia inhibitory factor, etc. might be important mediators of acute-phase protein synthesis in IBD. This needs to be clarified in future studies.

SOLUBLE CYTOKINE RECEPTORS

Cytokines exert their effects by binding to specific cell surface receptors. During recent years molecular cloning has allowed identification of a large number of specific cytokine receptors. Interestingly, besides the membrane-bound form of these receptors, soluble receptor proteins were detected for many cytokines. Soluble receptors have been identified for IL-1[79], IL-2[80], IL-4[81], IL-5[82], IL-6[83], IL-7[84], IFN-γ[83,85], G-CSF[86], and nerve growth factor[87]. Soluble cytokine receptors may be generated by different mechanisms. One possibility is that different splicing leads to different mRNA species of a receptor molecule, one of which lacks the hydrophobic transmembrane domain and encodes for a soluble form of the receptor. This is the case for IL-4, IL-5, IL-7, and G-CSF. Another mechanism is shedding of the soluble extracellular domain of a receptor, which presumably occurs in the case of soluble IL-2 and TNF receptors. The concentrations of soluble cytokine receptors in body fluids are remarkably high, generally in the range of several ng/ml, whereas the respective cytokine concentrations are generally much lower, i.e. in the range of pg/ml.

Soluble cytokine receptors may exert different effects. In the case of IL-6 it has been found that binding of IL-6 to the soluble IL-6 receptor leads to association of the complex with the 130 kDa membrane signal transducing glycoprotein, which mediates IL-6 activity[60,88]. In many other cases soluble receptors impair cytokine activities by forming soluble cytokine–receptor complexes, thus interfering with the binding of the cytokines to their cellular receptors. Inhibitory activities of soluble receptors have been described for IL-1[89], IL-2[90], IL-4[91] and TNF[92]. Since IL-1, IL-2 and TNF are important mediators in IBD, the study of their soluble receptors is of special interest.

Soluble IL-1 receptor[79,93] can be detected in culture supernatants of human cells or in human plasma. Recombinant soluble forms of the soluble IL-1 receptor have profound inhibitory effects and impair different forms of *in vivo* alloreactivity[89]. Thus far no data on soluble IL-1 receptor in patients with IBD are available.

The human IL-2 receptor consists of a low-affinity 55 kDa α chain and an intermediate-affinity 75 kDa β chain which form a dimeric, biologically active high-affinity IL-2 receptor complex[94-97]. The soluble IL-2 receptor does not appear to be the product of a unique post-transcriptional splicing event. Even in the absence of any post-translational modifications soluble IL-2 receptor is most probably generated by proteolytic cleavage of the α-chain[98,99]. Although the affinity of the soluble IL-2 receptor to IL-2 is much lower than that of the high-affinity cellular receptor (100–1000 times less), *in vitro* experiments show that soluble IL-2 receptor may limit the availability of free IL-2 to lymphocytes and down-regulate T-cell responses. Soluble IL-2 receptor does not directly affect the number or function of the cell-bound high-affinity IL-2 receptor[90]. It has been suggested that this mechanism may also play a role in human diseases[100,101]; however, direct evidence for this assumption has not yet been provided.

In human IBD increased concentrations of soluble IL-2 receptors have been described[102-108]. These studies were mostly done with patients with Crohn's disease. Mean serum concentrations in patients with inactive disease were around 500 U/ml, in patients with active disease around 800 U/ml, and in patients with highly active disease around 1100 U/ml. In our own study of patients with IBD (70 unselected patients with Crohn's disease, 23 unselected patients with ulcerative colitis) mean soluble IL-2 receptor concentrations were 898 ± 558 U/ml (mean $\pm$ SD) in patients with active Crohn's disease and 754 ± 389 U/ml in patients with inactive Crohn's disease, as defined by the severity activity index of Goebell[109] (Fig. 2). This indicates that soluble IL-2 receptor levels are significantly increased in both groups of patients with Crohn's disease (normal 273 U/ml, upper limit 477 U/ml). This is in accordance with the observations of other investigators who also found increased soluble IL-2 receptor concentrations in patients with inactive Crohn's disease[103,105,106]. In contrast to patients with Crohn's disease unselected patients with ulcerative colitis have no significantly increased soluble IL-2 receptor levels (281 ± 92, and 322 ± 168 U/ml, respectively). If only patients with highly active IBD are selected, and studied before and after successful corticosteroid therapy, increased soluble IL-2 receptor levels are also found in ulcerative colitis. Successful steroid therapy leads to a reduction in serum soluble IL-2 receptor concentrations within a few weeks (Table 2).

There is general consensus that increased serum levels of soluble IL-2 receptor are a marker for disease activity in patients with IBD. When Crohn's disease and ulcerative colitis are compared, soluble IL-2 receptors are increased not only in patients with active Crohn's disease but also in those with inactive disease. This is not the case in ulcerative colitis. This reflects a continuous activation of the immune system in patients with Crohn's disease in contrast to patients with ulcerative colitis.

Concerning the source of soluble IL-2 receptor in IBD an increased *in vitro* release has been demonstrated by colonic lamina propria mononuclear cells by Schreiber *et al.*[107], and increased concentrations of soluble IL-2 receptors have been determined in endoscopic mucosal biopsy specimens of patients with active IBD[108]. Whether soluble IL-2 receptor has a role at the

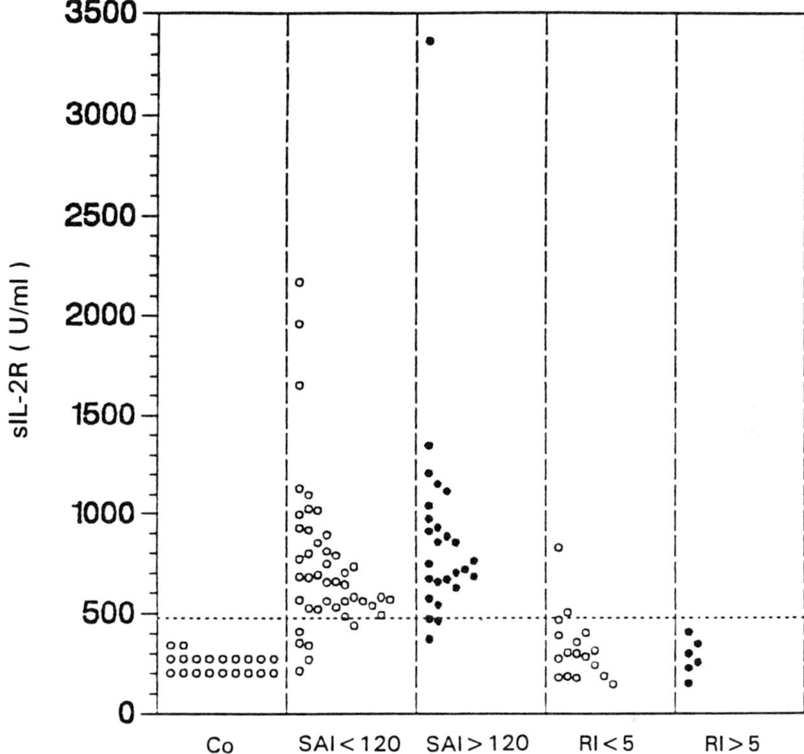

Fig. 2 Serum concentrations of soluble IL-2 receptor in patients with IBD. Soluble IL-2 receptor was determined in the serum of 70 patients with Crohn's disease and 23 patients with ulcerative colitis by ELISA (R&D Systems, Minneapaolis). The severity of Crohn's disease was assessed by the severity–activity index of Goebell[109], the severity of ulcerative colitis by the Rachmilewitz index[110]

gut level as a down-regulator of T-cell functions by binding free IL-2 is not clear.

There are two distinct TNF receptors (TNF-Rs) with molecular masses of 55 kDa (p55) and 75 kDa (p75)[112]. Soluble inhibitory TNF-Rs derived from the membrane-bound proteins with molecular masses of about 30 kDa have been found in human serum and urine[113]. Soluble TNF-Rs are released by activated neutrophils, mononuclear blood cells, fibroblasts, and cell lines such as HL-60. The release of sTNF-Rs from human neutrophils is increased by FMLP, C5a, GM-CSF, PMA and A23187, the release of sTNF-Rs from HL-60 was stimulated by TNF-α, TNF-β and PMA. The most likely mechanism for the release of sTNF-Rs is proteolytic processing, which leads to a shedding of sTNF-Rs from the cell membranes.

The effect of sTNF-Rs on the bioavailability of TNF is complex. Three molecules of the sTNF-R p55 bind to one trimer of TNF-α or TNF-β. Both sTNF-Rs inhibit binding of TNF to its cellular receptors and reduce the biological effects of TNF in a dose-dependent manner[92]. However, recently

Table 2 Serum concentrations of soluble IL-2 receptor in patients with highly active inflammatory bowel disease

	Before therapy	*After therapy*
Crohn's disease ($n = 27$)		
CDAI	284 ± 121	106 ± 69
SAI	219 ± 68	130 ± 59
sIL-2R (U/ml)	903 ± 682	772 ± 533
Ulcerative colitis ($n = 12$)		
Rachmilewitz index	12.3 ± 4.4	4.9 ± 5.3
sIL-2R (U/ml)	1130 ± 673	674 ± 294

All data are means $\pm$ SD. Soluble IL-2 receptor was determined by ELISA (R&D Systems, Minneapolis), CDAI, Crohn's disease activity index[111]; SAI, severity activity index[109]; Rachmilewitz index[110].

it has been shown that low concentrations of sTNF-Rs (resulting in sTNF-R/TNF ratios of up to 20) stabilize the trimeric structure and activity of TNF *in vitro*[114]. Therefore it was proposed that sTNF-Rs may act as carriers for TNF, or may even augment the effect of TNF by prolonging its function in closed compartments where clearance of the TNF–sTNF-R complexes is slow[114]. The finding that intra-articular injection of $1\,\mu$g of sTNF-R acts as an anti-inflammatory in a rat antigen-induced arthritis model[115] indicates that high concentrations of sTNF-R inhibit the function of TNF *in vivo* even in compartments such as the synovial space.

The modulatory function of sTNF-Rs may be an important, protective, physiological regulatory mechanism, which minimizes tissue destruction caused by an overproduction of TNF during acute inflammation. Although TNF usually contributes to the protection of the organism against infectious agents and to healing from injury, high concentrations of this powerful proinflammatory cytokine become pernicious in certain pathological situations such as septic shock, resulting in a more severe destruction than that induced by the pathogen itself. Regulators of the biological activity of TNF, such as the detected sTNF-Rs, which counteract potentially harmful effects of TNF, are therefore essential to maintain physiological homeostasis during infections.

Only limited data on soluble TNF receptors in patients with inflammatory bowel disease are available. When soluble TNF receptors were determined in plasma from seven patients with active Crohn's disease (CDAI 289 ± 101, mean $\pm$ SD), and in five patients with active ulcerative colitis (Rachmilewitz index 10.4 ± 4.3), patients with active Crohn's disease and active ulcerative colitis had elevated plasma concentrations of soluble TNF receptor p55 (4.2 ± 2.4 and $3.9 \pm 1.9\,$ng/ml). The plasma concentrations of soluble TNF receptor p75, however, remained normal in most patients with active Crohn's disease ($0.8 \pm 0.8\,$ng/ml) or active ulcerative colitis ($1.5 \pm 0.9\,$ng/ml). Systemic corticosteroid treatment led to a reduction of the disease activity and, concomitantly, the plasma concentrations of soluble TNF receptor p55 also decreased ($2.6 \pm 1.5\,$ng/ml in Crohn's disease; $2.2 \pm 0.6\,$ng/ml in ulcerative colitis) (Table 3). When soluble TNF receptor levels were serially determined in individual patients with IBD during therapy a reduction of soluble TNF

Table 3 Soluble TNF receptor levels in plasma of patients with inflammatory bowel disease

	Before therapy	*After therapy*
Crohn's disease ($n = 7$)		
CDAI	289 ± 101	80 ± 71
sTNF-R p55 (ng/ml)	4.16 ± 2.42	2.62 ± 1.51
sTNF-R p75 (ng/ml)	0.79 ± 0.79	0.69 ± 0.75
Ulcerative colitis ($n = 5$)		
Rachmilewitz index	10.4 ± 4.3	2.6 ± 2.3
sTNF-R p55 (ng/ml)	3.90 ± 1.88	2.23 ± 0.58
sTNF-R p75 (ng/ml)	1.46 ± 0.85	1.02 ± 0.73

All data are means ± SD. Normal values for both soluble TNF receptor p55 (sTNF-R p55) and soluble TNF receptor p75 (sTNF-R p75) are <1.5 ng/ml. Soluble TNF receptors were determined by ELIBA (F. Hoffmann La Roche AG, Basel). CDAI, Crohn's disease acitivity index[111]; Rachmilewitz index[110].

receptor p55, but not of p75, concomitantly with decreased disease activity could be observed (Fig. 3).

It may be concluded that soluble TNF receptor p55 levels are 2–3-fold increased in patients with active Crohn's disease or ulcerative colitis, whereas soluble TNF receptor p75 levels remain unaffected. In contrast to patients with IBD, patients with viral hepatitis or patients with decompensated liver cirrhosis and ascites show primarily an increase in soluble TNF receptor p75[116,117]. The different up-regulation of soluble TNF receptor p55 versus p75 in patients with IBD may indicate differences in the immunoregulation in these diseases, or may represent a defect of the defence.

CYTOKINE RECEPTOR ANTAGONISTS

A specific receptor antagonist exists for IL-1[118–120]. IL-1 receptor antagonist (IL-1ra), first discovered in the urine of febrile patients, is now available as recombinant protein. IL-1ra is synthesized by human monocytes. It has 19% and 26% homology with IL-1α and IL-1β, respectively. IL-1ra competes with IL-1 for type I and type II IL-1 receptors. When IL-1 occupies either receptor, signal transduction takes place, when IL-1ra occupies either receptor, no signal transduction occurs[121]. IL-1ra blocks the biological activity of IL-1 *in vitro* and *in vivo*, e.g. it inhibits IL-1-induced hypotension in rabbits and baboons, IL-1-induced fever in rabbits, IL-1-induced hepatic acute-phase protein synthesis, IL-1-induced increase in corticosterone in mice, IL-1-induced neutrophilia in mice, IL-1-induced lymphocyte proliferation, IL-1-induced collagenase production by rabbit chondrocytes, IL-1-induced synthesis of IL-1, TNF, IL-6, and GM-CSF in monocytes, and IL-1-induced nitric oxide production in human smooth muscle cells (reviewed in ref. 122).

In experimental immune complex colitis in rabbits IL-1ra decreased tissue injury[123]. Similarly, IL-1ra has been shown to inhibit both acute and chronic relapsing peptidoglycan–polysaccharide polymer-induced enterocolitis and

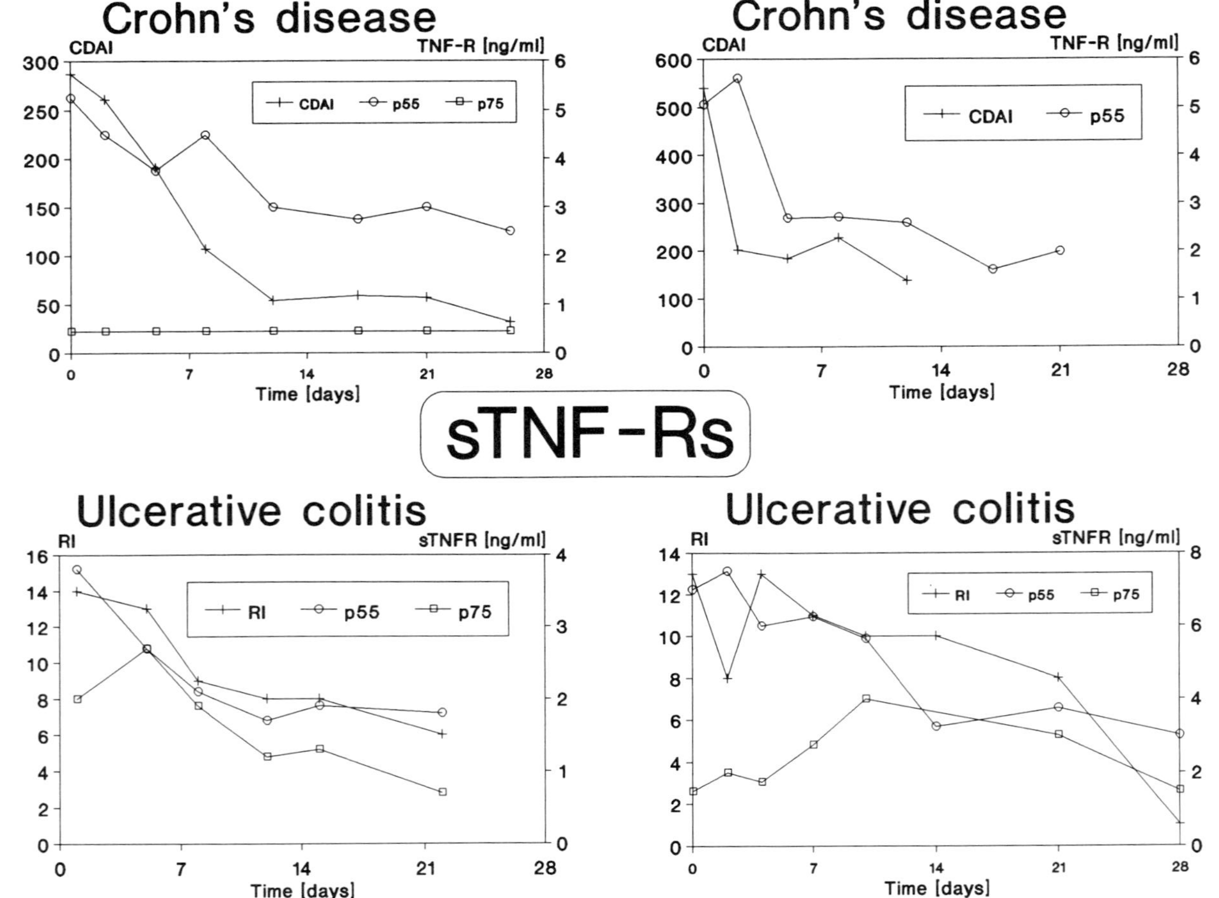

Fig. 3 Soluble TNF receptor p55 levels in individual patients with IBD during therapy. Soluble TNF receptor p55 was repeatedly determined by ELIBA (F. Hoffmann La Roche AG, Basel) in the plasma of patients with Crohn's disease (CD) or ulcerative colitis (UC) before and during corticosteroid therapy

its associated arthritis in rats, and to accelerate healing of indomethacin-induced enterocolitis[124]. The anti-inflammatory and protective effects of IL-1ra are both dependent on the time of administration and on the dose. Administration during early stages of experimental inflammation and high doses increase the protective effects of IL-1ra.

IL-1ra is synthesized by human monocytes upon adherence to IgG[120,125]. It may be induced in THP-1 cells by PMA[126]. IL-1ra may furthermore be induced in monocytes by LPS[127], GM-CFS[128], CSF 1[129], or TGF-β[130]. It may furthermore be expressed by intestinal epithelial cells (F. Cominelli, personal communication).

Interestingly, IL-1ra can be converted into an IL-1 agonist by site-specific mutagenesis by a single amino acid substitution (Lys 145-Asp)[131].

There is evidence for an increased synthesis of IL-1ra in patients with IBD. When IL-1ra levels were determined in 20 patients with highly active Crohn's disease and five patients with highly active ulcerative colitis before and after systemic corticosteroid therapy all patients showed 2–10-fold increased levels of IL-1ra during active disease with no difference between Crohn's disease or ulcerative colitis. Typical courses of IL-1ra are shown in Fig. 4. However, there was a wide variation in IL-1ra concentrations between individual patients. It is therefore not possible to determine any cut-off values which allow discrimination between patients with active or inactive disease. The increased IL-1ra levels in patients with active IBD may at least in part explain a well-known phenomenon, i.e. that patients with active Crohn's disease have an IL-1 antagonistic serum activity[32].

An increased expression of IL-1ra mRNA has been measured in acute and chronically inflamed bowel of rats after induction of experimental enterocolitis[133], indicating that the diseased bowel is an important source of IL-1ra. However, when the balance of IL-1 and IL-1ra was studied in the intestinal mucosa of Crohn's disease and ulcerative colitis patients[134] a significantly decreased ratio between IL-1ra and IL-1 was found in patients with inflammatory bowel disease as compared to surgical controls. In spite of its increased synthesis there might therefore be a relative lack of IL-1ra in IBD, at least at the mucosal level.

CONCLUSION AND PERSPECTIVES

There are several naturally occurring anti-inflammatory mechanisms in patients with IBD:

1. cytokines with anti-inflammatory effects,
2. acute-phase proteins,
3. soluble cytokine receptors,
4. cytokine receptor antagonists.

To further elucidate on these points:

1. Different cytokines may exhibit opposing biological effects on specific target cells. Well-described examples for this kind of mechanism are the

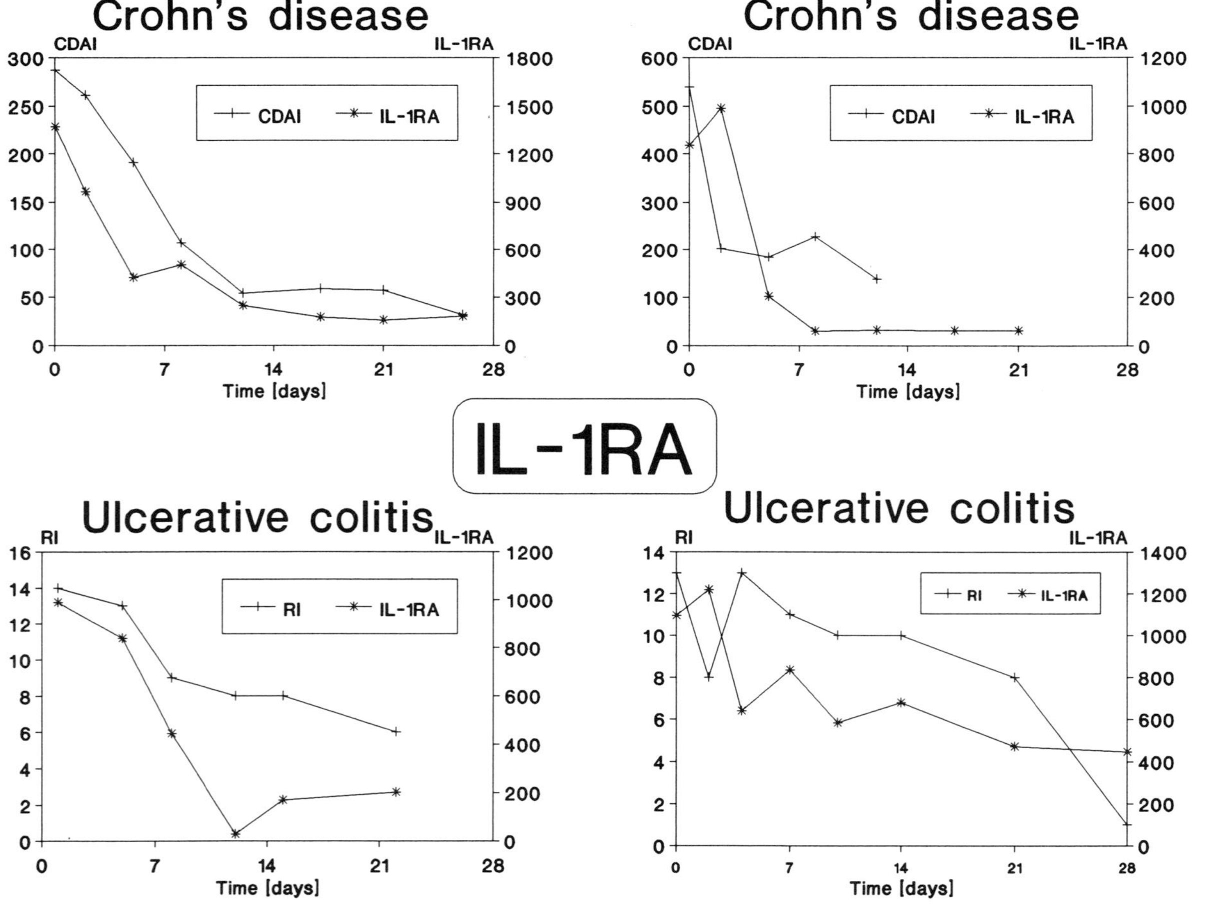

Fig. 4 IL-1 receptor antagonist in patients with IBD. Serum concentrations of IL-1ra were repeatedly determined by ELISA (R&D Systems, Minneapolis) in patients with highly active Crohn's disease or ulcerative colitis during acute-phase corticosteroid therapy

140

inhibition of monocyte activation by IL-4, IL-6, and TGF-β. IL-10 functions as an inhibitor of Th-1 cell activation. There is evidence for an increased synthesis of IL-4 and IL-6 in IBD.

2. Several cytokines, i.e. IL-1, IL-6, IL-11, TNF-α, IFN-γ, leukaemia inhibitory factor, oncostatin M, EGF, and TGF-β up-regulate the synthesis of acute-phase proteins in the liver, IL-6 being presumably the most important inducer. Since inhibition of proteinases and scavenging of oxygen radicals are major functions of acute-phase proteins they may reduce tissue injury caused by activated inflammatory cells. Increased acute-phase protein synthesis is a well-known phenomenon in active IBD.

3. Soluble receptors have been identified for several cytokines. In IBD soluble IL-2 receptors (sIL-2 R) and soluble TNF receptors (sTNF-Rs) are of special interest. Soluble receptors may act as specific cytokine inhibitors by forming soluble cytokine–receptor complexes. It has to be considered, however, that the effects of soluble receptors may vary depending on the concentration of the cytokine, the concentration of the soluble receptor, and the number and affinity of the respective cellular receptors. A 2–3-fold increase in sIL-2 R has been demonstrated in patients with active IBD. In patients with Crohn's disease sIL-2 R levels are also increased when the disease is clinically not active. In the case of sTNF-Rs a 2–3-fold increase of sTNF-R p55, but not of sTNF-R p75, can be observed in active Crohn's disease as well as in active ulcerative colitis.

4. A naturally occurring receptor antagonist synthesized by activated human monocytes exists for IL-1. IL-1 receptor antagonist (IL-1ra) has now become available as recombinant protein. Studies of several groups have shown that IL-1ra has the potential to impair experimental colitis in animals. In human IBD serum IL-1ra levels are increased 2–10-fold during active disease, with large variations between individual patients.

The reviewed data show that not only proinflammatory but also anti-inflammatory mechanisms are activated in patients with IBD. These anti-inflammatory mechanisms might protect the body from systemic injuries resulting from local inflammation. At the inflammatory site there may well be an imbalance between 'aggressive' and 'protective' factors, as shown in the case of IL-1 and IL-1ra. Future research is needed to reveal whether the administration of 'pharmacologically' active doses of any of the naturally occurring anti-inflammatory mechanisms might be of value for the treatment or prophylaxis of IBD.

References

1. Billiau A, Vandekerckhove F. Cytokines and their interactions with other inflammatory mediators in the pathogenesis of sepsis and septic shock. Eur J Clin Invest. 1991;21:559–73.
2. Cerami A. Inflammatory cytokines. Clin Immunol Immunopathol. 1992;62:3–10.
3. Crawford RM, Finbloom DS, Ohara J, Paul WE, Meltzer MS. B cell stimulatory factor-1 (interleukin 4) activates macrophages for increased tumoricidal activity and expression of Ia antigens. J Immunol. 1987;139:135–41.
4. Jansens JH, Wientjens GH, Fibbe WE, Willemze R, Kluin-Nelemans HC. Inhibition of human macrophage colony formation by interleukin 4. J Exp Med. 1989;170:577–82.

5. Lehn M, Weisner WY, Engelhorn S, Gillis S, Remold HG. IL-4 inhibits H_2O_2 production and antileishmanial capacity of human cultured monocytes mediated by IFN-gamma. J Immunol. 1989;143:3020–4.
6. May LT, Chrayel J, Santhanam V, Tatter SB, Sthoeger Z, Helfgott DC, Chiorazzi N, Grieninger G, Sehgal PB. Synthesis and secretion of multiple forms of β_2-interferon/B-cell differentiation factor 2/hepatocyte-stimulating factor by human fibroblasts and monocytes. J Biol Chem. 1988;263:7760–6.
7. Bauer J, Ganter U, Geiger T, Jacobshagen V, Hirano T, Matsuda T, Kishimoto T, Andus T, Acs G, Gerok W, Ciliberto G. Regulation of interleukin-6 expression in cultured human blood monocytes and monocyte-derived macrophages. Blood. 1988;72:1134–40.
8. Gross V, Andus T, Castell J, vom Berg D, Heinrich PC, Gerok W. O- and N-glycosylation lead to different molecular mass forms of human monocyte interleukin-6. FEBS Lett. 1989;247:323–6.
9. Defilipi P, Poupart P, Tavernier J, Fiers W, Content J. Induction and regulation of mRNA encoding 26 kDa protein in human cell lines treated with recombinant human tumor necrosis factor. Proc Natl Acad Sci USA. 1987;84:4557–61.
10. Walther Z, May LT, Seghal PR. Transcriptional regulation of the interferon $\beta2$/B-cell differentiation factor BSF-2/hepatocyte-stimulating factor gene in human fibroblasts by other cytokines. J Immunol. 1988;140:974–7.
11. Zhang Y, Lin J-X, Keung Y, Vilcek J. Enhancement of cAMP levels of protein kinase activity by tumor necrosis factor and interleukin-1 in human fibroblasts: Role in the induction of interleukin-6. Proc Natl Acad Sci USA. 1988;85:6802–5.
12. Seghal PB, Helfgott DC, Santhanam V, Tatter SB, Clarick RH, Ghrayel J, May LF. Regulation of the acute phase and immune responses in viral disease. J Exp Med. 1988;167:1951–2.
13. Jirik FR, Podor TJ, Hirano T, Kishimoto T, Loskutoff DJ, Carson DA, Lotz M. Bacterial lipopolysaccharide and inflammatory mediators augment IL-6 secretion by human endothelial cells. J Immunol. 1989;142:144–7.
14. Sironi M, Breviaris F, Prosperio P, Biondi A, Vecchi A, van Damme J, Dejana E, Mantovani A. IL-1 stimulates IL-6 production in endothelial cells. J Immunol. 1989;142:549–53.
15. Horii Y, Maraguchi A, Suematsu S, Matsuda T, Yoshizaki K, Hirano T, Kishimoto T. Regulation of BSF-2/IL-6 production by human mononuclear cells. Macrophage-dependent synthesis of BSF-2/IL-6 by T cells. J Immunol. 1988;141:1529–35.
16. Schindler R, Mancilla J, Endres S, Ghorbani R, Clark SC, Dinarello CA. Correlations and interactions in the production of interleukin-6 (IL-6), IL-1 and tumor necrosis factor (TNF) in human blood mononuclear cells: IL-6 suppresses IL-1 and TNF. Blood. 1990;75:40–7.
17. Aderka D, Le J, Vilcek J. IL-6 inhibits lipopolysaccharide-induced TNF production in cultured human monocytes, U937 cells, and in mice. J Immunol. 1989;143:3517–23.
18. Naitoh Y, Fukata J, Tominaga T, Nakai Y, Tamai S, Mori K, Imura H. Interleukin-6 stimulates the secretion of adrenocorticotropic hormone in conscious freely moving rats. Biochem Biophys Res Commun. 1988;155:1459–63.
19. Wahl SM, Hunt DA, Wakefield M, McCartney-Francis N, Wahl LM, Roberts AB, Sporn MB. Transforming growth factor type beta induces monocyte chemotaxis and growth factor production. Proc Natl Acad Sci USA. 1987;84:5788–92.
20. Postlethwaite AE, Keske-Oja J, Moses HL, Kang AH. Stimulation of the chemotactic migration of human fibroblasts by transforming growth factor beta. J Exp Med. 1987;165:251–6.
21. Welch G, Wong H, Wahl SM. Selective induction of FC gamma RIII on human monocytes by transforming growth factor-beta. J Immunol. 1990;144:3444–8.
22. Espevik T, Figari IS, Shalaby MR, Lackides GA, Lewis GD, Shepard HM, Palladino MA. Inhibition of cytokine production by cyclosporin A and transforming growth factor beta. J Exp Med. 1987;166:571–6.
23. Espevik T, Figari IS, Ranges GE, Palladino MA. Transforming growth factor-beta 1 (TGF-beta 1) and recombinant human tumor necrosis factor-alpha reciprocally regulate the generation of lymphokine-activated killer cell activity. J Immunol. 1988;140:2312–16.
24. Czarniecki CW, Chiu HH, Wong GHW, McCabe SM, Palladino MA. Transforming

growth factor beta 1 modulates the expression of class II histocompatibility antigens on human cells. J Immunol. 1988;140:4217–23.

25. Wahl SM, McCartney-Francis N, Mergenhagen SE. Inflammatory and immunoregulatory roles of TGF-beta. Immunol Today. 1989;10:258–61.

26. Sher A, Fiorentino D, Caspar P, Pearce E, Mosmann T. Production of IL-10 by CD4+ T lymphocytes correlates with down-regulation of Th1 cytokine synthesis in helminth infection. J Immunol. 1991;15:2713–16.

27. O'Garra A, Stapleton G, Dhar V, Pearce M, Schumacher J, Rugo H, Barbis D, Stall A, Cupp J, Moore K, et al. Production of cytokines by mouse B cells: B lymphomas and normal B cells produce interleukin 10. Int. Immunol. 1990;2:821–32.

28. Mosmann TR. Cytokine secretion patterns and cross-regulation of T cell subsets. Immunol Res. 1991;10:183–8.

29. Mosmann TR. Role of a new cytokine, interleukin-10, in the cross-regulation of T helper cells. Ann NY Acad Sci. 1991;628:337–44.

30. de Waal Malefyt R, Haanen J, Spits H, Roncarolo MG, te Velde A, Figdor C, Johnson K, Kastelein R, Ysel H, de Vries JE. Interleukin 10 (IL-10) and viral IL-10 strongly reduce antigen-specific human T cell proliferation by diminishing the antigen-presenting capacity of monocytes via downregulation of class II major histocompatibility complex expression. J Exp Med. 1991;174:915–24.

31. Fiorentino DF, Zlotnik A, Mosmann TR, Howard M, O'Garra A. IL-10 inhibits cytokine production by activated macrophages. J Immunol. 1991;147:3815–22.

32. Gross V, Andus T, Caesar I, Roth M, Schölmerich J. Evidence for continuous stimulation of interleukin-6 production in Crohn's disease. Gastroenterology. 1992;102:514–19.

33. Mahida YR, Kurlac L, Gallagher A, Hawkey CJ. High circulating concentrations of interleukin-6 in active Crohn's disease but not ulcerative colitis. Gut. 1991;32:1531–4.

34. Mahida YR, Kurlak L, Gallagher A, Hawkey CJ. Circulating and tissue interleukin-6 (IL-6) levels in inflammatory bowel disease. Gastroenterology. 1990;89:A461.

35. Andus T, Gross V, Cäsar I, Krumm D. Hosp J, David M, Schölmerich J. Activatation of monocytes during inflammatory bowel disease. Pathobiology. 1991;59:166–70.

36. Stevens C, Walz G, Zanker B, Singaram C, Lipmann M, Strom TB. Interleukin-6 (IL-6), interleukin-1β (IL-1β) and tumor necrosis factor α (TNFα) expression in inflammatory bowel disease (IBD). Gastroenterology. 1990;98:A475.

37. Raedler A, Steffen M, Reinecker C, Witthöft T, Schreiber S, MacDermott RP. Lamina propria mononuclear cells in patients with inflammatory bowel disease secrete enhanced levels of IL-1β, TNF-α and IL-6. Gastroenterology. 1992;102:A68.

38. Sinclair SB, Baca-Estrada ME, Croitoru K, Lea R, Clark DA, Riddell RH, Ernst PB. TGF-β production by eosinophils in inflamed human intestine. Gastroenterology. 1992;102:A696.

39. Malech HL, Gallin JI. Neutrophils in human diseases. N Engl J Med. 1987;317:687–94.

40. Weiss SJ. Tissue destruction by neutrophils. N Engl J Med. 1989;320:365–76.

41. Koj A. Function of acute phase proteins. In Gordon A and Koj A (eds). The acute phase response to injury and infection. Amsterdam: Elsevier; 1985;10:139–232.

42. Kushner I. The phenomenon of the acute phase response. Ann NY Acad Sci. 1982;389:39–48.

43. Carrell RW, Jeppson JO, Laurell CB, Brennan SO, Owen MC, Vaughan L, Boswell DR. Structure and variation of human α1-antitrypsin. Nature. 1982;298:329–34.

44. Walz G, Aruffo A, Kolanus W, Bevilacqua M, Seed B. Recognition by ELAM-1 of the sialyl-Lex determinant on myeloid and tumor cells. Science. 1990;250:1132–5.

45. Heinrich PC, Castell JV, Andus T. Interleukin-6 and the acute phase response. Biochem J. 1990;265:621–36.

46. Miller LL, Bly CG, Watson ML, Bal WF. The dominant role of the liver in plasma protein synthesis. J Exp Med. 1951;94:431–53.

47. Fey GH, Fuller GM. Regulation of acute phase gene expression by inflammatory mediators. Mol Biol Med. 1987;4:323–38.

48. Ramadori G, Sipe JD, Mizel SB, Dinarello CA, Colten HR. Pretranslational modulation of acute phase hepatic protein synthesis by murine recombinant interleukin-1 (IL-1) and purified human IL-1. J Exp Med. 1985;162:930–42.

49. Geiger T, Andus T, Northoff H, Heinrich PC. Induction of α_1-acid glycoprotein by recombinant human interleukin-1 in rat hepatoma cells. J Biol Chem. 1988;263:7141–6.

50. Gauldie J, Richards C, Harnish D, Lansdorp P, Baumman H. Interferon β_2/B-cell stimulatory factor type 2 shares identity with monocyte-derived hepatocyte-stimulating factor and regulates the major acute phase protein response in liver cells. Proc Natl Acad Sci. 1987;84:7251–5.
51. Andus T, Geiger T, Hirano T, Northoff H, Ganter U, Bauer J, KIishimoto T, Heinrich PC. Recombinant human B cell stimulatory factor 2 (BSF-2/IFN-β2) regulates β-fibronogen and albumin mRNA levels in Fao-9 cells. FEBS Lett. 1987;221:18–22.
52. Baumann H, Schendel P. Interleukin-11 regulates the hepatic expression of the same plasma protein genes as interleukin-6. J Biol Chem. 1991;266:20424–7.
53. Darlington GJ, Wilson DR, Lachman LR. Monocyte-conditioned medium, interleukin-1 and tumor necrosis factor stimulate the acute phase response in human hepatoma cells *in vitro*. J Cell Biol. 1986;103:787–93.
54. Perlmutter DH, Dinarello CA, Punsal PI, Colten HR. Cachectin/tumor necrosis factor regulates hepatic acute phase gene expression. J Clin Invest. 1986;78:1349–54.
55. Zuraw BL, Lotz M. Regulation of the hepatic synthesis of C1 inhibitor by the hepatocyte stimulating factors interleukin-6 and interferon-gamma. J Biol Chem. 1990;265:12664–70.
56. Baumann H, Wong GG. Hepatocyte stimulating factor III shares structural and functional identity with leukemia-inhibitory factor. J Immunol. 1989;143:1163–7.
57. Richards CD, Brown TJ, Shoyab M, Baumann H, Gauldie J. Recombinant oncostatin M stimulates the production of acute phase proteins in HepG2 cells and rat primary hepatocytes *in vitro*. J Immunol. 1992;148:1731–6.
58. Baumann H, Won KA, Jahreis GP. Human hepatocyte stimulating factor III and interleukin-6 are structurally and immunologically distinct but regulate the production of the same acute phase plasma proteins. J Biol Chem. 1989;264:8046–51.
59. Machiewicz A, Ganapathi M, Schultz C, Brabenec A, Weinstein J, Kelley M, Kushner I. Transforming growth factor β1 regulates production of acute phase proteins. Proc Natl Acad Sci. 1990;87:1491–5.
60. Taga T, Hibi M, Hirata Y, Yasukawa K, Matsuda T, Hirano T, Kishimoto T. Interleukin-6 triggers the association of its receptor with a possible signal transducer, gp130. Cell. 1989;58:573–81.
61. Nishimoto N, Yoshizaki K, Tagoh H, Monden M, Kishimoto S, Hirano T, Kishimoto T. Elevation of serum interleukin-6 prior to acute phase proteins on the inflammation by surgical operation. Clin Immunol Immunopathol. 1989;50:339–401.
62. Skenkin A, Fraser WD, Series J, Winstanley FP, McCartney AC, Burns HJG, van Damme J. The serum interleukin-6 response to elective surgery. Lymphokine Res. 1989;8:123–7.
63. Nijisten MW, DeGroot ER, TenDuis HJ, Hack CE, Aarden LA. Serum levels of interleukin-6 and acute phase response. Lancet. 1987;2:921.
64. Waage A, Bradtzaeg P, Halstensen A, Kierulf P, Espevik T. The complex shock. Association between interleukin-6, interleukin-1, and fatal outcome. J Exp Med. 1989;169:333–8.
65. Helfgott DC, Tatter SB, Santhanam U, Clarick RH, Bhardwaj N, May LT, Sehgal PB. Multiple forms of IFN-β_2/IL-6 in serum and body fluids during acute bacterial infection. J Immunol. 1989;142:948–53.
66. Leser HG, Gross V, Scheibenbogen C, Heinisch A, Salm R, Lausen M, Rüchauer K, Andreesen R, Farthmann EH, Gerok W, Schölmerich J. Elevation of serum interleukin-6 precedes acute-phase response and reflects severity in acute pancreatitis. Gastroenterology. 1991;101:782–5.
67. Cooke WT, Fowler DI, Cox EV, Gaddie R, Meynell M. The clinical significance of seromucoids in regional ileitis and ulcerative colitis. Gastroenterology. 1958;34:910–19.
68. Weeke B, Jarnum S. Serum concentration of 19 serum proteins in Crohn's disease and ulcerative colitis. Gut. 1971;12:297–302.
69. Marner JL, Friborg S, Simonson E. Disease activity and serum proteins in ulcerative colitis. Immunochemical quantitation. Scand J Gastroenterol. 1975;10:537–44.
70. Descos L, Andre C, Beorchia S, Vincent C, Revillard JP. Serum levels of β_2-microglobulin – a new marker of activity in Crohn's disease. N Engl J Med. 1979;301:440–1.
71. Buckell NA, Lennard-Jones JE, Hernandez MA, Kohn J, Riches PG, Wadsworth J. Measurements of serum proteins during attacks of ulcerative colitis as a guide to patient management. Gut. 1979;20:22–7.

72. Andre C, Descos C, Landais P, Fermanian J. Assessment of appropriate laboratory measurements to supplement the Crohn's disease activity index. Gut. 1981;22:571–4.
73. Fagan EA, Dyck RF, Maton PN. Serum levels of C-reactive protein in Crohn's disease and ulcerative colitis. Eur J Clin Invest. 1982;12:351–9.
74. Brignola C, Lanfranchi GA, Campieri M, Bazzocchi G, Devoto M, Boni P, Farruggia P, Vegetti S, Tragnmone A. Importance of laboratory parameters in the evaluation of Crohn's disease activity. J Clin Gastroenterol. 1986;8:245–8.
75. Chambers RE, Stross P, Barry RE, Whicher JT. Serum amyloid. A protein compared with C-reactive protein, α_1-antichymotrypsin and α_1-acid glycoprotein as a monitor of inflammatory bowel disease. Eur J Clin Invest. 1987;17:460–7.
76. Prantera C, Davoli M, Lorenzetti R, Pallone F, Marcheggioano A, Jannoni C, Mariotti S. Clinical and laboratorys indicators of extent of ulcerative colitis. J Clin Gastroenterol. 1988;10:41–5.
77. Boirivant M, Leoni M, Tariciotti D, Fais S, Squarcia O, Pallone F. The clinical significance of serum C-reactive protein levels in Crohn's disease. J Clin Gastroenterol. 1988;10:401–5.
78. Castell JV, Geiger T, Gross V, Andus T, Walter E, Hirano T, Kishimoto T, Heinrich PC. Plasma clearance, organ distribution and target cells of interleukin-6/hepatocyte-stimulating factor in the rat. Eur J Biochem. 1988;177:357–61.
79. Giri JG, Newton RC, Horuk R. Identification of soluble interleukin-1 receptor. J Biol Chem. 1990;265:17416–19.
80. Rubin LA, Kurman CC, Fritz ME, Giddison WE, Boutin B, Yarchoan R, Nelson DL. Soluble interleukin-2 receptors are released from activated human lymphoid cells *in vitro*. J Immunol. 1985;135:3172–7.
81. Mosley B, Beckmann MP, March CJ, Idzerda RL, Gimpel SD, Vandebos T, Friend D, Alpert A, Anderson DM, Jackson J, Wignall JM, Smith C, Gallis B, Sims JE, Urdal DI, Widmer Mv, Cosman D, Park LS. The murine interleukin-4 receptor: molecular cloning and characterisation of secreted and membrane-bound forms. Cell. 1989;59:335–48.
82. Takaki S, Tominaga A, Hitoshi Y, Mita S, Sonoda E, Yamaguchi N, Takatsu K. Molecular cloning and expression of the murine interleukin-5 receptor. EMBO J. 1990;9:4367–74.
83. Novick D, Engelmann H, Wallach D, Rubinstein M. Soluble cytokine receptors are present in normal human urine. J Exp Med. 1989;170:1409–14.
84. Goodwin RG, Friend D, Ziegler SF, Jerzys R, Falk BA, Gimpel S, Cosman D, Dower SK, March CJ, Namen AE, Park LS. Cloning of the human and murine in interleukin-7 receptors. Demonstration of a soluble form and homology to a new receptor superfamily. Cell. 1990;60:941–51.
85. Novick D, Engelmann H, Wallach D, Revel M, Rubinstein M. Purification of soluble cytokine receptors from normal human urine by ligand affinity and immunoaffinity chromatography. J Chromatogr. 1990;510:331–7.
86. Fukunaga R, Seto Y, Mizushima S, Nagata S. Three different mRNAs encoding human granulocyte colony-stimulating factor receptor. Proc Natl Acad Sci USA. 1990;87:8702–6.
87. DiStefano PS, Johnson EM. Identification of a truncated form of the nerve growth factor receptor. Proc Natl Acad Sci USA. 1988;85:270–4.
88. Hibi M, Murakami M, Saito M, Hirano T, Taga T, Kishimoto T. Molecular cloning and expression of an IL-6 signal transducer, gp130. Cell. 1990;264:14927–34.
89. Fanslow WC, Sims JE, Sassenfeld H, Morrissey PJ, Gillis S, Dower SK, Widmer MB. Regulation of alloreactivity *in vivo* by a soluble form of the interleukin-1 receptor. Science. 1990;248:739–42.
90. Chopra RK, Powers DC, Kendig NE, Adler WH, Nagel JE. Soluble interleukin-2 receptors released from mitogen stimulated human peripheral blood lymphocytes bind interleukin-2 and inhibit IL-2 dependent cell proliferation. Immunol Invest. 1989;18:961–73.
91. Dower SK, Smith CA, Park LS. Human cytokine receptors. J Clin Immunol. 1990;10:289–99.
92. Loetscher H, Gentz R, Zulauf M, Lustig A, Tabuchi H, Schlaeger EJ, Brockhaus M, Gallati H, Manneberg M, Lesslauer W. Recombinant 55-kDa tumor necrosis factor (TNF) receptor. Stoichiometry of binding to TNF alpha and TNF beta and inhibition of TNF activity. J Biol Chem. 1991;266:18324–9.
93. Eastgate JA, Symons JA, Duff GW. Identification of an interleukin-1 beta binding protein in human plasma. FEBS Lett. 1990;260:213–16.

94. Tsudo M, Kozak RW, Goldman CK, Waldman TA. Demonstration of a non-Tac peptide that binds interleukin 2: a potential participant in multichain interleukin 2 receptor complex. Proc Natl Acad Sci. 1986;83:9694–8.
95. Sharon M, Klausner RD, Cullen BR, Chizzonite R, Leonard WJ. Novel interleukin-2 receptor subunit detected by crosslinking under high-affinity conditions. Science. 1986;234:859–63.
96. Teshigawara K, Wang, Kato K, Smith SA. Interleukin 2 high-affinity receptor expression requires two distinct binding proteins. J Exp Med. 1986;165:223–38.
97. Fujii M, Sogamura K, Sabno K, Nakai M, Sugita K, Hinuma Y. High-affinity receptor-mediated internalization and degradation of interleukin 2 in human T-cells. J Exp Med. 1986;163:550–62.
98. Rubin LA, Galli F, Greene WC, Nelson DL, Jay G. The molecular basis for the generation of the human soluble interleukin 2 receptor. Cytokine. 1990;2:330–6.
99. Loughnan MS, Sanderson CJ, Nossal GJ. Soluble interleukin 2 receptors are released from the cell surface of normal murine B lymphocytes stimulated with interleukin 5. Proc Natl Acad Sci USA. 1988;85:3115–19.
100. Donati D, Degiannis D, Homer L, Gastaldi L, Raskova J, Raska K Jr. Immune deficience in uremia: interleukin-2 production and responsiveness and interleukin-2 receptor expression and release. Nephron. 1991;58:268–75.
101. Lissoni P, Tisi , Brivio F, Barni S, Rovelli F, Perego M, Tancini G. Increase in soluble interleukin-2 receptor and neopterin serum levels during immunotherapy of cancer with interleukin-2. Eur J Cancer. 1991;27:1014–6.
102. Brynskov J, Zvede N. Plasma interleukin-2 and a soluble/shed interleukin-2 receptor in serum of patients with Crohn's disease. Effect of cyclosporin. Gut. 1990;31:795–9.
103. Crabtree JE, Juby LD, Heatley RV, Lobo AJ, Bullimore DW, Axon ATR. Soluble interleukin-2 receptor in Crohn's disease: relation of serum concentration in disease activity. Gut. 1987;28:474–81.
104. Duclos B, Reimund JM, Lang JM, Coumaros G, Lehr L, Chamouard P. Elevated levels of soluble interleukin-2-receptors in Crohn's disease. Gastroenterol Clin Biol. 1990;14:104–5.
105. Mahida YR, Gallagher A, Kurlak L, Hawkey CJ. Plasma and tissue interleukin-2 receptor levels in inflammatory bowel disease. Clin Exp Immunol. 1990;82:75–80.
106. Mueller C, Knoflach P, Zielinski CC. T-cell activation in Crohn's disase. Increased levels of soluble interleukin-2 receptors in serum and in supernatants of stimulated peripheral blood mononuclear cells. Gastroenterology. 1990;98:639–46.
107. Schreiber S, Raedler A, Conn AR, Rombeau JL, MacDermott RP. Increased *in vitro* release of soluble interleukin 2 receptor by colonic lamina propria mononuclear cells in inflammatory bowel disease. Gut. 1992;33:236–41.
108. Brynskov J, Tvede N, Andersen CB, Vilien M. Increased concentrations of interleukin 1β, interleukin-2, and soluble interleukin-2 receptors in endoscopical mucosal biopsy specimens with active inflammatory bowel disease. Gut. 1992;33:55–8.
109. Goebell H. Different activity indices in Crohn's disease and their possible role. In: Goebell H, Peskar BM, Malchow H, editors. Inflammatory bowel diseases – basic research and clinical implications. Lancaster: MTP Press; 1988;253–8.
110. Rachmilewitz D. Coated mesalazine (5-amino-salicylic acid) versus suphasalazine in the treatment of active ulcerative colitis: a randomized trial. Br Med J. 1989;298:82–6.
111. Best WR, Becktel JM, Singelton JW, Kern F. Development of a Crohn's disease activity index: national co-operative Crohn's disease study. Gastroenterology. 1976;70:439–44.
112. Loetscher H, Schlaeger EJ, Lahm HW, Pan Y-CE, Lesslauer W, Brockhaus M. Purification and partial amino acid sequence analysis of two distinct tumor necrosis factor receptors from HL60 cells. J Biol Chem. 1990;265:20131–8.
113. Seckinger P, Isaaz S, Dayer J-M. Purification and biologic characterization of a specific tumor necrosis factor inhibitor. J Biol Chem. 1989;265:11966–73.
114. Aderka D, Engelmann H, Maor Y, Brakebysch C, Wallach D. Stabilization of the bioactivity of tumor necrosis factor by its soluble receptors. J Exp Med. 1992;175:323–9.
115. Mohler KM, Torrance DT, Young DM, Callis G, Roux ER, Jacobs CA. Immunotherapeutic potential of soluble cytokine receptors in inflammatory disease. FASEB J. 1992;6:A1086 (abstract).
116. Zachoval R, Spengler U, Gallati H, Jung MC, Hoffmann R, Zwiebel F, Pape GR,

Paumgartner G, Deinhardt F, Lösliche Tumor Nekrose Faktor Rezeptoren bei Virushepatitis während spontaner Auscheilung und unter Interferon Therapie. Z Gastroenterol. 1992;30:57 (abstract).

117. Andus T, Gross V, Holstege A, Ott M, Weber M, David M, Gallati H, Gerok W, Schölmerich J. High concentations of soluble tumor necrosis factor receptors in ascites. Hepatology. 1992;16:749–55.

118. Mazzei GJ, Seckinger PL, Dayer JM, Shaw AR. Purification and characterisation of a 26 kDa competitive inhibitor of interleukin 1. Eur J Immunol. 1990;20:683–9.

119. Carter DB, Deibel MR, Dunn CJ, Tomich CSC, Laborde AL, Slightom JL, Berger AE, Bienkowski MJ, Sun FF, McEwan RN, Harris PKW, Yem AW, Waszak GA, Chosay JG, Sieu LC, Hardee MM, Zurcher-Neely HA, Reardon IM, Heinrikson RL, Truesdell SE, Shelly JA, Eessalu TE, Taylor BM, Tracy DE. Purification, cloning, expression and biological characterisation of an interleukin-1 receptor antagonist protein. Nature. 1990;344:633–8.

120. Eisenberg SP, Evans RJ, Arend WP, Verderber E, Brewer MT, Hannum CH, Thompson RC. Primary structure and functional expression from complementary DNA of a human interleukin-1 receptor antagonist. Nature. 1990;343:341–6.

121. Hannum CH, Wilcox CJ, Arewnd WP, Joslin FG, Dripps BJ, Heimdal PL, Armes LG, Sommer A, Eisenberg SP, Thompson RC. Interleukin-1 receptor antagonist activity of a human interleukin-1 inhibitor. Nature. 1990;343:336–94.

122. Dinarello CA, Thompson RC. Block IL-1: interleukin 1 receptor antagonist *in vivo* and *in vitro*. Immunol Today. 1991;12:404–10.

123. Cominelli F, Nast CC, Clark BD, Schindler R, Ilerana R, Eysselein VE, Thompson RC, Dinarello CA. Interleukin-1 (IL-1) gene expression, synthesis, and effect of specific IL-1 receptor blockade in rabbit immune complex colitis. J Clin Invest. 1990;86:972–80.

124. Sartor RB, Holt LC, Bender DE, Murphy ME, McCall RD, Thompson RC. Prevention and treatment of experimental enterocolitis with a recombinant interleukin-1 receptor antagonist. Gastroenterology. 1991;100:A613.

125. Arend WP, Welgus HG, Thompson RC, Eisenberg SP. Biological properties of recombinant human monocyte-derived interleukin 1 receptor antagonist. J Clin Invest. 1990;85:1694–7.

126. Biekowski MJ, Eessalu TE, Berger AE, Truesdell SE, Shelly JA, Laborde AL, Zurcher-Neely HA, Reardon IM, Heinrikson RL, Chosay JG *et al*. Purification and characterization of interleukin-1 receptor level antagonist proteins from THP-1 cells. J Biol Chem. 1990;265:14505–11.

127. Arend WP, Smith MF Jr, Janson RW, Joslin FG. IL-1 receptor antagonist and IL-1 beta production in human monocytes are regulated differently. J Immunol. 1991;147:1530–6.

128. Poutsiaka DD, Clark BD, Vannier E, Dinarello CA. Production of interleukin-1 receptor antagonist and interleukin-1 beta by peripheral blood mononuclear cells is differentially regulated. Blood. 1991;78:1275–81.

129. Matsushime H, Roussel MF, Matsushima K, Hishinuma A, Sherr CJ. Cloning and expression of murine interleukin-1 receptor antagonist in macrophages stimulated by colony-stimulating factor 1. Blood. 1991;78:616–23.

130. Turner M, Chantry D, Katsikis P, Berger A, Brennan FM, Feldmann M. Induction of the interleukin 1 receptor antagonist protein by transforming growth factor-beta. Eur J Immunol. 1991;21:1635–9.

131. Ju G, Labriola-Tompkins E, Campen CA, Benjamin WR, Karas J, Plocinski J, Biondi D, Kaffka KL, Kilian PL, Eisenberg SP. Conversion of the interleukin 1 receptor antagonist into an agonist by site-specific mutagenesis. Proc Natl Acad Sci USA. 1991;88:2658–62.

132. Brynskov J, Hansen MB, Reimert C, Bendtzen K. Inhibitor of interleukin-1α and interleukin-1β-induced T-cell activation in serum of patients with active Crohn's disease. Dig Dis Sci. 1991;36:737–742.

133. McCall RD, Haskill JS, Sartor RB. Interleukin-1 and IL-1 receptor antagonist gene expression correlate with activity of inflammation in spontaneously relapsing enterocolitis in rats. Gastroenterology. 1991;100:A598.

134. Cominelli F, Fiocchi C, Eisenberg SP, Bortolami M. Imbalance of IL-1 and IL-1 receptor antagonist synthesis in the intestinal mucosa of Crohn's disease and ulcerative colitis patients: a novel pathogenetic mechanism. Gastroenterology. 1992;102:A609.

13
Sensory neuropeptides: inflammation and tissue healing

V. E. EYSSELEIN, M. REINSHAGEN AND A. PATEL

INTRODUCTION

The sensory nervous system plays a pivotal role in maintaining the integrity of the body in response to injury. The afferent function of the sensory nervous system – transmission of information about site and kind of injury to the central nervous system – is well recognized; however the efferent function is less well understood. Enhancement of the inflammatory tissue response after injury (termed 'neurogenic inflammation') and promotion of tissue healing are examples of the efferent function. The fact that in sensory nerve fibres the majority of sensory neuropeptides is transported to the periphery[1] underlines the importance of the efferent function of sensory nerves. The 'trophic' action of sensory neuropeptides on peripheral tissues represents a particular form of efferent function. It is hypothesized that the sensory nervous system operates tonically in a way that sensory stimuli produce a continuous outflow of signalling molecules whose action maintains the integrity of the tissue[2,3].

There are several examples of neurogenic inflammation. In the eye, electrical stimulation of the trigeminal nerves causes an inflammatory reaction[4-6] which is predominantly mediated by two released neuropeptides, substance P and calcitonin gene-related peptide (CGRP)[4-9]. Similar actions of sensory nerves have been described in the skin where the release of the sensory neuropeptides SP and CGRP results in a long-lasting wheal (oedema due to increased vascular permeability) and spreading flare (vasodilation via antidromic axon reflexes) response which occurs in response to irritation or trauma[10-13]. A proinflammatory action of sensory nerves seems also to be present during joint inflammation[14-16].

As mentioned, sensory nerve stimulation results not only in neurogenic inflammation but seems also to be important for tissue protection after injury. To study the function of sensory nerves, capsaicin (8-methyl-*N*-vanillyl-6-nonenamide), the major pungent ingredient of hot peppers of the plant genus *Capsicum*, has been used in many studies[17]. Capsaicin is a neurotoxin specific for small-diameter sensory nerves and causes first acute depletion of the nerve terminals followed by functional damage in adult rats and guinea pigs[2,3,17–20]. When capsaicin is administered in neonatal rats, permanent sensory nerve damage occurs. Rats treated as newborns by the sensory neurotoxin capsaicin show signs of cutaneous lesions and dystrophia[21]. Disturbed wound healing of the cornea has been demonstrated after sensory denervation in experimental animals[22,23]. Proliferation of basal layer epithelial cells and the normal geometry of cell renewal were severely impaired after capsaicin pretreatment[23]. Decreased wound healing of skin–muscle flaps was observed in capsaicin-pretreated rats[24]. In rat lungs, capsaicin pretreatment depleted substance P, a peptide found in a high proportion of sensory nerve fibres, and these animals exhibited a markedly higher pulmonary injury (bronchial epithelial cell exfoliation and ulceration) and mortality in response to pulmonary injury by hydrogen sulphide than control animals[25].

The phenomenon of neurogenic inflammation induced by sensory neurones seems to be contradictory to their wound healing promoting action. However, it is conceivable that sensory nerves are needed to defend injury of any kind first by modulating an inflammatory response which is needed for the subsequent healing process[3]. An inflammatory response is needed for subsequent wound healing. An imbalance between the inflammatory response and the healing promoting action of sensory nerves may lead to chronic inflammation.

The mechanisms and mediators of the wound healing promoting action of sensory nerves are poorly understood. As mentioned above, an inflammatory response seems to be necessary as a first defence mechanism. Sensory nerves presumably play a role in this phase. Important factors for subsequent healing supposedly include blood flow[3] and proliferation of connective tissue cells and epithelial cells[26]. Sensory nerves have a potent vasodilatory action[3]. Substance P is one important mediator of this effect. CGRP is colocalized with substance P in a majority of sensory nerve fibres[20] and co-released[4,5] with substance P upon sensory nerve stimulation. It potentiates the vasodilatory action of substance P resulting in the skin in a long-lasting erythema[13]. In the eye, substance P and CGRP can account for most of the changes seen after sensory nerve stimulation[4,6,7,9]

In the gastrointestinal tract, the function of sensory nerves during inflammation and tissue healing is poorly understood. The extrinsic nervous system of the gut is responsible for transmission of sensory stimuli[18]. The peripheral axons of the extrinsic sensory neurones, located in the dorsal root ganglia, reach the intestine via the mesenteric nerves passing through the prevertebral ganglia (where axon collaterals exist) and terminating at all layers of the gut, predominantly supplying blood vessels (for review see ref. 18). Central axons reach the dorsal horn of the spinal cord. Polysynaptic connections and interneurones exist within the central nervous system which may allow pain sensations to be transmitted from the periphery to the motoneurone system, the sympathetic and the higher brain centres. CGRP is expressed in a large population of sensory neurones supplying the gut which also contain substance P[20]. The cell bodies of these neurones are located mostly in the dorsal root ganglia and to much lower extent in the nodose ganglia of the vagus[27,28]. A good proportion of CGRP afferents innervating the gut also express substance P[27,28]. Sensory nerve fibres within the vagus seem not to be involved in the sensory innervation of the distal colon as shown by retrograde tracing experiments in the rat[27]. In the intrinsic enteric nervous system CGRP is synthesized in distinct cell bodies within the myenteric and submucosal plexus along the entire length of the gut. Interestingly, the intrinsic neurones seem to be not sensitive to capsaicin[2]. CGRP and SP fibres originating from intrinsic neurones in the myenteric and submucous plexus supply also the mucosa–submucosa[29]. It is not known whether CGRP released from intrinsic neurones can alter inflammatory reactions in the mucosal/submucosal layers.

Capsaicin has been used to unravel the function of sensory nerves in the gastrointestinal tract. Capsaicin given either parenterally[19] in neonatal rats, or applied topically to sensory nerve fibres in the prevertebral ganglia supplying the gut[30], reduces CGRP immunoreactivity in the stomach by up to 95%, and this decrease is due to loss of sensory nerve fibres containing CGRP. Capsaicin-sensitive sensory nerves have a protective function in experimental rat gastric ulcer models[31], and there is evidence that CGRP is the mediator by its potent vasodilatory action[32]. It thus appears that the sensory neuropeptide CGRP is an important mediator of the protective effect of sensory nerves in experimentally induced gastric ulcers. It is not known whether CGRP has a protective action also in the small and large intestine. Available data on the action of sensory nerves on healing of intestinal ulcerations are controversial. Evangelista et al.[33] used a rat hypersensitivity model of colitis (induced by rectal enemas containing trinitrobenzene sulphonic acid) to show that healing was considerably impaired 1 week after induction of colitis in animals whose sensory nervous system was functionally destroyed by the sensory neurotoxin capsaicin. When acetic acid was given to induce acute colitis there was no difference between capsaicin-pretreated animals and controls[33]. No data are available on the function of sensory nerves during chronic inflammation.

STUDIES IN ANIMALS WITH EXPERIMENTAL COLITIS

Content of substance P and CGRP in colon layers before and after induction of colitis

These studies were designed to answer the question whether sensory neuropeptides (substance P and CGRP) are released during inflammation. We hypothesized that a rapid decrease of substance P and CGRP in the colon layers after induction of colitis would indicate release of these neuropeptides from nerve fibres.

Acute colitis was induced in rabbits using a formalin–immune complex model as described by us[34,35]. Briefly, anaesthetized rabbits received 4 ml of 0.6% (v/v) formalin as rectal enema followed by i.v. administration of 1 ml immune complex 1 h later. Animals were sacrificed at various time points after induction of inflammation (see Table 1) and colonic tissue was obtained for histology to determine the inflammatory index (amount of neutrophil infiltration) and percentage necrosis, for radioimmunoassay to determine substance P and CGRP contents, and for substance P and CGRP immunohistochemistry. Formalin enemas combined with i.v. administration of immune complex induced an ulcerative colitis, which was predominantly limited to the mucosal–submucosal layers. The inflammatory index rose significantly after 4 h and reached a maximum after 24 h (Table 1). Mild mucosal necrosis was seen in some animals 4 h after induction of inflammation; severe mucosal–submucosal necrosis was evident after 24 h. The contents of immunoreactive CGRP decreased in a time-dependent fashion in the colonic extracts after induction of inflammation (Table 1). The decrease in immunoreactive CGRP was significant after only 4 h and reached a maximum 48 h after induction of inflammation. Immunoreactive CGRP decreased both in extracts of the mucosal–submucosal and muscle layers of the inflamed colon. There was also a time-dependent substance P decrease in the muscle layer (Table 1). Amounts of substance P in the mucosal–submucosal layer were too low for accurate measurements.

Immunohistochemical studies demonstrated that CGRP immunoreactivities are present in intrinsic neurones and nerve fibres distributed to all layers of the colon in both control and experimental animals[35]. In normal colon, CGRP-containing fibres were numerous in enteric plexus and in association with the vasculature. A moderate density of fibres was found in the mucosa, sometimes forming discrete networks towards the luminal aspect. Occasionally, small bundles of fibres were seen running through the muscle layers; usually a few fibres were present within the smooth muscle. In inflamed colon the CGRP innervation patterns were comparable to those described for the normal colon; however, there was a decrease in both the density and intensity of the staining at 48 h after induction of inflammation[35]. Substance

Table 1 Inflammatory parameters and concentrations† of immunoreactive substance P and calcitonin gene-related peptide (CGRP) in colitis tissue layers

| | | | | CGRP | |
| | *Inflammatory* | *Necrosis* | *Substance P* | | |
Hours	*index*	*%*	*Muscle*	*Muscle*	*Mucosa–submucosa*
0‡	0.7 ± 0.1	0 ± 0	8.6 ± 2.2	9.9 ± 1.5	10.7 ± 1.6
4	$1.9 \pm 0.4^*$	$11 \pm 6^*$	4.8 ± 1.6	$4.4 \pm 1.0^*$	$6.7 \pm 0.5^*$
8	$2.6 \pm 0.2^*$	$14 \pm 10^*$	6.5 ± 0.5	$5.0 \pm 0.9^*$	$4.3 \pm 1.2^*$
12	$2.2 \pm 0.4^*$	$13 \pm 7^*$	$3.4 \pm 0.9^*$	$3.2 \pm 0.9^*$	$5.7 \pm 0.6^*$
24	$2.2 \pm 0.5^*$	$49 \pm 13^*$	$1.9 \pm 1.1^*$	$2.0 \pm 1.1^*$	$2.7 \pm 1.4^*$
48	$2.6 \pm 0.5^*$	$18 \pm 6^*$	$3.2 \pm 0.7^*$	$1.9 \pm 0.4^*$	$2.1 \pm 0.6^*$

Results are means $\pm$ SE; $n = 4$ for 4–24 h, $n = 15$ for 48 h; $^*p < 0.05$
†Concentrations are expressed in nmol/g tissue protein
‡Controls

P immunoreactivity was predominantly present in the muscle layer and was descreased 48 h after incution of colitis[35].

These studies show that CGRP and substance P contents decrease early in the colon during development of colitis. We assume that release of CGRP during inflammation leads to diminished neuropeptide content in the nerve fibres. Toxic damage to the neurones cannot be excluded. However, when we determined the mRNA for another neuropeptide, substance P, in intrinsic neurones of the gut or in the dorsal root ganglia no decrease in message was detected 48 h after induction of colitis, indicating that the neurones were still viable[36].

Effect of sensory denervation on severity of colitis

Studies in the acute rabbit immune complex model

Capsaicin was dissolved in 10% ethanol (v/v), 10% Tween 80 (v/v) in 0.9% NaCl, resulting in a final concentration of 1% capsaicin. Capsaicin or vehicle was given subcutaneously to anaesthetized adult rabbits weighing 2–2.5 kg. The animals received 25, 50, 50 and 75 mg twice on the first, second, third and fourth day, respectively. On the first and second day the animals received, 15 min prior to the capsaicin treatment, atropine (0.2 mg/kg), benadryl (5 mg/kg), isoproterenol (20 µg/kg) and theophylline (1 mg/kg) given intramuscularily to reduce the side-effects of capsaicin (bronchoconstriction, hypotension). After capsaicin treatment of the adult rabbits the blepharospasm after instillation of one drop 0.1 N NaOH into one rabbit eye was completely abolished, and the inflammatory reaction in the conjunctiva and the wiping reflex were markedly diminished. These *in vivo* tests were used to assure that sufficient amounts of capsaicin had been administered. In addition, the immunoreactive CGRP content in extracts of the dorsal root ganglia (L4–S3) was determined in capsaicin-treated animals and controls. After capsaicin pretreatment CGRP decreased by about 50% in these extracts.

In a pilot study we investigated whether capsaicin treatment alone caused inflammation or ulcerations in the intestine. We showed in six animals that 5 days after the capsaicin pretreatment no inflammation or ulcerations were present as determined by histology.

Colitis was induced 5 days after completion of the capsaicin treatment. Formalin was given in a concentration of 0.4% followed by 0.85 ml immune complex causing a moderate colitis. The inflammatory response in the colonic tissue was investigated 48 and 96 h after induction of colitis in capsaicin-pretreated animals and in controls who received only the vehicle ($n = 6$, each group). The animals were sacrificed by an overdose of pentobarbital. The distal colon was removed and cut along the longitudinal axis. The severity of the colitis was determined macroscopically using a damage index: 10 cm of the distal colon were evaluated. A scale of 1 to 5 was used to quantitate percentage oedema, erosions and ulcerations in this area. Oedema: $1 = <50\%$, $2 = >50\%$; erosions: $1 = <25\%$, $2 = <50\%$, $3 = <75\%$, $4 = >75\%$; ulcerations: $3 = <25\%$, $4 = <50\%$, $5 = <75\%$, $6 = >75\%$. Representative longitudinal sections of the distal colon were obtained for histology.

As previously reported[37], the macroscopic damage score was, 48 h after induction of colitis, 8.33 ± 0.3 in the capsaicin-pretreated group and 3.2 ± 0.8 in the controls group, respectively (Fig. 1). By histology (Fig. 1), $63 \pm 13\%$ ulcerations were seen in the capsaicin-pretreated group, but only $3 \pm 3\%$ in the control group (means $\pm$ SE, $n = 6$). The inflammatory index was also significantly ($p < 0.05$) increased in the capsaicin-pretreated group (4.3 ± 0.7 vs 1.8 ± 0.5, respectively). When the animals were studied 96 h after induction of colitis, macroscopic damage score, ulcerations and inflammatory index were still higher in the capsaicin-pretreated group compared to the control group, being 3.4 ± 0.7 vs 0.8 ± 0.4, 20 ± 8.4 vs 1.5 ± 1.1, and 2.6 ± 0.6 vs 1.7 ± 0.3, respectively.

These results indicate that capsaicin pretreatment increases the severity of the ulcerating colitis. Diminished defence and impaired healing might be the result of sensory denervation of the intestine.

Studies in the chronic rat TNB colitis model

Since it was not known whether sensory nerves participate in tissue healing during chronic inflammation, the rat TNB model was used to study the effect of sensory denervation on colitis. Sensory denervation was achieved by pretreatment with capsaicin (125 mg/kg s.c.). Immunohistochemistry for substance P and CGRP showed a marked decrease in the dorsal root ganglia compared to vehicle-treated rats. In the trachea, substance P content decreased by 90%, and in the stomach, where CGRP fibres are predominantly of extrinsic origin, CGRP content decreased by over 95% compared to controls. These data showed that the capsaicin treatment was effective. Colitis was induced 1 week after capsaicin or vehicle pretreatment by giving trinitrobenze sulphonic acid (TNB) (50 mg/kg in 50% ethanol) as enema. Groups of six rats were studied 1 and 3 weeks after induction of colitis. Interestingly, 1 week after induction of colitis the severity (macroscopic damage score) was increased by 100% in the capsaicin-pretreated animals compared to the controls, and inflammation, determined by myeloperoxidase index, was also more severe (by 50%) in the capsaicin-treated group. In contrast to the 1-week study, 3 weeks after induction of colitis there was no

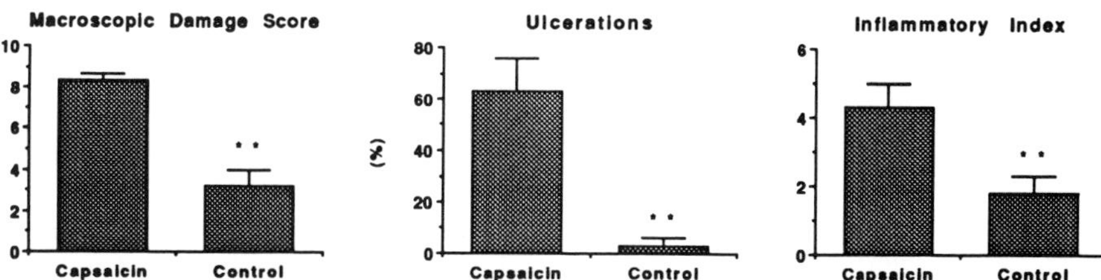

Fig. 1   Effect of capsaicin pretreatment on severity of experimental colitis. Macroscopic damage score, percentage necrosis (by histology) and inflammatory index (by histology) in animals pretreated with capsaicin were compared to control animals which received only the vehicle ($n = 6$, each). Colitis, induced in rabbits with formalin immune complex, was studied 48 h after induction of inflammation

difference in macroscopic damage score and inflammation between the capsaicin-pretreated and the vehicle group.

These data indicate that sensory nerves have a protective and healing promoting function during the acute phase of inflammation (1 week). During chronic inflammation (3 weeks) other factors (e.g. growth factors) may be more important for tissue healing. Indeed, in the chronic rat TNB model we could improve healing at 3 weeks by epidermal growth factor administered s.c.[38].

POSSIBLE IMPLICATIONS FOR INFLAMMATORY BOWEL DISEASE

The strongest evidence that sensory nerves containing substance P could participate in the inflammatory reactions in patients with IBD is presented by Mantyh *et al.*, who showed that binding sites for substance P are highly up-regulated around small blood vessels in the inflamed intestine of patients with IBD compared to controls[39,40]. Interestingly, lymph nodules also contained high binding sites, suggesting that substance P may interact with the immune system. It can be hypothesized that increased substance P binding sites during inflammation indicate enhanced tissue responsiveness to substance P. Tissue concentrations of sensory neuropeptides in inflamed tissues do not provide sufficient evidence for neuropeptide actions. It is difficult to study sensory neuropeptide actions in patients with IBD since no reagents are available altering sensory nerve function which could be used in humans. *In vitro* data suggest that substance P could act as a proinflammatory neuropeptide at neutrophils, macrophages, B- and T-cells. However, no *in vivo* data supporting the concepts obtained *in vitro* are available. Whether sensory nerves have also a protective and healing promoting action *in vivo* in humans as shown in our animal studies is unknown. Substance P stimulates *in vitro* fibroblasts and smooth muscle cells[26], thereby possibly inducing tissue healing. Substance P could also stimulate tissue healing by release of interleukin-1 (IL-1) from macrophages (see above). IL-1 could then up-regulate the receptors for epidermal growth factor on epithelial cells. We have previously shown that IL-1 up-regulates epidermal growth factor receptors on human colonic T84 cells *in vitro*[41], a growth factor shown to improve healing in our colitis model[38]. Thus, interactions between sensory neuropeptides, cytokines and growth factors during inflammation and tissue healing are likely to occur.

SUMMARY AND CONCLUSIONS

The action of sensory nerves on inflammation and tissue healing varies between different organ systems. In the skin, the eyes and the joints sensory nerves promote an inflammatory response via induction of 'neurogenic inflammation'. In the gut, the protective function of sensory nerves seems to be predominant. During the acute phase after tissue injury, sensory nerves protect the tissue, possibly by increasing the blood flow at the site of injury. CGRP, released from sensory nerve endings, may be at least in rabbits and rats the responsible mediator for this action. Sensory nerves may not only be protective but may also participate in subsequent tissue healing after injury. Again, increased blood flow and stimulation of tissue growth could account for this action. Interactions between sensory nerves, inflammatory mediators and growth factors during these processes are postulated to exist. In IBD, sensory nerves may modulate the inflammatory process since the inflamed intestine could be more responsive to substance P due to up-regulation of its binding site near blood vessels and lymph nodules.

We hypothesize that the action of sensory nerves depends on the cells present, and modulation of inflammation and tissue healing are key features of sensory nerve actions. To unravel the multiple interactions between sensory neuropeptides, inflammatory mediators, the immune system and growth factors will be a challenging task for the future.

References

1. Brimijoin S, Lundberg JM, Brodin E, Hoekfelt T, Nilsson G. Axonal transport of substance P in the vagus and sciatic nerves of the guinea pig. Brain Res. 1980;191:443–57.
2. Maggi CA, Meli A. The sensory–efferent function of capsaicin-sensitive sensory neurons. Gen Pharmacol. 1988;19:1–43.
3. Holzer P. Local effector functions of capsaicin-sensitive sensory nerve endings: involvement of tachykinins, calcitonin gene-related peptide and other neuropeptides. Neuroscience. 1988;24:739–68.
4. Wahlestedt C, Beding B, Ekaman R, Oksala O, Stiernschantz J, Hakanson R. Calcitonin gene-related peptide in the eye: release by sensory nerve stimulation and effects associated with neurogenic inflammation. Regul Pept. 1986;16:107–15.
5. Bill A, Stjernschantz J, Mandahl A, Brodin E, Nilsson G. Substance P release on trigeminal nerve stimulation, effects in the eye. Acta Physiol Scand. 1979;106:371–3.
6. Stiernschantz J, Sears M, Mishima H. Role of substance P in the antidromic vasodilatation, neurogenic plasma extravasation and disruption of the blood-aqueous barrier in the rabbit eye. Naunyn-Schmiedebergs Arch Pharmacol. 1982;321:329–35.
7. Holmdahl R, Hakanson R, Leander S, Rosell S, Folkers K, Sundler F. A substance P antagonist (D-Pro2,D-Trp7,9), SP, inhibits inflammatory responses in the rabbit eye. Nature. 1981;214:1029–31.
8. Camras CB, Bito LZ. The pathophysiological effects of nitrogen mustard on the rabbit eye. II. The inhibition of the initial hypertensive phase by capsaicin and the apparent role of substance P. Invest Ophthalmol Vis Sci. 1980;19:423–8.
9. Krootila K. CGRP in relation to neurogenic inflammation and cAMP in the rabbit eye. Exp Eye Res. 1988;47:307–16.
10. Haegermark Oe, Hoekfelt T, Pernow P. Flare and itch induced by substance P in human skin. J Invest Dermatol. 1978;71:233.
11. Brain SD, Williams TJ. Substance P regulates the vasodilator activity of calcitonin gene-related peptide. Nature. 1988;335:73–5.
12. Foremann JC. Substance P and calcitonin gene-related peptide: effects on mast cells and in human skin. Int Arch Allergy Appl Immunol. 1987;82:366–71.
13. Gamse R, Saria A. Potentiation of tachykinin-induced plasma protein extravasation by calcitonin gene-related peptide. Eur J Pharmacol. 1985;114:61–6.
14. Levine JD, Clark R, Devor M, Helms C, Moskowitz MA, Basbaum AI. Intraneuronal substance P contributes to the severity of experimental arthritis. Science. 1984;226:547–9.
15. Devillier P, Weill B, Renoux M, Menkes C, Pradelles P. Elevated levels of tachykinin-like immunoreactivity in joint fluids from patients with rheumatic inflammatory diseases. N Engl J Med. 1987;314:1323.

16. Inman RD, Chiu B, Rabinovich S, Marshall W. Neuromodulation of synovitis: capsaicin effect on severity of experimental arthritis. J Neuroimmunol. 1989;24:17–22.
17. Buck S, Burks T. The neuropharmacology of capsaicin: review of some recent observations. Pharmacol Rev. 1986;38:179–226.
18. Pernow B. Substance P. Pharmacol Rev. 1983;35:85–141.
19. Sternini C, Reeve JR Jr, Brecha N. Distribution and characterization of calcitonin gene related peptide immunoreactivity in the digestive system of normal and capsaicin-treated rats. Gastroenterology. 1987;93:852–62.
20. Gibbins IL, Furness JB, Costa M, MacIntyre I, Hillyard CJ, Girgis S. Colocalization of calcitonin gene-related peptide-like immunoreactivity with substance P in cutaneous, vascular and visceral sensory neurons of guinea pigs. Neurosci Lett. 1985;57:125–30.
21. Gamse R, Lachner D, Gamse G, Leeman S. Effect of capsaicin pretreatment on capsaicin-evoked release of immunoreactive somatostatin and substance P from primary sensory neurons. Naunyn Schmiedebergs Arch Pharmacol. 1982;316:38–41.
22. Beuerman RW, Schimmelpfennig B. Sensory denervation of the rabbit cornea affects epithelial properties. Exp Neurol. 1980;69:196–201.
23. Fujita S, Shimizu T, Izumi K, Fukuda T, Sameshima M, Ohba N. Capsaicin-induced neuroparalytic keratitis-like corneal changes in the mouse. Exp Eye Res. 1984;38:165–75.
24. Kjartansson J, Dalsgaard C-J, Jonsson C-E. Decreased survival of experimental critical flaps in rats after sensory denervation with capsaicin. Plastic Reconstr Surg. 1987;79:218–21.
25. Prior M, Green F, Lopez A, Balu A, DeSanctis GT, Fick G. Capsaicin pretreatment modifies hydrogen sulphide-induced pulmonary injury in rats. Toxicol Pharmacol. 1990;18:279–88.
26. Nilsson J, von Euler AM, Dalsgaard C-J. Stimulation of connective tissue cell growth by substance P and substance K. Nature. 1985;315:61–3.
27. Su HC, Bishop AE, Power RF, Hamada Y, Polak JM. Dual intrinsic and extrinsic origins of CGRP- and NPY-immunoreactive nerves of rat gut and pancreas. J Neurosci. 1987;7:2674–87.
28. Sternini C. Neurochemistry of spinal afferent supplying the gastrointestinal tract and pancreas. In: Tache Y, Wingate D, editors. Brain and gut interactions. Boca Raton, FL: CRC Press (In press).
29. Costa M, Furness JB, Llewellyn-Smith IJ. Histochemistry of the enteric nervous system. In: Johnson LR, editor. Physiology of the gastrointestinal tract. New York: Raven Press; 1986;1–40.
30. Raybould HE, Holzer P, Eysselein VE, Sternini C. Selective ablation of spinal sensory neurons containing CGRP inhibits the increase in rat gastric mucosal blood flow due to acid back-diffusion. Gastroenterology. 1990;94:A198.
31. Holzer P, Pabst MA, Lippe ITh. Intragastric capsaicin protects against aspirin-induced lesion formation and bleeding in the rat gastric mucosa. Gastroenterology. 1989;96:1425–33.
32. Lippe ITh, Holzer P. Close arterial infusion of calcitonin gene-related peptide into the rat stomach inhibits aspirin- and ethanol-induced hemorrhagic damage. Regul Pept. 1989;26:35–46.
33. Evangelista S, Meli A. Influence of capsaicin-sensitive fibres on experimentally-induced colitis in rats. J Pharm Pharmacol. 1989;41:574–5.
34. Cominelli F, Nast CC, Clark BD, Schindler R, Llerena R, Eysselein VE, Thompson RC, Dinarello ChA. Interleukin-1 (IL-1) gene expression, synthesis, and effect of specific IL-1 receptor blockade in rabbit immune complex colitis. J Clin Invest. 1990;86:972–80.
35. Eysselein VE, Reinshagen M, Cominelli F, Sternini C, Davis W, Patel A, Nast CC, Bernstein D, Anderson K, Khan H, Snape WJ, Jr. Calcitonin gene-related peptide and substance P decrease in rabbit colon during colitis: a time study. Gastroenterology. 1991;101:1211–19.
36. Reinshagen M, Patel A, Sottili M, Davis W, Eysselein VE. Regulation of substance P gene expression in experimental colitis. Gastroenterology. 1992;102:A505.
37. Reinshagen M, Patel A, Sottili M, Davis W, Mueller K, Nast C, Sternini C, Eysselein VE. Protective function of extrinsic sensory neurons in the rabbit colon. Gastroenterology. 1992;102:A505.
38. Patel A, Reinshagen M, Sottili M, Cox J, Xie YN, Eysselein VE. A healing role of epidermal growth factor (EGF) in the trinitrobenzenesulfonic acid (TNB) induced chronic colitis. Gastroenterology. 1992;102:A750.

39. Mantyh CR, Gates TS, Zimmermann RP, Welton ML, Passaro EP, Vigna SR, Maggio JE, Kruger L, Mantyh PW. Receptor binding sites for substance P, but not substance K or neuromedin K, are expressed in high concentrations by arterioles, venules, and lymph nodules in surgical specimens obtained from patients with ulcerative colitis and Crohn disease. Proc Natl Acad Sci USA. 1988;85:3235–9.
40. Mantyh PW, Catton MD, Boehmer CG, Welton ML, Passaro EP, Maggio JE, Vigna SR. Receptors for sensory neuropeptides in human inflammatory bowel diseases: implications for the effector role of sensory neurons. Peptides. 1989;10:627–45.
41. Sottili M, McRoberts JA, Reinshagen M, Patel A, Lezoche E, Eysselein VE. Up-regulation of the epidermal growth factor/transforming growth factor-alpha receptor in T84 colonic epithelial cells by interleukin-I beta. Gastroenterology. 1992;102:A758.

14
Regulation of collagen synthesis

A. STALLMACH, H. MATTHES and E. O. RIECKEN

INTRODUCTION

Crohn's disease is a chronic progressive disease of the gastrointestinal tract with an unknown aetiology. It is characterized by transmural inflammation of all layers of the bowel wall. The formation of stenoses and strictures is a common phenomenon in this disease, which causes abdominal pain, anorexia and weight loss. Approximately 50% of Crohn's disease patients undergo surgery for this type of complication during a 10-year course of the disease; however, the recurrence rate after surgery is high. In contrast, ulcerative colitis rarely causes intestinal stenosis[1,2]. Despite the significant morbidity associated with strictures in Crohn's disease, the mechanisms whereby the inflammation leads to stricturing of the intestinal tract are unknown.

Collagen synthesis in fibroblasts is physiologically induced during wound healing or after inflammatory tissue damage. However, inadequate collagen production can lead to fibrosis and severe organ dysfunction. An increased and qualitatively abnormal deposition of collagen type III during the fibrotic process is well documented in different tissues such as liver[3], pancreas[4] and lung[5]. Recent studies suggest that the development of intestinal strictures is frequently associated with altered collagen metabolism, resulting in deposition of interstitial collagens (mainly type III and V, to a lesser extent types I and VI) in the mucosal and muscular layers[6,7].

Cytokines released from inflammatory cells have long been implicated in the pathogenesis of fibrosis. In addition to the ability of cytokines to stimulate proliferation of mesenchymal cells, these mediators can also regulate the synthesis of extracellular matrix components by mesenchymal cells[8]. The literature suggests that many cytokines can alter fibroblast growth and metabolism, while a more limited set plays a role in the induction of fibrosis[9]. Transforming growth factor beta (TGF-β) has been identified as one of the cytokines that specifically induces a fibrotic response. TGF-β exists in several isoforms referred to as TGF-β_1, TGF-β_2 and TGF-$\beta_{1.2}$ (the latter being a heterodimeric protein consisting of either one chain of TGF-β_1 or one of TGF-β_2)[10]. All isoforms of TGF-β exhibit a variety of biological effects that are consistent with their proposed role in tumorigenesis, embryonic development and wound healing. TGF-β_1 has been shown to increase collagen synthesis in several *in vitro* systems[11], including cell cultures of intestinal smooth muscle cells[12]. However, the problem remains as to why inflammation of the intestinal tract leads to the development of segmental strictures in some cases but not in others. We hypothesize that differences in the synthesis or degradation of collagens may be an important factor in the pathogenesis of localized intestinal fibrosis. This report will focus on two major aspects of collagen metabolism in inflammatory bowel disease: (1) analyses of collagen synthesis with regard to state of inflammation and entity of inflammatory bowel disease; (2) investigation of the effect of cytokines on the *in vitro* production of collagens by lamina propria fibroblasts from strictured, non-strictured but inflamed or normal intestinal tissue of patients with inflammatory bowel disease.

COLLAGEN SYNTHESIS IN INFLAMMATORY BOWEL DISEASE

To analyse the synthesis of collagens *in vivo*, we used the method of *in situ* hybridization with single-stranded, [^{35}S]-labelled RNA probes specific for $\alpha_1(I)$, $\alpha_1(III)$, $\alpha_1(IV)$, and $\alpha_2(V)$ procollagen gene transcripts[7]. The aim of the study was to investigate intestinal tissues from patients with Crohn's disease, ulcerative colitis and patients with adenocarcinomas serving as controls.

Low steady-state levels of procollagen mRNA transcripts were present in histological normal intestinal tissues. Transcripts of the interstitial $\alpha_1(I)$, $\alpha_1(III)$, and $\alpha_2(V)$ procollagen, and also of the basement membrane $\alpha_1(IV)$ procollagen genes, were primarily present in lamina propria mesenchymal cells located directly beneath the epithelial layer or in the muscularis mucosae and propria (Fig. 1A). In active Crohn's disease, $\alpha_1(I)$ procollagen gene transcript levels were markedly increased in lamina propria cells. The number of labelled cells was higher than in control tissues and correlated with the cellular density of the inflammatory infiltrate. The $\alpha_1(III)$ and $\alpha_2(V)$ procollagen gene transcripts were colocalized with $\alpha_1(I)$ procollagen mRNA, although signal intensities of the latter were weaker. However, in this respect the lamina muscularis mucosae was unique as $\alpha_1(III)$ and $\alpha_2(V)$ transcripts were increased overproportionally compared to control tissues (Fig. 1B). Crohn's disease specimens hybridized with the $\alpha_1(IV)$ procollagen mRNA antisense probe showed a moderate increase of grains in the lamina propria. In the muscular layer there was an increase of both the signal intensity and the number of cells labelled for procollagen type IV mRNA.

Interestingly, in Crohn's disease the relative increase of $\alpha_1(III)$ transcripts in relation to $\alpha_1(I)$ and $\alpha_2(V)$ transcripts was significantly greater in fibrotic areas or stenoses compared to inflamed specimens (Fig. 1C).

Ulcerative colitis specimens showed highly elevated steady-state levels of $\alpha_1(I)$ procollagen transcripts in the lamina propria, particularly in subepithelial

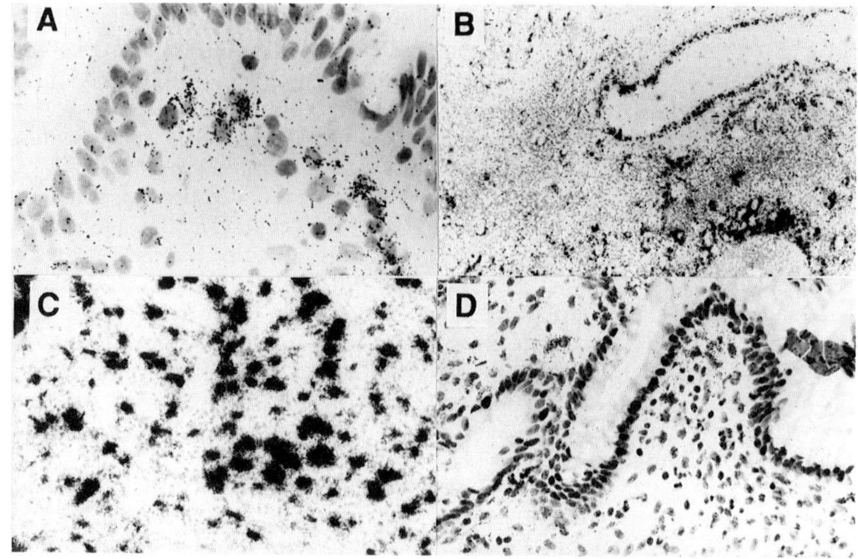

Fig. 1 *In situ* hybridization with [^{35}S]-labelled α_1(III) procollagen anti-sense RNA probe on colonic tissue with mild inflammation (control) (**A**), Crohn's disease (**B, C**), and ulcerative colitis (**D**). In control tissue the autoradiographic signal is mainly restricted to subepithelial mesenchymal cells (**A**). In Crohn's disease, both the number of grains and labelled cells is increased predominantly in the muscularis mucosae and in the muscularis propria (**B**). In a strictured specimen from the ileum of a patient with Crohn's disease, signal intensity and the number of labelled cells are strongly enhanced in the lamina propria compared to inflamed areas. In ulcerative colitis (**D**) the signal intensity and the number of labelled cells are also increased. Exposure times 28 days (**A**), 10 days (**B, C, D**). Original magnification ×400 (**A, B**), ×500 (**C**), and ×800 (**D**)

or – in the case of ulceration – in superficial stromal layers. Cells of the muscularis propria displayed an increased autoradiographic signal as well, but the proportion of significantly labelled cells was only moderately increased when compared with normal tissue. The α_1(III) and α_2(V) procollagen gene probes revealed patterns comparable in distribution to the α_1(I) probe; however, the label intensity was weaker (Fig. 1D). Procollagen α_1(IV) transcript steady-state levels were enhanced more in the lamina propria, particularly in subepithelial layers, both in terms of number of positive cells and signal intensity.

In summary, both in Crohn's disease and ulcerative colitis, the intensity of the autoradiographic procollagen-specific signals was positively correlated to the cellular density of the inflammatory infiltrate. In contrast to ulcerative colitis, in which the superficial lamina propria was the major site of procollagen gene expression, procollagen gene expression in Crohn's disease was predominant in the muscular layer. The main difference between inflamed and strictured areas in Crohn's disease was a relative increase of type III procollagen transcripts typical for stenoses.

In situ-hybridization experiments showed that mesenchymal cells of the lamina propria are mainly responsible for the synthesis of collagens in the intestinal tract. Furthermore, in order to investigate collagen synthesis by lamina propria fibroblasts in inflammatory bowel disease, cell culture studies were performed. Resected specimens from patients with Crohn's disease, ulcerative colitis and as controls from patients with adenocarcinomas of the colon were minced mechanically and digested by enzymatic treatment. The fragments were cultured *in vitro*, outgrowth of fibroblasts was observed after 2–3 days, and after 1 week a dense monolayer of intestinal fibroblasts surrounded the primary explants. Then monolayers were subcultured. To analyse the synthesis of collagens intestinal fibroblasts were incubated in serum-free medium containing ^{3}H-proline. After labelling, the cells were homogenized, precipitated, and placed in scintillation vials to be counted for radioactivity. The amount of non-collagenous protein synthesis was measured after treatment with collagenase as described above. The rate of collagen synthesis in each culture was determined by subtracting the 'counts per minute' (cpm) of non-collagenous protein from the cpm representing total protein synthesis. Using this experimental protocol we could demonstrate that human intestinal lamina propria fibroblasts isolated from strictures of patients with Crohn's disease produced significantly more total collagen than fibroblasts from inflamed or uninvolved mucosa obtained from the same patients ($p < 0.01$) (Fig. 2). Collagen synthesis in fibroblasts isolated from inflamed areas of patients with inflammatory bowel disease other than Crohn's disease was not statistically different from that in fibroblasts of inflamed areas in Crohn's disease.

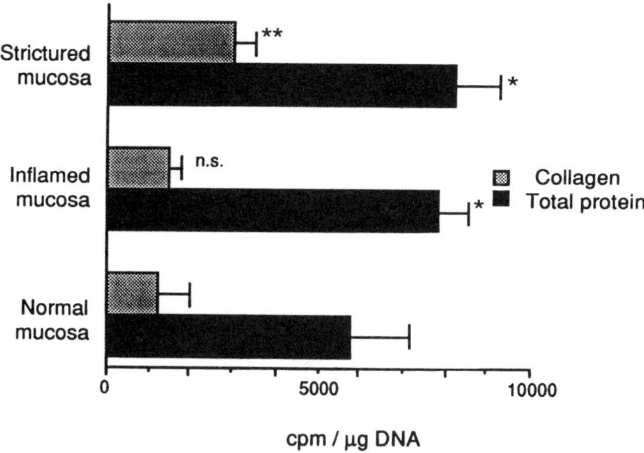

Fig. 2 Synthesis of collagen and total proteins by human intestinal lamina propria fibroblasts isolated from strictured, non-strictured but inflamed, and macroscopically normal specimens. *Note*: Collagen and total protein synthesis in human intestinal lamina propria fibroblasts isolated from strictured, non-strictured but inflamed, and macroscopically normal intestinal tissue of Crohn's disease. Collagen and total protein synthesis were assessed using the ^{3}H-proline incorporation method. n.s. = Non-significant vs normal mucosa; *$p < 0.05$ vs normal mucosa; **$p < 0.01$ vs normal mucosa

Since synthesis of type III collagen is increased in inflammatory bowel disease, especially in fibrotic areas in Crohn's disease, we analysed type III collagen synthesis by lamina propria fibroblast using a radioimmunoassay for the aminoterminal procollagen type III propeptide (PIIIP). PIIIP in cell cultures is quantitatively linked to the collagen type III triple helix and is thus proportional to type III procollagen synthesis. The concentration of PIIIP in cell lysates of intestinal fibroblasts isolated from strictures was significantly higher (32.2 ng/µg DNA; range 3.5–81.6) than that of intestinal fibroblasts from inflamed but non-strictured specimens (12.0 ng/µg DNA; range: 0.7–22.1), or of fibroblasts from uninvolved mucosa (2.3 ng/µg DNA; range: 0.7–13.4; $p < 0.05$ and $p < 0.01$, respectively) (Fig. 3). Normalized to DNA content, intestinal fibroblasts from strictures produced three times more type III procollagen than fibroblasts from inflamed mucosa and more than 10 times the amount compared to fibroblasts from uninvolved mucosa (Fig. 3).

Eﬀct of cytokines on collagen synthesis

Considering the importance of cytokines in the pathogenesis of fibrosis, we wanted to analyse the regulatory influence of two cytokines on type III collagen synthesis which are potentially involved in the development of intestinal fibrosis. TGF-β has been shown to stimulate the expression of collagen and fibronectin and to increase protein production[11,12]. In contrast, the platelet-derived growth factor (PDGF) has only marginal effects on collagen synthesis by human lung fibroblasts[13]. PDGF is a basic 30 kDa

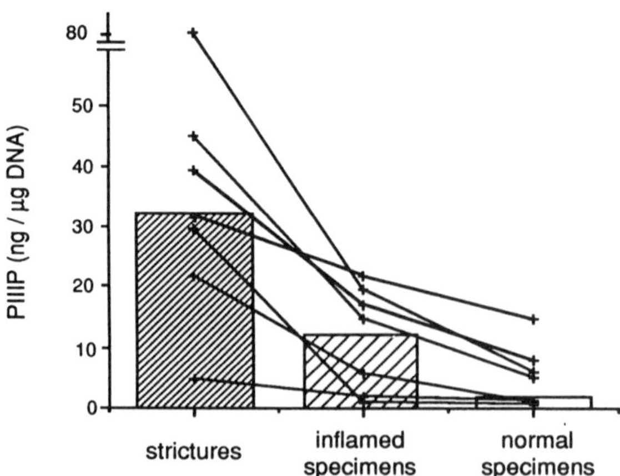

Fig. 3 Synthesis of PIIIP by human intestinal lamina propria fibroblasts isolated from strictured, non-strictured but inflamed, and macroscopically normal specimens. *Note*: Bars represent the median of analysed cultures. Graphs connect the interindividual values for PIIIP synthesized by lamina propria fibroblast isolated from strictured, inflamed but non-strictured, and macroscopically normal specimens obtained from the same patient

protein that was initially isolated from α granules of platelets. It consists of two subunits, A and B, which are linked by disulphide bonds forming a dimer. PDGF is secreted by a variety of cells including fibroblasts, smooth muscle cells and activated macrophages, leading to the suggestion that it plays an important role in the control of connective tissue production in wound healing.

Having characterized the type III collagen synthesis by isolated lamina propria fibroblasts of patients with chronic inflammatory bowel disease *in vitro* (see above), we now use this model to characterize the effects of these cytokines on type III collagen synthesis in inflammatory bowel disease. Interestingly, the effects of TGF-β_1 and PDGF on type III collagen synthesis by lamina propria fibroblasts isolated from strictures were different from those exerted on type III collagen synthesis by lamina propria fibroblasts isolated from merely inflamed specimens of the same patients. In a dose-dependent manner, TGF-β_1 stimulated synthesis of total proteins, collagen and PIIIP. In Crohn's disease the effect of TGF-β_1 on type III collagen synthesis in fibroblasts from strictures was significantly higher than that on type III collagen synthesis in fibroblasts of inflamed specimens of the same patients (Fig. 4). In contrast, the addition of PDGF to stricture-derived lamina propria fibroblasts resulted in decreased synthesis of PIIIP in a dose-dependent manner. On the other hand, PDGF stimulated non-collagen protein synthesis. In fibroblasts isolated from non-strictured but inflamed tissue of Crohn's disease, PDGF, even in high concentrations, did not

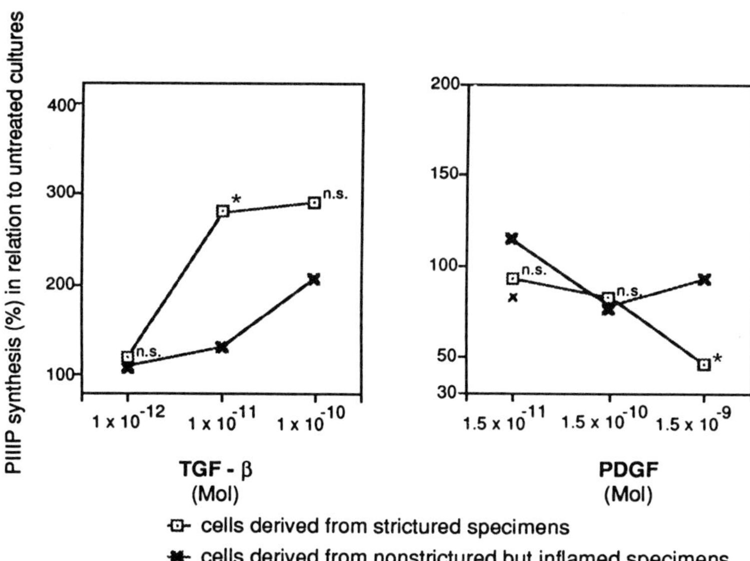

Fig. 4 Effect of TGF-β_1 and PDGF on PIIIP synthesis by lamina propria fibroblasts derived from strictured and non-strictured but inflamed Crohn's disease specimens. *Note*: Results are expressed as median and range of PIIIP synthesis. The amount of PIIIP (ng/µg DNA) in the cultures exposed to TGF-β_1 and PDGF is expressed relative to unstimulated controls (100%). Non-significant differences at the 5% level (n.s.); $*p \leqslant 0.05$

significantly decrease synthesis of PIIIP (Fig. 4). It is tempting to speculate that subsets of fibroblast in Crohn's disease are different concerning reactivity to cytokines than those from patients with other inflammatory bowel diseases or controls. This difference may be responsible for the formation of stenoses and strictures in the intestinal tract.

CONCLUSION

Transmural fibrosis and development of strictures due to massive deposition of collagen are frequent complications of Crohn's disease, whereas such complications are rarely seen in ulcerative colitis[1,2]. The present data show changes that reflect the altered collagen metabolism of intestinal lamina propria fibroblasts in Crohn's disease. First, *in situ* hybridization studies semiquantitatively revealed an increase of procollagen transcripts in inflammatory bowel disease. In Crohn's disease, signal intensity and number of labelled cells were significantly increased in all layers of the intestinal tract. A positive correlation was found between collagen mRNA transcripts and inflammatory infiltrates. Corresponding to the results of biochemical analyses and immunohistological studies using specific antibodies to analyse the distribution of collagens on the protein level[6,7], strictured specimens were characterized by an overproportional increase of type III, and to a lesser extent of type V procollagen transcripts in all layers of the bowel compared to inflamed areas. In contrast, in ulcerative colitis, type I, III, IV and V procollagen-transcript positive cells were concentrated in the lamina propria, particularly in the subepithelial intestinal layers. However, despite a significantly increased expression of collagen transcripts in ulcerative colitis, the deposition of collagens in the intestinal tract was not increased when compared to control sections.

Secondly, using an established cell culture model, we could show that intestinal lamina propria fibroblasts from strictures of Crohn's disease patients produce significantly more type III collagen than fibroblasts from inflamed or uninvolved mucosa of the same patients or inflamed mucosa of patients with ulcerative colitis. The increase of type III collagen synthesis by fibroblasts from strictures in Crohn's disease may have significant relevance in the pathogenesis of the disease. Recently, we could demonstrate that type III collagen stimulates proliferation of lamina fibroblasts *in vitro*[14]. Therefore it is tempting to speculate that an increase of type III collagen synthesis by lamina propria fibroblasts may be a contributing factor in the development of strictures in Crohn's disease.

Having characterized the collagen synthesis of human intestinal lamina propria fibroblasts *in vitro*, we used this model to analyse the effects of inflammatory mediators on fibroblasts isolated from strictured and inflamed specimens of Crohn's disease patients. It was found that there was a remarkable difference. Fibroblasts isolated from strictures or inflamed areas differed in their reactivity to cytokine exposure in type III collagen synthesis. TGF-β_1 mediated an overproportional increase of type III collagen synthesis by fibroblasts from strictures in Crohn's disease in comparison to unchanged type III collagen synthesis by fibroblasts from inflamed specimens of the same patient. In contrast, PDGF decreased collagen type III synthesis in lamina propria fibroblasts derived from strictures compared to fibroblasts from non-strictured but inflamed tissue. It is concluded that differences in the cytokine reactivity of fibroblasts from patients with Crohn's disease compared to fibroblasts from controls or patients with other inflammatory bowel diseases are responsible for the formation of stenoses and strictures in the intestinal tract. Similar differences have been reported between normal dermal skin fibroblasts, granulation tissue fibroblasts and mature scar tissue-derived fibroblasts in terms of glycosaminoglycan metabolism and response to interleukin 1[15], supporting our hypothesis of differences between the so-called normal intestinal lamina propria fibroblasts and lamina propria fibroblasts in intestinal disease.

However, it remains unclear whether differences in cytokine-induced collagen synthesis are invariably linked to different expression patterns. A differential – primarily or secondarily acquired – sensitivity of myofibroblasts to various cytokines might result in increased collagen synthesis in stenoses but not in non-strictured inflamed areas in Crohn's disease. Based on this hypothesis, differential sensitivity in collagen synthesis by cytokine stimulation might be a specific feature of intestinal strictures. Other explanations imply a different set of cytokines in strictured and non-strictured but inflamed areas, which induce a fibrotic response after injury. However, the latter speculation did not explain the observed differences in collagen synthesis. Therefore, further studies are required to characterize collagen metabolism of mesenchymal cells in inflammatory bowel disease. In the future this may result in the development of specific pharmacological inhibition of enhanced collagen synthesis and deposition in intestinal fibrosis.

References

1. Alexander WJ. Surgical aspects of inflammatory bowel disease. Scand J Gastroenterol. (Suppl.) 1990;172:39–42.
2. Pritchard TJ, Schoetz DJ, Caushaj FP *et al.* Strictureplasty of the small bowel in patients with Crohn's disease. An effective surgical option. Arch Surg. 1990;125:715–17.
3. Hahn EG, Schuppan D. Ethanol and fibrogenesis in the liver. In: Seitz HK, Kommerell B, editors. Alcohol related disease in gastroenterology. Berlin, Heidelberg: Springer Verlag; 1985:124–53.
4. Uscanga L, Kennedy RH, Choux R, Drugmont M, Grimand JA, Sarles H. Sequential connective tissue matrix changes in experimental acute pancreatitis. An immunohistochemical and biochemical assessment in the rat. Int J Panc. 1987;2:33–45.
5. Cantin AM, Boileau R, Begin R. Increased procollagen III aminoterminal peptide related antigens and fibroblastic growth signals in the lungs of patients with idiopathic pulmonary fibrosis. Am Rev Respir Dis. 1988;137:572–8.
6. Graham MF, Diegelmann RF, Elson CO, Lindblad WJ, Gotschalk N, Gay S, Gay R. Collagen content and types in the intestinal strictures of Crohn's disease. Gastroenterology. 1988;94:257–65.
7. Matthes H, Herbst H, Schuppan D, Stallmach A, Milani S, Stein H, Riecken EO. Cellular Localization of Procollagen Gene Transcripts in Inflammatory Bowel Disease. Gastroenterology. 1992;102:431–42.
8. Wahl SM. The role of lymphokines and monokines in fibrosis. Ann NY Acad Sci. 1985;460:224–31.

9. Kovacs EJ. Fibrogenic cytokines: the role of immune mediators in the development of scar tissue. Immunol Today. 1991;12:17–23.
10. Sporn MB, Roberts AB, Wakefield LM, de Crombugghe B. Some recent advances in the chemistry and biology of transforming growth factor-β. J Cell Biol. 1987;105:1039–45.
11. Ignotz RA, Massague J. Transforming growth factor-β stimulates the expression of fibronectin and collagen and their incorporation into the extracellular matrix. J Biol Chem. 1986;261:4337–45.
12. Graham MF, Bryson GR, Diegelmann RF. Transforming growth factor β_1 selectively augments collagen synthesis by human intestinal smooth muscle cells. Gastroenterology. 1990;99:447–53.
13. Morinex J-F, Martinet Y, Yamauchi K, et al. Spontaneous expression of the C-Sis gene and release of a platelet-derived growth factor-like molecule by human alvedar macrophages. J Clin Invest. 1986;78:61–6.
14. Stallmach A, Schuppan D, Lazar D, Riese HH, Riecken EO. Increased collagen type III synthesis by lamina propria fibroblasts from strictures in Crohn's disease. Gastroenterology. 1992;102:1900–6.
15. Bronson RC, Argenta JG, Bertolami CHN. Interleukin-1-induced changes in extracellular glycosaminoglycan composition of cutaneous scar-derived fibroblasts in culture. Collagen Rel Res. 1988;8:199–208.

15

Cytokines – implications for treatment

W. F. DOE

INTRODUCTION

Cytokines are low molecular weight glycopeptides that mediate potent biological functions at very low concentrations in a restricted microenvironment. The network of cytokines that effects immune and inflammatory responses is directly or indirectly implicated in the pathogenesis of inflammatory bowel disease (IBD)[1]. The biological roles of these cytokines are extremely complex. The purpose of this chapter is to discuss the therapeutic implications of modulating particular groups of cytokines that are involved in the chronic relapsing inflammatory events that attend IBD. The focus will be on cytokines that are involved in attracting and activating inflammatory cells, regulating the proinflammatory response and mediating tissue injury (Tables 1 and 2).

The mucosal lesion in IBD is characterized by a dense inflammatory cell infiltrate comprising neutrophils, mononuclear phagocytes and lymphocytes. Radiolabelled autologous phagocyte scanning has shown that the rapid and substantial migration of neutrophils from peripheral blood to sites of inflamed intestinal mucosa provides an objective measure of disease activity[2]. More recently, studies using purified radiolabelled blood monocytes have demonstrated

Table 1 Chemotactic cytokines

	Target cell		Target cell
IL-8	T-lymphocytes	IL-5	Eosinophils
	Neutrophils		Neutrophils
	Basophils		Monocytes
MCAF	Monocytes	GM-CSF	Eosinophils
Lymphotoxin (TNF-β)	Monocytes	G-CSF	Neutrophils

Table 2 Proinflammatory cytokines

TNF-α	GM-CSF
IL-1	G-CSF
IL-6	M-CSF
Lymphotoxin (TNF-β)	TGF-β
IL-10	

that there is also a high turnover of monocytes in the mucosal lesion of IBD, indicating that the mucosal mononuclear phagocytes that accumulate in IBD mucosa are derived from recruitment of peripheral blood monocytes and not lamina propria macrophages[3]. Amongst the chemotactic signals (Table 1) that generate the inflammatory cell infiltrate are cytokines that belong to a newly recognized supergene family comprising interleukin-8 (previously called monocyte-derived neutrophil chemotactic factor or MDNCF) and monocyte chemotactic and activating factor (MCAF) (also called monocyte chemotactic protein MCP-1) and related genes[4]. Foremost amongst its many functions, IL-8 activates and attracts neutrophils, basophils and T lymphocytes and activates 5α-lipoxygenase to release leukotriene B4, another powerful chemoattractant for neutrophils[5]. Secondly the MCAF subfamily both activates and attracts monocytes into tissue. Lymphotoxin (LT), also called tumour necrosis factor β (TNF-β), is a product of activated T lymphocytes that is strongly chemotactic for monocytes. Cytokine products of lymphocytes and monocytes also include the colony-stimulating factors (CSF), granulocyte–monocyte (GM-CSF) and granulocyte (G-CSF) which not only activate mature neutrophils, eosinophils and monocytes but also generate chemotactic activity, induce phagocytic activity, granulocyte cytotoxicity, superoxide generation and release of leukotrienes and prostaglandins. Lamina propria (LP) cells isolated from IBD mucosa produce significantly more CSF than LP cells from normal intestine, mainly due to increased levels of G-CSF associated with increased expression of the specific mRNA for G-CSF[6].

The proinflammatory cytokines include interleukins 1 and 6, tumour necrosis factor α (TFN-α), LT (TNF-β), GM-CSF, G-CSF, M-CSF and transforming growth factor β (TGF-β) (Table 2). Many of the proinflammatory cytokines induce IL-8 production, generate proinflammatory activity by activating granulocytes and monocytes and produce the local, systemic and catabolic features of inflammation. Increased levels of interleukin-1 (IL-1)[6], IL-6[7] and IL-8[8] activity and of mucosal mRNA expression for G-CSF, GM-CSF[6] IL-1, IL-6 and TNF-α[9] have been found in actively inflamed mucosa from IBD patients.

The therapeutic implications of the involvement of chemotactic and proinflammatory cytokines in the pathogenesis of the mucosal lesion of IBD are significant for the development of new treatment strategies. One strategy is to prevent migration of monocytes, lymphocytes and neutrophils, basophils and eosinophils into the acutely inflamed bowel, thereby offering the prospect of resolving the inflammatory response and preventing the development of chronic mucosal inflammation. A second strategy is to inhibit the salient proinflammatory cytokines that activate other effector cells and mediate tissue injury.

The predominant chemotactic cytokines and their specificities are shown in Table 1. Many of the current therapies for IBD including corticosteroids and 5-aminosalicylic acid at therapeutic concentrations profoundly decrease CSF production by LP cells during culture, suggesting that their therapeutic efficacy may be due in part to down-regulation of cytokine production in the inflamed mucosa[6]. There is significant therapeutic potential in being able to block IL-8 and MCAF production in the inflamed mucosa because of their marked effects on neutrophil, monocyte, lymphocyte and basophil migration both directly and by the induction of 5α-lipoxygenase activity to generate chemotactic leukotriene B4 and 5-HETE[4,5]. The biological activities of the IL-8/MCAF supergene family are set out in Table 3. IL-8 binds with high affinity to unique receptors on myelomonocytic cells and on T lymphocytes. The IL-8 receptor (IL-8) has been recently characterized as a glycoprotein. Although there are no known specific peptide antagonists for the IL-8 receptors, the lectin, wheat germ agglutinin (WGA), strongly inhibits IL-8 binding to human neutrophils, indicating binding recognition for N-acetylglucosamine and N-acetyl neuraminic acid. WGA-mediated inhibition of IL-8 binding to neutrophils is prevented by addition of N-acetyl-D-glucosamine, but not by other sugars, confirming that sugar recognition mediates the WGA-induced inhibition[10]. These studies encourage exploration of the therapeutic potential for using sugars to block IL-8 receptors on neutrophils, T-lymphocytes and basophils and serve as a paradigm for similar approaches to the specific receptors for other chemotactic cytokines. Both IL-8 and MCAF synthesis are suppressed by corticosteroids, and IL-8 is also affected by 1,25-dihydroxyvitamin D and by 5α-lipoxygenase inhibitors[4].

The inhibition of the proinflammatory cytokines represents a second therapeutic approach to preventing cytokine-induced tissue injury. Corticosteroids, 5-ASA and cyclosporin A markedly decrease IL-2 and CSF production by intestinal LP cells *in vitro* at therapeutic concentrations[6]. Recently, naturally occurring peptides that inhibit TNF-α and LT have been reported. Truncated TNF receptor (TNFR) molecules, lacking the transmembrane or cytoplasmic domains, have been isolated from urine and serum and function

Table 3 Biological activities of IL-8

In vivo	Neutrophilia
	Chemoattractant for neutrophils
	T-lymphocytes
	basophils
	Induces vascular permeability
	Destruction of synovial membrane and alveoli associated with neutrophil and lymphocyte infiltration
In vitro	Increases LT B4 and 5-HETE production
	Induces histamine and leukotriene release from basophils
	Decreases neutrophil adherence to cytokine-activated endothelial cells
	Increases adherence to unstimulated endothelial monolayers
	Increases CRI
	Increases granulocyte adhesion molecule (CD11)
	Induces histamine and leukotriene release from basophils

as TNF inhibitors[11]. Soluble truncated TNFR proteins, however, are unstable *in vivo*. Moreover, because they are univalent, TNFR proteins lack the avidity of a bivalent ligand and recombinant truncated receptor protein is difficult to produce in an active form in large amounts[12]. These studies – and the evidence that the extracellular portion of CD4, the receptor for the human immunodeficiency virus, can be linked to the IgG heavy chain to create a bivalent protein with a markedly longer plasma half-life than the soluble extracellular portion of CD4[13] – encouraged the development of an analogous chimeric protein for the TNFR. A potent TNF antagonist was constructed by recombinant methods by fusing the genes for the extracellular portion of human type I TNFR and the constant domains of human IgG heavy chain[14]. This chimeric protein functions as a TNFR immunoadhesin and displays 6–8-fold higher affinity for TNF-α than cell surface or soluble TNFR. TNFR-IgG completely blocks the cytolytic effects of TNF-α and LT (TNF-β) on susceptible target cells with much greater efficiency than either soluble TNFR molecules or monoclonal antibodies specific for TNF-α. TNFR-IgG also markedly inhibits LPS-induced lethality in mice in a dose-dependent manner[14]. The therapeutic potential for constructing chimeric proteins comprising the extracellular portion of a cytokine receptor and the IgG heavy chain therefore indicates another useful direction to explore.

The blocking of cell surface receptors for cytokines represents another means of therapeutic attack on proinflammatory cytokines in IBD. The potential for using the lectin WGA to block the IL-8 receptor has already been discussed. Recent reports describe a naturally occurring polypeptide that is a potent and specific IL-1 antagonist. It blocks the action of IL-1 by binding to IL-1 receptors with similar affinity to IL-1 but has no IL-1 activity. This molecule, called IL-1 receptor antagonist (IL-1ra), is produced by the same cells as those that produce IL-1, strongly suggesting that IL-1ra is a physiologically significant regulator of IL-1 activity[15]. Preliminary studies using recombinant IL-1ra in the rabbit immune complex model of colitis indicated its potential for therapy in IBD. When IL-1ra was given before or during the first 33 h after administration of immune complexes, there was marked reduction of inflammation in the colonic mucosa as measured histologically, suggesting that blockade of the IL-1 response may modify mucosal inflammation in IBD[16]. There are also preliminary data suggesting that an IL-1 response modifier (RO31-3948) inhibits the spontaneous and LPS-induced release of IL-1 and TNF-α from blood monocytes from IBD patients but not from controls[17].

The use of antibodies to block cytokine receptors has also been studied, particularly for TNF. The two TNFR, TNFR-1 and TNFR-2, both bind TNF-α and LT (TNF-β), but there are no significant homologies between the intracytoplasmic portions of the two TNFRs, suggesting either that each receptor activates a different intracellular signalling pathway or that some unidentified protein acts as a signal transducer as reported for the IL-6 receptor[18]. Antibodies specific for TNFR-1 and for TNFR-2 have been produced that block TNF-α and LT binding. Monoclonal antibodies (mAbs) against human TNFR-1 for example, block the binding of TNF-α, and LT to TNFR-1 and antagonize TNF effects including cytotoxicity, antiviral activity, fibroblast proliferation and induction of enzymes such as manganese superoxide dismutase[19] and neutralizing antibodies to TNF-α have provided protection against septic shock. But murine mAbs generate anti-murine antibodies in humans which compromise their efficacy if administered repeatedly or for prolonged periods.

While our knowledge of the role of cytokines in the pathogenesis of the mucosal lesion in IBD remains limited, rapid further progress may be possible when the critical pathways of cytokine-induced tissue injury are elucidated. Preliminary exploration of strategies to inhibit cytokines or to block their receptors encourage further research into developing these new approaches to the treatment of IBD.

References

1. Fiocchi C. Cytokines. In: MacDermott R, Stenson WF, editors. Inflammatory bowel disease. Amsterdam: Elsevier; 1991;137–62.
2. Pullman WE, Sullivan PJ, Barratt PJ, Lising J, Booth JA, Doe WF. Assessment of inflammatory bowel disease activity by Technetium 99m phagocyte scanning. Gastroenterology. 1988;95:989–96.
3. Grimm M, Pullman WE, Sullivan PJ, Doe WF. 99m Technetium-labelled monocyte scanning in inflammatory bowel disease. Aust NZ J Med. 1991;21:557 (abstract).
4. Matushima K, Baldwin ET, Mukaida N. Interleukin 8 and MCAF: novel leucocyte recruitment and activating cytokines. In: Kishimoto T, editor. Interleukins: molecular biology and immunology. Basel: Karger; 1992:51:236–65.
5. Lobos EA, Sharon P, Stenson WF. Chemotactic activity in inflammatory bowel disease. Role of leukotriene B4. Dig Dis Sci. 1987;32:1380–8.
6. Pullman WE, Elsbury S, Kobayashi M, Hapel AH, Doe WF. Enhanced mucosal cytokine production in inflammatory bowel disease. Gastroenterology. 1992;102:529–37.
7. Kitsuyama K, Sakasi E, Toyonaga A, Ikoda H, Tsuruta O, Irie A, Arima N, Oriishi T, Horada K, Fujisaki K, Sata M, Tanikawa Kawa K. Colonic Mucosal interleukin-6 in inflammatory bowel disease. Digestion. 1991;50:104–11.
8. Mahida YR, Ceska M, Effenberger F, Kurlak L, Lindley I, Hawkey CJ. Enhanced synthesis of neutrophil-activating peptide-1/interleukin-8 in active ulcerative colitis. Clin Sci. 1992;82:273–5.
9. Stevens C, Walz G, Zarker B, Sigaram C, Lipman M, Strom TB. Interleukin-6 (IL-6), interleukin-1 beta (IL-1$_\beta$) and tumor necrosis factor alpha (TNFα) expression in inflammatory bowel disease (IBD). Gastroenterology. 1990;98:A47S.
10. Grob PM, David E, Warren TE, DeLeon RP, Farina PR, Homon CA. Characterization of a receptor for human monocyte-derived neutrophil chemotactic factor/interleukin 8. J Biol Chem. 1990;265:8311–16.
11. Engelmann H, Aderka D, Rubenstein M, Rotman D, Wallach D. A tumor necrosis factor-binding protein purified to homogeneity from human urine protects cells from tumor necrosis factor toxicity. J Biol Chem. 1989;264:11974–80.
12. Peppel K, Crawford I, Beutler B. A tumor necrosis factor (TNF) receptor-IgG heavy chain chimeric protein as a bivalent antagonist of TNF activity. J Exp Med. 1991;174:1483–9.
13. Capon DJ, Chamow SM, Mordenti J, Marsters SA, Gregory TJ, Mitsuya H, Byrn RA, Lucas C, Wurm FM, Groopman Jr, Smith DH. Designing CD4 adhesins for AIDS therapy. Nature (Lond). 1989;337:525–31.
14. Ashkenazi A, Marsters SA, Capon DJ, Chamow SM, Figari IS, Pennica D, Goeddel DV, Palladino MA, Smith DH. Protection against endotoxic shock by a tumor necrosis factor receptor immunoadhesin. Proc Natl Acad Sci USA. 1991;88:10535–9.
15. Hannum CH, Wilcox CJ, Arend WP, Joslin FG, Dripps DJ, Heindal PL, Armes LG, Sommer A, Eisenberg SP, Thompson RC. Interleukin-1 receptor antagonist activity of human interleukin-1 inhibitor. Nature (Lond). 1990;343:336–40.

16. Cominelli F, Nast CC, Dinarello CA, Gentilini P, Zipser RD. Regulation of eicosanoid production in rabbit colon by interleukin-1. Gastroenterology. 1989;97:1400–5.
17. Leser HG, Andus T, Gross V, Fenner H, Gerok W, Scholmerich J. Inhibitory effects of a new interleukin-1 response modifier (RO31–3948) on cytokine release by monocytes from patients with inflammatory bowel disease. Gastroenterology. 1991;100:A593.
18. Toga T, Hibi M, Murakami M, Saito M, Yawata H, Narazaki M, Hirata Y, Sugita T, Yasakawa K, Hirano T, Kishimoto T. Interleukin-6 receptor and signals. In: Kishimoto T, editor. Interleukins: molecular biology and immunology. Chem Immunol. Basel: Karger; 1992;51:181–204.
19. Tartaglia LA, Goeddel DV. Two TNF receptors. Immunol Today. 1992;13:151–3.

Section IV
Pathophysiology – Microbiology, metabolism, motility and permeability

16

Role of the intestinal microflora in pathogenesis and complications

R. B. SARTOR

INTRODUCTION

Crohn's disease and ulcerative colitis appear to be the result of an unrestrained immune response, but antigen(s) initiating and perpetuating inflammation remain unknown. The fundamental question of whether these disorders result from a normal response to a pathogenic agent or from an abnormal host response to ubiquitous antigens remains controversial. However, considerable clinical and experimental evidence incriminates luminal bacteria and their products in the pathogenesis of these disorders (Table 1)[1,2]. This review will discuss the role of pathogenic and normal enteric microflora in idiopathic inflammatory bowel disease (IBD) and will present the hypothesis that IBD

Table 1 Evidence that luminal microflora are involved in IBD

A. Clinical
1. Distal ileum and colon have highest bacterial concentrations
2. Resemblance of IBD to enterocolonic infections
3. Improvement of Crohn's disease when luminal bacterial concentrations are decreased
4. Reactivation by intestinal and respiratory infections
5. Frequent suppurative complications
6. Enteric infections induce extraintestinal inflammation

B. Experimental
1. Increased anaerobic bacteria in Crohn's disease
2. Abnormal functional properties of aerobic bacteria in ulcerative colitis
3. Bacterial cell wall polymers induce intestinal and systemic inflammation
4. Indigenous bacteria and cell wall polymers potentiate experimental enterocolitis
5. Small intestinal bacterial overgrowth causes hepatobiliary inflammation and reactivates arthritis

is caused by a genetically determined overly aggressive immune response to the constituents of commensal bacteria.

ROLE OF LUMINAL BACTERIA AND BACTERIAL PRODUCTS IN INDUCTION AND PERPETUATION OF INTESTINAL INFLAMMATION

The distal ileum and colon contain 10^8 and 10^{11} predominantly anaerobic bacteria per gram of luminal contents respectively. These indigenous bacteria cause suppurative complications if they cross the epithelium and produce substances with well-documented proinflammatory properties[1-3]. Formylated oligopeptides – F-met-leu-phe (FMLP) and cell wall polymers – endotoxin or lipopolysaccharide (LPS) and peptidoglycan–polysaccharide (PG-PS) activate immunoregulatory and effector immune cells, activate the complement and kallikrein–kinin cascades and stimulate production of proinflammatory cytokines and eicosanoids. These bacterial products have synergistic activities, such that a phagocytic cell primed by LPS can be triggered by low doses of FMLP or PG-PS and an inflammatory focus previously injured by PG-PS can be reactivated by a low dose of LPS or PG-PS.

Induction of clinical and experimental enterocolitis by microbial agents

A small but reproducible number of patients develop classic ulcerative colitis or Crohn's disease following epidemics of *Shigella*, *Salmonella* or *Yersinia*, and IBD patients not infrequently report onset of chronic symptoms following apparently typical traveller's diarrhoea or amoebiasis[4]. Careful studies show no evidence of active infection in these patients, suggesting that transient infection in a predisposed patient may initiate a cascade of inflammatory events culminating in idiopathic IBD. These observations illustrate the possibility that factors initiating and perpetuating inflammation in IBD may be entirely separate. Investigation of tissues resected many years after onset of symptoms is unlikely to yield an aetiologic agent if this 'hit-and-run' hypothesis is correct.

Products of endogenous as well as pathogenic bacteria induce acute experimental intestinal inflammation which can progress to chronic enterocolitis in genetically susceptible hosts. FMLP in high concentrations induces experimental colitis[5], and at more physiological doses produces enhanced vascular and mucosal permeability in the small intestine, with a predilection for the distal ileum[6]. Intravenous LPS causes acute haemorrhagic injury of the mid-small intestine, which is mediated by tumour necrosis factor and platelet activating factor[7]. PG-PS injected intramurally (subserosally) into the distal ileum, caecum or distal colon induces acute local inflammation which progresses to more diffuse chronic granulomatous enterocolitis in the Lewis rat[8]. Submucosal fibrosis, a chronic time course (6 months), and spontaneous reactivation of inflammation are prominent features of this model which make it particularly relevant to IBD. Acute and chronic phases of PG-PS-induced enterocolitis are mediated in part by interleukin-1 (IL-1)[9] and are dependent on persistence of poorly biodegradable PG-PS within the inflamed tissues. Chronic granulomatous enterocolitis has been induced in rats by PG-PS derived from group A and D (enterococcus) streptococci[8], while chronic arthritis develops after systemic administration of PG-PS from certain Eubacterial strains, *Streptococcus faecium* and *Lactobacillus casei*[10]. PG-PS from a variety of common intestinal bacteria produce transient inflammation, clearly demonstrating the inflammatory potential of cell wall polymers from normal intestinal bacteria.

Perpetuation of clinical and experimental enterocolitis by microbial agents

Crohn's disease, but not ulcerative colitis, clinicaly improves when luminal bacterial concentrations are decreased by a variety of methods[11]. Metronidazole is superior to placebo[12] and equal to sulphasalazine in therapy of active Crohn's colitis and ileocolitis, but is not effective for isolated small intestinal disease. Non-absorbable antibiotics in combination with elemental diet were equal to prednisolone in inducing remission in active Crohn's disease and also dramatically diminished faecal FMLP concentrations[13]. Similarly, intestinal lavage plus 5-ASA hastened improvement and cleared endotoxaemia in patients with active Crohn's disease treated with parenteral nutrition and steroids[14]. In a provocative preliminary study Rutgeerts *et al.*[15] reported that metronidazole diminished the recurrence rate of Crohn's disease after ileal resection and primary ileocolonic anastomosis.

Bowel rest with total parenteral nutrition or elemental diets induce remissions in 60–80% of patients with active Crohn's disease (ileitis > colitis) but do not reproducibly help patients with ulcerative colitis. Similarly, faecal diversion with split ileostomy diminishes clinical activity in 95% of patients with Crohn's colitis, but not ulcerative colitis, although symptoms reappear in most patients when intestinal continuity is re-established or the bypassed colon is challenged with ileostomy effluent[16]. Recently Rutgeerts and colleagues[17] demonstrated that ileal diversion prevented recurrence of Crohn's disease after resection of all grossly active disease. While the relative importance of luminal bacterial versus dietary antigens in induction of remission with bowel rest is unclear, several lines of evidence incriminate bacterial influences. The relapse rate following resection of Crohn's disease is substantially lower with an end ileostomy than with an ileocolonic anastomosis, even though both ileal segments are exposed to identical dietary components. Reactivation of symptoms occurs in Crohn's patients with split ileostomies when the bypassed colon is challenged with unfractionated ileal effluents, but not 22 nm filtrates[16].

Endogenous intestinal flora exacerbate experimental enterocolitis of diverse aetiologies. In a well-studied model, germ-free rats treated with subcutaneous indomethacin have attenuated small intestinal ulcers and do not develop caecal ulceration which is clearly evident in littermates conventionalized with pathogen-free rat faecal flora[8,18]. Indomethacin-induced small intestinal ulcers almost return to numbers seen in conventional rats when germ-free rats are fed purified PG-PS, but caecal ulcers do not develop. These results suggest that viable bacteria are important for development of caecal ulcers but that purified bacterial cell wall polymers can potentiate small intestinal ulcers. Luminal PG-PS has been shown to exacerbate to a modest degree acetic acid-induced colitis[19], demonstrating that once colonic ulceration occurs, inflammation can be perpetuated by luminal cell wall polymers. Although broad-spectrum and anaerobic antibiotics diminish small intestinal ulcers in rats treated with indomethacin[8], caecal ulceration is affected to a greater extent (R. B. Sartor, unpublished observations). Similarly, germ-free and metronidazole-treated guinea pigs fail to develop carrageenan-induced colitis, which is dependent on *Bacteroides vulgatus* colonization[8,33].

Reactivation of IBD by microbial agents

Exacerbation of symptoms which closely mimic spontaneous relapses of IBD can be induced by a number of enteric pathogens, including *Campylobacter*, *Cytomegalovirus*, *Aeromonas*, toxigenic *E. coli*, mycobacteria and *Clostridium difficile*. The latter is particularly prevalent in hospitalized patients and those receiving antibiotics, including sulphasalazine. Upper respiratory tract infections frequently precede exacerbations of IBD, although mechanisms remain speculative. Kangro *et al.*[20] reported that 24% of clinical flares of IBD were temporally associated with viral or *Mycoplasma* infections, and that 44% of upper respiratory tract infections were associated with increased intestinal symptoms. Isgar *et al.*[21] found an approximate 50% relapse rate of ulcerative colitis following diarrhoea resulting from foreign travel, gastroenteritis or antibiotic therapy.

ROLE OF BACTERIA AND BACTERIAL PRODUCTS IN COMPLICATIONS OF IBD

Intestinal complications

Luminal bacteria produce the frequent septic complications of IBD, which are particularly frequent in Crohn's disease (Table 2). Keighley *et al.*[22] found grossly detectable abscesses in 10% of Crohn's disease patients undergoing intestinal resection, of which over half were clinically unsuspected. Postoperative abscesses occurred in 14% of these patients. *E. coli*, *Bacteroides fragilis*, enterococci and viridans streptococci were the principal isolates. Chronic metronidazole therapy improves approximately two-thirds of perianal fistulae, and ciprofloxacin has been reported to heal complex intestinal fistulae[11]. Small bowel bacterial overgrowth, a result of partial obstruction, loss of the

Table 2 Infectious complications of Crohn's disease

Intra-abdominal, perirectal and hepatic abscess
Intestinal and perianal fistulae
Small intestinal bacterial overgrowth
Postoperative infections

ileocaecal valve or enterocolonic fistula, usually responds to metronidazole, tetracycline or ciprofloxacin therapy. Pouchitis complicating ileal pouch–anal anastomosis following colectomy for ulcerative colitis responds to metronidazole, suggesting that anaerobic bacteria are involved, although the exact mechanism of injury remains to be defined.

Extraintestinal complications

A subset of patients with *Yersinia*, *Salmonella* and *Shigella* enteritis develop erythema nodosum, anterior uveitis and non-deforming, migratory poly-arthritis[3]. The frequency of these same extraintestinal complications of IBD correlates with the extent and activity of the underlying bowel disease, and they are more common in patients with colonic Crohn's disease than those with isolated small intestinal involvement[3]. These clinical observations suggest that systemic uptake of colonic (predominantly anaerobic) bacteria or their products are involved in the pathogenesis of skin, joint and eye complications of IBD. An anaerobic bacterial origin of systemic complications of intestinal injury is further supported by the prompt improvement in hepatobiliary, skin and joint inflammation accompanying jejunoileal bypass for morbid obesity with metronidazole therapy and recovery of bacterial antigens from circulating immune complexes in these patients[23].

Abundant experimental evidence demonstrates the ability of luminal bacteria and bacterial components to induce and reactivate systemic inflammation which closely resembles the extraintestinal manifestations of IBD[3]. Subserosal injection of PG-PS polymers into the ileum and caecum of Lewis rats induces chronic polyarthritis, granulomatous hepatitis and anaemia[8]. Small intestinal overgrowth by anaerobic bacteria induced by a self-filling blind loop causes hepatobiliary inflammation which resembles sclerosing cholangitis in genetically susceptible rats[24]. This inflammation is mediated by systemic absorption of PG-PS polymers from intestinal anaerobic bacteria, as indicated by prevention and treatment with metronidazole, tetracycline and mutanolysin, which is an enzyme whose sole known activity is to degrade peptidoglycan, and failure to recover viable bacteria from the inflamed liver. Further evidence incriminating PG-PS in the pathogenesis of experimental hepatobiliary disease is increased plasma antibodies to PG and demonstration of an enterohepatic circulation of luminal PG-PS[3].

Once arthritis has been induced by PG-PS it can be reactivated by local or systemic injections of PG-PS, LPS, bacterial superantigens and several proinflammatory cytokines or experimental intestinal bacterial overgrowth[3]. Similar mechanisms may be involved in recurrences of arthritis, skin lesions and uveitis during exacerbations of IBD.

UPTAKE OF LUMINAL BACTERIA AND BACTERIAL PRODUCTS IN INTESTINAL INFLAMMATION

As illustrated in Fig. 1, patients with IBD, especially Crohn's disease, have increased absorption of luminal bacterial and dietary antigens, toxic bacterial

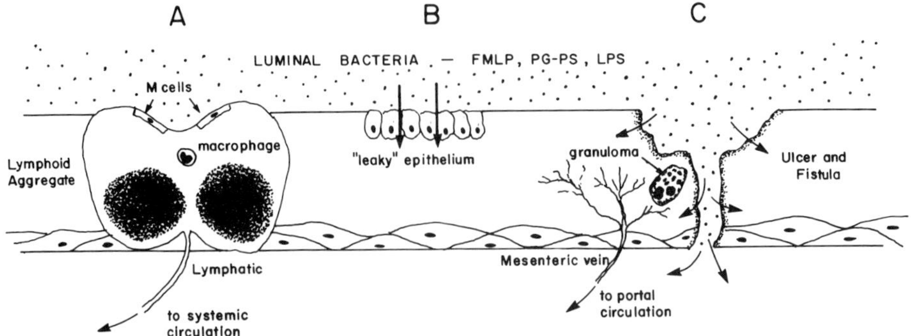

Fig. 1   Mechanisms of mucosal uptake of bacteria and bacterial products (*n*-formyl-methionyl-leucyl-phenyladamine (FMLP), lipopolysaccharide (LPS) and peptidoglycan–polysaccharide (PG-PS) polymers) present in high concentrations in the distal ileal and colonic lumen. **A**: Specialized epithelial cells (M cells) over Peyer's patches and organized lymphoid follicles preferentially transport luminal macromolecules in the normal state, initiating a normal, controlled mucosal immune response. **B**: Normally the intact epithelium provides a relatively impenetrable barrier, but with non-ulcerative inflammation, NSAID treatment or perhaps subclinical IBD, the epithelium is 'leaky', permitting enhanced uptake of luminal bacterial products. **C**: With intestinal ulceration there is secondary invasion of viable bacteria and unrestricted uptake of bacterial products and antigens, further intensifying inflammation. (Reproduced with permission from Sartor RB, Powell DW. In: Field M, (ed) *Controversies in Gastroenterology Diarrheal Diseases*. New York: Elsevier, 1991, pp. 75–114)

products and secondary invasion of mucosal ulcers and fistulae by viable bacteria. Patients with Crohn's disease have increased serum IgG antibodies to a number of commensal and pathogenic enteric organisms, which demonstrates that bacterial antigens are stimulating an immune response which could lead to local or systemic deposition of immune complexes and activate complement[3]. Plasma LPS is detectable in approximately 10% of ambulatory and 94% of hospitalized patients with active Crohn's disease[2,14]. Crohn's disease patients have increased antibodies to LPS and PG-PS, while ulcerative colitis patients have modestly elevated values[3]. Recently Chadwick and colleagues[25] demonstrated circulating FMLP in the majority of patients with active ulcerative colitis, Crohn's disease and sclerosing cholangitis, but not in normals or controls with systemic infections or rheumatoid arthritis. Both FMLP and PG-PS have been shown to undergo enterohepatic circulation.

Patients with active Crohn's disease have secondary invasion of mucosal ulcers and fistula by normal flora bacteria[26] with evidence of local and systemic dissemination. Ambrose *et al.*[27] cultured enteric bacteria from the serosa or mesenteric lymph nodes of 56% of resected tissues from Crohn's disease patients but only 17% of controls. Portal vein bacteraemia has been reported in up to 27% of ulcerative colitis patients[3], while the vast majority of ulcerative colitis patients undergoing colectomy have detectable FMLP in their portal vein blood[25]. Increased mucosal permeability correlates with degree of inflammation in experimental colitis and permits enhanced uptake of viable bacteria and bacterial products. Translocation of viable enteric bacteria occurs in experimental enterocolitis (Yamada, Grisham and Sartor, submitted) and small intestinal bacterial overgrowth[24]. Luminal PG-PS is transported to peripheral blood, liver and spleen following acetic acid-induced colitis[19] and small intestinal bacterial overgrowth, and undergoes enterohepatic circulation[3]. Colonic absorption and biliary excretion of FMLP is increased 8-fold following induction of experimental colitis[2].

MECHANISMS OF MICROBIAL INJURY IN IBD

These studies document with a considerable degree of confidence that phlogistic bacterial products and replicating enteric bacteria cross the mucosal barrier in active, and possibly in clinically quiescent, stages of IBD. Furthermore, endogenous bacteria and bacterial products can initiate and perpetuate local and systemic inflammation in genetically susceptible hosts. It remains to be determined whether idopathic ulcerative colitis and Crohn's disease are the result of a chronic but appropriate immune response to pathogenic or altered microbial agents or due to a dysregulated immune response to ubiquitous luminal flora. Potential mechanisms of intestinal and systemic injury by microbial agents are outlined in Table 3 and discussed below.

Toxic response to luminal contents

Specific infectious pathogens or pathogenic alterations in composition or function of commensal bacteria could lead to chronic intestinal inflammation in otherwise normal hosts.

Specific microbial pathogen

The simplest explanation for intestinal injury and the mechanism most amenable to therapy is that IBD arises from infection by a single pathogenic organism. No consistent epidemiological, clinical, microbiological, immunological or therapeutic evidence supports this hypothesis as a cause for the majority of cases of ulcerative colitis or Crohn's disease. However, it is possible that a specific, poorly cultivatable or novel pathogen is responsible for a subset of patients with this disease. *Mycobacterium paratuberculosis* is the only agent currently being actively investigated. This interest is based on the recovery of identical *M. paratuberculosis* strains from approximately 10 Crohn's disease patients but no controls on several different continents.

Table 3 Mechanisms of intestinal injury by microbial agents

Toxic response to luminal contents
    Specific microbial pathogen
    Abnormal composition of luminal bacteria
    Abnormal functional properties of endogenous bacteria
    Defective mucosal barrier to luminal macromolecules

Inappropriate immunological response to normal constituents

Induction of autoimmunity

This pathogen causes granulomatous enterocolitis in ruminents (Johne's disease) and a human isolate has induced asymptomatic ileal granulomas when inoculated into a neonatal goat[28]. A mycobacterial cause of Crohn's disease is plausible because of the resemblance of this disease to ileocaecal tuberculosis; however, no convincing evidence incriminates this organism in the majority of Crohn's disease cases. Attempts to detect mycobacterial antigens or DNA in resected tissue have been negative; no consistent evidence of a cellular or humoral immune response to *M. paratuberculosis* exists and antituberculous therapeutic trials have yielded inconsistent results[11]. Although analogy has been made to the lepromatous phase of mycobacterial infection, in which organisms are very rare and anergy exists, the lack of transmission to close contacts and improvement with immunosuppressive therapy make this theory less attractive.

Abnormal composition of luminal bacteria

An altered composition of normal intestinal bacteria could change ratios of short-chain fatty acids or increase production of toxic bacterial components, which could have profound effects on epithelial and lamina propria cell function. Faecal concentrations and serum antibodies to anaerobic bacteria, especially *Bacteroides vulgatus*[29] and Gram-positive coccoid rods (*Eubacteria, Peptostreptococci* and *Coprococcus*)[30] are increased in Crohn's disease and group D streptococci (enterococci) are increased in ulcerative colitis[31]. Metronidazole chronically decreases luminal *Bacteroides* concentrations and response to therapy correlates with faecal *Bacteroides* levels[32]. *Bacteroides vulgatus* has been incriminated in the pathogenesis of carrageenan colitis[33], further emphasizing that this organism should be targeted for future studies in IBD. Profiles of luminal bacteria appear to be genetically regulated. In a provocative prospective study van de Merwe *et al.*[30] demonstrated that one-third of asymptomatic children of Crohn's disease patients had increased concentrations of anaerobic bacteria which appeared to be a risk factor for later development of Crohn's disease, since three of nine children with abnormal flora later developed intestinal symptoms. Some but not all strains of *Eubacteria* produce PG-PS which induces chronic inflammation[10], demonstrating that subtle alterations in anaerobic bacteria can have profound implications for disease pathogenesis.

Abnormal functional properties of endogenous bacteria

Similarly, functional changes in virulence factors or enzyme or toxin production by endogenous bacteria could induce chronic inflammation. Such alterations would never be detected by standard clinical micobiological testing. *E. coli* isolated from ulcerative colitis and Crohn's disease patients exhibit enhanced binding to epithelial cells, which differs from adherence mechanisms of enteropathogenic *E. coli*[34]. *E. coli* isolated from several patients with active ulcerative colitis have been shown to produce verotoxin, *Shiga*-like toxin or necrotoxins[35]. Group D streptococci (enterococci) from ulcerative colitis patients produce hyaluronidase, while those from normals do not[31]. These enterococci and *Bacteroides vulgatus* have the ability to degrade mucin[31,36], which can result in enhanced uptake of macromolecules including FMLP[2]. Production of bacterial superantigens and heat shock proteins has not yet been investigated in IBD patients, but has great potential relevance to this field.

Defective mucosal barrier to luminal macromolecules

Increased mucosal permeability is a universal feature of active Crohn's disease but is less well documented in ulcerative colitis. Whether this abnormality is a primary or secondary event remains controversial[37], but the net effect is enhanced uptake of dietary and bacterial antigens, bacterial chemotactic peptides and cell wall polymers, which could continuously stimulate the lamina propria immunocytes to maintain active inflammation.

Inappropriate immunological response to normal luminal constituents

An alternative explanation compatible with the failure to find specific pathogenic agents is that IBD is the result of an inappropriately aggressive response or defect in down-regulation of the immune response to normal luminal constituents. This hypothesis is supported by the differential susceptibility of inbred rat strains to PG-PS[3,8]. Lewis rats injected subserosally into the distal ileum and caecum with PG-PS develop chronic, spontaneously relapsing, granulomatous enterocolitis with associated polyarthritis, granulomatous hepatitis and anaemia. Buffalo or Fischer F344 (MHC compatible with Lewis) rats exhibit only transient inflammation at the site of injection, but no chronic enterocolitis or extraintestinal manifestations with identical exposure to PG-PS. Similarly, Lewis rats, but not Buffalo or Fischer rats, develop chronic, fibrotic hepatobiliary inflammation following experimental small intestinal overgrowth of anaerobic bacteria despite very similar luminal bacterial concentrations in the three rat strains[24]. Immunological mechanisms to explain the differential susceptibility of these inbred rat strains are not yet fully determined, but we have reported in preliminary studies that Lewis rats have an increased IL-1/IL-1 receptor antagonist (IL-1ra) ratio in both acute and chronic phases of PG-PS-induced colitis compared with Buffalo rats[9], suggesting a defective down-regulation of the immune response in Lewis rats. We have found a similar increase in the IL-1/IL-1ra ratio in colonic biopsies and resected tissues from Crohn's disease patients[38], and demonstrated altered IL-1 and IL-8 secretion in monocytes of Crohn's disease patients stimulated with PG-PS and LPS[39]. These findings, although preliminary, suggest that Crohn's disease patients have an overly aggressive response to luminal bacterial products, possibly mediated by defective immunosuppressive mechanisms.

Induction of autoimmunity

A humoral or cellular immune response to luminal microbial antigens which share homology with epithelial cell components provides an attractive mechanism for cellular injury in ulcerative colitis. Serum antibodies which react with both Enterobacteriaceae and colonic epithelial cells are present in patients with ulcerative colitis. Molecular mimicry, or shared epitopes between mammalian and microbial antigens, is displayed by homology between bacterial and mammalian heat shock proteins; *Klebsiella pneumoniae* nitrogenase reductase and HLA-B27; and cartilage matrix proteins and PG-PS[3]. The expression of at least one heat shock protein is increased in ulcerative colitis epithelial cells[40], although intraepithelial and peripheral blood lymphocytes from Crohn's disease patients do not react abnormally to this protein[41].

CONCLUSIONS

Factors initiating inflammation in ulcerative colitis and Crohn's disease remain unclear. Multiple, relatively non-specific events may initially injure the mucosa, while specific genetically determined immunoregulatory factors which govern the inflammatory response to the ubiquitous microbial flora may determine the chronicity of inflammation and development of systemic complications. Endogenous anaerobic bacteria and their cell wall constituents appear to be important in perpetuating Crohn's disease, especially colonic involvement, probably initiate and maintain extraintestinal inflammation in both Crohn's disease and ulcerative colitis, and mediate pouchitis. Ulcerative colitis could be a result of either abnormal virulence factors of aerobic bacteria or an autoimmune response mediated by crossreacting epitopes shared by commensal bacteria and epithelial cells. Ulcerative colitis and Crohn's disease are separate and distinct entities; it is probable that each disorder is composed of groups of heterogeneous diseases linked by common inflammatory mediators and limited mechanisms of intestinal response to injury. Furthermore, small intestinal and colonic Crohn's disease appear to have different responses to luminal constituents.

The distal intestine contains viable bacteria, bacterial enzymes, metabolic products, antigens, chemotactic peptides and cell wall polymers capable of initiating and perpetuating intestinal and systemic injury. The critical issue is why intense distal intestinal inflammation does not develop in everyone? The answer to this question will provide important insights into the pathogenesis of IBD. We propose that in the normal state the delicate balance between proinflammatory luminal constituents and mucosal protective forces (Fig. 2) is tipped towards protection. Injurious agents are excluded by a relatively impermeable epithelial barrier, and suppression of inflammation is mediated by down-regulation of the immune response. This balance can be perturbed by environmental and genetic factors which alter luminal contents, decrease epithelial barrier function and diminish host resistance. A better understanding of basic mechanisms of down-regulation of inflammation,

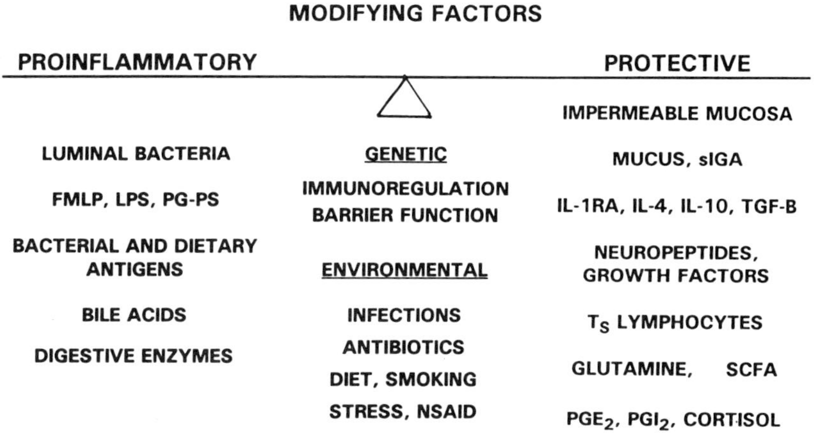

MODIFYING FACTORS

PROINFLAMMATORY		PROTECTIVE
		IMPERMEABLE MUCOSA
LUMINAL BACTERIA	GENETIC	MUCUS, sIGA
FMLP, LPS, PG-PS	IMMUNOREGULATION BARRIER FUNCTION	IL-1RA, IL-4, IL-10, TGF-B
BACTERIAL AND DIETARY ANTIGENS	ENVIRONMENTAL	NEUROPEPTIDES, GROWTH FACTORS
BILE ACIDS	INFECTIONS	T_S LYMPHOCYTES
DIGESTIVE ENZYMES	ANTIBIOTICS DIET, SMOKING	GLUTAMINE, SCFA
	STRESS, NSAID	PGE_2, PGI_2, CORTISOL

Fig. 2 The balance between luminal proinflammatory factors and mucosal protective mechanisms. The genetically determined immune response to bacterial products and epithelial barrier function can influence host susceptibility to chronic inflammation while environmental factors can influence initial onset and spontaneous reactivation of inflammation. FMLP, n-formyl-methionyl-leucyl-phenylalanine; LPS, lipopolysaccharide; PG-PS, peptidoglycan–polysaccharide polymers; PG, prostaglandin; IL, interleukin; TGF-B, transforming growth factor-B; NSAID, non-steroidal anti-inflammatory drug; T_s, T suppressor lymphocytes; SCFA, short-chain fatty acids. (Adapted from Sartor RB. Can J Gastroenterol. 1990;4:271–7 and used with permission)

environmental triggers and genetically determined immunoregulatory defects of IBD will permit more careful characterization of subsets of patients with ulcerative colitis and Crohn's disease, so that rational and specific therapy can be designed and an individual's clinical course can be accurately predicted.

Acknowledgements

The author gratefully acknowledges the expert secretarial assistance of Shirley Willard. Original research described in this review was supported by NIH grants DK 40249 and DK 34987 and the Crohn's and Colitis Foundation of America.

References

1. Sartor RB. Role of intestinal microflora in initiation and perpetuation of inflammatory bowel disease. Can J Gastroenterol. 1990;4:271–7.
2. Chadwick VS, Anderson RP. Microorganisms and their products in inflammatory bowel disease. In: MacDermott RP, Stenson WF, editors. Inflammatory bowel disease. New York: Elsevier; 1992:241–58.
3. Sartor RB, Lichtman SN. Mechanisms of systemic inflammation associated with intestinal injury. In: Targan SR, Shanahan F, editors. Inflammatory bowel disease: From Bench to Bedside. Baltimore, MD: Williams & Wilkins; 1992: in press.
4. Powell SJ, Wilmont AJ. Ulcerative post-dysenteric colitis. Gut. 1966;7:438–43.
5. Chester JF, Ross JS, Malt RA, Weitzman SA. Acute colitis produced by chemotactic peptides in rats and mice. Am J Pathol. 1985;121:284–90.

6. von Ritter C, Sekizuka E, Grisham MB, Granger DN. The chemotactic peptide *N*-formyl methionyl-leucyl-phenylalanine increases mucosal permeability in the distal ileum of the rat. Gastroenterology. 1988;95:651–6.

7. Hsueh W, Gonzalez-Crussi F, Arroyave JL. Platelet-activating factor: an endogenous mediator for bowel necrosis in endotoxemia. FASEB J. 1987;1:403–5.

8. Sartor RB. Animal models of intestinal inflammation: relevance to IBD. In: MacDermott RP, Stenson W, editors. Inflammatory bowel disease. New York: Elsevier; 1992:337–54.

9. McCall RD, Haskill JS, Sartor RB. Interleukin-1 and IL-1 receptor antagonist gene expression correlate with activity of inflammation in spontaneously relapsing enterocolitis in rats. Gastroenterology. 1991;100:598A.

10. Severijnen AJ, van Kleef R, Hazenberg MP, van de Merwe JP. Chronic arthritis induced in rats by cell wall fragments of *Eubacterium* species from the human intestinal flora. Infect Immun. 1990;58:523–8.

11. Sartor RB. Antimicrobial agents in IBD: clinical and pathogenetic considerations. Can J Gastroenterol. 1992: in press.

12. Sutherland L, Singleton J, Sessions J *et al*. Double blind, placebo controlled trial of metronidazole in Crohn's disease. Gut. 1991;32:1071–5.

13. Saverymuttu S, Hodgson HJF, Chadwick VA. Controlled trial comparing prednisolone with an elemental diet plus non-absorbable antibiotics in active Crohn's disease. Gut. 1985;26:994–8.

14. Wellmann W, Fink PC, Benner F. Endotoxaemia in active Crohn's disease. Treatment with whole gut irrigation and 5-aminosalicylic acid. Gut. 1986;27:814–20.

15. Rutgeerts P, Peeters M, Hiele M *et al*. A placebo controlled trial of metronidazole for recurrence prevention of Crohn's disease after resection of the terminal ileum. Gastroenterology. 1992;102:A688.

16. Harper PH, Lee ECG, Kettlewell MGW *et al*. Role of the faecal stream in the maintenance of Crohn's colitis. Gut. 1985;26:279–84.

17. Rutgeerts P, Goboes K, Peeters M *et al*. Effect of faecal stream diversion on recurrence of Crohn's disease in the neoterminal ileum. Lancet. 1991;338:771–4.

18. Davis SW, Holt LC, Sartor RB. Luminal bacterial and bacterial polymers potentiate indomethacin-induced intestinal injury in the rat. Gastroenterology. 1990;98:444A.

19. Sartor RB, Bond TM, Schwab JH. Systemic uptake and intestinal inflammatory effects of luminal bacterial cell wall polymers in rats with acute colonic injury. Infect Immun. 1988;56:2101–8.

20. Kangro HO, Chong SKF, Hardiman A, Heath RB, Walker-Smith JA. A prospective study of viral and mycoplasma infections in chronic inflammatory bowel disease. Gastroenterology. 1990;98:549–53.

21. Isgar B, Harman M, Whorwell PJ. Factors preceding relapse of ulcerative colitis. Digestion. 1983;26:236–8.

22. Keighley MRB, Eastwood D, Ambrose NS, Allan RN, Burdon DW. Incidence and microbiology of abdominal and pelvic abscess in Crohn's disease. Gastroenterology. 1982;83:1271–5.

23. Wands JR, LaMont JT, Mann E, Isselbacher KJ. Arthritis associated with intestinal-bypass procedure for morbid obesity. N Engl J Med. 1976;294:121–4.

24. Lichtman SN, Sartor RB, Schwab JH, Keku J. Hepatic inflammation in rats with experimental small bowel bacterial overgrowth. Gastroenterology. 1990;98:414–23.

25. Anderson RP, Friend GM, Ferry DM, Chadwick VS. Formyl peptidemia in patients with inflammatory bowel disease and primary sclerosing cholangitis. Gastroenterology. 1991;100:A557.

26. Carton RW, Van Kruiningen HJ, Pederaca CA, Berman MM. Extending the search for microbial agents in Crohn's disease. Preliminary results. Gastroenterology. 1989;96:A75.

27. Ambrose NS, Johnson M, Burdon DW, Keighley MRB. Incidence of pathogenic bacteria from mesenteric lymph nodes and ileal serosa during Crohn's disease. Br J Surg. 1984;71:6623–5.

28. Chiodini RJ. Crohn's disease and the mycobacterioses: a review and comparison of two disease entities. Clin Microbiol Rev. 1990;2:90–117.

29. Ruseler-van Embden JGH, Both-Patoir HC. Anaerobic gram-negative faecal flora in patients with Crohn's disease and healthy subjects. Antonie van Leeuwenhoek. 1983;49:125–32.

30. van de Merwe JP, Schroder AM, Wensinck F, Hazenberg MP. The obligate anaerobic faecal flora of patients with Crohn's disease and their first-degree relatives. Scand J Gastroenterol. 1988;23:1125–31.
31. van der Wiel-Korstanje JAA, Winkler KC. The faecal flora in ulcerative colitis. J Med Microbiol. 1975;8:491–501.
32. Krok A, Jarnerot G, Danielsson D. Clinical effect of metronidazole and sulfasalazine on Crohn's disease in relation to changes in the fecal flora. Scand J Gastroenterol. 1981;16:569–75.
33. Breeling JL, Onderdonk AB, Cisneros RL. *Bacteroides vulgatus* outer membrane antigens associated with carrageenan-induced colitis in guinea pigs. Infect Immun. 1988;56:1754–9.
34. Burke DA, Axon ATR. Adhesive *Escherichia coli* in inflammatory bowel disease and infective diarrhoea. Br Med J. 1988;297:102–4.
35. von Wulffen H, Russman H, Karch H *et al.* Verocytotoxin producing *Escherichia coli* 02:H5 isolated from patients with ulcerative colitis. Lancet. 1989;1449–50.
36. Ruseler-van Embden JGH, van der Helm R, van Lieshout LMC. Degradation of intestinal glycoproteins by *Bacteroides vulgatus*. FEMS Microbiol Lett. 1989;58:37–42.
37. Katz DK, Hollander D, Vadheim CM. Intestinal permeability in patients with Crohn's disease and their healthy relatives. Gastroenterology. 1989;97:927–31.
38. Isaacs KL, Sartor RB, Haskill JS. Cytokine mRNA profiles in inflammatory bowel disease mucosa detected by PCR amplification. Gastroenterology. 1992;103:1587–95.
39. Fu RD, Izatani R, Muraski T, Sartor RB, MacDermott RP. Increased secretion of interleukin-8 from peripheral monocytes in patients with Crohn's disease. Gastroenterology. 1992;102:A624.
40. Mojedhi G, Winrow VR, Blake DR, Rampton DS. Immunohistological localisation of stress proteins in rectal mucosa. Gastroenterology. 1990;98:A464.
41. Baca-Estrada M, Gupta RS, Chiba N, Croitoru K. Comparison of mucosal and systemic lymphocyte reactivity to 65 kD human heat shock protein (HSP65) in Crohn's disease. Gastroenterology. 1991;100:A558.

17

Intestinal glutamine metabolism

F. HARTMANN, M. PLAUTH and A. RAIBLE

INTRODUCTION

Studies over the past 15–20 years point towards the important role of the small intestine in mammalians as a major site of glutamine metabolism.

Glutamine has emerged as a quantitatively more important respiratory fuel than glucose in the enterocytes of the small intestine. This observation started with Neptune's work in 1965[1] where it was shown that incubated intestinal slices produced large amounts of CO_2 from glutamine. More direct clues emerged from arteriovenous difference measurements across the non-hepatic splanchnic organs of dog, sheep, rat and humans[2–12]. Since the most numerous cells in the intestine, the enterocytes, have a dual source of nutrients, the intestinal lumen and arterial blood, viable preparations of intact intestine – isolated as well as *in situ* – allowed separate access to both sources and were particularly well suited for metabolic studies[5,13–16].

The pacemaker work in this field has been performed by Windmueller and Spaeth[10,17–20] as well as Hanson and Parsons[5] more than 10 years ago. From their experiments we will focus first on the metabolism of arterial glutamine, second on the metabolism of dietary glutamine from the lumen, and third on the relevant enzymes located in the enterocytes.

UTILIZATION OF ARTERIAL GLUTAMINE

Arteriovenous difference measurements of glutamine *in vivo* across the tissues drained by the superior mesenteric vein were found to be larger than those measured across all portal drained organs, which means that the uptake in the small intestine and proximal colon is most important[2,10,11,21,22]. As Windmueller and Spaeth pointed out, the glutamine uptake was entirely from the plasma fraction of the blood, since the glutamine concentration of erythrocytes passing through the intestine did not change[17].

The highest uptake and also the most extensive metabolism occurred in the enterocytes of the small intestine where after 20 seconds 80% of the glutamine carbon was already in metabolic products[10]. Surprisingly, despite the continuous high uptake of glutamine by the mucosal cells, their steady-state glutamine content was low, only 0.2 µmol/g tissue or 3% of the concentration found in liver cells and 6% of that in skeletal muscle[10]. This seemed to be related to the high substrate affinity of the intestinal phosphate dependent glutaminase[23].

Gut preparations from rats fasted overnight showed a net glutamine uptake of 74 µmol/h when sufficient glutamine was infused continuously into the perfusate to maintain the normal blood concentration[10] of about 0.6 mmol/l. The net rate of glutamine utilization by the perfused gut was concentration-dependent with a maximum near the normal blood concentration of 0.6 mmol/l.

As Schröck and Goldstein[24] showed, the glutamine uptake by the non-hepatic splanchnic vascular bed of the rat is sufficient to account for the entire glutamine output by skeletal muscle, the major site to release glutamine into the circulation.

In autoperfused intestinal segments of the rat *in vivo* again Windmueller and Spaeth confirmed these results[17]. A similar rate of glutamine utilization was found by Hanson and Parsons[5], again in an isolated rat preparation but with a high glutamine concentration, namely 1.5 mmol.

In rats not fasted, intestinal segments rinsed free of diet residue, utilized arterial glutamine and glucose at about twice the rates per unit weight of tissue as observed in fasted animals. The rate of glutamine metabolism was also unaffected by perfusing the lumen with up to 70 mmol/l glucose which was readily transported with only 3% being metabolized during the arbsorption[19]. Glutamine and glucose utilization were not further increased when the lumen of the segment was perfused with non-metabolized luminal substrates like 3-*O*-methyl-D-glucose and several amino acids[19].

The influence of the additional absorption of metabolized luminal substrates such as glucose might be different. Weber[25] demonstrated a significant increase of arterial glutamine uptake and elevation of ammonia release into mesenteric venous blood when 50 mmol/l glucose was offered on the luminal side of *in situ*-perfused intestinal segments of anaesthetized fasted dogs. If this observation holds true in humans, it might be of considerable clinical importance as cirrhotic patients are usually treated with a diet rich in carbohydrates and low in protein.

In conclusion, the utilization rate of arterial glutamine is concentration-dependent, it is approximately equal to the rate of glucose utilization, it is reduced by fasting and it is not increased by carrier-mediated transport of non-metabolized luminal substrates.

These data have been confirmed in recent human studies with measurement of glutamine concentration in portal venous and systemic blood samples or enterectomized patients[26,27].

LUMINAL GLUTAMINE UTILIZATION

When ^{14}C-labeled glutamine was given intraluminally in autoperfused jejunal segments at a concentration of 6 mmol/l, which is close to the postprandial luminal levels, almost all of the radioactivity was recovered in the collected venous blood within 60 min[17]. About one-third of the ^{14}C remained in glutamine, the remainder was distributed among a group of metabolites which resembled those observed after arterial glutamine administration[10,17]. Following the luminal application of glutamine the venous output of ammonia, alanine, citrulline and proline was also increased. Apparently, the metabolism of the luminally absorbed glutamine depends on the luminal concentration administered: according to Windmueller and Spaeth at 6 mmol/l only 34% of the glutamine was translocated intact to the vascular side, in contrast to 70% at 45 mmol/l luminal concentration[17].

As no glutamate was released during the luminal perfusion with either 6 or 45 mmol/l glutamine[17] the rate-limiting step for glutamine catabolism presumably is its deamidation, and not the metabolism of the resulting glutamate. Perfusion experiments with glutamate on the luminal side exhibited the same ^{14}C-labelled products on the venous side as observed upon the luminal administration of glutamine[17].

Windmueller and Spaeth[17], as well as Hanson and Parsons[5], showed that the presence of glutamine or glutamate in the lumen does reduce the rate of glutamine utilization from the blood; nevertheless the total rate of glutamine metabolized when offered from both sides was significantly increased. These studies emphasize again the large capacity of the small intestine to metabolize glutamine.

METABOLIC FATE

In the small intestine glutamine carbon may be metabolized via two principal routes either forming α^1-pyrroline-5-carboxylate[28,29] or via α-ketoglutarate as Krebs-cycle intermediate. The former pathway leads to the formation of proline, ornithine and citrulline, which are released from small intestine, accounting for 10% of glutamine carbon utilized[10]. Another 10–15% of glutamine carbon is incorporated into tissue protein[10]. Thus the major proportion (75%) is being metabolized via the Krebs cycle, spinning off at different levels. More than half (55%) of glutamine carbon taken up is being oxidized to CO_2, thus serving as a respiratory fuel[10]. The share of glutamine carbon in gut respiration ranges from 33% in the isolated perfused organ from starved animals[10] to about 70% in autoperfused isolated segments of fed animals[19]. The remaining 20% of glutamine carbon is recovered as citrate, lactate, other organic acids and glucose[10,17,18].

The product distribution of the glutamine carbons is similar whether conventional or germ-free rats are used, thus precluding the intestinal microflora as a source for any of these metabolic products[10]. The same products have been detected in different rat gut preparations by other groups as well as *in vivo* in dog, sheep, and humans[2–7,9–11]. In contrast to *in vitro* experiments with intestinal slices and isolated enterocytes almost no glutamate escaped unmetabolized into the vascular medium[17].

Complete oxidation of glutamine carbon would yield almost as much energy as complete oxidation of glucose. However, complete oxidation of glutamine in the small intestine has not yet been demonstrated convincingly. Using uniformly labelled glutamine the measured ^{14}(C)-CO_2 production does not necessarily reflect the further degradation of pyruvate via pyruvate dehydrogenase[30]. As the intestinal mucosa does exhibit pyruvate carboxylase activity[31] labelled CO_2 might derive from a redistribution of pyruvate via oxaloacetate and further metabolic degradation of this molecule in the Krebs cycle.

Using differentially labelled ^{14}(C) succinate Mallet *et al.*[32] demonstrated a rather partial than complete glutamine oxidation and conservation of three carbon units in rat enterocytes. These results support previous observations by Watford *et al.*[9] that alanine carbon may be provided from glutamine. In analogy to the partial oxidation of glucose to lactate, known as glycolysis, the term glutaminolysis has been proposed to describe the partial oxidation of glutamine in rapidly proliferating tissues[33].

ENZYMOLOGY

High activity of glutaminase (3–6 µmol/h per mg protein) has been demonstrated in duodenal, jejunal, and ileal mucosa of rat, dog, cat, hamster, rabbit, and monkey[10]. Glutaminase activity was found in mature villous tip cells as well as in the rapidly dividing mucosal crypt cells[23]. The high substrate affinity of the glutaminase is consistent with the low tissue levels of glutamine. The apparent K_m of the intestinal glutaminase is about 2.2 mmol/l for glutamine, thus only 10% that of liver glutaminase[17,23]. Nearly all the intestinal glutaminase is associated with the mitochondria and is membrane-bound[23]. The apparent $K_{0.5}$ for activation by phosphate is 22 mmol/l[23]. The crude intestinal glutaminase resembles the glutaminase of kidney, brain, and ascites cells in many of its properties, but is different from the liver enzyme[23].

In addition to glutaminase all of the other enzymes involved in the proposed metabolic pathways of glutamine carbon and nitrogen have been demonstrated individually in cell-free mucosal preparations of small intestine by various laboratories.

INTESTINAL GLUTAMINE TRANSPORT

Bradford and McGivan described a sodium-dependent, ouabain, and methyl-aminoisobutyrate inhibited system A-like mechanism for glutamine and alanine transport into isolated rat enterocytes[34]. No localization as to the apical or the basolateral membrane was possible in their experimental design. Apparently, glutamine is transported into isolated rat colonocytes by an almost identical carrier system[35]. Although the presence of two Na-independent and three Na-dependent carrier-mediated pathways for a number of amino acids has been observed in rabbit jejunal brush border vesicles[36], glutamine transport, unfortunately, was not measured. The authors are also not aware of any investigation regarding glutamine transport across the mitochondrial membrane of enterocytes.

POSTABSORPTIVE STATE

In the postabsorptive state with an almost empty intestinal lumen glutamine is taken up at high rates across the basolateral membrane of the enterocyte[2-6,8-10]. In this state the release of alanine and glutamine from the skeletal muscle[37] is matched by the splanchnic uptake[3,4,38]. While alanine serves as direct substrate for hepatic gluconeogenesis and possibly also intestinal gluconeogenesis, most of the glutamine is taken up by the small intestine[24,38-40] and processed for further metabolism in the liver and in the kidney.

POSTPRANDIAL STATE

In the postprandial state the pattern of amino acids cr related compounds in portal blood is characterized by the absence of glutamic and aspartic acid, as well as disproportionately elevated levels of alanine, ammonia and, at least in the rat, glycine[2,11,12,41-43]. Glutamine applied from the luminal side at concentrations comparable to the postprandial situation is utilized at rates equal to glutamine taken up from the bloodstream[17,19]. Ammonia and alanine are formed[5,17,19], alanine probably at higher proportions as from glutamine taken up from the vascular side[5].

STARVATION

Prolonged fasting is accompanied by adaptive changes in intestinal glutamine metabolism at various levels. Glutaminase activity decreases after 48 h or more of fasting[5,44,45] with no change of specific activity, however[5,44]. In chronically catheterized dogs after 96 h of fasting Cersosimo[46] observed a doubling of gut glutamine uptake with a corresponding increase of NH_3 output and a 40% drop in alanine release. Obviously alterations in extraction rate, or more likely intestinal blood flow, must have occurred as arterial glutamine levels were found unaltered in this study[46], although reported as elevated in a previous communication from the same group[47]. The observed shift in nitrogenous products from glutamine metabolism may reflect recruitment of oxidative glutamate deamination via the glutamate dehydrogenase pathway as shown operative in renal tubules from acidotic rats[48]. Moreover, the adaptive changes seen in both starvation[46,47] and chronic acidosis[39,49] may well result from acidosis at least in part, as mild metabolic acidosis was found in dogs starved for 96 h[46].

ACIDOSIS

Regarding the small intestinal contribution to glutamine metabolism in acidosis controversies do exist. There are reports on increased[6,21], decreased[49] and unaltered[5,24,44,49] intestinal glutamine metabolism in the literature.

DIABETES

The most striking change of intestinal glutamine flux has been observed in streptozotocin-induced diabetic rats. Arterial glutamine removal by the intestine was sharply reduced or ceased completely together with a concomitant reduction of citrulline and alanine release[50,51]. These changes might be due to extremely low plasma levels of arterial glutamine[52]. Interestingly, arterial glutamine was lowered also in diabetic humans[3]. The capacity to handle glutamine may vary in the course of the disease. In rats, after 6 weeks of uncontrolled diabetes normal[53] as well as a 10-fold rise[51] of glutaminase activity were found associated with profound visceral hyperplasia[51,53]. On the other hand, a decrease of jejunal glutaminase as a result of inactivated enzyme protein was observed 48 h after streptozotocin administration[49]. However, a reduction of similar magnitude has been demonstrated after 48 h starvation[5,43-45].

TRAUMA

In conscious dogs after trauma Souba and Wilmore[40] reported a 75% increase in intestinal glutamine uptake on the second postoperative day returning towards normal on the fourth postoperative day. Alanine release was reduced in a reciprocal manner. Unfortunately ammonia was not measured, but may have risen as in acidosis[49] and starvation[46]. In enterectomized rats[22,54] and dogs[55] an accelerated intestinal glutamine consumption characteristic for catabolic illness contributed to low arterial glutamine levels in these stress states.

Contrary to chronic acidosis, when intestinal glutamine uptake appeared to be reduced only moderately due to lowered arterial levels[39,49,56-58], after trauma glutamine uptake by the gut almost doubled despite reduction of arterial levels and reduced portal blood flow[40]. These observations in starvation[46] and trauma[40] are in contrast to Newsholme's proposal[59] of glutamine flux regulation by glutamine availability.

Recent human data in a small number of patients with multisystem trauma confirm these results[26].

GLUCOCORTICOIDS

As glucocorticoids are thought to mediate at least in part the net breakdown of muscle protein in catabolic states[38], there are several reports describing the influence of dexamethasone on the intestinal glutamine utilization in sheep[6], everted segments of rat small intestine[60] and the conscious dog[38].

Souba and Wilmore[38] observed a significant increase in intestinal glutamine uptake, accompanied by a doubled alanine release. In contrast to the post-traumatic state[40] dexamethasone elevated both portal blood flow and arteriovenous differences. An earlier study in sheep produced controversial results[6]. In both studies direct and indirect effects of dexamethasone cannot be differentiated.

In rats, pretreatment with intramuscular dexamethasone (0.6 mg/100 g) led to a 50% increase of glutamine uptake and a 25% reduction of protein content of everted intestinal segments[60].

In order to eliminate severe artifacts due to ischaemia of the intestinal mucosa[16] we examined the uptake of arterial glutamine in an isolated vascularly and luminally perfused rat small intestine[15]. The addition of dexamethasone (250 μg/dl) to the vascular perfusion medium neither increased intestinal glutamine utilization nor alanine release. Also, ammonia production remained unaltered.

EFFECT OF LACTULOSE AND PAROMOMYCIN/NEOMYCIN ON AMMONIAGENESIS

With the recent appreciation of a significant endogenous intestinal ammoniagenesis the question arose whether the beneficial effect of lactulose and neomycin in the treatment of hepatic encephalopathy might result from their influence on intestinal glutamine utilization. Van Leeuwen[61], from the results obtained with incubated intestinal slices[62], measurements of arterioportal differences in germ-free rats[61] and selectively decontaminated and gnotobiotic animals[63] concluded that lactulose and neomycin decreased intestinal glutamine uptake, thus reducing endogenous ammonia production.

In the vascularly and luminally perfused isolated rat small intestine we were unable to confirm any effect of lactulose or paromomycin on ammonia formation and glutamine uptake when glutamine was supplied from the vascular side at physiological concentrations[64]. Clearly, pharmacodynamic effects of lactulose and neomycin/paromomycin on brush-border glutamine transport need to be investigated.

GLUTAMINE AND MUCOSAL BARRIER

Recent investigations exhibited an important role for glutamine concerning the maintenance of gut barrier function. Survival after experimentally induced enteritis (radiation injury, methotrexate-induced enterocolitis) is significantly improved by glutamine. Gut immune function as measured in bacterial translocation or response to endotoxin is also well preserved with a glutamine-supplemented enteral or parenteral nitrition[65-69].

CONCLUSION

The small intestine shows a uniquely high uptake of glutamine from the lumen and from arterial blood. The small intestine is the predominant site of glutamine catabolism in various physiological and pathophysiological states. There is evidence for an active adaptation of intestinal glutamine metabolism to various metabolic conditions. Moreover, an active cooperation in glutamine metabolism between small intestine and liver apparently plays a key role in maintaining nitrogen homeostasis of the whole organism, but little is known about the regulation of these events. The addition of glutamine to enteral or parenteral nutritional regimens might prove to become very important for patients treated with cytostatic drugs, patients after trauma and patients with chronic inflammatory bowel disease.

References

1. Neptune EM. Respiration and oxidation of various substrates by ileum in vitro. Am J Physiol. 1965;209:329–33.
2. Elwyn DH, Parikh HC, Shoemaker WC. Amino acid movements between gut liver and periphery in unanaesthetized dogs. Am J Physiol. 1968;215:1260–75.
3. Felig P, Wahren J, Karl I et al. Glutamine and glutamate metabolism in normal and diabetic subjects. Diabetes. 1973;22:573–6.
4. Felig P, Wahren J, Räf L. Evidence of inter-organ amino acid transport by blood cells in humans. Proc Natl Acad Sci USA. 1973;70:1775–9.
5. Hanson PJ, Parsons DS. Metabolism and transport of glutamine and glucose in vascularly perfused rat small intestine. Biochem J. 1977;166:509–19.
6. Heitmann RN, Bergmann AE. Glutamine metabolism inter-organ transport and glucogenicity in the sheep. Am J Physiol. 1978;234:E197–E203.
7. Matsutaka H, Aikawa T, Yamamoto H et al. Gluconeogenesis and amino acid metabolism III. Uptake of glutamine and output of alanine and ammonia by non-hepatic splanchnic organs of fasted rats and their metabolic significance. J. Biochem. 1973;74:1019–29.
8. Owen OE, Reichle FA, Mozzoli MA et al. Hepatic gut and renal substrate flux rates in patients with hepatic cirrhosis. J Clin Invest. 1981;68:240–52.
9. Watford M, Lund P, Krebs HA. Isolation and metabolic charactertistics of rat and chicken enterocytes. Biochem J. 1979;178:589–96.
10. Windmueller HG, Spaeth AE. Uptake and metabolism of plasma glutamine by the small intestine. J Biol Chem. 1974;249:5070–9.
11. Wolff JE, Berman EN, Williams HH. Net metabolism of plasma amino acids by liver and portal-drained viscera of fed sheep. Am J Physiol. 1972;223:438–46.
12. Yamamoto H, Aikawa T, Matsutaka H et al. Interorganal relationship of amino acid metabolism in fed rats. Am J Physiol. 1974; 226:1428–33.
13. Kavin H, Levin NW, Stanley MM. Isolated perfused rat small bowel technic studies of viability glucose absorption. J Appl Physiol. 1967;22:604–11.
14. Windmueller HG, Spaeth AE, Ganote CE. Vascular perfusion of isolated rat gut: Norepinephrine and glucocorticoid requirement. Am J Physiol. 1970;218:197–204.
15. Hartmann F, Vieillard-Baron D, Heinrich R. Isolated perfusion of the small intestine using perfluorotributylamine as artificial oxygen carrier. Adv Exp Med Biol. 1984;180:711–20.
16. Plumb JA, Burston D, Baker TG, Gardner MLG. A comparison of the structural integrity of several commonly used preparations of rat small intestine in vitro. Clin Sci. 1987;73:53–9.
17. Windmueller HG, Spaeth AE. Intestinal metabolism of glutamine and glutamate from the lumen as compared to glutamine from blood. Arch Biophys Biochem. 1975;171:662–72.
18. Windmueller HG, Spaeth AE. Identification of ketone bodies and glutamine as the respiratory fuels in vivo for postabsorptive rate small intestine. J Biol Chem. 1978;253:69–76.

19. Windmueller HG, Spaeth AE. Respiratory fuels and nitrogen metabolism in vivo in small intestine of fed rats. Quantitative importance of glutamine, glutamate and aspartate. J Biol Chem. 1980;255:107–12.
20. Windmueller HG, Spaeth AE. Source and fate of circulating citrulline. Am J Physiol. 1981;241:E473–80.
21. Addae SK, Lotspeich WD. Relation between glutamine utilization and production in metabolic acidosis. Am J Physiol. 1968;215:269–77.
22. Ishikawa E, Aikawa T, Matsutaka H. The roles of alanine as a major precursor among amino acids for hepatic gluconeogenesis and as major end product of the degradation of amino acids in rat tissue. J Biochem. 1972;71:1097–9.
23. Pinkus LM, Windmueller HG. Phosphate-dependent glutaminase of small intestine: localization and role in intestinal glutamine metabolism. Arch Biochem Biophys. 1977;182:506–17.
24. Schrock H, Goldstein L. Interorgan relationships for glutamine metabolism in normal acidotic rats. Am J Physiol. 1981;240:E519–25.
25. Weber FL, Veach G, Friedman DW. Stimulation of ammonia production from glutamine by intraluminal glucose in small intestine of dogs. Am J Physiol. 1982;242:G552–7.
26. McAnenea OJ, Moore FA, Moore EE, Jones TN, Parsons P. Selective uptake of glutamine in the gastrointestinal tract: Confirmation in a human study. Br J Surg. 1991;78:480–2.
27. Darmaun D, Messing B, Just B, Rongier M, Desjeux JF. Glutamine metabolism after small intestinal resection in humans. Metabol Clin Exp. 1991;40:42–4.
28. Herzfeld A, Raper SM. Enzymes of ornithine metabolism in adult and developing rat intestine. Biochim Biophys Acta. 1976;428:600–10.
29. Wakabayashi Y, Jones ME. Pyrroline-5-carboxylate synthesis from glutamate by rat intestinal mucosa. J Biol Chem. 1983;258:3865–72.
30. Myles DD, Strong P, Sugden MC: Errors arising from the use of [1-^{14}C]pyruvate to measure flux through the liver pyruvate dehydrogenase complex. Biochem J. 1984;218:997–8.
31. Anderson JW. Pyruvate carboxylase and phosphoenolpyruvate carboxykinase in rat intestinal mucosa. Biochim Biophys Acta. 1970;208:165–7.
32. Mallet RT, Kellerer JK, Jackson MJ. Substrate metabolism of isolated jejunal epithelium: conservation of three-carbon units. Am J Physiol. 1986;250:C191–C198.
33. McKeehan WL. Glycolysis glutaminolysis and cell proliferation. Cell Biol Int Rep. 1982;6:635–47.
34. Bradford NN, McGiven JD. The transport of alanine and glutamine into isolated rat intestinal epithelial cells. Biochim Biophys Acta. 1982;689:55–62.
35. Ardawi MSM. The transport of glutamine and alanine into rat colonocytes. Biochem J. 1986;238:131–5.
36. Stevens BR, Ross HJ, Wright EM. Multiple transport pathways for neutral amino acids in rabbit jejunal brush border vesicles. J Membrane Biol. 1982;66:213–25.
37. Felig P. Amino acid metabolism in man. Ann Rev Biochem. 1975;44:933–55.
38. Souba WW, Smith RJ, Wilmore DW. Effects of glucocorticoids on glutamine metabolism in visceral organs. Metabolism. 1985;34:450–6.
39. Phjromphetcharat V, Jackson A, Dass PD et al. Ammonia partitioning between glutamine and urea: interorgan participation in metabolic acidosis. Kidney Int. 1981;20:598–605.
40. Souba WW, Wilmore DW. Postoperative alterations of arteriovenous exchange of amino acids across the gastrointestinal tract. Surgery. 1983;94:342–50.
41. Matthews DM, Wiseman G. Transamination by the small intestine of the rat. J Physiol. 1953;120:55P.
42. Neame KD, Wiseman G. The transamination of glutamic and aspartic acids during absorption by the small intestine of the dog in vivo. J. Physiol. 1957;135:442–50.
43. Neame KD, Wiseman G. The alanine and oxo acid concentrations in mesenteric blood during the absorption of L-glutamic acid by the small intestine of the dog, cat and rabbit in vivo. J Physiol. 1958;140:148–55.
44. Budohoski L, Challis RAI, Newsholme EA. Effects of starvation on the maximal activities of some glycolytic and citric acid-cycle enzymes and glutaminase in mucosa of the small intestine of the rat. Biochem J. 1982;206:169–72.
45. Nagy LE, Kretchmer N. Effect of diabetic ketoacidosis on jejunal glutaminase. Arch Biochem Biophys. 1986;248:80–8.

46. Cersosimo E, Williams PE, Radosevich PM *et al.* Role of glutamine in adaptations in nitrogen metabolism during fasting. Am J Physiol. 1986;250:E622–E628.
47. Miller BM, Cersosimo E, McRae J *et al.* Interorgan relationship of alanine and glutamine during fasting in the conscious dog. J Surg Res. 1983;35:310–18.
48. Nissam I, Yudkoff M, Segal S. Metabolism of glutamine and glutamate by rat renal tubules study with ^{15}N and gas chromatography-mass spectrometry. J Biol Chem. 1985;260:13955–67.
49. Lund P, Watford M. Glutamine as a precursor of urea. In: Grisolia S, Baguena R, Mayor F, editors. The urea cycle. New York: Wiley; 1976:479–88.
50. Brosnan JT, Man K-C, Hall DE *et al.* Interorgan metabolism of amino acids in streptozotocin-diabetic ketoacidotic rat. Am J Physiol. 1983;244:E151–E158.
51. Watford M, Smith EM, Erbelding EJ. The regulation of phosphate-activated glutaminase activity and glutamine metabolism in the streptozotocin-diabetic rat. Biochem J. 1984;224:207–14.
52. Erbelding EJ, Watford M. Glutamine metabolism in the diabetic rat small intestine. Fed Proc. 1985;44:1213.
53. Ardawi MSM. The maximal activity of phosphate-dependent glutaminase and glutamine metabolism in the colon and the small intestine of streptozotocin-diabetic rats. Diabetologia. 1987;30:109–14.
54. Aikawa T, Matsutaka H, Yamamoto H, Okuda T, Ishikawa E, Kawano T, Matsumura E. Gluconeogenesis and amino acid metabolism. II Interorganal relations and roles of glutamine and alanine in the amino acid metabolism of fasted rats. J Biochem. 1973;74:1003–17.
55. Souba WW, Roughneen PT, Goldwater DL, Williams JC, Rowlands BJ. Postoperative alterations in interorgan glutamine exchange in enterectomized dogs. J Surg Res. 1987;42:117–25.
56. Squires EJ, Hall DE, Brosnan JT. Arteriovenous differences for amino acids and lactate across kidney of normal and acidotic rats. Biochem J. 1976;160:125–8.
57. Tizianello A, deFerrari D, Garibotto G *et al.* Effects of chronic renal insufficiency and metabolic acidosis on glutamine metabolism in man. Clin Sci Molec Med. 1978;55:391–7.
58. Welbourne TC. Effect of metabolic acidosis on hindquarter glutamine and alanine release. Metabolism. 1986;35:614–18.
59. Newsholme EA, Crabtree B, Ardawi MSM. Glutamine metabolism in lymphocytes: Its biochemical physiological and clinical importance. J Exp Physiol. 1985;70:473–89.
60. Souba WW, Smith RJ, Wilmore DW. Glucocorticoids regulate intestinal glutamine consumption. Curr Surg. 1985;42:385–8.
61. VanLeeuwen PAM, vdBogaard EJ, Janssen MA *et al.* Ammonia production and glutamine metabolism in the small and large intestine of the rat and the influence of lactulose and neomycine. In: Kleinberger G *et al.*, editors. Advances in hepatic encephalopathy and urea cycle diseases. Basel: Karger; 1984;154–62.
62. VanLeeuwen PAM, Janssen MA, deBoer JEG *et al.* The effect of lactulose and neomycine on metabolic ammonia generation in small and large bowel in vitro in male Wistar rats. In: Kleinberger G *et al.*, editors. Advances in hepatic encephalopathy and urea cycle diseases. Basel: Karger; 1984:163–8.
63. Soeters PB, vanLeeuwen PAM, Janssen MA *et al.* Metabolic generation of ammonia and amino acids in the intestinal wall and the influence of neomycine and lactulose. In: Kleiberger G *et al.*, editors. Advances in hepatic encephalopathy and urea cycle diseases. Basel: Karger; 1984:147–53.
64. Plauth M, Graser TA, Vieillard-Baron D, Bauder D, Fürst P, Hartmann F. Influence of lactulose and paromomycine on the endogenous intestinal ammoniagenesis – correlation of glutamine consumption and ammonia formation. In: Soeters PB, Wilson JHP, Meijer AJ, Holm E, editors. Advances in ammonia metabolism and hepatic encephalopathy. Amsterdam: Elsevier; 1988:170–6.
65. Barber AE, Jones WG, Minei JP, Fahey TJ, Moldawer LL, Rayburn JL, Fischer E, Keogh CV, Shires GT, Lowry SF. Glutamine or fiber supplementation of a defined formula diet: Impact on bacterial translocation, tissue composition and response to toxin. J Parent Ent Nutr. 1990;14:335–43.
66. Burke DJ, Alverdy JC, Aoys E, Moss GS. Glutamine-supplemented total parenteral nutrition improves gut immune function. Arch Surg. 1989;124:1396–9.

67. Klimberg VS, Souba WW, Dolson DJ. Prophylactic glutamine protects the intestinal mucosa from radiation injury. Cancer. 1990;66:62–8.
68. Shou J, Lieberman MD, Hoffman K, Leon P, Redmond HP, Davies H, Daly JM. Dietary manipulation of methotrexate-induced enterocolitis. J Parent Ent Nutr. 1991;15:307–12.
69. Souba WW, Klimberg VS, Hautamaki RD. Oral glutamine reduces bacterial translocation following abdominal radiation. J Surg Res. 1990;48:1–5.

18

Role of reactive oxygen metabolites in the microvascular response to inflammation

M. M. SLOCUM, B. J. ZIMMERMAN and D. N. GRANGER

INTRODUCTION

There is a large body of evidence indicating that reactive oxygen metabolites play an important role in mediating the microvascular response to inflammation. The results of studies from our laboratory and by others indicate inflammation is associated with oxygen radical-mediated changes in blood flow, microvascular fluid exchange, and leucocyte–endothelial cell adhesion. The objective of this chapter is to summarize the available data on the contribution of reactive oxygen metabolites to the microvascular alterations observed in the inflamed bowel.

OXYGEN RADICALS AND INFLAMMATION-INDUCED ALTERATIONS IN BLOOD FLOW

Several studies have recently implicated nitric oxide (NO) as an important mediator of microvascular vasodilation[1]. NO is a product of the reaction of NO synthase with its substrate, L-arginine. NO is produced by a variety of cell types, including inflammatory cells and microvascular endothelium. NO directly activates guanylate cyclase to produce cGMP, which modulates the tone of vascular smooth muscle. The importance of endothelium-derived nitric oxide as an intrinsic modulator of tissue blood flow is exemplified by observations that inhibition of NO production with the L-arginine analogue N^G-nitrio-L-arginine methyl ester (L-NAME) results in arteriolar vasoconstriction and a reduction in erythrocyte velocity[2]. It is now well recognized that the potent vasodilatory effect of NO is influenced by superoxide, inasmuch as NO is rapidly inactivated by superoxide[3,4]. This contention is supported by reports that describe an enhancement of vasodilation with superoxide dismutase[1] or an attenuation of NO-induced vasodilation when endogenous SOD activity is inhibited[5,6]. Thus, conditions associated with enhanced formation of superoxide (e.g. inflammation) should be accompanied by vasoconstriction and a decline in blood flow. Recently, De Kimpe et al.[7] have demonstrated that addition of polymorphonuclear leucocytes to isolated bovine mesenteric arteries resulted in an increased sensitivity of noradrenaline, and this increase in vascular tone was inhibited by the addition of superoxide dismutase. These results suggest that generation of superoxide by the neutrophil may lead to inactivation of the potent vasodilator NO and cause a decrease in blood flow in inflamed tissue.

In contrast to the aforementioned studies, experiments which examine the direct effect of reactive oxygen metabolites on the microvasculature often demonstrate a superoxide-induced vasodilation. Okabe et al.[8] have shown that generation of oxygen radicals by the reaction of hypoxanthine (HX) and xanthine oxidase (XO) resulted in sustained arteriolar vasodilation in feline mesentery. This vasodilatory effect was reversed by the addition of superoxide dismutase (SOD). Del Maestro et al.[9] have demonstrated that superfusion of the hamster cheek pouch with HX-XO results in a dramatic rise in venular red blood cell velocity, which is also attenuated by administration of superoxide dismutase. The discrepancy between the results obtained from studies utilizing extravascular generation of superoxide and the nitric oxide data may be explained by superoxide-mediated injury to microvascular smooth muscle (which leads to vasodilation) in the experiments where HX-XO is superfused on the surface of the microvasculature.

It is well known that inflammatory conditions of the intestine, including inflammatory bowel disease, are associated with an intense hyperaemia in the inflamed tissue. The substances responsible for the inflammation-induced hyperaemia remain undefined; however, several mediators have been proposed to explain colitis-induced intestinal hyperaemia. Because of the large number of resident and infiltrating granulocytes in the mucosa of the inflamed colon, it is possible that the mediators of colitis-induced hyperaemia are derived from these phagocytic leucocytes. In addition to superoxide, it is well known that the leukotrienes and prostaglandins produced by activated leucocytes are vasodilatory[10]. We examined the relationship between neutrophil infiltration and blood flow in a rat model of acetic acid-induced colitis in order to test the hypothesis that neutrophil-derived products mediate the hyperaemia observed in this model[11]. Animals rendered neutropenic by administration of antiserum directed against rat neutrophils completely prevented the large increase in tissue myeloperoxidase activity (an index of the number of neutrophils) normally observed following the induction of colitis. However, the intensity of the hyperaemic response and the extent of mucosal ulceration were not affected by neutrophil depletion. These findings indicate that neutrophil-derived substances probably do not mediate the hyperaemic response elicited by inflammation of the colon.

OXYGEN RADICALS AND MICROVASCULAR PROTEIN EXCHANGE

Reactive oxygen metabolites also appear to contribute to the increased microvascular permeability and interstitial oedema that are characteristic of an acute inflammatory response. We have demonstrated that oxygen radicals generated by local intra-arterial infusion of hypoxanthine–xanthine oxidase are capable of increasing intestinal vascular permeability to plasma proteins[12]. This increase in microvascular permeability was largely prevented by treatment with either SOD or dimethylsulphoxide (a hydroxyl radical scavenger). It has also been demonstrated in the hamster cheek pouch by Del Maestro et al.[13] that superfusion with xanthine oxidase resulted in a dramatic increase in the number of leakage sites in postcapillary venules. They showed that topical application of either superoxide dismutase, catalase, or dimethyl sulphoxide prior to the administration of xanthine oxidase reduced the number of leakage sites elicited by HX-XO. Therefore, these studies suggest that enhanced oxygen radical production may account for at least part of the increased microvascular permeability and interstitial oedema that accompanies an acute inflammatory response.

Although exogenously administered oxygen radicals have been repeatedly shown to increase microvascular permeability, less is known about the contribution of reactive oxygen metabolites to the microvascular and mucosal dysfunction observed in models of acute intestinal inflammation. One model of acute intestinal inflammation which has been extensively characterized relative to oxygen radical-mediated microvascular dysfunction is ischaemia–reperfusion[14]. It has been demonstrated that the dramatic rise in vascular permeability observed following 1 h of partial intestinal ischaemia (blood flow reduced to 20% of control) is significantly attenuated by pretreatment with superoxide dismutase[15]. Agents which scavenge either hydrogen peroxide (catalase) or hydroxyl radicals (dimethylsulphoxide), or which chelate iron are also effective in ablating the reperfusion-induced rise in microvascular permeability[16–18]. These observations are consistent with the view that hydroxyl radicals, generated via the iron-catalysed Haber–Weiss reaction, ultimately mediate the microvascular dysfunction associated with superoxide and hydrogen peroxide production in post-ischaemic intestine. The source of reactive oxygen metabolites in the reperfused intestine appears to be the enzyme xanthine oxidase, rather than activated neutrophils.

OXYGEN RADICALS AND MODULATION OF LEUCOCYTE–ENDOTHELIAL CELL ADHESION

While it appears that reactive oxygen metabolites mediate the microvascular dysfunction induced by acute inflammatory stimuli such as ischaemia–reperfusion (I/R) recent studies indicate that oxygen radicals generated by endothelial and/or parenchymal cells may play a more important role in initiating the formation of substances that attract, activate, and promote the adherence of leucocytes to microvascular endothelium. We have employed the technique of intravital microscopy in our laboratory to monitor leucocyte adherence and emigration in the cat mesenteric microcirculation. Mesenteric venules (25–45 µm diameter) were observed using a video camera mounted on a microscope, thus allowing the image to be displayed on a monitor and recorded on videotape for subsequent analysis. Adherence (stationary for ≥ 30 s) and emigration of leucocytes into the perivascular interstitium were among the parameters quantitated using this technique[19]. We have demonstrated that 1 h of partial ischaemia (blood flow 20% of control) resulted in significant increases in leucocyte adherence (4.4-fold) and emigration 3.4-fold), while 1 h of reperfusion resulted in further increments in leucocyte adherence (7-fold) and emigration (8-fold).

The first evidence that superoxide might be an important modulator of leucocyte–endothelial cell adhesive interactions came from Del Maestro *et al.*[9]. They found that oxygen radicals, generated by superfusion of the hamster cheek pouch with hypoxanthine and xanthine oxidase, attenuated leucocyte rolling velocity by 50% and increased the number of adherent leucocytes in postcapillary venules. These HX-XO alterations in leucocyte–endothelial cell adhesion were completely prevented by superoxide dismutase, but neither catalase nor L-methionine had an effect, indicating that superoxide promotes leucocyte–endothelial cell adhesion.

Based on the findings of Del Maestro, and a large body of evidence which suggests that XO-derived superoxide plays a significant role in I/R injury, it was postulated that the leucocyte adhesion initiated by I/R may be mediated by XO-derived reactive oxygen metabolites. This hypothesis was tested by observing the leucocyte adherence and emigration response to I/R in animals pretreated with either allopurinol or SOD. During the ischaemic period, SOD significantly decreased leucocyte adhesion and emigration, while allopurinol did not. However, both agents attenuated the increased leucocyte adherence and emigration that occurred during reperfusion. The decrease in reperfusion-induced leucocyte emigration observed in SOD- and allopurinol-treated animals appears to be due to interference of leucocyte–endothelial cell adhesion rather than interference with emigration *per se*, because the linear relationships between leucocyte emigration and adhesion in allopurinol and SOD-treated animals were not different from the relationship derived from untreated controls[19].

The aforementioned studies established that superoxide plays a role in I/R-induced leucocyte adherence, but it was not clear whether superoxide merely initiated the adhesive interactions or if it was responsible for the sustained leucocyte adherence observed long after reperfusion. To address this issue, experiments were performed in which SOD was administered 1 h after reperfusion. Administration of human recombinant CuZn-SOD (hSOD) reduced reperfusion-induced leucocyte adhesion by 35–45% within 10 min of intravenous administration. The ratio of leucocyte rolling velocity to erythrocyte velocity was increased after administration of hSOD, indicating that rolling, as well as leucocyte adhesion, are modulated by superoxide. In contrast, MoAb IB$_4$, which is directed against the common β-subunit (CD18) of the leucocyte adhesion glycoprotein CD11/CD18, reduced reperfusion-induced leucocyte adhesion by 75%; however, it did not affect leucocyte rolling velocity[20].

Additional studies utilizing *in vitro* models of I/R (anoxia/reoxygenation) have demonstrated that exposure of cultured microvascular endothelium to 30 min of anoxia and 60 min of reoxygenation results in a significant increase in neutrophil adhesion[20]. The effect of the addition of neutrophils in the presence of hSOD (4 and 8 mg/kg), peroxide-inactivated hSOD, or MoAB IB$_4$ paralleled that observed in the *in vivo* experiments. hSOD decreased adherence by 19% (low dose) and 27% (high dose), MoAb IB$_4$ decreased adherence by 38%, while inactive hSOD had no effect. In addition, MoAb IB$_4$ completely prevented neutrophil adherence to a biologically inert surface (plastic) while hSOD had no effect[20]. From these results four conclusions can be drawn: (1) the catalytic activity of hSOD appears to be responsible for the anti-adherence properties of the enzyme; (2) leucocyte rolling appears to be modulated by superoxide but not by the leucocyte adhesion glycoprotein CD11/CD18; (3) the presence of endothelial cells appears to be necessary for superoxide-mediated neutrophil adherence; and (4) I/R-induced leucocyte adherence is influenced both by superoxide and CD11/CD18.

Because SOD has been shown to attenuate I/R-induced leucocyte adhesion and emigration, the possibility that other agents which either scavenge or prevent the production of reactive oxygen metabolites may also attenuate leucocyte adhesion to venular endothelium was examined[21]. This was accomplished by determining whether catalase, desferoxamine, or oxypurinol alter the I/R-induced increase in leucocyte–endothelial cell adhesion. Administration of either catalase or oxypurinol significantly decreased leucocyte adhesion when given 1 h after reperfusion; however, neither inactive catalase nor desferoxamine altered leucocyte adhesion. These results suggest that at least part of the protective effect of catalase and oxypurinol observed in models of acute inflammation may be attributed to the ability of these agents to attenuate leucocyte adhesion, while any protection observed with desferoxamine cannot. Thus, these results indicate that xanthine oxidase and hydrogen peroxide also play an important role in modulating leucocyte–endothelial cell adhesion in inflamed tissue.

The anti-adhesive action of catalase implicates hydrogen peroxide as a mediator of leucocyte adherence; however, it remains uncertain whether hydrogen peroxide *per se* or myeloperoxidase-derived oxidants such as hypochlorous acid (HOCl) and/or monochloramine (NH$_2$Cl) are responsible for the anti-adhesive properties of catalase. It has been estimated that most of the hydrogen peroxide produced by activated neutrophils is consumed by myeloperoxidase (MPO), which is released into extracellular fluid from azurophilic granules. MPO catalyses the oxidation of chloride by hydrogen peroxide to yield HOCl, which in turn rapidly reacts with primary amines to yield *N*-chloramines, such as monochloramine and taurine monochloramine. HOCl and *N*-chloramines are highly reactive oxidants which may be more or less cytotoxic than hydrogen peroxide, depending on the lipophilicity of the compound. In order to address the possible role of neutrophil-derived oxidants in the modulation of leucocyte adhesion we determined whether H$_2$O$_2$, HOCl, and NH$_2$Cl, at concentrations produced by activated neutrophils, promote leucocyte adherence to microvascular endothelium in postcapillary venules[22]. The results of these experiments indicate that H$_2$O$_2$ and NH$_2$Cl, but not HOCl, promote leucocyte adhesion to venular endothelium. The leucocyte adherence induced by either H_2O_2 or NH_2Cl was largely prevented by the CD18-specific monoclonal antibody IB_4. A platelet-activating factor receptor antagonist prevented the leucocyte adhesion mediated by H_2O_2 but not by NH_4Cl. In addition, *in vitro* studies (flow cytometry) indicate that incubation of isolated cat neutrophils with H_2O_2 results in an increased expression of CD11/CD18 on the leucocyte surface. These results indicate that both NH_2Cl and H_2O_2 promote leucocyte adherence at physiologically relevant concentrations, and that the adhesion results from up-regulation and/or activation of CD11/CD18.

Although SOD has been shown to reduce leucocyte adhesion in postcapillary venules, the exact mechanism by which superoxide anion promotes leucocyte adhesion remains unclear. The possibilities include superoxide-induced formation of inflammatory mediators, increased expression of leucocyte and endothelial cell adhesion molecules, or inactivation of an endothelial cell-derived anti-adhesive substance. The possibility that NO might be an endogenous anti-adhesion molecule has recently been addressed in our laboratory[2]. Inasmuch as NO is inactivated by superoxide, we hypothesized that if NO normally attenuates leucocyte adhesion to vascular endothelium, then conditions associated with an enhanced formation of superoxide should lead to increased leucocyte adhesion. In order to test this hypothesis we examined the influence of inhibitors of nitric oxide production on leucocyte adherence in normal postcapillary venules. L-NAME and N^G-monomethyl-L-arginine (L-NMMA), analogues of L-arginine that inhibit NO production, were superfused onto the surface of cat mesentery. Both inhibitors significantly increased both leucocyte adherence and emigration. Administration of a CD18-specific antibody abolished the leucocyte adherence induced by both L-NAME and L-NMMA. Also, administration of L-arginine, but not D-arginine (the biologically inactive enantiomer) significantly attenuated the L-NAME-induced leucocyte adherence. Although these results suggest that inhibition of nitric oxide results in an increase in leucocyte adhesion, administration of L-NMMA also caused a 50% reduction in red blood cell velocity resulting in a dramatic decrease in shear rate. Consequently, additional tests were performed in which partial arterial occlusion was used to decrease venular shear rate. The results from these experiments indicate that reduced shear rates cannot explain the increased leucocyte adherence observed during L-NAME treatment[2]. Overall, the results of these studies suggest that NO may be an important endogenous inhibitor of leucocyte adherence in postcapillary venules, and that inactivation of NO by superoxide may contribute to the increased leucocyte adherence observed in conditions associated with enhanced production of superoxide by endothelial cells and/or neutrophils.

SUMMARY

There is a growing body of evidence which implicates reactive oxygen metabolites as mediators of the vascular and parenchymal cell responses to

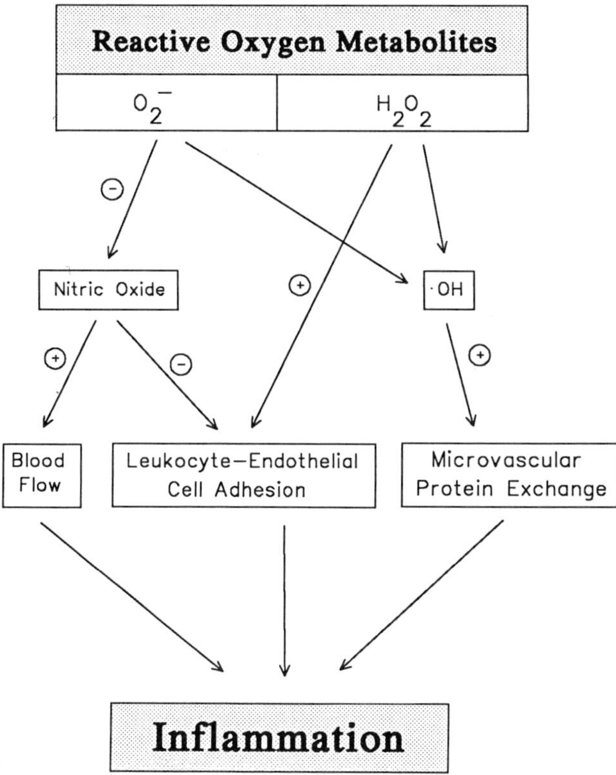

Fig. 1 Synopsis of the role of reactive oxygen metabolites in inflammation. Blood flow is enhanced by endothelial-derived nitric oxide (NO), but in the presence of superoxide, NO is rapidly inactivated resulting in a decrease in blood flow. Leucocyte–endothelial cell adhesion is promoted directly by hydrogen peroxide. NO is inhibitory to adhesion, but this inhibitory effect is lost in the presence of superoxide. Microvascular protein exhange is mediated by the hydroxyl radical produced from superoxide and hydrogen peroxide via the Haber–Weiss reaction. These alterations in blood flow, microvascular protein leakage, and leucocyte–endothelial cell adhesion are a part of the broad spectrum of inflammation

acute and chronic inflammation. While much emphasis has been placed on the potential of oxygen radicals to directly mediate organ dysfunction and tissue injury, it is now recognized that these highly reactive species also contribute to the haemodynamic and local immune responses of the gut to inflammatory stimuli. Superoxide appears to contribute to inflammatory responses elicited in both the arterial (vasodilation) and venous (leucocyte adherence and emigration) segments of the microcirculation. These effects appear to result, in large part, from an ability of superoxide to inactivate nitric oxide, which is normally produced and released by microvascular endothelium.

Hydrogen peroxide also participates in local inflammatory responses, yet part of the proinflammatory effect of this oxidant results from its ability to stimulate the formation of platelet-activating factor, which is capable of both altering blood flow and recruiting granulocytes. The net result of these biological actions of superoxide and hydrogen peroxide is an amplification of the inflammatory response by products of neutrophil activation. Consequently, reactive oxygen metabolites may play a more important role in allowing recruited granulocytes to sustain an inflammatory response than as mediators of tissue injury. There are a number of unresolved issues and areas of controversy concerning the contribution of reactive oxygen metabolites to intestinal inflammation. Thus, additional experimentation is needed in different models of gut inflammation before decisions can be reached regarding the potential therapeutic efficacy of radical scavengers in the treatment of inflammatory bowel diseases.

References

1. Ignarro LJ. Biological actions and properties of endothelium-derived nitric oxide formed and released from artery and vein. Circ Res. 1989;65:1–21.
2. Kubes P, Suzuki M, Granger DN. Nitric oxide: an endogenous modulator of leukocyte adhesion. Proc Natl Acad Sci USA. 1991;88:4651–5.
3. Gryglewski RJ, Palmer RM, Moncada S. Superoxide anion is involved in the breakdown of endothelium-derived vascular relaxing factor. Nature. 1986;320:454–6.
4. Rubanyi G, Vanhoutte PM. Superoxide anions and hyperoxia inactivate endothelium-derived relaxing factor. Am J Physiol. 1986;19:250:H822–7.
5. Cherry PD, Omar HA, Farrell KA, Stuart JS, Wolin MS. Superoxide anion inhibits cGMP-associated bovine pulmonary arterial relaxation. Am J Physiol. 1990;259:H1267–73.
6. Omar H, Cherry PD, Wolin MS. Modulation of cGMP-associated and endothelium-dependent coronary arterial relaxation by inhibition of superoxide dismutase. Circ Res. 1989;80:275–80.
7. De Kimpe SJ, Van Heuven-Nolsen D, Nijkamp FP. Bovine polymorphonuclear leukocytes increase sensitivity to noradrenaline in isolated mesenteric arteries. Br J Pharmacol. 1992;105:581–6.
8. Okabe E, Todoki K, Odajima C, Ito H. Free radicals induced changes in mesenteric microvascular dimensions in the anesthetized cat. Jpn J Pharmacol. 1983;33:1233–9.
9. Del Maestro RF, Planker M, Arfors KE. Evidence for the participation of superoxide anion radical in altering the adhesive interaction between granulocytes and endothelium, *in vivo*. Int J Microcirc: Clin Exp. 1982;1:105–20.
10. Bisgaard H, Kristersen J, Sondergaard J. The effect of leukotriene C4 and D4 on cutaneous blood flow in humans. Prostaglandins. 1982;23:797–801.
11. Sekizuka E, Grisham MB, Deitch EA, Granger DN. Inflammation-induced intestinal hyperemia in the rat: role of neutrophils. Gastroenterology. 1988;95:1528–34.
12. Parks DA, Shah AK, Granger DN. Oxygen radicals: effects on intestinal vascular permeability. Am J Physiol. 1984;247:10:G167–70.
13. Del Maestro RF, Bjork J, Arfors KE. Increase in microvascular permeability induced by enzymatically generated free radicals. II. Role of superoxide anion radical, hydrogen peroxide, and hydroxyl radical. Microvasc Res. 1981;22:255–70.
14. Granger DN. Role of xanthine oxidase and granulocytes in ischemia-reperfusion injury. Am J Physiol. 1988;255:H1269–75.
15. Granger DN, Rutili G, McCord JM. Superoxide radicals in feline intestinal ischemia. Gastroenterology. 1981;81:22–9.
16. Parks DA, Granger DN. Role of hydrogen peroxide in ischemic injury to the small intestine. Gastroenterology. 1984;86:1207.
17. Parks DA, Granger DN. Ischemia-induced vascular changes: role of xanthine oxidase and hydroxyl radicals. Am J Physiol. 1983;245:G285–9.
18. Hernandez LA, Grisham MB, Granger DN. A role for iron in oxidant-mediated ischemic injury to intestinal microvasculature. Am J Physiol. 1987;253:G49–53.

19. Granger DN, Benoit JN, Suzuki M, Grisham MB. Leukocyte adherence to venular endothelium during ischemia–reperfusion. Am J Physiol. 1989;257:20:G683–8.
20. Suzuki M, Inauen W, Kvietys PR, Grisham MB, Meininger C, Schelling ME, Granger HJ, Granger DN. Superoxide mediates reperfusion-induced leukocyte-endothelial cell interactions. Am J Physiol. 1989;257:26:H1740–5.
21. Suzuki M, Grisham MB, Granger DN. Leukocyte–endothelial cell adhesive interactions: role of xanthine oxidase-derived oxidants. J Leuk Biol. 1991;50:488–94.
22. Suzuki M, Asako H, Kubes P, Jennings S, Grisham MB, Granger DN. Neutrophil-derived oxidants promote leukocyte adherence in postcapillary venules. Microvasc Res. 1991;42:125–38.

19

Non-steroid anti-inflammatory drugs and Crohn's disease

I. BJARNASON, A. J. S. MACPHERSON, S. SOMASUNDARAM and K. TEAHON

INTRODUCTION

Non-steroidal anti-inflammatory drugs (NSAIDs) are a common cause of gastroduodenal damage. In the United Kingdom it is estimated that NSAID-induced gastric and duodenal ulcers, with their complications of perforation and massive haemorrhage, are directly responsible for 30 000–40 000 hospital admisssions annually[1-3]. NSAIDs are, however, increasingly recognized as adversely affecting the whole of the gastrointestinal tract. In the colon NSAID ingestion is associated with an aggressive form of diverticulitis, occasionally colitis (particularly mefenamic acid) and ulceration with perforation and haemorrhage[4-18]. Rectally administered NSAIDs frequently cause distressing local side-effects with histological changes that may resemble chronic inflammatory bowel disease[19-23]. More recently it has become apparent that NSAIDs may cause small intestinal damage[24-31]. Historically this was first evident in premature infants who developed small intestinal perforation as a consequence of indomethacin treatment for closure of a persistent ductus arteriosus[32-34]. NSAIDs were purported to cause malabsorption but there are only a few reports of significant morphological damage in the small intestine due to these drugs[35-38]. Small intestinal ulcers, strictures, perforations and haemorrhage are described but are so rare that they represent a medical curiosity rather than a clinical problem[30,39-47]. However, when studied systematically it is clear that NSAIDs have a major subtle effect on small intestinal function and integrity[24-31], as indeed should have been predicted from animal experiments[48]. NSAIDs have a specific and a selective biochemical effect which leads to disruption of mucosal integrity[49-51]. There then follows an interesting interplay between luminal aggressive factors and mucosal defence which leads to small intestinal inflammation in 60–70% of patients on NSAIDs. NSAID enteropathy, defined on the basis of the faecal excretion of indium-111-labelled leucocytes, appears to be a disease entity in its own right, with its complications of blood and protein loss which may contribute to management problems in patients receiving these drugs.

At first sight there would not seem to be any important connection between NSAIDs and Crohn's disease. The observation of high prostaglandin levels in rectal mucosa and dialysate in patients with inflammatory bowel disease suggested that NSAIDs might be therapeutically useful in these patients, via their effect to inhibit cyclooxygenase[52-54]. On the contrary it was found that NSAIDs increased the activity of the disease[55]. Moreover there are isolated reports of NSAIDs causing relapse of quiescent inflammatory bowel disease[56-58]. Studying the self-evident Riley *et al.* concluded that NSAIDs are not the most frequent cause of relapse in patients with inflammatory bowel disease[59]. No room for optimism here.

A number of relatively non-invasive techniques have recently been introduced for the specific assessment of intestinal inflammation and permeability in humans which have increased our knowledge and appreciation of the specificity, function and importance of the intestinal barrier and neutrophils in the pathogenesis of small and large intestinal disease. Furthermore the simultaneous, sequential assessment of two or more related functions and their response to simple therapeutic measures has allowed an insight into pathophysiological processes which is not possible using the techniques by themselves in isolation. Their application in patients on NSAIDs and volunteers taking NSAIDs in the short term, extrapolation from reliable data from animal studies, substituting indium-111 leucocyte assessment of disease activity for the clinical disease activity scores and sequential studies in patients with Crohn's disease achieving clinical remission from disease with the use of elemental diets has allowed insight into the possible mechanism of relapse in Crohn's disease. At the same time the results suggest a common final pathway for the pathogenesis of many small intestinal diseases which is amiable for further testing.

PATHOGENESIS OF NSAID ENTEROPATHY

The great advantage of studying the pathogenesis of NSAID-induced gastrointestinal damage is the availability of patients, the reproducibility of damage and the natural occurrence of the damage in experimental animals which appears to resemble the human disease in many respects.

The pathogenesis of NSAID enteropathy has been detailed elsewhere[50,60]. It has been suggested that the pathogenesis can be divided into two separate steps as shown in Fig. 1[60].

Stage 1 is the summation of the specific, sequential, biochemical actions of NSAIDs. These do not differ fundamentally between NSAIDs, and require a high local concentration of drug which may explain why damage is so common in the stomach, duodenum and small intestine whilst the colon is only rarely adversely affected.

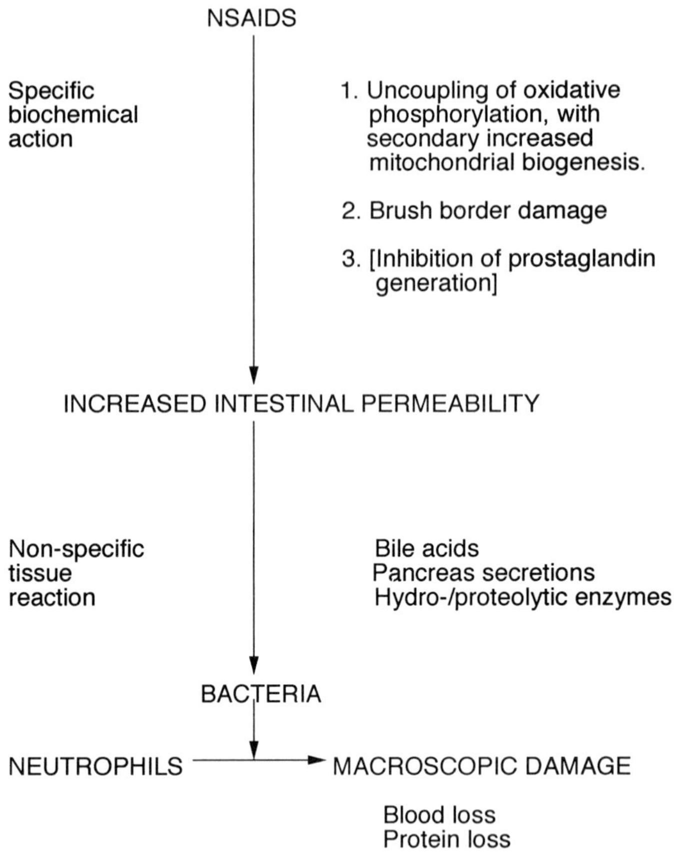

Fig. 1 Pathogenesis of NSAID enteropathy. It is suggested that NSAID-induced intestinal damage is a two-step pathogenic event. The first stage is characterized by NSAID specific biochemical damage to the enterocyte mitochondria and brush border. The consequence is an increase in intestinal permeability which calls into play an interaction between luminal aggressive factors and mucosal defence, which appears to be the final common pathway of a number of diseases. Only when bacteria or their degradation products elicit a neutrophil chemotactic response is there evidence of significant macroscopic damage, and hence the complications of inflammation, namely blood and protein loss

The early adverse effect of NSAIDs is uncoupling of mitochondrial oxidative phosphorylation, as demonstrated by electron microscopy[51]. This happens in the small intestine within 1 h of NSAID administration to rats. The precise mechanism requires further study but it may simply occur by virtue of the low pK of NSAIDs. Following this, and still long before macroscopic damage is evident, there is in addition biochemical evidence of damage to the brush border in the form of reduced activities of alkaline phosphatase[19,50]. The precise mechanism of the damage to the brush border is uncertain and the available data are fraught with difficulties of experimental design[50]. At the same time there is increased activity of succinate dehydrogenase acid α-glucosidase, markers of mitochondria and endoplasmic reticulum, respectively. Histochemical activity stains of citrate synthase (tricarboxylic and cycle enzyme), succinate dehydrogenase and cytochrome C oxidase (respiratory chain) suggests that the increased activity is an appropriate compensatory response (mitochondrial biogenesis) to the initial effect of uncoupling of oxidative phosphorylation[51]. Depletion of enterocyte (and in principle gastric and duodenal) ATP, if of sufficient severity, leads to secondary organelle dysfunction and eventually cell death. These abnormalities are reflected functionally on a tissue level by increased intestinal permeability[61–69] which triggers off the non-specific second stage of NSAID damage which indeed may be the common final pathogenic pathway for many diseases. Because of the action of NSAIDs to inhibit cyclooxygenase, thereby effectively preventing the generation of reparative prostaglandins, the increased intestinal permeability is much more prolonged following NSAIDs than other agents that alter intestinal integrity, such as hyperosmolarity, alcohol or detergents.

According to this framework, and unlike previous suggestions, the NSAID inhibition of cyclooxygenase is not a primary event. On the contrary it is suggested that it represents a late, albeit biochemically specific occurrence, in the first stage of the damage. This is in agreement with the finding of Whittle, who showed an absence of a temporal relationship between cyclooxygenase inhibition and the development of macroscopic damage due to NSAIDs[70].

The second-stage mechanisms are more site-dependent but are the inevitable consequence of the interplay of mucosal defence and luminal aggressive factors. NSAIDs action in increasing intestinal permeability relates in part to NSAID potency in inhibiting cyclooxygenase, is dependent on an active NSAID (pro-drugs do not appear to increase intestinal permeability), and can be partially prevented by concomitant ingestion of synthetic prostaglandins in large doses and with a glucose-citrate formulation which may counteract some of the early biochemical changes[61–63,67,68]. The permeability changes occur within hours of NSAID ingestion. In the stomach and duodenum the aggressive factors are pepsin, acid and to some extent bile acids that may reflux into the stomach. The luminal aggressive factors in the small intestine are equally well defined, although the relative importance of each (bile acids, pancreas secretion, ingested food, bacteria and their degradation products, hydrolytic and proteolytic enzymes) is by and large unknown. A part of the uncertainty may have arisen by failure to consider why the damage is site-specific.

Thus as bile acids are released in response to food ingestion they have limited access to the mucosa initially because of mixing. As the food is digested and absorbed the luminal concentration of bile acids increases progressively and then decreases again as they are themselves absorbed in the ileum. The mid-small intestine may therefore be exposed to the highest concentration of bile acids. Similarly bacterial counts increase progressively from stomach to colon. The role of ingested food is controversial. Re-feeding undoubtedly potentiates NSAID damage to the small intestine, but the problem is dissociating any specific effect of food from the inevitable release of bile acids, etc. It is noticeable that in coeliac disease, where the mucosa is indeed leaky, there is a noticeable lack of neutrophils which might have been attracted if food was indeed harmful. In rats the importance of bacteria, feeding and bile acids in NSAID-induced small intestinal damage is undoubted[71-75]. The uncertainty is again their precise role in the pathogenesis. It is possible that the role of bile acids is predominantly to perturbate cell membranes, and particularly so in cells that might have been on the verge of recovery following the first-stage assault of NSAIDs. Alternatively, and not mutually exclusive, the biliary excreted conjugates of NSAIDs (20–70% of intravenously administered NSAIDs are excreted in bile) may be toxic following bacterial deconjugation, effectively providing a mechanism for delivery of NSAIDs in high cncentration to the distal small intestine. Indomethacin certainly potentiates the damage of bile acids.

The latter pathogenic stage of NSAID enteropathy involves neutrophil chemotaxis, and this is where bacteria may be particularly important. The consensus is that macroscopic damage does not occur, or is greatly diminished in germ-free rats[72]. Curiously pre- or post-treatment of animals with antimicrobials does not prevent damage or accelerate healing[71]. Nevertheless, in humans metronidazole reduces the inflammation and blood loss while intestinal permeability is not affected[76]. Neutrophils are now recognized as the main effector cell in various diseases[77-82], and certainly the main cell by which activity is defined histologically in inflammatory bowel disease. Neutrophil chemoattraction involves a complex (locomotion, aggregation, adherence, migration) but co-ordinated response to specific chemoattractants[83,84]. The neutrophil movement is uniquely suited for quantitation by the use of indium-111-labelled leucocytes, and utlizes the specific chemoattractive properties of the neutrophil. It is shown that 60–70% of patients taking NSAIDs for over 6 months have small intestinal inflammation[24-31]. This is unrelated to type of NSAID, age or gender. The localization is similar to that in experimental animals, namely predominantly in the mid-small intestine as shown by kinetic studies of neutrophil accumulation and by direct visualization by enteroscopy demonstrating a range of macroscopic pathology from erythematous blebs to frank ulceration[28]. When in contact with the chemoattractant the neutrophil responds in a predetermined predictable fashion with a burst of generation of oxygen radical species and internalization of the chemoattractant with subsequent lysosomal enzyme release into the immediate vicinity of the neutrophil[81,82,84]. There is considerable evidence that this is the main mechanism of the macroscopic damage in NSAID enteropathy, the preceding events simply paving the way for the bacterial–neutrophil interaction. Hence neutropenia, inhibition of neutrophil adherence and locomotion minimize the macroscopic damage following NSAIDs in rats, and indeed in some other forms of experimental enteropathies[77-80].

Another important aspect of neutrophil-induced damage is the precise site at which activation of the neutrophil occurs. If the neutrophil is simply seeking a luminal chemoattractant there will be minimal tissue damage. However, if the chemoattractant is within the gastrointestinal mucosa there will be far greater tissue damage. It is possible to localize the site of neutrophil chemoattractants in humans[85]. If there is a significant correlation between the intensity of the acute inflammatory reaction, as assessed by the 4-day faecal excretion of indium-111 leucocytes and the tissue damage as assessed by the daily faecal blood loss of chromium-51-labelled red cells (or labelled albumin) this indicates that the neutrophils are activated within the mucosa. The lack of such a correlation, along with a disproportionately greater excretion of labelled neutrophils, is more in keeping with a luminal chemoattractant. Thus in NSAID enteropathy it seems likely that the protein loss and red cell loss is the direct consequence of neutrophil activation within the mucosa. Certainly inflammation and blood loss correlate significantly in patients on NSAIDs, and neither correlates in any way with macro- or microscopic findings on gastroduodenoscopy[27,85]. This also suggests that the main site of low-grade bleeding originates in the small intestine in patients with rheumatoid arthritis and not the stomach, which is important as over 50% of these patients with anaemia of chronic disease have co-existing iron deficiency.

The realization of a protein-losing enteropathy has particular clinical relevance as 10% of patients with rheumatoid arthritis admitted to hospital have hypoalbuminaemia. The above findings suggest a new therapeutic approach to this problem which has been so resistant to conventional treatment, based on the idea that hypoalbuminaemia in these patients was caused by reduced hepatic synthesis.

THE COMMON FINAL PATHWAY

The essential feature of the second-stage pathogenic framework for NSAID enteropathy is that of an agent-specific damage leading to increased intestinal permeability with secondary but unavoidable consequences of small intestinal inflammation. Extrapolation of this idea suggests that there may be various forms of enteropathies hitherto undefined or poorly characterized. In general, and in the simplest form, these might be predominantly brought about by a breach in intestinal permeability, an increase in the luminal aggressive factors or reduced mucosal defence. These three are clearly interactive and interrelated, so that an alteration in one leads to a predictable response in the other.

Intestinal permeability breakers

NSAID-induced small intestinal damage is the prototype of a barrier breaker. There are a number of other agents that have a striking and predominant effect on intestinal permeability, but in many cases an enteropathy has not yet been sought. We have, however, recently studied patients with chronic renal failure (unpublished). Clinically this group of patients has many similarities with patients with rheumatoid arthritis. They often develop iron deficiency associated with the anaemia of chronic disease. There is loss of appetite, and various gastrointestinal symptoms which are often ascribed to uraemic gastritis. Still most do not have significant findings on endoscopy that explain the symptoms adequately. To date we have studied nine patients with long-standing renal failure not treated with haemo- or peritoneal dialysis. They were studied simultaneously with indium-111 leucocytes and chromium-51 red cells to assess intestinal inflammation and blood loss, respectively. The results showed that those with creatinine levels above 600 µmol/l had an enteropathy of a similar severity to that seen in patients on NSAIDs. The blood loss in these patients was likewise increased. It is suggested that uraemia causes damage to enterocytes with increased intestinal permeability and the cascade of events detailed above. Further comparative studies assessing intestinal permeability and the response to treatment with metronidazole in patients with uraemic enteropathy will be of major interest and importance.

Alcoholic patients and patients with diabetes mellitus have striking increases in intestinal permeability but an enteropathy has not been sought[86,87]. Many chemotherapeutic agents increase intestinal permeability and the gastrointestinal toxicity may be one of the major factors limiting the dosage given[88–92]. As these drugs may also compromise immune function it would seem probable, providing that the hypothesis is right, that many of them will have an enteropathy if sought.

Luminal aggressive factors

The small intestinal mucosa is well equipped to deal with the 'normal' luminal aggressive factors. Whilst bile acid spillover into the colon may cause diarrhoea and inflammation there are no reports of small intestinal damage due to hypersecretion of bile or pancreas secretions. The most common aggressive factors causing small intestinal disease are infections. These may be endogenous, such as that seen following intestinal bypass surgery for morbid obesity, or exogenous with *Giardia lamblia*, *Campylobacter jejuni*, *Salmonella*, *Shigella* or *Yersinia*.

Intestinal permeability has not been assessed systematically in patients with small intestinal infections except in hepatitis A and rotaviral infections, where it was found to be uniformly increased[93,94]. *Giardia* (unpublished) increases intestinal permeability in some patients but there are few data in other infections. Kardossis *et al.* studied 18 patients with gastroenteritis of various causes with indium-111 leucocytes[95]. Many had abnormal scintigrams and the faecal excretion of labelled cells (over 3 days) was raised in most. Quantitatively the majority had excretion levels between 1% and 9%, similar to that seen in NSAID and uraemic enteropathy. Similarly a patient with *Yersinia* was reported to have small intestinal inflammation with the indium-111 technique and we have seen three patients with a faecal excretion of 1.2–3.7%, which is much lower than that expected in Crohn's disease of similar clinical severity.

Reduced mucosal defence

Patients with primary hypogammaglobulinaemia (common variable or X-linked) often have diarrhoea and wasting[96-99]. Morphological changes in the small intestine were common as were infections with *Giardia*. *Giardia* is, however, rarely a problem, since these patients are now treated with intravenous gammaglobulins. Still the gastrointestinal symptoms persist in many patients. In a systematic study of such patients we found an enteropathy with the use of indium-111 leucocytes[100]. The 4-day faecal excretion varied between 0.5% and 9% with a mean of 4%, again resembling the diseases discussed above. Intestinal permeability was increased, but jejunal morphological alterations were much less severe than previously reported. Most patients, however, had a lymphocytic colitis which is a variant of microscopic colitis. A few patients came to surgery with small intestinal obstruction. The histology was non-specific, but clearly distinguishable from Crohn's disease. Moreover, five patients were treated with an elemental diet and they improved both clinically with loss of cachexia, tiredness, diarrhoea and weight gain and reduced intestinal inflammation, although the latter was less impressive than that seen in Crohn's disease.

Human immune deficiency virus (HIV) infected individuals are prone to a similar clinical problem as patients with hypogammaglobulinaemia. There is, however, a marked difference in the pathogens found in these patients. HIV-positive patients are purported to have major jejunal abnormalities, although this has not been the British experience. Many have increased intestinal permeability and we (unpublished) have documented ($n = 12$) an enteropathy with a faecal excretion in the range of 0.5–5.0%. The localization in the mid-small intestine is similar to the above diseases. Similar to the patients with hypogammaglobulinaemia the enteropathy responds predictably, but only partially, to elemental diets.

CROHN'S DISEASE

From the above it would seem that there is a similar quantitative increase in intestinal permeability and indium-111 neutrophil flux in all of these disorders, regardless of whether the pathogenesis involves a primary change in intestinal permeability, alterations in luminal aggressive factors or mucosal immunity. So where does Crohn's disease fit into this framework?

Intestinal permeability is increased in patients with small intestinal Crohn's disease and it relates quantitatively to the activity and the extent of the disease[101-111]. While a given permeability result will not be particularly helpful clinically, serial measurements may be used as a rapidly obtainable objective index of disease activity. Nevertheless the increased intestinal permeability in Crohn's disease is similar to that seen in the aforementioned enteropathies. Previous claims of a genetically determined, primary increase in intestinal permeability as a co-cause or a prerequisite for the disease is no longer tenable[112-114].

The neutrophil flux to the intestine is uniformly increased in active disease (the defining histological feature) with a 4-day faecal excretion of labelled neutrophils of 5–60% and a mean of 20% in small intestinal Crohn's disease. This is an order of magnitude higher than seen in the other group of enteropathies. This could be due to increased immune responsiveness to a common antigen or an appropriate response to a unique one. Interestingly, in remission the faecal excretion of neutrophils rarely returns to control levels, and many patients in full clinical remission have an excretion of 2–6%, similar to that seen in the other enteropathies.

It is the treatment of active Crohn's disease with an elemental diet with sequential measurement of intestinal permeability and inflammation which has been most informative. There is a consistent reduction in both parameters with successful treatment, both occurring within 2 weeks of treatment, but patients are treated empirically for a further 2 weeks[115]. At the same time there is no significant change in the serum levels of soluble interleukin-2 receptor levels, indicating a continuous ongoing activation of T lymphocytes[116].

Elemental diets reduce luminal aggressive factors, that is bile acid and pancreas secretions, and alter bacterial flora. There is also a reduction in ingested antigens as no normal food is allowed during the treatment period. It is therefore conceivable that the beneficial effect of elemental diet is simply caused by an action to reduce the luminal aggressive factors, and the relapse would therefore represent an exaggerated response. The continuous T cell activation is certainly in keeping with this, but further studies are needed.

Interestingly, all the known causes of relapse of Crohn's disease – NSAIDs, infections, alcohol binges and stress – have in common an action to increase intestinal permeability or a potential (stress) to do so[61–69,86,93,117–119]. Following treatment with an elemental diet those with normal intestinal permeability have significantly longer remissions than those who do not (relapse within 6 months) despite an exclusion diet (unpublished). Neutrophils from patients with Crohn's disease have increased numbers of F-meth receptors and are more responsive to N-formyl-methonyl-oligopeptides of intestinal microbial origin suggesting a specific neutrophil chemoattractive signal[120,121]. Macpherson et al. (unpublished) have isolated mucosal immunoglobulin G (IgG) from patients with Crohn's disease. The amount of IgG relates to activity of disease and were found to be primarily directed towards normal intestinal bacterial constituents. Thus the two most specific immunological responses are directed against bacteria or their products, and relate to the relapse. This leads us to believe that Crohn's disease and its relapse are two separate pathophysiological processes. The relapse centres around the intestinal permeability barrier, identical to the second stage of the pathogenic framework for NSAID enteropathy, allowing mucosal exposure to non-specific luminal aggressive factors. The local immune response findings support this, as do the neutrophil studies, and both represent an appropriate response to a breach in mucosal integrity. The inappropriateness in patients with inflammatory bowel disease is the magnitude of the response.

These conclusions are in keeping with the known importance of luminal factors in Crohn's disease which distinguishes it in some fundamental way from ulcerative colitis. Thus bypass surgery, total parenteral nutrition and elemental diet, all of which have a major effect on the luminal milieu to reduce luminal aggressive factors, are as consistently useful in reducing disease activity in Crohn's disease as they are useless for patients with ulcerative colitis. Furthermore, by using the double-isotopic technique to localize the site of neutrophil chemoattractants, Teahon *et al.* have provided further support for this, and showed a significant correlation between intestinal inflammation and blood loss in patients with active ulcerative colitis, suggesting a mucosal chemoattractant. The inflammation was disproportionally much greater than the blood loss in patients with active Crohn's disease and there was no significant correlation between the two[121]. Indeed, in the patients with Crohn's disease the blood loss was no more than seen in NSAID enteropathy despite 10-fold greater inflammation[122]. This suggests a luminal chemoattractant in Crohn's disease in keeping with the above.

The highlights of the hypothesis of Crohn's disease and its common pathway mechanism for the relapse are the realization of a multistage pathogenic mechanism with implications for research workers interested in the aetiology and pathogenesis of the relapse. It emphasizes that an integrated approach must be made to study the problem, rather than using a single-technique, single-component (i.e. vascular) one that in realistic terms has got us nowhere and diverts scarce research funds.

The practical aspects of the framework relate towards the possible lines of treatment and their chance of success. Thus if workers want to develop agents such as leukotriene inhibitors, that mechanistically work at the very late stages of the inflammatory cascade, so be it; but these would not be predicted, from the above, to have any significant advantages over the current forms of treatment. However, those interested in establishing better forms of treatment than that currently available will reason that we should be targeting therapy on the early pathogenic events. Recent proposals for a combination of agents, known to be useful for the relapse of disease, to alter the natural history of the disease would appear to be doomed if the above proposals are correct. A disease-modifying treatment strategy (second-line agents) such as that used in patients with rheumatoid arthritis may be the immediate first goal at this stage, to prevent the number of relapses, and this may have been inadvertently introduced into inflammatory bowel disease in the form of mercaptopurine, but it will be noted that these agents will not necessarily be particularly effective for the relapse itself.

References

1. Beardon PHG, Brown SV, McDevitt DG. Gastrointestinal events in patients prescribed NSAIDs: a controlled study using record linkage in Tayside. Q J Med. 1989;71:497–505.
2. Cockel R. NSAIDs – should every prescription carry a government health warning? Gut. 1987;28:515–18.
3. Armstrong CP, Blower AC. Non-steroidal anti-inflammatory drugs and life threatening complications of peptic ulceration. Gut. 1987;28:527–32.
4. Ravi S, Keat AC, Keat ECB. Colitis caused by NSAID. Postgrad Med J. 1986;62:773–6.
5. Clements D, Williams GT, Rhodes J. Colitis associated with ibuprofen. Br Med J. 1990;301:987.
6. Tanner AR, Raghunat H. Colonic inflammation and NSAID administration. Digestion. 1988;41:116–20.

7. Pearson DJ, Stones NA, Bentley SJ, Reid H. Proctocolitis induced by salicylate and associated with asthma and recurrent nasal polyps. Br Med J. 1983;287:1675.
8. Rutherford D, Stockdill G, Hammer-Hodges DW, Ferguson A. Proctocolitis induced by salicylates. Br Med J. 1984;288:794.
9. Phillips MS, Fehilly B, Stewart S, Dronfield WM. Enteritis and colitis associated with mefenamic acid. Br Med J. 1983;287:1626–7.
10. Edwards AL, Heagerty AM, Bing RF. Enteritis and colitis associated with mefenamic acid. Br Med J. 1983;287:1627.
11. Rampton DS, Trapping PJ. Enteritis and colitis associated with mefenamic acid. Br Med J. 1983;287:1627.
12. Hall RI, Petty AH, Cobden I, Lendrum R. Enteritis and colitis associated with mefenamic acid. Br Med J. 1983;287:1182.
13. Isaacs PET, Sladen GGE, Filipie I. Mefenamic acid enteropathy. J Clin Pathol. 1987;40:121–7.
14. Williams R, Glazier G. Enteritis and colitis associated with mefenamic acid. Br Med J. 1983;287:1627.
15. Langman MJS, Morgan L, Worrall A. Use of anti-inflammatory drugs by patients with small or large bowel perforation and haemorrhage. Br Med J. 1985;290:347–9.
16. Corder A. Steroids, NSAID and serious septic complications of diverticular disease. Br Med J. 1987;295:1238.
17. Finkelstein JA, Jamieson CG. An association between anti-inflammatory medication and internal pelvic fistulas. Dis Colon Rectum. 1987;30:168–70.
18. Wilson RG, Smith AN, Macintyre IMC. Complications of diverticular disease and NSAID: a prospective study. Br J Surg. 1990;77:1103–4.
19. Woolf DL. Indomethacin suppositories. Br Med J. 1965;1:1497.
20. Berry H, Seinson D, Jones H, Hamilton EBD. Indomethacin and naproxen suppositories in the treatment of rheumatoid arthritis. Ann Rheum Dis. 1978;37:370–2.
21. Wright V, Hopkins R. A note on indomethacin suppositories in rheumatic conditions. Rheumatol Rehab. 1979;18:186–7.
22. Levy N, Gaspar E. Rectal bleeding and indomethacin suppositories. Lancet. 1975;1:577.
23. Lanthier P, Detry R, Debongnie JC, Mahieu P, Vanheuverzwyn R. Solitary rectal lesions due to suppositories containing acetylsalicylic acid and paracetamol. Gastroenterol Clin Biol. 1987;11:250–3.
24. Bjarnason I, Williams P, So A, Zanelli G, Levi AJ, Gumpel MJ, Peters TJ, Ansell B. Intestinal inflammation and permeability in rheumatoid arthritis; effects of non-steroidal anti-inflammatory drug. Lancet 1984;2:1171–4.
25. Bjarnason I, Zanelli G, Smith T, Prouse P, De Lacey G, Gumpel MJ, Levi AJ. Nonsteroidal anti-inflammatory drug induced inflammation in humans. Gastroenterology. 1987;93:480–9.
26. Bjarnason I, Macpherson A. The changing gastrointestinal side effect profile of a new problem. Scand J Gastroenterol. 1989;24(suppl. 163):56–64.
27. Bjarnason I, Smethurst P, Hayllar J, Levi AJ. NSAID enteropathy; The main site of chronic blood loss in patients on NSAIDs. Gut. 1990;91:A1203.
28. Morris J, Madhok R, Sturrock RD, Capell HA, Mackenzie JF. Enteroscopic diagnosis of small bowel ulceration in patients receiving non-steroidal anti-inflammatory drugs. Lancet. 1991;337:520.
29. Bjarnason I, Zanelli G, Prouse P, Smethurst P, Smith T, Levi S, Gumpel MJ, Levi AJ. Blood and protein loss via small intestinal inflammation induced by non-steroidal anti-inflammatory drugs. Lancet. 1987;2:711–14.
30. Lang J, Price AB, Levi AJ, Burk M, Gumpel JM, Bjarnason I. Diaphragm disease: the pathology of non-steroidal anti-inflammatory drug induced small intestinal strictures. J Clin Pathol. 1988;51:516–26.
31. Bjarnason I. Non-steroidal anti-inflammatory drug induced small intestinal inflammation in man. In: Pounder R, editor. Recent advances in Gastroenterology, vol. 7. London: Churchill Livingstone; 1988:23–46.
32. Nagaraj HS, Sandhu AS, Cook LN, Buchuno JT, Groff DB. Gastrointestinal perforation following indomethacin in very low birth weight infants. J Paediat Surg. 1981;16:1003–7.
33. Alpan G, Eyal F, Vinograd I, Udasin R, Amir G, Mogle P, Blick B. Localized intestinal perforation after enteral administration of indomethacin in premature infants. J Pediatr. 1985;106:277–81.

34. Marshall TA. Intestinal perforation following enteral administration of indomethacin. J Pediatr. 1985;107:484–5.
35. Kendall MJ, Hawkins CF. Xylose test; effects of aspirin and indomethacin. Br Med J. 1971;1:533–5.
36. Dyer NH, Kendall MJ, Hawkins CF. Malabsorption in rheumatoid arthritis. Ann Rheum Dis. 1971;30:626–30.
37. Freeman HJ. Sulindac-associated small bowel lesion. J Clin Gastroenterol. 1986;8:569–71.
38. Lewis JH. Gastrointestinal injury due to medicinal agents. Am J Gastroenterol. 1986;81:819–34.
39. Sturges HF, Krone CL. Ulcers and strictures of the jejunum in a patient on long term indomethacin therapy. Am J Gastroenterol. 1973;59:162–9.
40. Venturatos SG, Hines C, Blalock JB. Ulceration of the small intestine in a patient with coeliac disease. South Med J. 1984;77:520–2.
41. Neoptolemos JP, Lockie TJ. Recurrent and small bowel obstruction associated with phenylbutazone. Br J Surg. 1983;70:244–5.
42. Madhok R, Mackenzie JA, Lee FD, Bruckner FE, Terry TR, Sturrock RD. Small bowel ulceration in patients receiving NSAIDs for rheumatoid arthritis. Q J Med. 1986;58:53–8.
43. Saverymuttu SH, Thomas A, Grundy A, Maxwell JD. Ileal stricturing after long term indomethacin treatment. Postgrad Med J. 1986;62:267–8.
44. Sukumar L. Recurrent small bowel obstruction with piroxicam. Br J Surg. 1987;74:186.
45. Johnson F. Recurrent small bowel obstruction with piroxicam. Br J Surg. 1987;74:654.
46. Bjarnason I, Price AB, Zanelli G, Smethurst P, Burke M, Gumpel MJ, Levi AJ. Clinicopathological features of nonsteroidal anti-inflammatory drug-induced small intestinal strictures. Gastroenterology. 1988;94:1070–4.
47. Huber T, Ruchti C, Halter F. Nonsteroidal anti-inflammatory drug-induced colonic strictures: a case report. Gastroenterology. 1991;100:1119–22.
48. Kent TH, Cardeli RM, Stanier FU. Small intestinal ulcers and intestinal flora in rats given indomethacin. Am J Pathol. 1969;54:237–45.
49. Hayllar J, Somasundaram S, Saathchandra P, Levi AJ, Bjarnason I. Early cellular events in the pathogenesis of NSAID enteropathy in the rat. Gastroenterology. 1991;100:A216.
50. Somaqsundaram S, Hayllar J, Macpherson A, Bjarnason I. The biochemical basis of intestinal damage due to NSAIDs. A review and a hypothesis. (Submitted).
51. Somasundaram S, Macpherson AJ, Hayllar J, Saratchandra P, Bjarnason I. Enterocyte mitochondrial damage due to NSAID in the rat. Gut. 1992;33(Suppl):S5.
52. Campieri M, Franchi LGA, Bazzocchi G, Brignola C, Benatia B, Boccia S et al. Prostaglandins, indomethacin and ulcerative colitis. Gastroenterology. 1980;79:193.
53. Hawkey CJ, Rampton DS. Prostaglandins and the gastrointestinal mucosa: are they important in its function, disease or treatment? Gastroenterology. 1985;89:1162–88.
54. Rask-Madsen J, Bukhave K, Laursen LS, Lauritsen K. Eicosanoids in inflammatory bowel disease – physiology and pathology. In Peters TJ, editor. The cell biology of inflammation in the gastrointestinal tract. Hull: Corners Publication; 1990:255–71.
55. Rampton DS, Sladen G. Prostaglandin synthesis inhibition in ulcerative colitis. Flurbiprofen compared with conventional treatment. Prostaglandins. 1981;21:417–25.
56. Kaufman HJ, Taubin HL. NSAID activate quiescent inflammatory bowel disease. Ann Intern Med. 1987;107:513–16.
57. Rampton DS, Sladen GE. Relapse of ulcerative proctocolitis during treatment with NSAID. Postgrad Med J. 1981;57:297–9.
58. Rampton DS, McNeil NI, Sarner M. Analgesic ingestion and other factors preceding relapse in ulcerative colitis. Gut. 1983;24:187–9.
59. Riley SA, Mani V, Goodman MJ, Lucas S. Why do patients with ulcerative colitis relapse? Gut. 190;31:179–83.
60. Bjarnason I, Macpherson AJS, Teahon K. Nonsteroidal anti-inflammatory drugs and inflammatory bowel disease. Can J Gastroenterol. 1992: in press.
61. Bjarnason I, Williams P, Smethurst P, Peters TJ, Levi AJ. The effects of NSAID and prostaglandins on the permeability of the human small bowel. Gut. 1986;27:1292–7.
62. Bjarnason I, Smethurst P, Clarke P, Menzies IS, Levi AJ, Peters TJ. Effect of prostaglandins on indomethacin-induced increased intestinal permeability in man. Scand J Gastroenterol. 1989;29(Suppl. 164):97–103.

63. Bjarnason I, Smethurst P, Fenn CG, Lee CF, Menzies IS, Levi AJ. Misoprostol reduces indomethacin induced changes in human small intestinal permeability. Dig Dis Sci. 1989;34:407–11.
64. Jenkins RT, Rooney PJ, Jones DB, Bienenstock J, Goodacre RC. Increased intestinal permeability in patients with rheumatoid arthritis: a side effect of oral NSAID therapy? Br J Rheumatol. 1987;26:103–7.
65. Auer IO, Habscheid W, Hiller S, Gerhards W, Eilles C. Nicht-steroidale antiphlogistika erohen die darmpermeabilitat. Deutsche Med Woschenschr. 1987;112:1032–7.
66. Asabakken C, Osnes M. 51-Cr ethylenediaminetetraacetic acid absorption test. Effects of naproxen, a NSAID. Scand J Gastroenterol. 1990;25:917–24.
67. Bjarnason I, Fehilly B, Smethurst P, Menzies IS, Levi AJ. The importance of local versus systemic effects of NSAID to increase small intestinal permeability in man. Gut. 1991;32:275–7.
68. Bjarnason I, Smethurst P, Walker F, Macpherson A, McElnay SC, Pearson P, Menzies IS. Glucose and citrate reduce the permeability changes caused by indomethacin. Gastroenterology. 1992;102:1546–50.
69. Bjarnason I. Intestinal permeability barriers. In: Peters TJ, editor. The cell biology of inflammation in the gastrointestinal tract. Hull: Corner's Publication; 1990:127–42.
70. Whittle BJR. Temporal relationship between cyclooxygenase inhibition, as measured by prostacyclin biosynthesis, and gastrointestinal damage induced by indomethacin in the rat. Gastroenterology. 1981;80:94–8.
71. Robert A. Cytoprotection by prostaglandins. Gastroenterology. 1975;77:761–7.
72. Robert A, Asano T. Resistance of germ free rats to indomethacin-induced intestinal lesions. Prostaglandins. 1977;14:331–41.
73. Satoh H, Guth PH, Grossman MI. Role of bacteria in gastric ulceration produced by indomethacin in the rat: cytoprotective action of antibiotics. Gatroenterology. 1983;84:483–9.
74. Del Soldato P, Foschi D, Benoni G, Velo GP. Early and late phases in the formation by anti-inflammatory drugs of intestinal lesions in the rat. In: Rainsford KD, Velo GP, editors. Side effects of antinflammatory drugs. Lancaster: MTP Press; 1987:67–81.
75. Brodie DA, Cook PG, Bauer BJ, Dagleg E. Indomethacin-induced intestinal lesions in the rat. Toxicol Appl. Pharmacol. 1970;17:615–24.
76. Wallace JL, Kennan CM, Granger DN. Gastric ulceration induced by nonsteroidal antiinflammatory drugs is a neutrophil dependent process. Am J Physiol. 1990;259:G462–7.
77. Bjarnason I, Hayllar J, Smethurst P, Price AB, Gumpel MJ. Metronidazole reduces intestinal inflammation and blood loss in non-steroidal anti-inflammatory drug induced enteropathy. Gut. 1992: in press.
78. Wallace JL, Arfors KE, McKnight GW. A monoclonal antibody against the CD 18 leucocyte adhesion molecule prevents indomethacin-induced gastric damage in the rabbit. Gastroenterology. 1991;100:878–83.
79. Granger DN, Benoit JN, Suzuki M, Grisham MB. Leucocyte adherence to venular endothelium during ischemia perfusion. Am J Physiol. 1985;257:G683–8.
80. Granger DN, Zimmerman BJ, Seikizuka E, Grisham MB. Intestinal microvascular exchange in the rat during luminal perfusion with N-formyl-methionyl-leucyl-phenylalanin. Gastroenterology. 1988;94:673–81.
81. Malech MI, Callin JI. Neutrophils in human disease. N Engl J Med. 1987;317:687–94.
82. Weiss SJ. Tissue destruction by neutrophils. N Engl J Med. 1989;320:365–76.
83. Wilkinson PC. Leucocyte locomotion: determinants of locomotor capacity, chemotaxis and chemokinesis. In: Peters TJ, editors. The cell biology of inflammation in the gastrointestinal tract. Hull: Corner Publication; 1990:15–27.
84. Segall AW. The electron transport chain of the microbicidal oxidase of phagocytic cells and its involvement in the molecular pathology of chronic granulomatous disease. In: Peters TJ, editor. The cell biology of inflammation in the gastrointestinal tract. Hull: Corner Publication; 1990:51–73.
85. Teahon K, Bjarnason I. Site of neutrophil chemoattractants in inflammatory bowel disease. Gastroenterology. 1991;100:A254.
86. Bjarnason I, Ward K, Peters TJ. The leaky gut of alcoholism; a route of entry for toxic compounds. Lancet 1984;1:179–82.
87. Cooper GR, Mayer RJ, Levin MJ. Increased gastrointestinal absorption of large molecules in patients after 5-fluorouracil therapy for metastatic colon carcinoma. Cancer Res.

1980;40:3430–6.

89. Selby P, McElwain TJ, Crofts M, Lopes N, Mundy J. 51EDTA test for intestinal permeability. Lancet 1984;2:31.

90. Pearson ADJ, Craft AW, Pledger JV, Eastham EJ, Laker MF, Pearson CS. Small bowel function in acute lymphoblastic leukaemia. Arch Dis Childh. 1984;59:460–5.

91. Pledger JV, Pearson ADJ, Craft AW, Laker MF, Eastham EJ. Intestinal permeability during chemotherapy for childhood tumors. Eur J Pediatr. 1988;147:123–7.

92. Selby PJ, Lopes N, Mundy J, Crofts M, Millar JL, McElvain TJ. Cyclophosphamide priming reduces intestinal damage in man following high dose melphalan chemotherapy. Br J Cancer. 1987;55:531–3.

93. Noone C, Menzies IS, Banatvala JE, Scopes JW. Intestinal permeability and lactose hydrolysis in human rotaviral gastroenteritis assessed simultaneously by non-invasive differential sugar permeation. Eur J Clin Invest. 1986;6:217–25.

94. Parrili G, Cuomo R, Nardone G, Maio G, Izzo CM, Budillon G. Investigation of intestinal function during acute viral hepatitis using combined sugar oral loads. Gut. 1987;28:1439–44.

95. Kordossis T, Joseph AEA, Gane JN, Bridges CE, Griffin GE. Fecal leukocytosis, Indium-111-labelled autologous polymorphonuclear leucocyte abdominal scanning, and quantitative fecal indium-111 excretion in acute gastroenteritis and enteropathogen carriage. Dig Dis Sci. 1988;33:1383–90.

96. Hermans PE, Diaz-Buxo JA, Stobo JD. Idiopathic late onset immunoglobulin deficiency. Clinical observations in 50 patients. Am J Med. 1976;61:221–37.

97. Ament ME, Ochs HD, Davis SD. Structure and function of the gastrointestinal tract in primary immunodeficiency syndromes. A study of 39 patients. Medicine. 1973;52:227–48.

98. Johnson RL, Van-Arsdel PP, Tobe AD, Ching Y. Adult hypogammaglobulinaemia with malabsorption and iron deficiency anaemia. Am J Med. 1967;43:935–43.

99. Diaz-Buxo JA, Hermans PE, Huizenga KA. Gastrointestinal dysfunction in immunoglobulin deficiency. Effects of corticosteroid and tetracyclin. J Am Med Assoc. 1975;233:1189–91.

100. Teahon K, Webster D, Price AB, Bjarnason I. Studies of gastrointestinal structure and function in patients with primary hypogammaglobulinaemia. Submitted.

101. Ukabam SO, Clamp JR, Cooper BT. Abnormal small intestinal permeability to sugars in patients with Crohn's disease of the terminal ileum and colon. Digestion. 1983;27:70–4.

102. Andre F, Andre C, Emery Y, Foricon J, Descos L, Minaire Y. Assessment of the lactulose-mannitol test in Crohn's disease. Gut. 1988;29:511–15.

103. Murphy MS, Eastham EJ, Nelson R, Pearson ADJ, Laker MF. Intestinal permeability in Crohn's disease. Arch Dis Child. 1989;64:321–5.

104. Pearson ADJ, Eastham EJ, Laker MF, Ceaft AW, Nelson R. Intestinal permeability in children with Crohn's disease and coeliac disease. Br Med J. 1982;285:20–21.

105. Sanderson IR, Boulton P, Menzies IS, Walker-Smith JA. Improvement of abnormal lactulose/rhamnose permeability in active Crohn's disease of small bowel by elemental diet. Gut. 1987;28:1073–6.

106. Bjarnason I, O'Morain C, Levi AJ, Peters TJ. Absorption of 51-Chromium-labelled ethylenediaminetetraacetate in inflammatory bowel disease. Gastroenterology. 1983;85:318–22.

107. O'Morain C, Abelow CA, Cheru LR, Fleischner GM, Das KM. 51-CrEDTA test: A useful test in the assessment of inflammatory bowel disease. J Lab Clin Med. 1986;108:430–5.

108. Casellas F, Aguade S, Soriano B, Accarino A, Molero J, Guarner L. Intestinal permeability to 99mTc-diethylenetetriaminopentaacetic acid in inflammatory bowel disease. Am J Gastroenterol. 1986;81:767–70.

109. Pironi L, Migliolti M, Ruggeri E, Levorato M, Dallasta MA, Corbelli C, Nibali MG, Barbara L. Relationship between intestinal permeability to 51 Cr EDTA and inflammatory activity in asymptomatic patients with Crohn's disease. Dig Dis Sci. 1990;35:582–8.

110. Jenkins RT, Ramage JK, Jones DB, Collins SM, Hunt RH. Small bowel and colonic permeability to 51Cr EDTA in patients with active inflammatory bowel disease. Clin Invest Med. 1988;11:151–5.

111. Resnik RH, Royal H, Marshall W, Barron R, Werth T. Intestinal permeability in gastrointestinal disorders. Use of 99m Tc DTPA. Dig Dis Sci. 1990;35:205–211.

112. Hollander D. Crohn's disease – A permeability disorder of tight junctions. Gut. 1988;29:1621–4.

113. Hollander D, Vadheim CM, Breththotz E, Peterson GM, Delahunty TJ, Rutter J. Increased intestinal permeability in Crohn's disease patients and their first degree relatives: an etiologic factor? Ann Intern Med. 1986;105:883–5.
114. Teahon K, Smethurst P, Levi AJ, Menzies IS, Bjarnason I. Intestinal permeability in patients with Crohn's disease and their first degree relatives. Gut. 1992;33:320–3.
115. Teahon K, Smethurst P, Pearson M, Levi AJ, Bjarnason I. The effect of elemental diet on intestinal permeability and inflammation in Crohn's disease. Gastroenterology. 1991;101:84–9.
116. Duane PD, Teahon K, Crabtree JE, Levi AJ, Heatley RV, Bjarnason I. The relationship between nutritional status and serum soluble interleukin 2 receptor concentrations in patients with Crohn's disease treated with elemental diet. Clin Nutr. 1991;10:222–7.
117. MacQueen G, Marshall J, Perdue M, Siegel S, Bienenstock J. Pavlovian conditioning of rat mucosal mast cells to secrete rat mast cell protease. II. Science. 1989;243:83–5.
118. D'Inca R, Ramage J, Hunt RH, Perdue MH. Antigen-induced mucosal damage and restitution in the small intestine of the immunised rat. Int Arch Allergy Appl. Immunol. 1990;91:270–7.
119. Crowe SE, Sestini P, Perdue MH. Allergenic reactions of rat jejunal mucosa. Gastroenterology. 1990;99:74–82.
120. Sartor RB. The role of intestinal bacteria in initiation and perpetuation of inflammatory bowel disease. In: Williams CN, editor. Trends in inflammatory bowel disease. Falk Symposium 56. Dordrecht: Kluwer; 1991:17–27.
121. Anton PA, Targan SR, Shanahan F. Increased neutrophil receptors for and response to the proinflammatory bacterial peptide formyl-methionyl-leucyl-phenylalanine in Crohn's disease. Gastroenterology. 1989;97:20–8.
122. Teahon K, Levi AJ, Bjarnason I. Intestinal inflammation and bleeding in NSAID enteropathy and inflammatory bowel disease. Gut. 1990;31:A593.

20

Treatment implications for *Mycobacterium paratuberculosis* in Crohn's disease

W. R. THAYER, Jr

INTRODUCTION

When Crohn and colleagues reported what is considered to be the landmark article describing the illness which bears Crohn's name[1], a very important reference was omitted. Published in the 1913 *British Medical Journal*, Dalziel clearly described the disease[2], and noted its resemblance to intestinal tuberculosis, or Johne's disease (an illness of cattle and sheep caused by *Mycobacterium paratuberculosis*).

In the mid-1980s Chiodini *et al.* isolated *M. paratuberculosis* from some patients with Crohn's disease (CD)[3]. Since this organism does not replicate outside the intestinal tract, its presence in CD intestine appeared to be of great importance. They also showed that a number of other cultures from CD tissue, but not from controls or ulcerative colitis (UC) tissue, had cell wall defective organisms[4]. Although these organisms would agglutinate with antibodies to the *M. paratuberculosis* bacillary strain, they would not grow, and could not otherwise be identified. These findings were confirmed by others, but only small number(s) of *M. paratuberculosis* isolates were found[5,6].

McFadden *et al.*, working in the laboratory of Dr Hermon-Taylor in 1989, extracted genomic DNA from one of our isolates – 'Ben' – cloned it into a plasmid vector which was, in turn, screened against genomic DNA from various mycobacterial species. In this manner a number of hybridizing clones were identified. Using these clones as probes, the investigators identified restrictive fragment length polymorphism which distinguished between mycobacterial species[7,8]. One clone showed multiple banding patterns when used to probe Southern blots of *M. paratuberculosis* DNA, suggesting the

"

presence of a repetitive sequence within the paratuberculous genome. This insertion element was designated as IS-900 and has been found in all Crohn's *M. paratuberculosis* isolates, as well as in wild types of *M. paratuberculosis*[9].

When this signal was sought using polymerase chain reaction (PCR) in our cultures, 38% (10 of 26) were positive for *M. paratuberculosis*, as were 33% (6 of 16) of Dr Graham's cultures[10], indicating that some of these unidentified cell wall defective organisms are, indeed, *M. paratuberculosis*. This technology was then used to detect IS-900 in tissue biopsies; its presence was confirmed in 65% (26 of 40) CD patients[11]. UC patients and controls had far fewer detections. These findings, suggesting that one-third of CD mycobacterial cultures and two-thirds of CD tissue biopsies show evidence of *M. paratuberculosis*, heightens the possibility that this organism might be responsible for some cases of CD.

Antibacterial therapy might then be useful in controlling this organism. Unfortunately, things are not quite that simple. Johne's disease has resisted therapy and, although antibiotics reduce the number of organisms and prolong life, animals ultimately succumb to the illness[12].

Several medical journal 'Letters to the Editor' suggested that antimycobacterial therapy could induce remission in CD[13-15]; on the other hand, control trials with chemotherapy active against mycobacteria have been ineffective[16-19]. In an uncontrolled trial, Hampson *et al.* treated 20 CD cases with quadruple antibacterial therapy using rifampin, ethambutol, isoniazid, and either pyrazinamide or clofazamine. Seventy-one per cent had significant improvement in the Crohn's Disease Activity Index, and 90% were totally withdrawn from steroids[20]. Wirotsko *et al.*, treating uveitis of CD with rifampin, noted coincidental improvement of intestinal disease. Rifampin withdrawal was associated with an exacerbation of both conditions[21]. Several French reports suggest antimycobacterial therapy could cause significant improvement in CD[22,23]. Dapsone, a drug used to treat leprosy, has been shown to have some effect in CD[24], while clofazamine, an antimycobacterial drug also used in leprosy, seems ineffective, although it was used for only a short time[25]. In a recently reported controlled trial of rifampin, ethambutol, dapsone, and clofazamine Kohn *et al.* showed definite improvement in the actively treated group[26].

There is considerable evidence that effective treatment of mycobacteria requires two or more drugs[27]. Even the most effective bactericidal antimycobacterial drugs, if used alone, lead to the emergence of resistant variants before a therapeutic endpoint is reached. Although there is no published evidence on *M. paratuberculosis* resistance, considerable evidence exists that resistance is a common problem in the closely related *Mycobacterium avium* complex of mycobacteria.

Chiodini carried out *in vivo* and *in vitro* studies of antibiotic sensitivity to *M. paratuberculosis* isolates of CD. Initial *in vitro* results indicate that rifabutin, ciprofloxacin, streptomycin, amikacin, and clofazamine had significant antimicrobial activity with attainable therapeutic levels against this organism[28,29]. However, since the use of single agents often leads to therapy failure and drug resistance, various combinations of antimicrobial agents were tested[30]. Bacterial synergism, reflected in a fractional bactericidal concentration (FBC_{50}) of 0.5 or less, was observed with rifabutin and ethambutol, rifabutin and clofazamine, and rifabutin and cefazolin. *In vivo* data using rifabutin alone to treat *M. paratuberculosis* infection of mice did not correlate well with *in vitro* data, however (unpublished data). Bactericidal levels occurred only with the highest concentrations, which exceeded the recommended human doses. Combination therapy, on the other hand, might alleviate the need for higher doses. Studies performed on monkeys naturally infected with *M. paratuberculosis* confirm that complete recovery and bacterial elimination occurred when combination antimycobacterial therapy (rifabutin and kanamycin) was employed[31] (unpublished data). Although one very ill animal died, the remaining three improved. Following 1 year of therapy the drugs were discontinued. Laparatomy 1 year later showed healing; cultures of intestinal biopsies showed no growth. These animals remain well into their fifth year.

The United States Food and Drug Administration would not allow this combination of drugs in our human patients. Streptomycin was substituted for kanamycin in a dose of 1 g/day for 5 days/week for 8 weeks[32]; because frequent relapses occurred following cessation of therapy, streptomycin usage was extended to 16 weeks. Rifabutin was administered in an oral dose of 300 mg/day for an indefinite period; the drug was stopped only on patient request, or if significant side-effects occurred.

Eighteen patients were studied because of severe refractory CD[8], prolonged steroid dependency with serious side-effects[5], extensive repetitive fistulization[8], and severe extracolonic manifestations[4]. Thirteen females and five males ranging in age from 19 to 50 were entered. Seven patients completed 1 year of therapy and no longer required medication to control their CD symptoms; five have remained on rifabutin for up to 5 years and continue to do well. Two elected to stop the medication: one relapsed several months later, and one continues to do well. Six patients initially showed improvement but the drug was discontinued because of side-effects (two), recurrence of symptoms (three), or pregnancy (one). The three with recurrent symptoms are, at present, doing well on low-dose steroids. The pregnant patient delivered a healthy baby; 4 months postpartum she moved out of the area and all contact with her has been lost.

Three individuals showed no response after an adequate course of therapy; two patients did not have adequate therapy.

Of eight patients entered for recurrent fistulae or abscess, seven showed initial healing; one failed to respond. However, five of the healed fistulae and abscess developed recurrence(s) even though the drug was maintained. Six patients with severe refractory illness unresponsive to steroids or to combination with 6-mercaptopurine, are off all therapy except rifabutin and are doing well. Four of five patients with prolonged steroid use and steroid side-effects were eventually weaned from steroids; two subsequently relapsed after cessation of rifabutin. Of note, all four patients with severe extracolonic manifestations – arthritis (three), pyoderma gangrenosum (three) – showed complete resolution.

These pilot study results suggest that antimycobacterial therapy can moderate the course of CD, and justifies the need for a double-blind trial to assess the contribution of these agents in the therapy of CD. Such a trial is currently in progress.

The mucosal barrier provides the mechanism that facilitates the absorption of nutrients but excludes the penetration and uptake of potentially toxic, infectious, or immunogenic substances. There appears to exist an altered gut permeability in CD; whether acquired as a result of disease[33,34], or as an inherited defect is unclear[35]. The specific role permeability plays in the genesis of this illness has not been determined. However, if *M. paratuberculosis* is responsible for some cases of CD, increased permeability early in life may prove to be the mechanism whereby the organism gains access. There exists an age-dependent resistance of ruminant animals to *M. paratuberculosis* infection[36]. The neonatal animal is easily infected, but resistance to the organism increases with age; adult animals are almost totally resistant. Although the mechanism of resistance is unclear, the neonatal and mammalian intestine is capable of taking up macromolecules and particulate matter by endocytic mechanisms[37]. This involves interaction between the particles and receptors on the mucous membrane surface triggering internalization by pinocytosis. Particulate matter contained within membrane-bound vesicles migrates to the supranuclear portion of the cell coalescing with lysosomes. Intracellular digestion takes place[38]. However, in neonatal animals much of this particulate matter is not digested, and is deposited into intracellular spaces. There is increasing evidence that bacteria and viruses may gain access during this time. In the perinatal period, and for some time thereafter, the intestinal mucosal barrier remains immature and porous until cells mature morphologically and functionally, and macromolecular uptake decreases – an event known as 'closure'. This perhaps explains why there is increased susceptibility to *M. paratuberculosis* in immature ruminants. If a similar phenomenon occurred in humans it might explain why the disease seems to develop in adolescence (presumably a latent period), and why spousal transmission does not occur.

The role of *M. paratuberculosis* in CD remains far from proven; however, the recent application of molecular biology raises this possibility above mere speculation. The comparison of CD with *M. paratuberculosis*, and to other atypical mycobacterial infections, underscores many similarities. In the end Dalziel's theory might be correct, but it looks as though it will take more than 80 years to prove.

References

1. Crohn B, Ginzburg L, Oppenheimer G. Regional ileitis: a pathologic and clinical entity. J Am Med Assoc. 1932;99:1323–9.
2. Dalziel T. Chronic intestinal enteritis. Br Med J. 1913;2:1068–70.
3. Chiodini R, VanKruiningen H, Thayer W *et al*. Possible role of mycobacteria in inflammatory bowel disease. 1. An unclassified *Mycobacterium* species isolated from patients with Crohn's disease. Dig Dis Sci. 1984;29:1073–9.
4. Chiodini R, VanKruiningen H, Thayer W *et al*. Spheroplastic phase of mycobacteria isolated from patients with Crohn's disease. J Clin Microbiol. 1986;24:357–63.

5. Markesich D, Graham D, Yoshimura H. Progress in culture and subculture of spheroplasts and fastidious acid-fast bacilli isolated from intestinal tissues. J Clin Microbiol. 1988;26:1600–3.
6. Gitnick G, Collins J, Beaman B *et al.* Prospective evaluation of mycobacterial infection in Crohn's disease; isolation and transmission studies. In: MacDermott R, editor. Inflammatory bowel disease: current status and future approach. New York: Elsevier; 1987:527–34.
7. McFadden J, Butcher P, Chiodini R *et al.* Crohn's disease: isolated mycobacteria are identical to *Mycobacerium paratuberculosis* as determined by DNA probes that distinguish between mycobacterial species. J Clin Microbiol. 1987;25:796–801.
8. McFadden J, Butcher P, Thompson J *et al.* The use of DNA probes identifying restriction-fragment-length polymorphism to examine the *Mycobacterium avium* complex. Mol Microbiol. 1987;56:283–91.
9. Moss M, Green E, Tizard M *et al.* Specific detection of *Mycobacterium paratuberculosis* by DNA hybridization with a fragment of the insertional element IS900. Gut. 1991;32:395–8.
10. Moss M, Sanderson M, Tizard M *et al.* Identification of *M. paratuberculosis* by PCR in longterm cultures of Crohn's disease tissue. Proc. 3rd Int Colloq Paratuberculosis. Int. Assoc. Paratuberculosis; 1991:208–13.
11. Sanderson J, Moss M, Tizard M *et al.* PCR detection of *Mycobacterium paratuberculosis* in Crohn's disease tissue DNA extracts. Proc 3rd Int Colloq Paratuberculosis. Int. Assoc. Paratuberculosis; 1991:201–7.
12. Farthing M, Butcher P. *Mycobacterium tuberculosis* and *paratuberculosis*. In: Farthing M and Keusch G, editors. Enteric infection: mechanisms, manifestations and management. New York: Raven Press; 1989:351–63.
13. Warren J, Rees H, Cox T. Remission of Crohn's disease with tuberculous chemotherapy. N Engl J Med. 1986;314:382.
14. Schultz M, Rieder M, Hersh T *et al.* Remission of Crohn's disease with antimycobacterial chemotherapy. Lancet. 1987;2:1391–2.
15. Picciotto A, Geser G, Schito G *et al.* Antimycobacterial chemotherapy in two cases of inflammatory bowel disease. Lancet. 1988;1:536–7.
16. Howell-Jones J, Lennard-Jones J. Corticosteroids and corticotrophin in the treatment of Crohn's disease. Gut. 1966;7:181–7.
17. Elliott P, Burnham W, Berghouse L *et al.* Sulphadoxine-pyrimethamine therapy in Crohn's disease. Digestion. 1982;23:132–4.
18. Shaffer J, Turnberg L. Does antituberculous chemotherapy for Crohn's disease provide longterm benefit? A five year follow-up study. Gut. 1989;30:A1480.
19. Rutgeerts P, Geboes K, Vantrappen G *et al.* Treatment of severe recurrence of Crohn's disease in the neoterminal ileum with rifabutin and ethambutol. J Clin Gastroenterol. 1992;15:24–8.
20. Hampson S, Parker M, Saverymutter S *et al.* Quadruple antimycobacterial chemotherapy in Crohn's disease; results of 9 months of a pilot study in 20 patients. Aliment Pharmacol Ther. 1989;3:343–52.
21. Wirotsko E, Johnson L, Wirostko B *et al.* Crohn's disease. Rifampin treatment of the occular and gut disease. Hepatogastroenterologica. 1987;34:90–3.
22. Paris J, Simon V, Paris J. Etude critique des effets de la medication antituberculeuse. Dans une serie de 52 cas de formes severes de la maladie de Crohn. Ann Gastroenterol Hepatol. 1977;13:427–33.
23. Toulet J, Rousselet J, Viteau J. La rifampicine dans le traitement de la maladie de Crohn. Gastroenterol Clin Biol. 1979;3:209–11.
24. Ward M, McManus J. Dapsone in Crohn's disease. Lancet. 1975;1:1236–7.
25. Afdhal N, Long A, Lennon J *et al.* Controlled trial of antimycobacterial therapy in Crohn's disease. Clofazamine versus placebo. Dig Dis Sci. 1991;36:449–53.
26. Kohn A, Prantera C, Mangiaroth R *et al.* Antimycobacterial therapy and Crohn's disease: a controlled randomized placebo controlled trial. Gastroenterology. 1992;102:A647.
27. Raleigh J. Chemotherapy of tuberculosis. In: Kubica G, Wayne L, editors. Mycobacteria: a source book. New York: Dekker; 1984;15:1007–20.
28. Chiodini R, VanKruiningen H, Thayer W *et al. In vitro* antimicrobial susceptibility of a *Mycobacterium* species isolated from patients with Crohn's disease. Antimicrob Agents Chemother. 1984;26:930–2.

29. Chiodini R. Bacterial activities of various antimicrobial agents against human and animal isolates of *Mycobacterium paratuberculosis*. Antimicrob Agents Chemother. 1990;34:366–9.
30. Chiodini R. Antimicrobial activity of rifabutin in combination with two and three other antimicrobial agents against strains of *Mycobacterium paratuberculosis*. J Antimicrob Chemother. 1991;27:171–6.
31. McClure H, Chiodini R, Anderson P *et al*. *Mycobacterium paratuberculosis* in a colony of stumptail macaques (Macaca arctoides). J Infect Dis. 1987;155:1011–19.
32. Thayer WR, Coutu J, Chiodini R *et al*. Use of rifabutin and streptomycin in the therapy of Crohn's disease – preliminary results. In: MacDermott R, editor. Inflammatory bowel disease: current status and future approach. New York: Elsevier; 1988:565–8.
33. Bjarnason I, O'Morain C, Levi A *et al*. Absorption of [51]chromium labeled ethylene diamine tetraacetate in inflammatory bowel disease. Gastroenterology. 1983;85:318–22.
34. Pironi L, Miglioli M, Ruggeri E *et al*. Relationship between intestinal permeability to [51Cr] EDTA and inflammatory activity in asymptomatic patients with Crohn's disease. Dig Dis Sci. 1990;35:582–8.
35. Hollander D, Vadheim C, Brettholz E *et al*. Increased intestinal permeability in patients with Crohn's disease and their relatives – a possible etiologic factor. Ann Intern Med. 1986;105:883–5.
36. Doyle T. Susceptibility to Johne disease in relation to age. Vet Rec. 1953;65:363–5.
37. Udall J, Pam K, Fritze L *et al*. Development of gastrointestinal mucosal barrier. I. The effect of age on intestinal permeability to macromolecules. Pediatr Res. 1981;15:241–4.
38. Walker W. Gastrointestinal host defense. Importance of gut closure in control of macromolecular transport. CIBA Fed Symp. 1979;70:201–9.

Section V
The diseased bowel – effects on other organ systems

21

Consequences of reduced absorption: stone and bone disease

H. FROMM

This discussion of stone and bone disease as consequences of reduced absorption focuses on pathophysiological and clinical aspects of several relatively common absorptive disturbances in inflammatory bowel disease (IBD), in particular of those in ileal Crohn's disease. Ileal disease is frequently complicated by a number of abnormalities which are either the direct result of ileal dysfunction or represent the consequence of the overall impact of IBD on the nutritional and metabolic status of the patient.

ABSORPTIVE ABNORMALITIES AS THE DIRECT RESULT OF ILEAL DYSFUNCTION

The terminal ileum represents the site for active bile acid and vitamin B_{12} absorption. Ileal dysfunction, which occurs as the result of either ileal disease or ileal resection, is therefore characterized by bile acid and vitamin B_{12} malabsorption[1,2]. Although the clinical expression and consequences of bile acid and vitamin B_{12} malabsorption vary considerably among patients, several therapeutically relevant predictions can be made with a reasonable degree of accuracy once the extent of the bowel involvement and/or length of ileal resection are known[1-3]. These predictions concern both the severity and pathophysiological role of the respective malabsorptive abnormality[4-9].

Types of diarrhoea in ileal disease or after ileal resection

Choleretic (bile acid-induced) diarrhoea

If their concentrations in the colon are increased, the dihydroxy bile acids, chenodeoxycholic and deoxycholic acids, and their glycine and taurine conjugates, are capable of inducing intestinal water and electrolyte secretion[5]. Concentrations high enough to induce diarrhoea are found only in cases of severe bile acid malabsorption due to ileal disease and/or resection.

Severe bile acid malabsorption and consequent loss of large quantities of bile acids into the colon are seldom found in Crohn's disease without ileal resection[3,4]. Usually a resection of at least 40 cm of distal ileum is required, before a major interruption of the enterohepatic circulation leads to severe bile acid malabsorption[1,6]. However, the increased amounts of bile acids passed into the colon induce diarrhoea only if the aqueous concentrations of chenodeoxycholic and/or deoxycholic acids are 1.5 mmol/l or higher[5]. In other words, the bile acids have not only to be present in increased concentrations, but also have to be solubilized in the aqueous phase. The key prerequisite for a sufficient solubility is a neutral or alkaline pH[6]. Chenodeoxycholic and deoxycholic acids become fully water-soluble only at pH levels above 6.6 and 7.0, respectively. Such pH conditions and consequent secretory bile acid concentrations are characteristically found in patients with severe bile acid malabsorption due to small ileal resection, i.e. a resection of less than 100 cm of terminal ileum[6]. Although the faecal pH in patients with diarrhoea and Crohn's disease without resection is usually also alkaline, bile acid malabsorption is, as mentioned above, seldom severe enough to allow the generation of secretory concentrations of bile acids.

It is only this type of diarrhoea – induced by high aqueous phase concentrations of bile acids in a neutral or an alkaline pH in the colon – which responds therapeutically to cholestyramine[6,9]. It is noteworthy that major steatorrhoea is *not* a feature of choleretic enteropathy. Faecal fat excretion[1,6,9] rarely exceeds 10–15 g/24 h.

Fatty acid-induced diarrhoea

If larger segments of distal ileum are resected (usually more than 100 cm)[1,6,9], steatorrhoea becomes a major feature, faecal pH drops below 6.6 and bile acids – present in large quantities in the colon – are virtually insoluble[6]. The diarrhoea in this condition is therefore not caused by bile acids[6]. It is assumed that, in this condition, steatorrhoea is responsible for the diarrhoea[8,9], since both fatty acids and hydroxy fatty acids are known to have a secretory effect on the intestinal mucosa[8]. The steatorrhoea in large ileal resection is the result of both a significant decrease in intestinal absorptional surface and a disturbance in the intraluminal micellar solubilization of fat due to a marked fall in bile acid concentrations in the upper small bowel. The faecal fat excretion on a 80–100 g fat diet usually exceeds 15–20 g/24 h. The diarrhoea may worsen if cholestyramine is given, since this drug further reduces, through its binding action, micellar bile acids, with resultant deterioration of fat absorption. The treatment is therefore aimed at reducing faecal fat, the substrate for the fatty acid-induced diarrhoea. A reduction in dietary fat – the majority of which consists of long-chain triglycerides – to about 10–15 g/day is usually effective in decreasing the diarrhoea to a tolerable level. A replacement of long-chain triglycerides by medium-chain triglycerides, which are not dependent on a micellar solubilization and are absorbed via the portal route, is used by some physicians in patients with massive small bowel resection (short bowel syndrome) in order to reduce the diarrhoea and supply calories in the form of lipids. However, replacement therapy with medium-chain triglycerides is expensive and inconvenient. A more practical approach would be a very low-fat diet.

Diarrhoea due to passage of large amounts of unabsorbed fluids from the small intestine into the colon

Although the colon has a considerable capacity for reabsorbing fluids, this capacity is exceeded by conditions in which there is massive fluid loss from the small bowel, due to either fluid secretion or limited absorption. The diarrhoea in jejunoileal bypass falls, in many instances, into the latter category[6,7]. The considerable reduction in the absorptional surface of the small bowel, which occurs after jejunoileal bypass surgery, results in the passage of large quantities of fluids into the colon. This explains the very high stool volume, often in the order of 2000–3000 g/day, and the resultant dilution of bile acids and fatty acids in the colon[6,7]. Bile acids play no role in the mechanism of diarrhoea in jejunoileal bypass[7]. Their aqueous concentrations are very low due to both the dilutional effect of the large volume of unabsorbed fluid in the colon and a low faecal pH. The treatment of diarrhoea in patients who have undergone a jejunoileal bypass operation for morbid obesity is often difficult because of the inability of the patient to control the composition of his diet, as well as the amount of food eaten. A discussion of the treatment would go beyond the scope of this chapter.

Diagnostic considerations in the management of diarrhoea in ileopathies

If the diarrhoea in a patient with ileal disease and/or resection does not improve by conventional therapeutic measures, several diagnostic tests should be performed. The presence and severity of bile acid malabsorption can be documented by the cholylglycine-1-^{14}C (bile acid) breath test in conjunction with the measurement of the bile acid label in stool[1]. In addition, faecal pH should be determined and faecal fat be quantitated. If the patient has severe bile acid malabsorption, à neutral or an alkaline faecal pH and no or only mild steatorrhoea (less than 15 g/day), the chances are good that the diarrhoea is caused by bile acids and that it promptly responds to cholestyramine therapy. If the bile acid breath test is not available to the physician, a treatment trial with cholestyramine could be carried out, especially if faecal pH is alkaline and steatorrhoea is absent. In contrast, the presence of significant steatorrhoea (more than 15 g/day) and of a low faecal pH (6 or lower) indicates that the diarrhoea is not caused by bile acids and that therapeutic measures other than cholestyramine have to be considered.

BONE AND STONE DISEASE AS CONSEQUENCES OF ABSORPTIVE AND NUTRITIONAL ABNORMALITIES

General comment

The type, number and severity of metabolic and nutritional disturbances in Crohn's disease differ greatly among patients due to considerable variations in the anatomical involvement of the intestine by the inflammatory, ulcerative process. In addition, major changes in digestion and absorption occur frequently after operative resection of functionally important parts of the intestine[1,10-12]. Crohn's disease may affect any part of the gastrointestinal tract and is characterized by a transmural involvement of the bowel wall. Operative resection of diseased bowel segments is followed by a high recurrence rate and frequently by an aggravation of absorptional and nutritional problems[13,14].

Absorptive and digestive abnormalities in Crohn's disease can also arise from bacterial overgrowth in the small intestine (stagnant loop syndrome) due to stenosis and strictures. Bacterial overgrowth may cause clinically significant vitamin B_{12} malabsorption as well as bile acid deconjugation with consequent malabsorption of fat and fat-soluble vitamins[15].

However, nutritional problems in Crohn's disease are frequently as much related to general metabolic and systemic manifestations of the disease (anorexia, abdominal pain, fever, etc., with resultant inadequate food intake) as they are the result of absorptive abnormalities. In other words, malnutrition in Crohn's disease is often multifactorial in origin rather than attributable to a single cause such as malabsorption.

Frequently, patients with Crohn's disease eat less because they have anorexia, or because food intake worsens symptoms such as abdominal pain and diarrhoea. Anorexia may be a sequela of the chronic disease state, especially if it is complicated by infection and abscess formation. In many cases, patients avoid food because they experience abdominal pain and distension due to intestinal obstruction. In other cases food intake is diminished in order to decrease bowel frequency, which is often a leading sign of the exacerbation of the disease.

Metabolic bone disease

Prevalence

Skeletal demineralization has been reported to be much more common in Crohn's disease than in both the general population and patients with ulcerative colitis[16]. Different authors have found evidence for metabolic bone disease in 30–45% of patients with Crohn's disease. However, in spite of this high prevalence of bone demineralization, clinical manifestations of bone disease are relatively uncommon. Fractures, bone pain and/or muscle weakness occur in less than 10% of Crohn's disease patients reported to show signs of metabolic bone disease.

Diagnostic parameters of metabolic bone disease

The most reliable method of documenting osteoporosis and osteomalacia involves the performance of transiliac needle bone biopsies. While osteoporosis is often defined as decreased volume of normally mineralized bone, the term osteomalacia is used by some authors to describe hyperosteoidosis without evidence of osteoclastosis, marrow fibrosis and woven bone[16]. Osteomalacia may also manifest low trabecular bone volume (osteopenia). A commonly used and relatively sensitive indicator of metabolic bone disease is the serum level of 25-hydroxycholecalciferol (25-OH-vitamin D)[16-20]. In many studies, single-photon absorptiometry, dual-photon absorptiometry, quantitative CT scan and/or X-rays (cortical area ratio of shaft of metacarpal bones) serve as non-invasive techniques for the assessment of bone mineralization.

Factors in the pathogenesis of metabolic bone disease in Crohn's disease

Demineralization of the bones in Crohn's disease is multifactorial in origin. Several authors found a correlation between the prevalence of metabolic bone disease and the activity of Crohn's disease[19], length of ileal resection[20], degree of malnutrition, degree of fat malabsorption and total dose of corticosteroids[21]. Other factors are oestrogen deficiency (in women), use of cholestyramine and lack of sufficient sun exposure. There is evidence that, normally, vitamin D undergoes an enterohepatic circulation which is disturbed in Crohn's disease. 25-OH-vitamin D has been shown to be better absorbed than its metabolic precursor, cholecalciferol (vitamin D)[20].

The exact mechanism of corticosteroid-induced bone disease is not known, but is thought to involve decreased calcium absorption, inhibition of osteoblast formation and a decrease in serum 25-OH-vitamin D. Prolonged administration of high doses of corticosteroids appears to be a major factor in the development of clinically manifest bone disease in Crohn's disease[21]. For example, all six Crohn's disease patients with vertebral fractures described by Compston *et al.* had been treated with corticosteroids for prolonged periods of time[22]. Amenorrhoea and oestrogen deficiency are additional factors which appear to promote metabolic bone disease. Cholestyramine, through its action as anionic exchange resin, binds vitamin D, thus promoting deficiency of this vitamin. In addition, cholestyramine compromises the fat-solubilizing function of bile acids in the small intestine, which may lead to decreased absorption of vitamin D. Last, but not least, sun exposure is a major modulator of metabolic bone disease in Crohn's disease. The prevalence of positive markers of metabolic bone disease, such as decreased serum levels of 25-OH-vitamin D, is much lower during the summer than in the winter. Measurements taken in the winter therefore provide a more sensitive indicator for the risk of metabolic bone disease than do those obtained in the summer.

Treatment of metabolic bone disease in Crohn's disease

While there is little question or controversy as to the need of therapy for the patients who have developed clinically manifest complications of metabolic bone disease, uncertainty exists regarding the management of the relatively large number of patients who, upon testing, are discovered to have subclinical abnormalities consistent with metabolic bone disease. There are few conclusive data in the literature which provide generally accepted guidelines for the management of subclinical bone demineralization. Studies by Driscoll *et al.*, which involved repeated bone biopsies, showed that treatment with an oral vitamin D preparation at a daily dose of 4000 IU led to a normalization of serum 25-OH-vitamin D and a significant improvement of the osteomalacia[16]. However, the response to vitamin D therapy varied. A small number of patients required very high doses of vitamin D, i.e. 25 000–50 000 IU per day, for prolonged periods of time. In some of the patients with low serum 25-OH-vitamin D levels osteoporosis was found on bone biopsy. The authors had no conclusive data as to whether or not the response to vitamin D therapy in osteoporosis is similar to that in osteomalacia. The effect of vitamin D therapy should be monitored by measuring serum 25-OH-vitamin D.

As mentioned above, 25-OH-vitamin D is better absorbed than is vitamin D^{20}. The difference in the absorbability of these two vitamin D forms is considerable in patients with severe fat malabsorption and/or large ileal resection. If serum 25-OH-vitamin D responds poorly to oral administration of vitamin D, oral therapy with 25-OH-vitamin D should be considered, although this treatment is more expensive than that using vitamin D.

Most authors agree that, in the management of patients at risk of developing complications from metabolic bone disease (i.e. those with large ileal resection, steatorrhoea, high disease activity and/or on high-dose corticosteroid therapy), long-term treatment with vitamin D, calcium and oestrogens (in women) should be considered, in addition to increased sun exposure.

Stone disease: enteric nephrolithiasis

Prevalence

The prevalence of nephrolithiasis in IBD is increased. According to several reports, 4–6% of patients with IBD have kidney stones[23–25]. The incidence is somewhat higher in Crohn's disease than in ulcerative colitis and it increases with ileal resection[23,24,26]. Most of the kidney stones in IBD consist of calcium oxalate.

Mechanism

Although kidney stones may simply form as the result of dehydration, which is often caused by diarrhoea in IBD, several other mechanisms are operative. The mechanism, which appears to be the most important one, relates to the development of *hyperoxaluria*. The urinary excretion of oxalate is significantly increased in patients with Crohn's disease[27,28]. The highest urinary oxalate values are seen in patients with extensive ileal resection[29]. However, hyperoxaluria is also seen in malabsorption syndromes unrelated to IBD and intestinal resection, such as sprue and pancreative insufficiency[28]. Furthermore, urinary oxalate excretion has been reported to be increased in patients with liver cirrhosis[28].

What causes hyperoxaluria in IBD and other intestinal disorders? The most common cause appears to be fat malabsorption. Normally, only 2–5% of the oxalate in the diet is absorbed, because insoluble calcium oxalate forms in the lumen of the intestine and is excreted in the stool. In the presence of fat malabsorption, the calcium in the lumen of the intestine is competitively bound to fatty acids with the formation of calcium soaps. Consequently, less calcium is available for the formation of calcium oxalate, leading to an increased absorption of soluble sodium oxalate[29–31].

The second cause of hyperoxaluria is bile acid malabsorption. Increased concentrations of bile acids, specifically of deoxycholate, induce marked enhancement of oxalate absorption in the colon[30,31]. The colon appears to be the main site for the intestinal absorption of oxalate[32,33]. Hyperoxaluria is therefore uncommon in patients after colectomy[29]. However, cases of hyperoxaluria and urolithiasis have been observed in ileostomy patients[28].

In addition to hyperoxaluria, *deficiencies of inhibitors of crystallization* in the urine play a critical role in the pathogenesis of kidney stones in IBD. In particular, citrate, magnesium and pyrophosphate are inhibitors of the formation and aggregation of crystals in the urine. Among the patients with gastrointestinal malabsorption described by Rudman *et al.* to have hypocitraturia were four with Crohn's disease, three of whom had a history of calcium oxalate stones[34]. The patients were also characterized by subnormal serum levels of serum citrate and magnesium.

Treatment

The preventive treatment of calcium oxalate kidney stones in IBD is directed at (1) decreasing the urinary oxalate excretion, and (2) normalizing the serum levels of citrate and magnesium.

The first goal, a decrease in urinary oxalate, can be accomplished by several measures. The most effective one consists of the elimination of dietary oxalate by the institution of a low-oxalate diet[35]. The intestinal absorption of oxalate can also be reduced by the ingestion of calcium (which increases the calcium available in the intestinal lumen for the formation of non-absorbable calcium oxalate) or cholestyramine (which binds oxalate)[32,35].

In addition to decreasing urinary oxalate excretion, it may also be necessary to correct the hypocitraturia which is frequently present in patients with severe IBD and ileal resection. Full correction of this disorder can be achieved by oral administration of citrate and intramuscular injection of magnesium[34]. Magnesium deficiency, which may develop as the result of diarrhoea in IBD, induces enhanced tubular reabsorption of citrate with consequent hypocitraturia. Magnesium chelates with citrate in the tubular urine and thereby diminishes the reabsorption of citrate in the tubule.

References

1. Fromm H, Thomas PF, Hofmann AF. Sensitivity and specificity in tests of distal ileal function: prospective comparison of bile acid and vitamin B_{12} absorption in ileal resection patients. Gastroenterology. 1973;64:1077–90.
2. Fromm H. Bile acid diarrhea: diagnosis and treatment of a clinical disorder of bile acid metabolism. In: Louhija A, Valtonen V, editors. Internal Medicine: 1976 topics. Basel: Karger; 1977:29–38.
3. Farivar S, Fromm H, Schindler D, Schmidt FW. Tests of bile acid and vitamin B_{12} metabolism in ileal Crohn's disease. Am J Clin Pathol. 1980;73:69–74.
4. Sarva RP, Farivar S, Fromm H, Bazzoli F, Wald A, Amin P. Comparative sensitivity of eight and 24-hour bile acid breath tests and Schilling test in ileopathies. Am J Gastroenterol. 1981;76:432–7.
5. Mekhjian HS, Phillips SF, Hofmann AF. Colonic secretion of water and electrolytes induced by bile acids: perfusion studies in man. J Clin Invest. 1971;50:1569–77.
6. McJunkin B, Fromm H, Sarva RP, Amin P. Factors in the mechanism of diarrhea in bile acid malabsorption: fecal pH – a key determinant. Gastroenterology. 1981;80:1454–64.
7. Fromm H, Sarva RP, Ravitch MM, McJunkin B, Farivar S, Amin P. Effects of jejunoileal bypass on the enterohepatic circulation of bile acids, bacterial flora in the upper small intestine and absorption of vitamin B_{12}. Metabolism. 1983;12:1133–41.
8. Ammon HV, Phillips SF. Inhibition of colonic water and electrolyte absorption by fatty acids in man. Gastroenterology. 1973;65:744–9.
9. Hofmann AF, Poley JR. Role of bile acid malabsorption in pathogenesis of diarrhea and statorrhea in patients with ileal resection. I. Response to cholestyramine or replacement of dietary long chain triglyceride by medium chain triglyceride. Gastroenterology. 1972;62:918–34.
10. Booth CC, MacIntyre I, Mollin DL. Nutritional problems associated with extensive lesions of the distal small intestine in man. Q J Med. 1964;33:401–20.
11. Stanley MM, Nemchausky B. Fecal C^{14}-bile acid excretion in normal subjects and patients with steroid-wasting syndromes secondary to ileal dysfunction. J Lab Clin Med. 1967;70:627–39.
12. Meihoff WE, Kern F, Jr. Bile salt malabsorption in regional ileitis, ileal resection, and mannitol-induced diarrhea. J Clin Invest. 1968;47:261–7.
13. Fromm H, Wilson FA, Rodgers JB, Balint JA. Granulomatous bowel (Crohn's) disease. A retrospective study of the course and treatment. Arch Intern Med. 1971;128:739–45.
14. Greenstein AJ, Sachar DB, Pasternack BS, Janowitz HD. Reoperation and recurrence in Crohn's colitis and ileocolitis. Crude and cumulative rates. N Engl J Med. 1975;293:685–90.
15. Donaldson RM Jr. Small bowel bacterial overgrowth. Adv Intern Med. 1970;16:191–212.
16. Driscoll RH, Meredith SC, Sitrin M, Rosenberg IH. Vitamin D deficiency and bone disease in patients with Crohn's disease. Gastroenterology. 1982;83:1252–8.
17. Compston JE, Creamer B. Plasma levels and intestinal absorption of 25-hydroxy vitamin D in patients with small bowel resection. Gut. 1977;18:171–5.
18. Sonnenberg A, Ehms H, Sonnenberg GE, Strohmeyer G. 25-Hydroxycholecalciferol serum levels in patients with Crohn's disease. Acta Hepatogastroenterol. 1977;24:293–5.
19. Harries AD, Brown R, Heatley RV, Williams LA, Woodhead JS, Rhodes J. Vitamin D status in Crohn's disease: association with nutrition and disease activity. Gut. 1985;26:1197–203.
20. Leichtmann G, Bengoa JM, Bolt MJG, Sitrin MD. Intestinal absorption of cholecalciferol and 25-hydroxycholecalciferol in patients with both Crohn's disease and intestinal resection. Am J Clin Nutr. 1991;54:548–52.
21. Hahn TJ. Drug-induced disorders of vitamin D and mineral metabolism. Clin Endocrinol Metab. 1980;9:107.
22. Compston JE, Judd D, Crawley EO, Evans WD, Evans C, Church HA, Reid EM, Rhodes J. Osteoporosis in patients with inflammatory bowel disease. Gut. 1987;28:410–15.
23. Deren JJ, Purush JG, Levitt MF, Khilnan MT. Nephrolithiasis as a complication of ulcerative colitis and regional enteritis. Ann Intern Med. 1962;56:843.
24. Gelzayd EA, Breuer RI, Kirsner JB. Nephrolithiasis in inflammatory bowel disease. Am J Dig Dis. 1968;13:1027.
25. Kern F Jr. Extraintestinal complications. In: Kirsner JB, Shorter RG, editors. Inflammatory bowel disease. Philadelphia: Lea & Febiger; 1975:309–22.

26. Knudsen L, Marcussen H, Fleckenstein P, Pedersen EB, Jarnum S. Urolithiasis in chronic inflammatory bowel disease. Scand J Gastroenterol. 1978;13:433–6.
27. Smith LH, Fromm H, Hofmann AF. Acquired hyperoxaluria, nephrolithiasis, and intestinal disease. Description of a syndrome. N Engl J Med. 1972;286:1371–5.
28. Ruge W, Kohler J, Fromm H, Schindler D, Canzler H. Hyperoxalurie bei Darm-und Lebererkrankungen. Z Gastroenterol. 1977;15:45–55.
29. Earnest DL, Johnson G, Williams HE, Admirand WH. Hyperoxaluria in patients with ileal resection: an abnormality in dietary oxalate absorption. Gastroenterology. 1974;66:1114–22.
30. Binder HJ. Intestinal oxalate absorption. Gastroenterology. 1974;67:441.
31. Dobbins JW, Binder HJ. Effect of bile salts and fatty acids on the colonic absorption of oxalate. Gastroenterology. 1976;70:1096–100.
32. Earnest DL, Johnson G, Williams HE, Admirand WH. Hyperoxaluria in patients with ileal resection: an abnormality in dietary oxalate absorption. Gastroenterology. 1974;66:1114–22.
33. Caspary WF. Erworbene Hyperoxalurie und Nephrolithiasis bei gastroenterologischen Erkrankungen (enterale Hyperoxalurie) Dtsch med Wochenschr. 1975;100:1509.
34. Rudman D, Dedonis JL, Fountain MT, Chandler JB, Gerron GG, Fleming GA, Kutner MH. Hypocitraturia in patients with gastrointestinal malabsorption. N Engl J Med. 1980;303:657–61.
35. Chadwick VS, Modha K, Dowling RH. Mechanism for hyperoxaluria in patients with ileal dysfunction. N Engl J Med. 1973;289:172–6.

22
Hepatobiliary abnormalities

W. J. TREMAINE

Diseases of the liver and bile ducts are the most common extra-intestinal conditions associated with inflammatory bowel disease. Abnormalities that occur in both ulcerative colitis and Crohn's disease are: primary sclerosing cholangitis, cholangiocarcinoma, chronic active hepatitis, and fatty infiltration. Other disorders found in association with Crohn's disease but not ulcerative colitis are: gallstones, granulomas, and amyloidosis.

PRIMARY SCLEROSING CHOLANGITIS

Primary sclerosing cholangitis, the most common hepatobiliary disorder associated with inflammatory bowel disease, is a syndrome of unknown cause characterized by chronic fibrosing inflammation of the bile ducts, usually affecting both the intrahepatic and extrahepatic biliary ductal systems[1]. In a recent population-based study from Sweden[2] the prevalence of primary sclerosing cholangitis was determined in 1500 patients with ulcerative colitis. In patients with colonic disease that extended higher than the splenic flexure, 5.5% had primary sclerosing cholangitis. If the colonic disease was distal to the splenic flexure, 0.5% of patients had primary sclerosing cholangitis. The male to female ratio with ulcerative colitis without primary sclerosing cholangitis was 1.13. In contrast, for patients with both ulcerative colitis and primary sclerosing cholangitis, the male to female ratio was 2.06. On average, in patients who developed both ulcerative colitis and primary sclerosing cholangitis, men developed each condition about 10 years earlier than women. The prevalence of ulcerative colitis among patients with primary sclerosing cholangitis is high, approximately 80%. In contrast, the prevalence of Crohn's disease among patients with primary sclerosing cholangitis is much lower, in the range of 4 to 13%[3].

240

PATHOGENESIS OF PRIMARY SCLEROSING CHOLANGITIS

The relationship of the hepatobiliary abnormalities to the intestinal disease in patients with primary sclerosing cholangitis and inflammatory bowel disease is unclear. Whether the hepatobiliary disease represents a second site of end-organ damage from a common pathogen that also attacks the intestine, or if the hepatobiliary disease results directly from the intestinal disorder is controversial. A relationship of primary sclerosing cholangitis to inflammatory bowel disease can be defined by similarities and differences according to a number of criteria: genetic, infectious, vascular, and immunological, as discussed next.

There is evidence for a genetic predisposition both for ulcerative colitis and primary sclerosing cholangitis. The HLA alleles HLA-DR3 and HLA-B8 have been found in some patients with ulcerative colitis[4]. A recent study[5] by Prochazka and colleagues in Los Angeles showed that some patients with primary sclerosing cholangitis in combination with ulcerative colitis have an extended haplotype of A1, B8, Cw7, DR3, DQw2, DRw52a. In this prospective study of patients awaiting liver transplantation, all 29 patients with primary sclerosing cholangitis who were studied had the HLA-DRw52a antigen, which is normally present in only 35% of the normal population. Fifteen of the patients had a single common haplotype: A1, B8, Cw7, DRw17, DQw2, DRw52a, and in the remaining 17 patients there was a difference in only one of the antigens. As HLA molecules play a key role in the generation and regulation of the immune response by binding foreign antigen on the surfaces of antigen-presenting cells, the finding of a common HLA haplotype has exciting implications for understanding the aetiology of these diseases[6]. However, a true cause and effect relationship of this genetic abnormality to the development of primary sclerosing cholangitis has not been proven.

The possible role of portal bacteraemia as the cause of primary sclerosing cholangitis has been raised. However, systemic and portal blood cultures taken at surgery in patients undergoing colonic resection for severe colitis have not demonstrated bacteraemia[7]. The possibility that toxic bile acids are reabsorbed from diseased mucosa in patients with ulcerative colitis and then cause damage to the liver via the portal system has been suggested, but no abnormal circulating bile acids have been found in patients with severe inflammatory bowel disease[8]. There is no apparent relationship between the severity of ulcerative colitis and the rate of progression of primary sclerosing cholangitis. Indeed, primary sclerosing cholangitis can develop years following proctocolectomy[9]. Conversely, ulcerative colitis can develop after liver transplantation for primary sclerosing cholangitis. These observations make it unlikely that primary sclerosing cholangitis occurs as a consequence of the bowel disease itself.

Viral causes for primary sclerosing cholangitis have been investigated. Hepatitis viruses A and B have been excluded[10]. To date, hepatitis C has not been rigorously studied. Reovirus type III has been associated with biliary atresia, even to the point of having histological similarities. However, there is no direct evidence for reovirus type III infection as a cause for primary sclerosing cholangitis[11]. Although cytomegalovirus may cause an obliterative cholangitis, the histological changes are not typical of those seen in patients with primary sclerosing cholangitis[12]. Patients with the human immunodeficiency virus who develop superimposed cryptosporidiosis or cytomegalovirus infection have histological and cholangiographic changes identical to those seen in patients with primary sclerosing cholangitis[13].

A vascular cause for primary sclerosing cholangitis has been suggested. Extrahepatic biliary disease resembling primary sclerosing cholangitis has been seen in patients with hepatic artery thrombosis after liver transplantation[14] and in patients who have received hepatic artery infusions of 5-fluorodeoxyuridine, probably on the basis of ischaemic injury[15].

Immunological mechanisms are important in the pathogenesis of primary sclerosing cholangitis and inflammatory bowel disease. Increased titres of the immunoglobulin G neutrophil antibodies, in combination with a perinuclear fluorescence pattern, has a sensitivity in the range of 60–65% and a specificity in the range of 94–100% for distinguishing ulcerative colitis from other types of colitides, and in identifying patients with primary sclerosing cholangitis and ulcerative colitis that occur in association[16,17]. The finding of this antibody may be more than simply an epiphenomenon, but its significance in relation to the pathogenesis of disease is yet to be defined.

CLINICAL FEATURES

Ulcerative colitis associated with primary sclerosing cholangitis is usually mildly active or quiescent. In recent series, between 20% and 30% of patients with primary sclerosing cholangitis were asymptomatic[18,19]. The symptoms of primary sclerosing cholangitis begin insidiously, with a gradual onset of fatigue, pruritus, and later jaundice. At the time of diagnosis of primary sclerosing cholangitis, many patients have abnormalities on physical examination, such as hepatomegaly, jaundice, or splenomegaly[1]. Biochemical studies typically show a cholestatic profile, but not invariably so. Cholangiography usually shows diffuse strictures of the intrahepatic and extrahepatic bile ducts. Although these X-ray findings are characteristic of primary sclerosing cholangitis, they are not diagnostic and may be mimicked by infectious or ischaemic causes, as noted previously. In the past, the term 'pericholangitis' was used for inflammatory lesions of the portal tract found in patients with inflammatory bowel disease. With the widespread use of endoscopic retrograde cholangiography it is apparent that most patients with pericholangitis actually have primary sclerosing cholangitis involving the small intrahepatic bile ducts[18]. With this in mind, the terms 'microscopic primary sclerosing cholangitis' or 'small duct primary sclerosing cholangitis' are more appropriate than 'pericholangitis', which is simply a descriptive, morphological term.

TREATMENT OPTIONS IN PRIMARY SCLEROSING CHOLANGITIS

Patients with primary sclerosing cholangitis who undergo colectomy for ulcerative colitis have no differences in the clinical findings, biochemical studies, histology, or survival data as compared with patients with primary sclerosing cholangitis who do not undergo colectomy. If a patient with primary sclerosing cholangitis and ulcerative colitis requires colectomy because of the activity of the colonic disease, an internal anastomosis such as an ileal reservoir to anal anastomosis, or an ileorectostomy is preferable to an end-ileostomy to avoid the potential complication of peristomal varices with the attendant risk of bleeding[20].

A variety of medications have been assessed for the treatment of primary sclerosing cholangitis. The slow progression of the disease, and the fluctuations that occur in the biochemical parameters, make it difficult to determine the value of a particular therapy[21]. Agents shown to be ineffective or toxic include: corticosteroids, azathioprine, antibiotics, penicillamine, colchicine, and cyclosporin. Patients with ulcerative colitis who are treated with cyclosporin, however, have less activity of the colitis while on treatment than do patients who receive placebo[22]. Currently being tested in controlled trials for treatment of primary sclerosing cholangitis are methotrexate and ursodeoxycholic acid.

Interventional procedures are used in primary sclerosing cholangitis to treat dominant strictures and biliary stones. Balloon dilatation of a dominant stricture, either by endoscopic or transhepatic methods, can improve the clinical status and biochemical values[23]. Biliary stones are found in about 25% of patients with primary sclerosing cholangitis, usually gallstones. Surgical intervention for biliary stones should be avoided if possible. Instead, endoscopic sphincterotomy can be performed for common bile duct obstruction to avoid the increased risk of ascending cholangitis that occurs in patients who undergo laparotomy and bile duct exploration.

Liver transplantation is the treatment of choice for patients with end-stage primary sclerosing cholangitis. The 2-year actuarial survival after transplantation for primary sclerosing cholangitis is in the range 57–83%[24].

RISKS OF MALIGNANCY

Cholangiocarcinoma is more common in patients with ulcerative colitis and in patients with Crohn's disease than in the general population[3,25]. Primary sclerosing cholangitis appears to be a prerequisite for the development of cholangiocarcinoma in patients who have inflammatory bowel disease[26]. There is a male predominance among inflammatory bowel disease patients with cholangiocarcinoma and the mean age is about 20 years younger than that of patients with cholangiocarcinoma in the general population[27]. Although the clinical features of cholangiocarcinoma and primary sclerosing cholangitis are similar, presentation of obstructive jaundice of short duration should raise the suspicion of bile duct carcinoma. The differentiation of primary sclerosing cholangitis and cholangiocarcinoma by endoscopic retrograde cholangiopancreatography, by bile duct cytology, and by histology on bile duct biopsies taken endoscopically can be difficult. In contrast to patients with cholangiocarcinoma who do not have inflammatory bowel disease, gallstones are rare in patients with inflammatory bowel disease who have bile duct cancer[27].

Primary sclerosing cholangitis appears to be a risk factor for the development of colonic dysplasia, DNA aneuploidy, and colon cancer in patients with ulcerative colitis[28]. In a Swedish study, among 72 patients with extensive ulcerative colitis (involvement proximal to the hepatic flexure) who were followed with surveillance biopsies during a 15-year period, 17 patients developed dysplasia, carcinoma, and/or DNA aneuploidy. Five (28%) of the 17 patients with these changes had primary sclerosing cholangitis and none of the 55 patients who did not have dysplasia (carcinoma) or DNA aneuploidy, had primary sclerosing cholangitis. When assessed by multivariant analysis, primary sclerosing cholangitis appeared to be an independent risk factor. Although the cause of this increased risk is unknown, one hypothesis concerns faecal bile acid concentrations that are higher in patients with ulcerative colitis who develop dysplasia or carcinoma as compared to patients without dysplasia or carcinoma[29]. Whether faecal bile acid abnormalities could play a role in patients with primary sclerosing cholangitis and colon cancer remains open to speculation.

OTHER HEPATIC DISORDERS ASSOCIATED WITH INFLAMMATORY BOWEL DISEASE

Chronic active hepatitis has been reported in patients with ulcerative colitis and less commonly in those with Crohn's disease. Since piecemeal necrosis may also occur in primary sclerosing cholangitis, it is important to exclude the latter before making the diagnosis[25]. The prevalence of post-transfusion hepatitis C in this group has not been established.

The majority of patients with inflammatory bowel disease who develop cirrhosis have primary sclerosing cholangitis. However, cirrhosis may be found in patients who have no evidence for bile duct disease or for an underlying viral cause. Of the 1–5% of patients with inflammatory bowel disease who develop cirrhosis, only a small percentage have this cryptogenic type[30].

Hepatic steatosis, usually microvesicular, occurs in up to 80% of patients with inflammatory bowel disease[31]. There are multiple potential aetiologies for fat accumulation, including malabsorption, drug effects, and bacterial toxins. In most cases the abnormality is asymptomatic.

Gallstones occur in about one-third of patients with Crohn's ileitis, as compared to a prevalence of up to 15% in the general population. There is a direct correlation between the extent and duration of ileal disease and the prevalence of gallstones[32].

Scattered hepatic granulomas are seen in the liver biopsies of patients with Crohn's disease, with or without an associated increase in the serum alkaline phosphatase. The granulomas may disappear after excision of the diseased bowel[30].

Hepatic amyloidosis occurs in up to 10% of patients with severe Crohn's disease[26], and there may be improvement after resection of diseased bowel. Coexisting renal amyloidosis is common.

SUMMARY

Patients with inflammatory bowel disease frequently have coexisting hepatobiliary abnormalities. Because the aetiology and pathogenesis of the intestinal disease and of the liver disease is unknown, the precise nature of the relationships of the hepatic to intestinal abnormalities is also unclear. Genetic and immunological changes that are found in patients with inflammatory bowel disease, with and without liver disease, may give important clues as to the cause of these disorders.

References

1. LaRusso NF, Wiesner RH, Ludwig J, MacCarty RL. Primary sclerosing cholangitis. N Engl J Med. 1984;310:899–903.
2. Olsson R, Danielsson A, Jarnerot G, Lindstrom E *et al.* Prevalence of primary sclerosing cholangitis in patients with ulcerative colitis. Gastroenterology. 1991;100:1319–23.
3. Aadland E, Schrumpf E, Fausa O *et al.* Primary sclerosing cholangitis: a long-term follow-up study. Scand J Gastroenterol. 1987;22:655–64.
4. Schrumpf E, Fausa O, Forre O, Dobloug JH, Ritland S, Thorsby E. HLA antigens and immunoregulatory T-cells in ulcerative colitis associated with hepatobiliary disease. Scand J Gastroenterol. 1982;17:187–91.
5. Prochazka EJ, Teresaki PI, Park MN, Goldstein LI, Busuttil RW. Association of primary sclerosing cholangitis with HLA-DRw52a. N Engl J Med. 1990;322:1842–4.
6. Segall M, Bach FH. HLA and disease: the perils of simplification. N Engl J Med. 1990;322:1879–80.
7. Palmer KR, Duerden BI, Holdsworth CD. Bacteriological and endotoxin studies in cases of ulcerative colitis submitted to surgery. Gut. 1980;21:1851–4.
8. Holzbach RT, Marsh ME, Freedman MR, Fazio VW, Lavery IC, Jagelman DA. Portal vein bile acids in patients with severe inflammatory bowel disease. Gut. 1980;21:428–35.
9. Cangemi JR, Wiesner RH, Beaver SJ, Ludwig J, MacCarty RL, Dozois RR, Zinsmeister AR, LaRusso NF. Effect of proctocolectomy for chronic ulcerative colitis on the natural history of primary sclerosing cholangitis. Gastroenterology. 1989;96:790–4.
10. Wiesner RH, LaRusso NF. Clinicopathologic features of the syndrome of primary sclerosing cholangitis. Gastroenterology. 1980;79:200–6.
11. Morecki R, Glaser JH, Cho S, Balistreri WF, Horwitz MS. Biliary atresia and reovirus type III infection. N Engl J Med. 1982;307:481–4.
12. Snover DC, Horwitz CA. Liver disease in cytomegalovirus mononucleosis: a light microscopical and immunoperoxidase study of six cases. Hepatology. 1984;4:408–12.
13. Cello JP. Acquired immunodeficiency syndrome cholangiopathy: spectrum of disease. Am J Med. 1989;86:539–46.
14. Zajko AB, Campbell WL, Logsdon GA *et al.* Cholangiographic findings in hepatic artery occlusion after liver transplantation. Am J Radiol. 1987;149:485–9.
15. Ludwig J, Kim CH, Wiesner RH, Krom RAF. Floxuridine-induced sclerosing cholangitis: an ischemic cholangiopathy. Hepatology. 1989;9:215–18.
16. Duerr RH, Targan SR, Landers CJ, LaRusso NF *et al.* Neutrophil cytoplasmic antibodies: a link between primary sclerosing cholangitis and ulcerative colitis. Gastroenterology. 1991;100:1385–91.
17. Duerr RH, Targan SR, Landers CJ *et al.* Anti-neutrophil cytoplasmic antibodies in ulcerative colitis. Gastroenterology. 1991;100:1590–6.

18. Porayko MK, LaRusso NF, Wiesner RH. Primary sclerosing cholangitis: a progressive disease? Semi Liver Dis. 1991;11(1):18–25.
19. Helzberg JH, Petersen JM, Boyer JL. Improved survival with primary sclerosing cholangitis: a review of clinicopathologic features and comparison of symptomatic and asymptomatic patients. Gastroenterology. 1987;92:1869–75.
20. Wiesner RH, LaRusso NF, Dozois RR, Beaver SJ. Peristomal varices after proctocolectomy in patients with primary sclerosing cholangitis. Gastroenterology. 1986;90:316–22.
21. Kaplan MM. Medical approaches to primary sclerosing cholangitis. Sem Liver Dis. 1991;11(1):56–63.
22. Sandborn WJ, Wiesner RH, LaRusso NF. Ulcerative colitis disease activity after treatment of associated primary sclerosing cholangitis with cyclosporine or placebo. Am J Gastroenterol. 1991;86:285 (abstr.).
23. May GR, Bender CE, LaRusso NF, Wiesner RH. Non-operative dilatation of dominant strictures in primary sclerosing cholangitis. Am J Radiol. 1985;145:1061–4.
24. Lindor KD, Wiesner RH, MacCarty RL, Ludwig J, LaRusso NF. Advances in primary sclerosing cholangitis. Am J Med. 1990;89:73–80.
25. Berman MD, Falchuck KR, Trey C. Carcinoma of the biliary tree complicating Crohn's disease. Dig Dis Sci. 1980;25:795–7.
26. van Erpecum KJ, van Berge Henegouwen KJ. Hepatobiliary abnormalities in inflammatory bowel disease. Neth J Med. 1989;35:S40–49.
27. Converse CF, Reagan JW, DeCosse JJ. Ulcerative colitis and carcinoma of the bile ducts. Am J Surg. 1971;121:39–45.
28. Broome U, Lindberg G, Loftberg R. Primary sclerosing cholangitis and ulcerative colitis – a risk factor for the development of dysplasia and DNA aneuploidy? Gastroenterology. 1992;102:1877–80.
29. Hill MJ, Lennard-Jones JE, Melville DM, Neale K, Ritchie JK. Fecal bile acids, dysplasia and carcinoma in ulcerative colitis. Lancet. 1987;2:185–6.
30. Eade MN, Cooke WT, Brooke BN, Thompson H. Liver disease in Crohn's colitis: a study of 21 consecutive patients having colectomy. Ann Intern Med. 1971;74:518–28.
31. Desmet J, Gebos K. Liver lesions in inflammatory bowel disorders. J Pathol. 1987;151:247.
32. Rankin GB. Extraintestinal and systemic manifestations of inflammatory bowel disease. Med Clin N Am. 1990;74(1):39–50.

23
Consequences of unknown cause: the skin as target organ

W. STOLZ, S. KÁRPÁTI and M. LANDTHALER

The skin and the gastrointestinal (GI) tract are closely related systems. Both are covered or lined by epithelium and both communicate with the external environment[1]. There are disorders which present with both skin and GI involvement and there are diseases of the gut and the skin that coexist more often than would be expected by chance[1,2].

It is frequently assumed that if both systems are involved, then the GI disease is the primary one[2]. However, the following possibilities exist:

1. GI disease is the cause of skin disease. On occasion skin lesions can provide clues to the underlying GI tract disease[1].
2. GI disease can be a risk factor for the development of a polyaetiologic skin disease.
3. Skin disease secondarily can also spread to the GI tract.
4. GI tract and skin are involved by the same systemic disorder.

GI DISEASE IS THE CAUSE OF A SKIN DISEASE

In patients with GI tract malignancy, cutaneous signs may occur as a paraneoplastic phenomenon or as a result of tumour infiltration of the skin via direct extension or metastatic spread[1].

Paraneoplastic signs relatively specific for GI tract malignancy are (the most common site of primary tumour is given in parentheses following the skin disease): acanthosis nigricans (stomach, colon); sudden appearance of seborrhoeic keratoses (sign of Leser–Trélat: adenocarcinoma of the stomach and colon); acrokeratosis paraneoplastica (Bazex syndrome: oesophagus); diffuse palmoplantar hyperkeratosis (Howel–Evans syndrome: oesophagus); flushing (carcinoid syndrome); necrolytic migratory erythema (glucagonoma in the tail of pancreas)[1]. In a review presenting data[3] of 724 patients with cutaneous metastases, 9% in women were secondary to adenocarcinoma of the GI tract, whereas in men 19% were of this origin. The metastases from GI tract cancer are most frequently located on the abdominal skin, and the majority are derived from colonic adenocarcinoma. Umbilical metastases in a patient with colon carcinoma are known under the term Sister Mary Joseph's nodule[1,2].

Malabsorption can lead to a dry and therefore itching skin similar to a mild type of dominantly inherited ichthyosis[2]. These changes are mainly found in patients with malabsorption due to malignant disease, but are not necessarily confined to this group. In addition, brittle nails, a reduction of the diameter of the hairs with liability to break, and hyperpigmentation of the skin can be found in these patients[2]. A defect in the absorption of zinc causes acrodermatitis enteropathica[4], a sharply demarcated scaling erythematous vesiculobullous eruption present at the orifices (mouth, genitoanal region) and distal extremities. Similar manifestations can be seen in patients receiving intravenous infusion therapy which lacks zinc salts[4].

In Crohn's disease specific lesions can be found on the skin demonstrating pathological features identical to those of GI disease[5]. The skin lesions in inflammatory bowel diseases are discussed in detail below. Recent concepts for the pathogenesis of dermatitis herpetiformis indicate that a mild gluten-sensitive enteropathy is necessary for the development of skin eruptions. A possible mechanism is also described below.

Severe vomiting attacks can lead to the appearance of purpura on the face and on the neck in predisposed patients.

GI DISEASE IS A RISK FACTOR FOR THE DEVELOPMENT OF A POLYAETIOLOGIC SKIN DISEASE

In inflammatory bowel diseases a variety of reactive skin lesions can develop, which will be described in detail below. Most frequent are pyoderma gangrenosum, erythema nodosum, and aphthous ulcers. However, these skin lesions can also be found in other internal diseases. The aphthous ulcers in Crohn's disease and Behçet's disease are sometimes difficult to differentiate[2].

SKIN DISEASES SECONDARILY INVOLVING THE GI TRACT

There are only a few skin diseases secondarily leading to GI lesions. In epidermolysis bullosa dystrophica, Hallopeau–Siemens type, characterized by a loss of anchoring fibrils in the sublamina densa zone, the oesophagus can also be involved. Moreover, mucosal lesions are found in epidermolysis bullosa dystrophica inversa, Gedde–Dahl type[4]. Decreased motility of the oesophagus can also be observed in progressive sclerosis. Patients with a congenital lack or impaired function of the C1-esterase inhibitor periodically develop deep oedema all over the body. Rarely also the GI tract can be involved, leading to the clinical symptoms of an acute abdomen. Inherited defects of connective tissue, such as Ehlers–Danlos syndrome and pseudoxanthoma elasticum can lead to GI symptoms such as bleeding, blockage, and perforation.

GI TRACT AND SKIN ARE INVOLVED BY THE SAME SYSTEMIC DISORDER

There are numerous disorders in which both the GI tract and the skin are involved. In various polyposis syndromes skin lesions may be present[1]: epidermoid cysts, alopecia, and nail defects can be detected in Gardner's syndrome, hyperpigmented macules and patches on the hands and arms in Cronkhite–Canada syndrome, pigmented labial macules in Peutz–Jeghers syndrome, facial trichilemmomas in Cowden's syndrome as well as multiple sebaceous adenomas and other skin tumours with sebaceous differentiation in Muir–Torre syndrome. In 25% of patients with neurofibromatosis, neurofibromas have been noted in the submucosa of the GI tract[1]. In Osler's disease GI tract bleeding due to angiomas located in the stomach and duodenum can be found in 13–40% of cases[5]. In blue rubber bleb naevus syndrome haemangiomas may be present in the large and small bowel[5]; 50–80% of patients with Kaposi's sarcoma on the skin and almost all patients with lesions within the mouth will have GI tract lesions. A majority of patients with Henoch–Schoenlein purpura have GI lesions and the most common complaints are crampy abdominal pain and bleeding[5].

In mastocytosis of the skin, characterized by circumscribed proliferations of benign mast cells, infiltration of the small bowel may occur. Diarrhoea and abdominal pain in these patients might be due not only to this specific involvement, but also to the liberation of histamine and related substances from cutaneous mast cells, which are pharmacologically active and can lead to abdominal pain and to diarrhoea[2].

SKIN LESIONS IN INFLAMMATORY BOWEL DISEASE

Whereas in most of the neoplastic GI disorders skin lesions are rare events, the inflammatory bowel diseases (IBD), ulcerative colitis (UC) and Crohn's disease (CD) are accompanied in 9–19% (UC) and 9–23% (CD) by cutaneous manifestations[5].

Mucocutaneous manifestations of IBD may be classified as specific lesions, reactive lesions, and lesions secondary to malabsorption or treatment (drug eruptions).

Specific lesions (fissures, oral and metastatic CD) are due to direct involvement of the skin by the same disease process that affects the GI tract. In contrast, reactive lesions (erythema nodosum, pyoderma gangrenosum, oral aphthous ulcers, vesiculopustular eruptions, pyoderma and pyostomatitis vegetans[6], necrotizing vasculitis, cutaneous periarteritis nodosa, and Sweet syndrome[7] show different pathological features, but represent a reaction to the underlying IBD. It is speculated that some of these diseases may be immunologically mediated via cross-antigenicity between the skin and the gut[1]. However, a variety of other internal diseases can also lead to these reactive lesions.

Fissures and fistulae are probably the most common cutaneous manifestations, and may be the presenting complaint in CD. The most common affected site is the perianal region. Oral lesions are characterized by oedema, a cobblestone appearance, and tiny nodules, predominantly found on the gingival and alveolar mucosa. Metastatic CD is rare and demonstrates nodules, plaques, or ulcerated lesions.

Erythema nodosum is characterized by painful nodules on the shins, mostly accompanied by weakness, raised temperature, and elevated sedimentation rate[4]. Pyoderma gangrenosum starts with sterile pustular foci, followed by ulcers, which peripherally spread. If, under the diagnosis of an abscess, surgical treatment is performed, a significant increase in the size of the ulcer can be seen. Treatment of choice is with oral corticosteroids, sometimes in combination with the antileprosy drug clofazimine.

Both erythema nodosum and pyoderma gangrenosum are present in about 4–5% of patients with UC and in 1–2% of patients with CD. About 50% of patients with pyoderma gangrenosum have UC. In children erythema nodosum may be the most common extracolonic manifestation of the disease[5]. Aphthous ulcers are present in about 6% and 8% of patients with CD and UC, respectively[2].

DERMATITIS HERPETIFORMIS: A POSSIBLE HYPOTHESIS FOR THE RELATIONSHIP BETWEEN GI TRACT AND SKIN

The reason behind the relationship between skin and GI tract has yet to be clarified in almost all the disorders involving both organs. However, in coeliac disease and dermatitis herpetiformis (DH) investigations by immunofluorescence and immunoelectron microscopy offered a possible explanation for the association between small bowel and skin[8-12].

Dermatitis herpetiformis is a polymorphous, itching dermatosis characterized by a simultaneous presence of erythema, papules, and vesicles distributed typically in a herpetiform pattern. Diagnosis of dermatitis herpetiformis is based on the detection of granular IgA antibodies in the dermal papillary skin; 70–80% of patients have circulating IgA antibodies, which, however, do not bind to normal papillary skin[12]. Recent investigations demonstrated that in 90% of patients with coeliac disease identical circulating IgA antibodies could be found on human fetal jejunum by immunofluorescence[8,9]. Binding studies using the ultrastructural immunogold technique revealed that these antijejunal antibodies may be similar to circulating antiendomysium and antireticulin antibodies also described in these two disorders[9], and that jejunal antibodies recognize binding sites in association with reticulin fibres in normal jejunum[11]. It was concluded that jejunal antibodies could be the target-organ-related autoantibodies in coeliac disease[9].

In dermatitis herpetiformis patients the presence of jejunal antibodies correlated with the presence of a mild variant of gluten-sensitive enteropathy, but not with the activity of skin disease[8,12]. Moreover, binding sites of these circulating IgA antibodies could not be detected in normal human skin. Immunoelectron microscopic investigations in diseased skin of dermatitis herpetiformis disclosed that the IgA deposits in the skin represent either IgA complexes bound to a non-fibrillar component of dermal connective tissue or immune complexes trapped in dermatitis herpetiformis skin[10]. Almost all coeliac patients have circulating IgA antibodies; however, the small bowel disease is not accompanied by skin rash. Only patients who have specific IgA deposition in the skin have the associated skin disease we recognize as dermatitis herpetiformis[10]. Due to the data outlined here, the following hypothesis for the pathogenesis of dermatititis herpetiformis was presented by Kárpáti[12].

Antijejunal antibodies are induced in association with immunologically mediated jejunal damage caused by the ingestion of wheat protein in patients with gluten-sensitive enteropathy.

Long-lasting mild mucosal damage may result in permanent autoantigen exposition, and this challenge might lead to immune complex formation. Patients with dermatitis herpetiformis and coeliac disease eliminate immune complexes poorly, which might enhance the possibility of immune complex disease developing under gluten intake. The detailed pathomechanism of how immune complexes in the skin lead to neutrophil activation and blister formation is not known. Environmental factors – e.g. daily gluten intake, iodine intake, unknown dietary antigens being absorbed by gluten damaged jejunum, and/or consecutive serum factors – might influence the activity of the skin disease[12].

CONCLUSION

Four possibilities for a relationship between GI tract and the skin exist: (1) GI disease can be the cause of skin disease; (2) GI disease can be a risk factor for the development of a polyaetiologic skin disease, which can also be due to other underlying diseases; (3) skin disease may secondarily spread to the GI tract; (4) both the skin and the GI tract can be involved by the same systemic disorder.

Whereas many diseases are present both in the skin and the gut, the reason behind the link between the GI tract and the skin has not yet been clarified. We outlined a hypothesis for the relationship between coeliac disease and dermatitis herpetiformis based on the production of immune complexes in the diseased uppermost bowel.

ACKNOWLEDGEMENT

This work was supported by a grant from the Humboldt-Stiftung for Sarolta Kárpáti.

References

1. Gregory B, Ho VC. Cutaneous manifestations of gastrointestinal disorders. Part I. J Am Acad Dermatol. 1992;26:153–66.
2. Marks J, Shuster S. The skin and disorders of the alimentary tract. In: Fitzpatrick TB, Eisen AZ, Wolff K, Freedberg IM, Austen KF, editors. Dermatology in general medicine. New York: McGraw-Hill; 1987:1965–76.
3. Brownstein MH, Helwig ER. Metastatic tumors of the skin. Cancer. 1972;29:1298–307.
4. Braun-Falco O, Plewig G, Wolff HH, Winkelmann RK. Dermatology. Heidelberg: Springer; 1991.
5. Gregory B, Ho VC. Cutaneous manifestations of gastrointestinal disorders. Part II. J Am Acad Dermatol. 1992;26:371–83.
6. Lobkowicz F, Eckert F, Braun-Falco O. Pyostomatitis vegetans. Ein spezifischer Marker für Morbus Crohn und Colitis ulcerosa. Hautarzt. 1991;42:92–5.
7. Schlegel Gómez R, Kiesewetter F, von den Driesch P, Hornstein OP. Sweet-Syndrom (akute febrile neutrophile Dermatose) und Erythema nodosum bei Morbus Crohn. Hautarzt. 1990;41:398–401.
8. Karpati S, Török E, Kosnai K. IgA class antibody against human jejunum in sera from children with dermatitis herpetiformis. J Invest Dermatol. 1986;87:703–6.
9. Karpati S, Bürgin-Wolff A, Krieg T, Meurer M, Stolz W, Braun-Falco O. Binding to human jejunum of serum IgA antibody from children with coeliac disease. Lancet. 1990;36:1335–8.
10. Karpati S, Meurer M, Stolz W, Schrallhammer K, Krieg T, Braun-Falco O. Dermatitis herpetiformis bodies. Ultrastructural study on the skin of patients using direct preembedding labeling. Arch Dermatol. 1990;126:1469–74.
11. Karpati S, Stolz W, Meurer M, Krieg T, Braun-Falco O. Extracellular binding sites of IgA anti-jejunal antibodies on normal small bowel detected by indirect immunoelectronmicroscopy. J Invest Dermatol. 1991;96:228–33.
12. Karpati S. Advances in pathophysiology of dermatitis herpetiformis. Eur J Dermatol. 1992;2:389–97.

24
Diseased bowel in an intact organism – implications for surgical treatment

M. STARLINGER and F. MAKOWIEC

Although chronic inflammatory bowel diseases, i.e. ulcerative colitis and Crohn's disease, are limited to the large bowel and the gastrointestinal tract respectively, both diseases, as in fact any chronic inflammatory process, indirectly affect the otherwise intact organism.

Two aspects of these effects of the diseased bowel on other organs primarily not affected by the disease itself, or on the whole organism, will be discussed here, namely the so-called extraintestinal manifestations and malnutrition. In both instances we will look into the question of whether the surgical removal of the diseased intestine cures or alleviates these secondary manifestations, and therefore whether they influence the indication for surgery.

EXTRAINTESTINAL MANIFESTATIONS OF CROHN'S DISEASE

The pathogenetic mechanisms which lead to the development of extraintestinal manifestations are still unclear[1]. An immunological dysregulation has been postulated. This is supported by the presence of circulating immune complexes in patients with IBD who have extraintestinal manifestations. However, these immune complexes are found not only in patients with extraintestinal manifestations, but also in patients without extraintestinal manifestations. Extraintestinal manifestations are present more frequently in patients with colonic involvement (ulcerative colitis and Crohn's colitis) but their correlation to intestinal disease activity is variable.

Extraintestinal manifestations with a chronic and aggressive course (e.g. ankylosing spondylitis, primary sclerosing cholangitis and pericholangitis) are almost independent of the course and therapy of intestinal disease[1,2].

Peripheral arthritis, erythema nodosum, stomatitis or uveitis in general show a close correlation to intestinal disease activity. However, these extraintestinal manifestations are self-limiting or respond well to medical treatment.

A pyoderma gangrenosum often appears independent of intestinal activity but only rarely after surgical treatment of the underlying intestinal disease. In patients with extensive colitis and high inflammatory activity, however, the additional occurrence of a pyoderma gangrenosum may be an important argument for surgical treatment of colitis.

MALNUTRITION

Three possible forms of disease course have been proposed by Binder *et al.*[3] For each year of observation, 45% of the patients had inactive disease, 35% intermittent and 20% continuous disease activity. Patients from the latter group frequently present symptoms of malnutrition[4], almost always the consequence of several factors:

Abdominal pain or anorexia may lead to decreased intake of food. Malabsorption may be the consequence of a reduction of absorptive intestinal surface by extensive inflammation or after surgical resection. Extensive inflammation, especially in the colon, or high-output fistulae, may lead to excessive loss of proteins, blood, fluid or electrolytes. Finally, caloric consumption may be increased by the presence of fever or sepsis.

As a consequence of malnutrition, anaemia, hypoalbuminaemia and reduced body weight are found clinically. Patients in general complain of decreased physical ability. As a result of these symptoms, approximately 20% of the patients in the study of Binder *et al.*[3] were not able to work.

In a study at our institution we examined the influence of intestinal activity on haemoglobin, albumin, blood sedimentation rate and body weight in 492 patients with Crohn's disease (mean follow-up 5.2 years). Inflammatory activity was further analysed by the frequencies of abdominal pain, disease flare-up and the need of hospitalization for therapy per observation-year. The comparison of patients who were operated later in the observation period and patients who were not operated during the study period revealed on average a significantly higher disease activity in patients who eventually came to surgery (Fig. 1). In general, patients who did not have surgery, and had no continuous disease activity, were in the normal ranges regarding haemoglobin, albumin and body weight; therefore, diseased bowel that does not require surgery has little or no influence on other organs, when bowel activity is well controlled by medical therapy.

In the same study[5], we analysed the influence of surgical therapy (resection) on the above-mentioned parameters of intestinal activity in the years before and after surgery ($n = 130$; Table 1). Following operation, all parameters improved significantly, indicating decreased overall disease activity. In addition, these improvements could be demonstrated over several years. These data clearly demonstrate that a resection of diseased or inflamed bowel

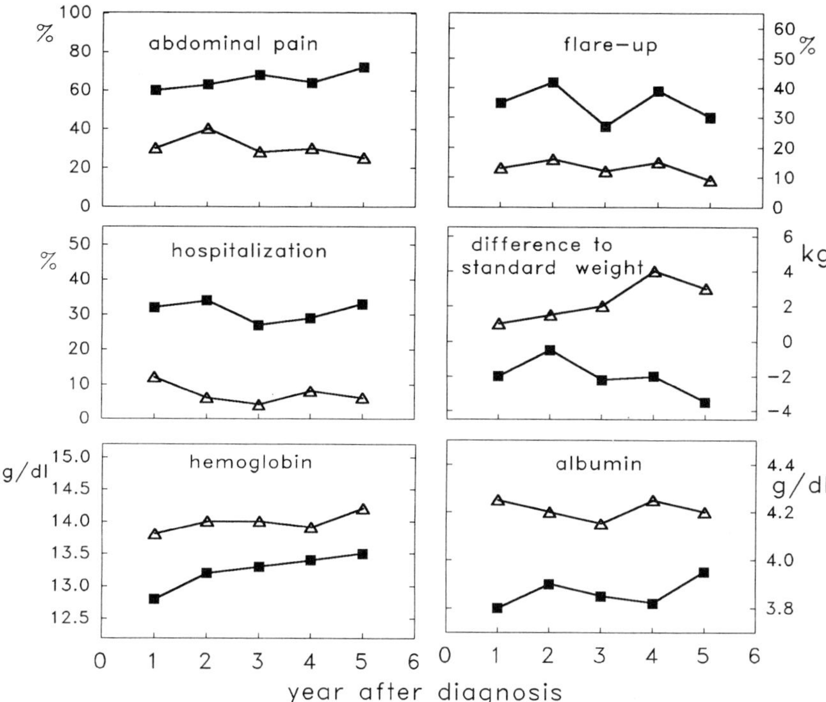

Fig. 1 Clinical and biochemical parameters for disease activity in the 5 years after diagnosis of Crohn's disease. The diagrams show different disease activity in patients who were operated later (filled square) and patients who were not operated during the study period (open triangle). The first three diagrams show the frequencies per year of the patients who at least once had abdominal pain, one disease flare-up and one hospitalization for therapy in the corresponding year. The three other curves show the mean values of weight, haemoglobin and albumin for the two different groups. The weight difference is the difference of actual body weight to a standard weight (Broca)

abolishes the negative influence of the inflamed bowel on other organ systems in most patients over a long period of time.

Despite this fact, almost all patients will develop an endoscopically visible recurrence early after surgery, as shown by Rutgeerts et al.[6] and by our group[5]. However, only 40% of the patients have increased disease activity and only 20% need a reoperation within 5 years after primary surgery[5]; therefore, only extensive inflammation intractable by medical therapy, or complications such as stenosis, fistulae or abscesses may have a relevant influence on the organism.

As shown in both examples, diseased bowel influences other organs or the whole organism. Extraintestinal manifestations are only exceptionally an indication for resectional intestinal surgery. Resection of diseased bowel segments has no influence on the natural course of some extraintestinal manifestations; other extraintestinal manifestations respond well to medical

Table 1 Clinical and biochemical parameters for disease activity in the years before and after surgery

Parameter	Preoperatively, year before surgery			Postoperatively, year after surgery		
	5 ($n = 22$)	3 ($n = 52$)	1 ($n = 118$)	1 ($n = 122$)	3 ($n = 76$)	5 ($n = 41$)
Haemoglobin (g/dl)	13.8	13.2	12.8	13.8[a]	14.2[b]	14.1
Albumin (g/dl)	4.2	3.9	3.8	4.25[a]	4.3[b]	4.2
ESR (mm at 1 h)	26	28	35	18[a]	19[b]	16[c]
Weight difference (kg)	−2.6	−2.8	−3	+1.5[a]	+2.5[b]	+3.4[c]
Flare-up (%)	9	27	41	11[a]	13[b]	7
Hospitalization (%)	6	14	70	20[a]	12[b]	8
Abdominal pain (%)	56	63	72	40[a]	34[b]	28[c]

[a] Significant improvement compared to year before surgery
[b] Significant improvement compared to 3rd year before surgery
[c] Significant improvement compared to 5th year before surgery
Quantitative values are mean values per year. Weight-difference is the difference of actual body-weight from a standard-weight (Broca). Frequencies are the number of patients who had at least once a flare-up, one hospitalization or once abdominal pain in the concerning year

treatment. However, the symptoms of malnutrition, the consequence of diseased bowel, respond well to surgery. In the case of malnutrition, resectional surgery should be considered early to improve the physical ability and therefore the quality of life in these mostly young patients.

References

1. O'Brian J. Extraintestinal manifestations of inflammatory bowel disease. In: MacDermott RP, Stenson WF, editors. Inflammatory bowel disease. New York: Elsevier; 1992:387–403.
2. White H, Peters M. Hepatobiliary disorders in inflammatory bowel disease. In: MacDermott RP, Stenson WF, editors. Inflammatory bowel disease. New York: Elsevier; 1992:405–17.
3. Binder V, Hendriksen C, Kreiner S. Prognosis in Crohn's disease – based on results from a regional patient group from the county of Copenhagen. Gut. 1985;26:146–50.
4. Alfonso JJ, Rombeau JL. Nutritional care for patients with Crohn's disease. Hepatogastroenterology. 1990;37:32–41.
5. Makowiec F, Köveker G, Weber P, Jenss H, Starlinger M. Morbus Crohn: Krankheitsaktivität und Rezidiv nach Operation. Dtsch Med Wochenschr. 1990;115:1659–64.
6. Rutgeerts P, Geboes K, Vantrappen G, Beyls J, Kerremans R, Hiele M. Predictability of the postoperative course of Crohn's disease. Gastroenterology. 1990;99:956–63.

25
Pathophysiology: facts, hopes and implications for treatment

C. FIOCCHI

Pathophysiology is a term used to describe a series of events, both normal and abnormal, that are involved in the cause, development, and mechanisms of disease. When all those events are known and understood, then it becomes possible to devise rational approaches whose purpose is to eliminate the cause, modify all abnormalities triggered by the aetiological factor, and devise strategies to re-establish physiological responses and restore health. This perfect series of circumstances is not commonly encountered in human diseases, and basic and clinical investigators must often content themselves with adopting the best therapeutic options available to them to relieve the patients' symptoms in spite of wide gaps in knowledge of the specific cause of an illness, the pathophysiological mechanisms involved, or both. Unfortunately, this less than ideal picture translates well the current status of inflammatory bowel disease (IBD), and applies with some variations to both Crohn's disease and ulcerative colitis.

There are several reasons why the pathophysiology of IBD is poorly understood. First, in regard to the aetiology, no unique agent, bacterium, virus or fungus, has ever been unmistakenly linked to the cause of Crohn's disease or ulcerative colitis. Second, in regard to the target of disease, it is unclear what specific cellular components of the gut are being attacked, even though it is accepted that the superficial mucosa is more involved in ulcerative colitis, whereas in Crohn's disease the inflammation involves both mucosal and submucosal structures. Third, there is general agreement that the mucosal immune system is the central mediator of inflammation and tissue injury. However, it is uncertain what activates it, why immune cells are recurrently turned on and off, and how many pathways of inflammation are responsible for tissue destruction[1]. An all-inclusive and realistic hypothesis is that the mucosal immune system, under the influence of genetic, dietary, and environmental factors, in addition to the enteric flora and perhaps a still unknown aetiological agent, is activated. This activation results in the stimulation of a variety of effector cells which release soluble substances: plasma cells may release antibodies that fix complement and cause cell death[2]; T cells could mediate lysis of target cells by recognizing cell surface antigens to which they have been previously sensitized, or through the release of cytotoxic cytokines[3]; macrophages could be non-specifically activated by bacterial antigens or cytokines and cause local injury by direct cytotoxicity or production of soluble mediators; finally, neutrophils could be locally recruited, and destroy surrounding tissue by direct lysis or through release of reactive oxygen metabolites[4]. None of these mechanisms has been definitively proven to act in IBD, but there is sufficient circumstantial evidence to strongly suggest that one or more of such pathways of inflammation are operative in Crohn's disease or ulcerative colitis.

Thus, it is fair to state that during the last decade, a period of time when the importance of mucosal immune responses has become the major focus of attention in IBD, many facts have been observed and described. The problem is that these facts are several, they are often confusing, and the actual importance of each one is yet to be elucidated. A key goal in the understanding of IBD pathophysiology is to establish beyond any doubt which facts are relevant, which translate pathophysiology, and which are epiphenomena. This is obviously a very difficult and extremely complex task. In this chapter an attempt will be made to comprehensively review current evidence (facts) relevant to IBD pathophysiology, mention ideal developments (hopes) to be expected from assessing these facts, and discuss what implications they may have for an improved therapy of Crohn's disease and ulcerative colitis.

FACTS – I – AETIOLOGY

It is still unknown whether each of the two clinical forms of IBD, Crohn's disease or ulcerative colitis, has a single or multiple aetiology. The heterogeneity of the clinical course and variability of the response to therapy tend to suggest that we may be dealing with syndromes rather than distinct entities, particularly in regard to Crohn's disease. This is very likely to remain an unresolved issue until specific agents or triggers are detected in essentially each case of the two types of IBD. At present one must be contented in searching for clues based on indirect evidence. In this section data derived from animal models of colitis, genetics and environmental/psychosocial factors will be discussed in proportion to their relative emphasis (Table 1).

Table 1 Pathophysiology of inflammatory bowel disease. Facts – I – aetiology

Animal models	Still lacking an ideal model
Genetics	Still defining markers with very strong association
Psychosocial factors	Influence of the environment, diet, social status, etc.?

Animal models

The search for an animal model of IBD has been pursued ever since ulcerative colitis and Crohn's disease were identified as clinical entities. Unfortunately, this search has been only partially successful, as an ideal animal model sharing with human patients the same cause, pathogenesis, pathological and clinical manifestations has yet to be found[5]. This had limited the appeal of the study of IBD animal models until recently, when a resurgence of interest in this topic was spurred by the utilization of experimental forms of colitis for screening of new drugs, more so than by the investigation of pathogenesis. A variety of substances and manoeuvres can be used to induce gut inflammation in laboratory animals, including irritants, chemicals, bacterial products, haptens, immune complexes, and immune manipulations, in addition to sporadic forms of spontaneous colitis (Table 2).

Most models reproduce acute or subacute colitides with little to moderate degree of resemblance to ulcerative colitis, and seldom Crohn's disease[6]. Nevertheless, they provide systems in which modulation of the gut inflammatory reaction can be achieved with a wide variety of agents, whose effectiveness and potential usefulness as new drugs can be assessed. Among the many substances that have an anti-inflammatory or healing effect on experimental colitis are prostaglandin analogues[7,8], thomboxane synthetase inhibitors[9,10], platelet-activating factor (PAF) inhibitors[11], 5-lipoxygenase inhibitors[12], eicosapentaenoic acid[13], verapamil[14], aminophenols[15], and inhibitors of leucocyte adhesion[16].

Far more interesting for the investigation of aetiopathogenesis are those rare animals that develop IBD spontaneously. The best prototype is the cotton-top tamarin (*Saguinus oedipus*), a South American non-human primate that develops an ulcerative colitis-like picture complicated by colorectal carcinoma in the chronic stage of the disease[17]. In spite of these similarities, the tamarin's colitis is probably quite different from the human counterpart, as recent evidence shows that these animals do not develop circulating anti-neutrophil cytoplasmic antibodies (ANCA), whose frequency is quite high in human patients[18]. Continued search in alternative models of IBD has led to the discovery of a new form of spontaneous murine colitis, obtained by repeated inbreeding of C3H/HeJ mice[19]. A preliminary report claims that

Table 2 Pathophysiology of inflammatory bowel disease – animal models

Irritants (ethanol, acetic acid)
Chemicals (NSAID[a], indomethacin)
Bacterial products (PG-PS)[b]
Immune complexes, TNBS[c]
Gastrointestinal infarction
Immunological (clonal deletion, transgenic)
Spontaneous (*S. oedipus* monkeys, C3H/HeJ mice)

[a] Non-steroidal anti-inflammatory drugs
[b] Peptidoglycan-polysaccharide
[c] Trinitrobenzene sulphonic acid

these animals develop a chronic and recurrent inflammation of the colon and rectum. If confirmed, this could be an invaluable model, considering the ease of manipulation, the low cost, and the tremendous potential for immunological investigation. Additional forms of immune-type colitis have been or are being developed. For instance, cyclosporin A-induced clonal deletion of thymocytes in young mice produces animals with autoimmune disease and large bowel inflammation[20]. However, the most innovative and exciting animal model of IBD has been reported by Hammer *et al.*[21]. These authors transfected rats with the human HLA-B27 gene, known to be expressed by almost all ankylosing spondylitis patients. The resulting transgenic animals develop florid arthropathies, and also chronic inflammation of the small and large bowel. Therefore, the level of sophistication reached by the study of IBD animal models has steadily increased, and it is possible to envision an even greater use of experimental models not solely for screening of anti-inflammatory agents, but also investigating in much greater detail the immunological and genetic components of IBD.

Genetics

The high familial incidence of Crohn's disease and ulcerative colitis is well established[22]. What is not established, however, is whether this phenomenon is due to genetic or environmental factors, and arguments in favour of one vs the other component have been presented[23,24]. Healthy relatives of patients with IBD may show immune or biochemical abnormalities that are associated with no apparent clinical manifestations, such as a high prevalence of serum antibodies to intestinal epithelial antigens and increased intestinal permeability[25,26]. However, the primary vs secondary nature of these findings, and their link to IBD pathogenesis, are unclear.

Classical associations of either forms of IBD with class I (HLA-A, B, C) or class II (HLA-DR, DQ, DP) histocompatibility antigens have been reported infrequently, and usually in genetically homogeneous populations, such as HLA-DR2 in Japanese subjects suffering from ulcerative colitis[27]. This lack of a consistent genetic link has led Rotter to propose the concept of genetic heterogeneity in IBD, in which subgroups of patients with Crohn's disease or ulcerative colitis may display susceptibilities restricted to different immunogenes, like those of the HLA complex, complement, immunoglobulin heavy chain allotypes, and T cell receptor[28]. A proposed association with polymorphism of the T cell receptor (TCR) α-chain and ulcerative colitis has not been confirmed[29]. In contrast, data gathered from North American populations have revealed a positive association of HLA-DR2 with ulcerative colitis and HLA-DR1/DQw5 with Crohn's disease[30].

Although statistically significant, such associations are still not very strong, perhaps due to the small samples studied or the fact that genetic heterogeneity limits the prevalence of each gene in any given population. Further support for the concept of genetic heterogeneity has been provided quite recently by family studies in ulcerative colitis, showing that unaffected relatives have unexpectedly high prevalence of ANCA, a proposed genetic marker of susceptibility for this condition[31]. At present only carefully planned studies in large and well-defined populations will answer the question of whether or not true genetic predisposition exists in IBD.

Environmental/psychosocial factors

This represents an extremely heterogeneous group of factors that have been linked to the appearance, incidence, and prevalence of IBD in various populations throughout the world. They include climate, social and economic status, living in urban vs rural areas, breast and early feeding, associated diseases, infections, smoking, pollutants, psychological status, etc. So far no real clue has emerged from any of these factors that has helped in formulating solid and testable hypotheses. Only long-term prospective studies in large populations may generate interpretable data, particularly the incidence and prevalence in countries where IBD was uncommon until a few decades ago, such as western and southern Europe, South America and Japan.

FACTS – II – IMMUNOLOGY

Immune cells

It is generally accepted that immune abnormalities are an intrinsic and essential component of the chronic inflammatory response of IBD, even though a specific defect associated with Crohn's disease, ulcerative colitis or both has yet to be identified. Nevertheless, there is enough evidence showing that immune cells display aberrant behaviour at both the systemic and mucosal levels to implicate them in the pathophysiology of IBD (Table 3). A multitude of functional defects of T cells, B cells, macrophages, and natural killer (NK) cells have been described and recently reviewed in detail[32]. Other cells that are potentially important to IBD are mucosal eosinophils, mast cells, and basophils, but their scant number in normal and diseased tissue, and their difficult isolation, have limited their investigation. Consequently, very little is known about their actual relevance to IBD, although they also appear to be in an activated state[33].

The evaluation of immune cells is becoming increasingly sophisticated with the help of molecular biological methodology, and researchers no longer rely solely on phenotypic and functional characteristics. Presently, a major area of emphasis is the TCR, a key structure which, together with class II antigens on the surface of antigen-presenting cells (macrophages, dendritic cells, etc.) and other accessory molecules, is responsible for the recognition and response of T lymphocytes to specific antigens. This is accomplished by the α and β

Table 3 Pathophysiology of inflammatory bowel disease. Facts – II – Immunology

Lymphocytes	Which are the critical ones? Are there critical ones?
Other immune cells	Are they more important?
Other cells (epithelial, mesenchymal)	How 'immune' are they?
Immune and 'non-immune' cells	Are they all important?

chains of the TCR which utilize different portions of their variable (V) regions depending on the unique molecular structure of each antigen. Therefore, the antigen recognition process by T cells can be investigated through the different types of V regions, and the frequency with which each of these regions is used. Several reports have shown that in some autoimmune diseases there is a definite over- or underutilization of specific V regions of the TCR, implying that a unique antigen is preferentially being seen by the T cells, or that these are being activated by superantigens[34,35]. Thus, defining the Vβ or α region utilization pattern can provide clues to the nature of the antigen or superantigen involved in T cell activation. An initial study found increased numbers of T cells expressing Vβ8 gene products in the mesenteric lymph nodes draining inflammatory lesions of Crohn's disease, but not among T cells in the affected mucosa[36]. Duchmann *et al.*[37] reported a decreased usage of the Vβ2 regions among T cells of the inflamed lamina propria of Crohn's disease and ulcerative colitis specimens, while Landau *et al.*[38] found an increased usage of Vδ3 region among intraepithelial lymphocytes isolated from ulcerative colitis-involved mucosa. Since the number of identifiable V regions is continuously expanding, a systematic approach to TCR utilization will be needed to explore all possibilities in IBD.

Non-immune cells

The intestinal mucosa is a complex structure with a variety of cell types anatomically arranged to serve special functions. The overwhelming emphasis devoted to the local immune system has until recently caused many 'non-immune' cell types to receive little attention by IBD investigators, but there is strong evidence indicating that such cells are also actively involved in intestinal immunity (Table 3). In IBD the epithelial cell has classically been considered as the passive target of an attack by local immune cells[39], or the source of neoplastic complications. In reality, gut epithelial cells probably play a much more dynamic role. It has been definitively proven that epithelial cells have an antigen-presenting capacity[40]. This function may be abnormal in IBD, where the epithelium expresses high levels of class II antigens[41], and activates preferentially helper rather than suppressor T cells, in contrast to what the normal epithelium does[42]. Ongoing studies also show that epithelial cells may produce potent mediators of inflammation, such as PAF, and that in ulcerative colitis this production is significantly elevated[43]. Thus, it appears that in IBD the gut epithelium is clearly not exerting a simple by-stander role subject to the events in the surrounding environment, but actually contributes to the conditioning of the local inflammatory response.

In addition to the epithelium, other non-immune cells appear to be involved in inflammation. The studies of Graham and collaborators have shown that muscularis propria cells are responsible for abundant collagen production in IBD[44]. Stallmach *et al.* have demonstrated that intestinal fibroblasts also contribute to collagen deposition, particularly when these cells derive from strictured areas of Crohn's disease[45]. Other mesenchymal-type cells are likely to be involved. A typical histological finding of IBD is a thickened muscularis mucosae layer[46]. Since this phenomenon is invariably associated with chronic inflammation, it is reasonable to assume that local hyperplastic or hypertrophic changes are due to the influence of the surrounding inflammatory cells and factors. To explore this possibility we recently conducted studies in our laboratory in which isolated human muscularis mucosae cells were exposed *in vitro* to recombinant cytokines or supernatants derived from cultures of lamina propria mononuclear cells[47]. The results of these experiments show that both stimuli induced a vigorous proliferative response from muscularis mucosae cells, suggesting an explanation for their excessive growth in IBD. Similar results were obtained with mucosal fibroblasts. Even more exciting are preliminary studies showing that when muscularis mucosae cells were exposed to interleukin-1β, a typical inflammatory mediator, there was induction of high levels of interleukin-6 (IL-6) and pro-collagen type III mRNA (Strong *et al.*, work in progress). These results are potentially important to IBD pathogenesis for several reasons. First, they clearly demonstrate that growth and gene induction of non-immune mucosal cells are regulated by cytokines. Second, they confirm the long-held suspicion that non-immune cells can produce inflammatory mediators. Third, they raise the question of how much of the local IBD response is actually due to classical inflammatory vs mesenchymal cells. Finally, they reinforce the concept of a mutual interaction between immune and non-immune cells that is fundamental to the mucosal cytokine network. Therefore, this should be expanded to include cells and soluble factors acting bi-directionally between mononuclear cells and each of the epithelial, endothelial, muscle and fibroblast cell types.

FACTS – III – CYTOKINES AND MEDIATORS

Among the many exciting areas of investigation of the normal and pathological immune response none has received as much attention as the study of cytokines and other soluble mediators. These include a wide array of factors from diverse cellular origins and with the capacity of triggering or modulating essentially any function of the immune system. Because of this broad definition and spectrum of activities, a practical approach to study cytokines and mediators can be based on their preferential immunoregulatory vs pro-inflammatory role. A detailed review of this topic in IBD has been recently published[48]. In this section we will adopt an even broader definition of soluble factors to include lipid mediators and neuropeptides (Table 4).

One of the most attractive features in the study of cytokines is the opportunity of using them not only to understand cell-to-cell communications and intimate mechanisms of pathogenesis, but also to diagnose, monitor, and even treat specific diseases. All this is based on the assumption that measurement of cytokine activities in the systemic circulation or affected tissues reflects the status and degree of immune activation at the site of disease (Fig. 1). There is good evidence to support this assumption. A representative example is provided by the assessment of serum levels of soluble IL-2 receptor (sIL-2R), one of the most commonly used parameters

Table 4 Pathophysiology of inflammatory bowel disease. Facts – III – Cytokines and mediators

Immunoregulatory cytokines: IL-2, IL-4, IL-10, IFN-γ, etc.[a]	Is there an imbalance?
Inflammatory cytokines: IL-1, IL-6, IL-8, TNF, etc.[b]	Are they all increased?
Lipid mediators: PG, TBX, LT, PAF, etc.[c]	Are they all important?
Neuropeptides: VIP, SP, somatostatin, etc.[d]	How important are they?

[a] Interleukins 2, 4, 10; interferon-γ
[b] Interleukins 1, 6, 8; tumour necrosis factor
[c] Prostaglandins, thromboxanes, leukotrienes, platelet-activating factor
[d] Vasoactive intestinal peptide, substance P

of immune activation[49]. The sIL-2R has been shown to be a potentially useful marker of clinical activity in IBD, and particularly Crohn's disease, where a positive correlation is observed between circulating sIL-2R levels and the score of the Crohn's disease activity index[50]. The production of sIL-2R in IBD-involved mucosa is also increased, but a correlation with peripheral levels is detected only in Crohn's disease and not ulcerative colitis[51]. Thus, although useful, caution should be exerted in the interpretation of cytokine levels, and before attributing them an excessive clinical value. The concentration of tumour necrosis factor α (TNF-α), another inflammatory cytokine, is elevated in both the circulation and the stools of IBD patients[52].

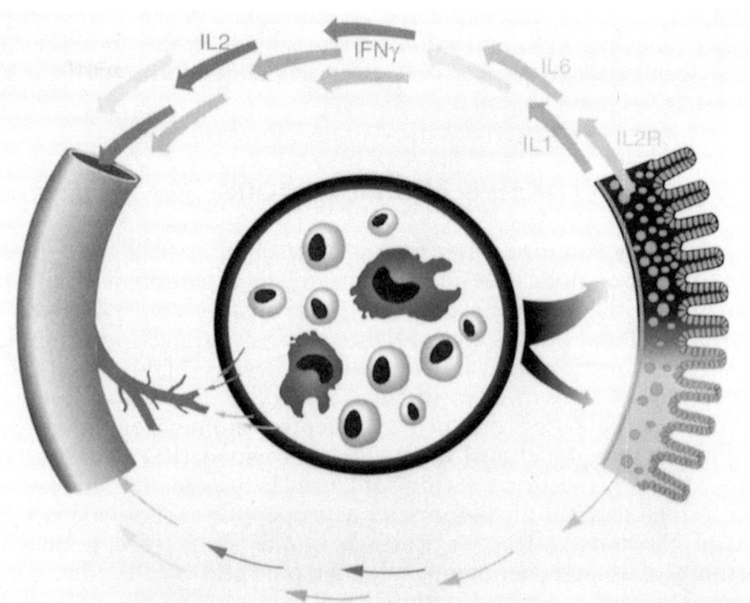

Fig. 1 Schematic representation of cytokine production in the intestinal immune system and subsequent transfer to the peripheral blood. Under physiological conditions, immune cells in the various compartments of the body (central circle) and the intestinal mucosa (right), produce low baseline levels of cytokines (thin arrows) which enter the systemic circulation (left). In inflammatory bowel disease both the number and state of activation of the local mononuclear cells are enhanced. These cells secrete high levels of cytokines which enter the circulation in larger amounts (thick arrows) and cause an elevation of their concentration in the serum

Additional inflammatory cytokines are also of interest, such as the reported elevation of serum interleukin-8 (IL-8) in ulcerative colitis[53], and of IL-6 in Crohn's disease but not ulcerative colitis[54,55], suggesting that these measurements may be helpful in the differential diagnosis of IBD.

Immunoregulatory cytokines

Previous attempts to define the immunoregulatory status of IBD patients based on the predominance of helper or suppressor cells or function were unsuccessful. Similarly, in spite of numerous reports on levels of various cytokines at the systemic and intestinal level of Crohn's disease and ulcerative colitis patients, a clear picture of immunoregulation in IBD has not been achieved yet. However, this situation is likely to be changed by dramatic advances in our understanding of what forces control the balance of the immune system. The fundamental contribution by Mossmann and Coffman of the concept of two distinct types of T helper cells has revolutionized the approach to cytokine-mediated immunoregulation[56]. These authors have demonstrated that within the CD4+ T helper (Th) cell population, there are at least two distinct cell subsets, Th-1 and Th-2. Each one of these subsets produces a certain spectrum of cytokines, some of them being mutually exclusive for each subset. Th-1 cells produce IL-2, interferon-γ (IFN-γ) and lymphotoxin, while Th-2 produce interleukins 4, 5, 6 and 10 (IL-4, IL-5, IL-6 and IL-10)[57]. These cytokines profiles establish and maintain an equilibrium between Th-1 and Th-2 cells, and it is postulated that under physiological circumstances an excess of activity of either subset is counterbalanced by the inhibitory control of the cytokines of the other Th subset.

There is substantial evidence from animal models that the Th-1/Th-2 balance is altered in disease states, as well exemplified by murine leishmaniasis. Mice resistant to the parasite produce high levels of IFN-γ and susceptible mice produce little IFN-γ but abundant IL-4, a picture consistent with opposing Th-1 and Th-2 patterns, respectively[58]. This situation is not found exclusively in experimental models, and there is convincing evidence that imbalances of Th-1- and Th-2-derived cytokines are also present in human diseases. T cell clones from atopic subjects produce preferentially IL-4, IL-5 and IL-6, whereas non-allergic subjects produce more IL-2 and IFN-γ[59,60]. Even in the same clinical entity the expression of cytokine profiles is altered, depending on whether the patients develop a strong or a weak immune response to the same antigen, as in leprosy[61]. It should not be surprising if a similar situation is found in IBD, not only conditioning Crohn's disease or ulcerative colititis, but also different clinical presentations in the same form of IBD. Therefore, defining the Th-1, Th-2, or Th-0 (mixed) profiles in gut tissues during the various stages of disease development seems to be of fundamental importance to understand IBD pathogenesis. Although the present knowledge of mucosal cytokine production does not fit in any clearly defined pattern[48], it still may be so, once more sensitive techniques (polymerase chain reaction – PCR) and specific cell types (CD4+ T cell clones) are carefully analysed.

Inflammatory cytokines

While immunoregulatory cytokines may determine the direction of an immune response, the effector phase of such response is usually mediated by an entirely different group of soluble factors. These are produced preferentially by cells of monocyte–macrophage lineage, in relatively larger amounts, and they usually share a proinflammatory, tissue damaging activity. Interleukin-1, IL-6, TNF-α and perhaps IL-8 fit into this category. Although they display common properties, each one of them tends to exhibit predominant activities, such as control of inflammation for IL-1, modulation of antibody synthesis for IL-6, and tumoricidal activity for TNF-α[62]. Current information on these cytokines in IBD has been discussed above[52–55].

Since they all contribute to inflammation, their blockade could have some effect on down-regulating or decreasing mucosal injury. In fact, preliminary evidence supports this potentially important and novel approach. Several receptors and proteins that specifically bind to and block the function of cytokines have been described[63]. One of them, the IL-1 receptor antagonist (IL-1ra), has been cloned, well characterized, and shown to have a profound inhibitory activity on most IL-1 functions[64]. Cominelli *et al.* have demonstrated that IL-1 is of primary importance in rabbit experimental colitis, suggesting that an imbalance of IL-1 and IL-1ra may be present in the inflamed mucosa[65]. Additionally, these authors presented preliminary evidence indicating that this imbalance occurs in the intestine of humans affected by Crohn's disease and ulcerative colitis[66]. If confirmed, this observation could open the door to a totally new approach to the treatment of IBD, i.e. the use of immunotherapeutic agents that block distinct pathways of the inflammatory cascade. The complete specificity of the substances used, such as IL-1ra, would prevent more general and potentially undesirable effects on other immunoregulatory circuits, and should be very safe, since the substances to be administered will be of human origin and therefore perfectly tolerated by the patients. The first double-blind, placebo-controlled clinical trial of IL-1ra in ulcerative colitis is now under way.

Lipid mediators

Before cytokines received so much attention, the pathway of arachidonic acid metabolism was the one on which most of the active research was focused. Initially, products of the cyclooxygenase pathway, such as prostaglandins, were thought to be important inflammatory mediators because of their elevated levels in IBD mucosa[67]. Their cytoprotective effect was recognized only later, as was the lack of effectiveness of PGE_2 synthesis inhibitors in reducing inflammation in ulcerative colitis[68]. Subsequently, the more potent and unequivocal inflammatory activity of the products of the lipoxygenase pathway, such as leukotriene B4 (LTB4), became established[69], as well as the role of PAF[70]. All these data confirmed the long-held suspicion that multiple lipid mediators are involved in IBD. However, it is not established which one of them, if any, is of central relevance[71]. Ongoing trials with lipoxygenase inhibitors and eicosapentaenoic acid (EPA – fish oil) should help in establishing the relative contribution of each mediator to mucosal inflammation[72,73].

Neuropeptides

Neuropeptides represent a totally different class of substances that may contribute to inflammation. The concept of 'neurogenic inflammation' is being increasingly associated with many inflammatory and autoimmune diseases, mostly due to the well-recognized input of several neuropeptides in immunoregulation[74]. The rich innervation of the intestinal mucosa and the intimate physical and functional relationship between the local nervous and immune systems have been well established[75]. Alterations of calcitonin gene-related peptide and substance P have been recently described in rabbit colitis[76], and several abnormalities of vasoactive intestinal peptide, substance P, somatostatin, or their receptors, have been reported in patients with IBD[77-81]. At present the primary vs secondary nature of the various neuropeptide abnormalities is being actively investigated, as is their relevance to IBD pathophysiology.

FACTS – IV – MICROBIOLOGY, METABOLISM, MOTILITY AND PERMEABILITY

In addition to the numerous pathophysiological facts discussed in the preceding sections, a whole host of other causes, factors, and theories have been proposed to explain IBD. To even enumerate all of them would be too time-consuming and fruitless, since quite a few are not based on solid scientific data. Thus, in this section we will limit our discussion to a brief overview of only the most recent facts based on concrete information (Table 5).

Microorganisms

Investigators of IBD have searched for specific aetiological microorganisms since Crohn's disease and ulcerative colitis were first described. Looking back at the history of this search is an exercise in excitement and disappointment, as one after another many different bacteria, viruses and fungi have ascended

Table 5 Pathophysiology of inflammatory bowel disease.
Facts – IV – Microbiology, metabolism, motility and permeability

Microorganisms	Specific or non-specific?
Microcirculation	Primary or secondary role?
Oxygen radicals	The final 'hit'?
Motility	What are the modulatory factors?
Permeability	Is it really abnormal?

to and descended from the hopes of researchers, clinicians and patients alike. The only survivor of a long list of candidate organisms is *Mycobacterium paratuberculosis*, initially proposed by Chiodini *et al.* as the possible cause for Crohn's disease[82]. The main problems encountered with this organism, that have prevented it from becoming a more convincing causative candidate, have been the extreme technical difficulty in its isolation, and the sporadic nature of positive culture from affected tissues[83]. Furthermore, the presence of this bacterium in normal and ulcerative colitis bowel, albeit at a lower rate than Crohn's disease tissues, also raises concerns, as *M. paratuberculosis* is considered an obligate pathogen. As in other instances, the power of molecular biology has been summoned to help investigators in finding this organism in the diseased tissue under the assumption that only very few copies are present, or that most of it is incorporated into the host's DNA. Initial investigations have been negative[84], but more recent data obtained by PCR showed a relatively high frequency (65%) of *M. paratuberculosis* DNA in Crohn's disease-affected intestine[85]. However, a small but significant proportion (12.5%) of normal control tissues also contained mycobacterial DNA, while other laboratories reported lower rates of recovery or completely negative results[86,87]. Although inconclusive so far, systematic application of PCR technology may help in characterizing unknown organisms and the role they may have in IBD[88].

Due to the inconsistency of the recovery of *M. paratuberculosis*, some investigators have proposed that perhaps only a subgroup of Crohn's disease patients have their illness caused by this agent. Based on this premise, several centres have tried antituberculous therapy with second- or third-generation antibiotics, with generally disappointing results. The most intriguing data have been cited by Khon and collaborators, who found a significantly lower recurrence rate in Crohn's disease subjects treated with anti-tuberculous drugs as compared to untreated patients followed for the same period of time[89]. Whether these results are caused by specific killing of *M. paratuberculosis*, or are due to a non-specific effect of the antibiotics on the gut flora, is not clear. There is little doubt that the intestinal microflora has a role in modulating intestinal immunity. For instance, bacterial components can cause gut inflammation in susceptible animals and probably influence the rate of recurrence in Crohn's disease patients[90,91]. Therefore, before the effect of antimicrobial agents in Crohn's disease is fully understood, more information of their action on the enteric microflora must be obtained.

Microcirculation

The notion that Crohn's disease could be caused by vascular abnormalities is not new, and this hypothesis has received renewed support by recent studies showing the presence of multifocal GI infarctions and granulomatous vasculitis in bowel involved by Crohn's disease[92,93]. A vasculopathy could explain the classical 'skip lesions' and would corroborate the negative effect of smoking and contraceptives on this disease[94]. Although intriguing, evidence implicating microvascular abnormalities as being of major pathophysiological relevance to granulomatous enteritis is still preliminary, and additional studies are needed.

Oxygen radicals

The overwhelming emphasis devoted to the role of classical immunity in triggering and conditioning IBD has caused the investigators to overlook what may be a critical component of the local inflammatory process, i.e. the polymorphonuclear neutrophil. This cell type is present in variable numbers during all stages of Crohn's disease and ulcerative colitis, and probably plays a prominent function in the efferent limb of the immune response[95]. In addition, neutrophil products are likely to be of importance in mucosal injury, an event mediated by a variety of reactive oxygen metabolites (ROM)[4]. These substances have been shown to be generated in the colon of animals subjected to experimental colitis[96], and they can damage fresh enterocytes as well as cultured intestinal epithelial cell monolayers[97,98]. The importance of ROM in intestinal injury is not restricted to artificial systems, and it probably represents a real pathogenic event in actively inflamed bowel of IBD patients, as confirmed by chemiluminescence probes[99,100]. Preliminary results of clinical trials using superoxide dismutase as an anti-oxidant in Crohn's disease have been encouraging[101].

Another compound that is receiving much attention is nitric oxide (NO), another biologically active radical with a multiplicity of physiological and toxic activities[102]. Among these, NO is an endogenous modulator of leucocyte adhesion, and therefore may represent another significant contributor to the complex inflammatory cascade of IBD[103]. However, since blocking NO may have both beneficial and detrimental effects, more detailed information is needed before considering this substance as a potential target for therapeutic agents in Crohn's disease or ulcerative colitis.

Motility

Abnormalities of bowel motility are some of the most classical manifestations in patients with IBD, even though their precise pathophysiology is still incompletely understood[104]. In the context of mucosal inflammation it is becoming increasingly evident that the immune system has a previously unrecognized and perhaps direct input on bowel motility. Studies in *Trichinella spiralis*-infected rats clearly show that some changes in intestinal smooth muscle function are T lymphocyte-dependent[105]. Therefore, an additional and unexpected immune component must be added to the already complex mechanisms of dismotility in IBD.

Permeability

It has been proposed that Crohn's disease may be the result of an increased permeability of the tight junction between epithelial cells, and such defect may represent a primary pathogenic factor, since it is also encountered in some healthy relatives of Crohn's disease patients[26]. Abnormal results seem to depend on the type and molecular size of the probe used, and the abnormal permeability hypothesis has been supported by some, but challenged by other, studies[106-108]. It will not be surprising if additional investigation proves that a defect of intestinal absorption is a secondary rather than primary event.

HOPES

All the facts discussed so far make up an impressive amount of data, but when all available evidence is put together it is difficult to construct a unifying and clear hypothesis to explain the pathophysiology of IBD. Almost certainly distinct mechanisms control Crohn's disease and ulcerative colitis, and although some overlap probably exists, separate pathogenic events are operative in each form of IBD. Faced with so many perspectives and possibilities to pursue, investigators are now waiting for the time when the cause, the exact pathogenesis, and the specific treatment for IBD will be known. While that time is coming, many hopes remain to be fulfilled (Table 6).

The discovery of two separate aetiological microorganisms for Crohn's disease and ulcerative colitis would definitely sanction these two entities as unequivocally distinct, and would allow specific treatment with antimicrobials. The finding of a highly sensitive and totally specific genetic marker would permit an intrauterine diagnosis, and theoretically prevention of IBD. If the myriad of environmental and psychosocial factors predisposing or conditioning the disease could be identified, they could be eliminated or avoided. Ideally, investigators of mucosal immunology could finally solve the 'immunology of IBD puzzle' with all the numerous pieces fitting tightly together to form a meaningful picture of immunoregulation, immune dysfunction, and immune-mediated injury amenable to immunotherapy. Prominent in the solution of this puzzle would be the complete enumeration of all inflammatory mediators, which could be clearly separated into the critical and the irrelevant ones. Consequently, once the critical mediators of inflammation are defined, then molecular biological techniques could be called in to engineer custom-made antibodies, antagonists, inhibitors or blockers that would specifically and totally shut down the intestinal inflammatory reaction of IBD. While we wait for these hopes to become actual facts, a less ambitious but more realistic and practical approach to the treatment of IBD based on current knowledge of pathophysiology is delineated in the following section.

Table 6 Pathophysiology of inflammatory bowel disease – Hopes

Discover a single aetiological microorganism
Identify a specific and sensitive genetic marker
Characterize all predisposing environmental factors
Solve the 'immunology of IBD puzzle'
Define the critical inflammatory mediators
Develop specific antagonists, inhibitors, blockers

IMPLICATIONS FOR TREATMENT

Facing the challenge of treating a patient suffering with IBD, the physician is confronted by several questions (Table 7). Some of them are easy to answer, such as when to intervene. Obviously, the sooner, the better. If asked how to intervene, what would be the best approach? A broad one where all possible inflammatory pathways are comprehensively and effectively blocked, or a narrow one, where only selected cells or soluble mediators are turned off? Most of the drugs that are commonly used in Crohn's disease or ulcerative colitis have a wide spectrum of activities, and this is probably one of the main reasons for their efficacy. Sulphasalazine is still one of the drugs of choice, and its spectrum of activities is incredibly broad, including down-modulation of arachidonic acid metabolism, scavenger activity for ROM, inhibition of myeloperoxidase activity, down-regulation of lymphocyte proliferation, inhibition of cytokine production, antibody production and cytotoxicity, to name a few[109]. While it can be advantageous to inhibit multiple inflammatory and immune pathways, it is also unlikely that all of them are suppressed to the same degree and with the same efficiency, resulting in an incomplete or short-lived response. The same is probably true for corticosteroids and immunosuppressive agents. The most difficult question to answer, however, is where to intervene in IBD: at the triggering, regulatory, amplification, or 'final hit' stage? From the initial to the ultimate events involved in the inflammatory cascade, the number of options is presently too large for a systematic approach[110]. In an attempt to briefly discuss most treatment modalities, these will be classified as past, present and future (Table 8). This arbitrary classification is not necessarily based on time, but

Table 7 Pathophysiology of inflammatory bowel disease – Implications for treatment

When to intervene	Early or late?
How to intervene	Broad or narrow approach?
Where to intervene	Triggering, regulation, amplification, or 'final hit' stage?

Table 8 Pathophysiology of inflammatory bowel disease – Treatment modalities

Past	*Present*	*Future*
Aminosalicylates	Soluble mediator blockade:	Anti-adhesion molecules?
Corticosteroids	inhibitors	Toxin-IL2 fusion protein?
Immunosuppressives	antagonists	Oral tolerance induction?
(6-MP, MTX, CyA,	receptor blockade	Genetic manipulation?
FK506)[a]	(leukotrienes, etc.)	
Antibiotics	Immune mediator blockade	
	(IL-1, IL-6, IL-8, TNF, PAF,	
Diet	etc.)[b]	
	Anti-CD4 monoclonal	
	antibodies	
	Oxygen radical scavengers	

[a] 6-mercaptopurine, methotrexate, cyclosporin A
[b] Interleukin-1, interleukin-6, interleukin-8, tumour necrosis factor, platelet-activating factor

rather on current and anticipated progress in IBD pathophysiology.

Past

Aminosalicylates and corticosteroids have been the drugs of choice for decades, and they still represent the most effective and reliable medications for the majority of IBD patients. Modifications of the molecular structure of sulphasalazine, such as elimination of the sulphapyridine component allowing administration of the active aminosalicylic acid moiety (5-ASA), or of the metabolism of corticosteroids improving removal through liver passage (budenoside), have decreased some undesirable side-effects, but have not increased their overall efficacy.

Old and new immunosuppressive agents, such as azathioprine, 6-mercaptopurine, methotrexate, cyclosporin A and FK506, are still restricted to particularly resistant or difficult patients. In addition, their toxicity will continue to be a serious limiting factor for routine clinical use. Antibiotics still do not have a clear role in IBD, unless the time comes when specific aetiological organisms are isolated in Crohn's disease or ulcerative colitis.

The possible role of diet in the management of IBD should deserve additional consideration. In Crohn's disease the antigenic load of the faecal stream is receiving increasing attention in the triggering or exacerbation of this disease[111]. In ulcerative colitis administration of fish oil alters the composition of colonic lipids, prostaglandin and thromboxane synthesis, and appears to decrease mucosal inflammation[72,112]. Although it is unlikely that dietary management alone will ever be used as a single treatment for IBD, it may improve the effectiveness of associated drug therapy, such as lipoxygenase inhibitors.

Present

What the clinician may consider future forms of IBD treatment, are actually already available from a pathophysiological point of view. We now have a better-than-ever understanding of the mechanisms of inflammation, and it is simply a matter of finding a practical way of applying this knowledge to jump from the past into the present. Two major differences exist between 'past' and 'present' therapies: first, past treatments are aimed at many targets, whereas the present ones have only a single or a few objectives; second, past treatments are non-specific, whereas the present ones are highly specific. These dramatic changes have been induced by the isolation, characterization, and cloning of unique molecules that are mediators of inflammation and/or their respective receptors. Once characterized in their function and molecular structure, it becomes feasible to systematically develop drugs that inhibit or antagonize them, or block their receptor occupancy, thus preventing them from triggering or sustaining inflammation. There is encouraging evidence for the effectiveness of anti-inflammatory agents, in both human and animal models. Lipoxygenase inhibitors selectively decrease the level of LTB4 in rectal dialysates in ulcerative colitis patients without significantly affecting

PGE$_2$ concentrations[113]. Recombinant IL-1ra blocks the inflammatory activity of IL-1 in experimental animal models of colitis[114]. In addition to these, other inhibitors are being investigated, including those for IL-6, IL-8, TNF-α, PAF, etc.

Two other novel approaches are also already available. First, T cell-targeted immunotherapy is becoming a reality with the use of peptides, antibodies, and vaccines[115]. Two preliminary trials with anti-CD4 monoclonal antibodies have been reported, with exciting results, particularly when a chimeric ('humanized') antibody was administered to eliminate the risk of forming autoantibodies to the foreign protein[116,117]. Second, anti-oxidants can be used based on the assumption that ROM-mediated bowel injury is a final step of many different pathways of inflammation. Several inhibitors for distinct ROM are available, and clinical trials are under way[101].

Future

The increasingly fast pace of research, and the bold application of *in vitro* findings to experimental animals, and from these to humans, constantly blur the line between present and future. Therefore, it is anticipated that several innovative approaches will soon be transferred from the bench to the bedside.

Cell-to-cell communication is essential to the triggering and amplification of inflammation. A large number of adhesion molecules scattered on the surface of neutrophils, lymphocytes, macrophages and endothelial cells help in establishing essential physical contacts among these cells and allow functional interactions to take place[118]. There is strong evidence that blocking such adhesion molecules causes enough disruption of cellular interactions to prevent immune responses. This approach has been suggested as a potentially useful tool in the diagnosis and treatment of inflammatory diseases[119]. The expression of adhesion molecules is remarkably enhanced in IBD-involved intestine[120,121]. This justifies the use of antibodies directed against them as potentially useful, and there is preliminary evidence for their effectiveness in models of experimental colitis[122]. Another way of suppressing inflammation could be through the elimination of activated immune cells. Although probably less specific, there are preliminary data showing that this is practically feasible[123].

The ultimate form of treatment would be the one which is the most specific, totally safe, and completely effective. It is difficult to envision how to achieve this goal in practice, but it is theoretically within reach. For instance, this could be done by the induction of oral tolerance, if and when the antigen(s) targeted by the mucosal immune system are identified in Crohn's disease and ulcerative colitis. Mice develop experimental autoimmune encephalomyelitis (EAE), a multiple sclerosis-like disease, after becoming sensitized to myelin basic protein (MBP). Prevention of EAE can be obtained by desensitizing animals by feeding them with MBP, and inducing a switch-off of the immune system exclusively for this antigen (oral tolerance). This is now being tried in human subjects suffering from multiple sclerosis[124]. Perhaps one day a similar system will be adopted for IBD patients. The ultimate treatment of

IBD, of course, will be its total prevention, and in the future this may also be feasible once the genetic codes that control this disease are deciphered.

SUMMARY AND CONCLUSIONS

The reality of the state-of-the-art of IBD pathophysiology still does not allow a satisfactory understanding of all causes and mechanisms of IBD in order to establish a meaningful treatment programme. This apparently less than optimal situation is abundantly compensated by the impressive amount of knowledge accumulated in the past decade when compared to all information gathered since the time when Crohn's disease and ulcerative colitis were originally described. Based on this cumulative knowledge, the following statements realistically reflect the status of IBD at present and in the immediate future:

1. Single or multiple aetiological organisms may exist, but it may be very difficult to prove their direct implication.
2. Predisposing genetic and environmental factors are probably too numerous, complex, and variable to be completely characterized.
3. The 'immunology of IBD puzzle' will require a very long time and effort before it is solved, but it will generate fundamental information on the cells and the soluble factors responsible for bowel inflammation.
4. Ultimately, a relatively restricted number of inflammatory mediators will be identified, and combination therapy with multiple specific inhibitors is likely to become highly effective. This will result in dramatic clinical benefits for the patients, even if the specific aetiology of IBD remains unknown.

ACKNOWLEDGEMENTS

The author wishes to thank Kouhei Fukushima, John S. Klein, Toshihiro Matsuura, Scott A. Strong, Gail A. West, and Kenneth R. Youngman for technical and scientific assistance. The cooperation of the members of the Department of Colon and Rectal Surgery, and Department of Pathology, Cleveland Clinic Foundation, is also appreciated. This work was supported by the National Institutes of Health (NIDDK), Bethesda, Maryland, and The Crohn's and Colitis Foundation of America, New York.

References

1. Fiocchi C. Pathogenesis and clinical implications: where do we stand, where do we go? In: Goebell H, Ewe K, Malchow H, Koelbel C, editors. Inflammatory bowel disease: progress in basic research and clinical implications. Lancaster: Kluwer; 1991:237–54.
2. Halstensen TS, Mollnes TE, Garred P, Fausa O, Brandtzaeg P. Epithelial deposition of immunoglobulin G1 and activated complement (C3b and terminal complement complex) in ulcerative colitis. Gastroenterology. 1990;98:1264–71.
3. Deem RL, Shanahan F, Targan SR. Triggered human mucosal T cells release tumor necrosis factor-α and interferon-γ which kill human colonic epithelial cells. Clin Exp Immunol. 1991;83:79–84.

4. Grisham MB, Granger DN. Neutrophil-mediated mucosal injury. Role of reactive oxygen metabolites. Dig Dis Sci. 1988;33:6S-15S.

5. Strober W. Animal models of inflammatory bowel disease – an overview. Dig Dis Sci. 1985;30:3S-10S.

6. Hudson M, Piasecki C, Sankey EA, Sim R, Wakefield AJ, More LJ, Sawyerr AF, Dhillon AP, Pounder RE. A ferret model of acute multifocal gastrointestinal infarction. Gastroenterology. 1992;102:1591-6.

7. Allgayer H, Deschryver K, Stenson WF. Treatment with 16,16'-dimethyl prostaglandin E2 before and after induction of colitis with trinitrobenzenesulfonic acid in rats decreases inflammation. Gastroenterology. 1989;96:1290-300.

8. Fedorak RN, Empey LR, MacArthur C, Jewell LD. Misoprostol provides a colonic mucosal protective effect during acetic acid-induced colitis in rats. Gastroenterology. 1990;98:615-25.

9. Vilaseca J, Salas A, Guarner F, Rodriguez R, Malagelada J-R. Participation of thromboxane and other eicosanoid synthesis in the course of experimental inflammatory colitis. Gastroenterology. 1990;98:269-77.

10. Banerjee AK, Peters TJ. Experimental non-steroidal anti-inflammatory drug-induced enteropathy in the rat: similarities to inflammatory bowel disease and effect of thromboxane synthetase inhibitors. Gut. 1990;31:1358-64.

11. Caplan MS, Sun W-M, Hsueh W. Hypoxia causes ischemic bowel necrosis in rats: the role of platelet-activating factor (PAF-acether). Gastroenterology. 1990;99:979-86.

12. Wallace JL, Keenan CM. An orally active inhibitor of leukotriene synthesis accelerates healing in a rat model of colitis. Am J Physiol. 1990;258:G527-34.

13. Kitsukawa Y, Saito H, Suzuki Y, Kasanuki J, Tamura Y, Yoshida S. Effect of ingestion of eicosapentaenoic acid ethyl ester on carrageenan-induced colitis in guinea pigs. Gastroenterology. 1992;102:1859-66.

14. Fedorak RN, Empey LR, Walker K. Verapamil alters eicosanoid synthesis and accelerates healing during experimental colitis in rats. Gastroenterology. 1992;102:1229-35.

15. Rachmilewitz D, Karmeli F, Schwartz LW, Simon PL. Effect of aminophenols (5-ASA and 4-ASA) on colonic interleukin-1 generation. Gut. 1992;33:929-32.

16. Asako H, Kubes P, Wallace J, Wolf RE, Granger DN. Modulation of leukocyte adhesion in rat mesenteric venules by aspirin and salicylate. Gastroenterology. 1992;103:146-52.

17. Madara JL, Podolsky DK, King NW, Seghal PK, Moore R, Winter HS. Characterization of spontaneous colitis in cotton-top tamarins (*Saguinus oedipus*) and its response to sulfasalazine. Gastroenterology. 1985;88:13-19.

18. Targan SR, Landers CJ, King NW, Podolsky DJ, Shanahan F. Ulcerative colitis-linked antineutrophil cytoplasmic antibody in the cotton-top tamarin model of colitis. Gastroenterology. 1992;102:1493-8.

19. Sundberg JP, Elson CO. A heritable form of colitis in mice. Gastroenterology. 1992;102:A596.

20. Bucy RP. Cyclosporin A-induced autoimmune disease in mice is inhibited by the presence of normal T cells. FASEB J. 1991;5:A648.

21. Hammer RD, Maika SD, Richardson JA, Tang J-P, Taurog JD. Spontaneous inflammatory disease in transgenic rats expressing HLA-B27 and human b2m: an animal model of HLA-B27-associated human disorders. Cell. 1990;63:1099-112.

22. Farmer RG, Michener WM. Association of inflammatory bowel disease in families. Front Gastrointest Res. 1986;11:17-26.

23. Orholm M, Munkholm P, Langholz E, Nielsen OH, Sorensen TIA, Binder V. Familial occurence of inflammatory bowel disease. N Engl J Med. 1991;324:84-8.

24. Ekbom A, Helmick C, Zack M, Adami H-O. The epidemiology of inflammatory bowel disease: a large, population-based study in Sweden. Gastroenterology. 1991;100:350-8.

25. Fiocchi C, Roche JK, Michener WM. High prevalence of antibodies to intestinal epithelial antigens in patients with inflammatory bowel disease and their relatives. Ann Intern Med. 1989;110:786-94.

26. Hollander D. Crohn's disease – a permeability disorder of the tight junction? Gut. 1988;29:1621-4.

27. Asakura H, Tsuchiya M, Aiso S, Watanabe M, Kokayashi K, Hibi T, Ando K, Takata H, Sekiguchi S. Association of the human lymphocyte-DR2 antigen with japanese ulcerative colitis. Gastroenterology. 1982;82:413-18.

28. Rotter JI. Immunogenetic susceptibilities in inflammatory bowel disease. Can J Gastroenterol.

1990;4:261–6.
29. Randolph LM, Toyoda H, McElree CK, Shanahan F, Targan SR, Rotter JI. Lack of an association between polymorphisms of the T-cell receptor α-chain and ulcerative colitis. Gastroenterology. 1989;97:1115–20.
30. Rotter JI, Wang S-J, Yang H, McElree C, Pressman S, Redford A, Magalong D, Tyan D, Shanahan F, Targan S, Toyoda H. Genetic heterogeneity between ulcerative colitis (UC) and Crohn's disease (CD) identified by molecular HLA class II association. Gastroenterology. 1992;102:A688.
31. Shanahan F, Duerr RH, Rotter JI, Yang H, Sutherland LR, McElree C, Landers CJ, Targan SR. Neutrophil autoantibodies in ulcerative colitis: familial aggregation and genetic heterogeneity. Gastroenterology. 1992;103:456–61.
32. MacDermott RP, Stenson WF. Alterations of the immune system in ulcerative colitis and Crohn's disease. Adv Immunol. 1988;42:285–328.
33. Fox CC, Lazenby AJ, Moore WC, Yardley JH, Bayless TM, Lichtenstein LM. Enhancement of human intestinal mast cell mediator release in active ulcerative colitis. Gastroenterology. 1990;99:119–24.
34. Paliard X, West SG, Lafferty JA, Clements JC, Kappler JW, Marrack P, Kotzin BL. Evidence for the effects of a superantigen in rheumatoid arthritis. Science. 1991;253:325–9.
35. Davies TF, Martin A, Concepcion ES, Graves P, Cohen L, Ben-Num A. Evidence of limited variability of antigen receptors on intrathyroidal T cells in autoimmune thyroid disease. N Engl J Med. 1991;325:238–44.
36. Posnett DN, Schmelkin I, Burton DA, August A, McGrath H, Mayer LF. T cell antigen receptor V gene usage. Increases in Vb8+ T cells in Crohn's disease. J Clin Invest. 1990;85:1770–6.
37. Duchmann R, Strober W, Fiocchi C, James SP. TCR Vβ2 gene expression is selective in control but not in IBD lamina propria lymphocytes. Gastroenterology. 1992;102:A617.
38. Landau SB, Balk SP, Yang L, Burke SK, Blumberg RS. T-cell receptor (TCR) δ variable region utilization is altered in ulcerative colitis. Gastroenterology. 1992;102:A650.
39. Shorter RG, McGill DB, Bahn RC. Cytotoxicity of mononuclear cells for autologous colonic epithelial cells in colonic diseases. Gastroenterology. 1984;86:13–22.
40. Mayer L, Shlien R. Evidence for function of Ia molecules on gut epithelial cells in man. J Exp Med. 1987;166:1471–83.
41. Mayer L, Eisenhardt D, Salomon P, Bauer W, Plous R, Piccinini L. Expression of class II molecules on intestinal epithelial cells in humans. Differences between normal and inflammatory bowel disease. Gastroenterology. 1991;100:3–12.
42. Mayer L, Eisenhardt D. Lack of induction of suppressor T cells by intestinal epithelial cells from patients with inflammatory bowel disease. J Clin Invest. 1990;86:1255–60.
43. Ferraris L, Klein J, Fiocchi C, Karmeli F, Eliakim R, Rachmilewitz D. Both epithelial and lamina propria mononuclear cells contribute to the enhanced platelet activating factor generation in inflammatory bowel disease. Gastroenterology. 1992;102:A622.
44. Graham MF, Drucker DEM, Diegelmann RF, Elson CO. Collagen synthesis by human intestinal smooth muscle cells in culture. Gastroenterology. 1987;92:400–5.
45. Stallmach A, Schuppan D, Riese HH, Matthes H, Rieken EO. Increased collagen type III synthesis by fibroblasts isolated from strictures of patients with Crohn's disease. Gastroenterology. 1992;102:1920–9.
46. Lee EY, Stenson WF, DeSchryver-Kecskemeti K. Thickening of muscularis mucosae in Crohn's disease. Mod Pathol. 1991;4:87–90.
47. Strong SA, West GA, Klein JS, Milsom JW, Fiocchi C. Inflammatory cytokines stimulate proliferation of intestinal mucosa mesenchymal cells. Gastroenterology. 1992;102:A701.
48. Fiocchi C. Cytokines. In: MacDermott RP, Stenson W, editors. Inflammatory bowel disease. New York: Elsevier; 1992:137–62.
49. Rubin LA, Nelson DL. The soluble interleukin-2 receptor: biology, function, and clinical application. Ann Intern Med. 1990;113:619–27.
50. Mueller C, Knoflach P, Zielinski CC. T-cell activation in Crohn's disease. Increased levels of soluble interleukin-2 receptor in serum and supernatants of stimulated peripheral blood mononuclear cells. Gastroenterology. 1990;98:639–46.
51. Matsuura T, West GA, Klein JS, Ferraris L, Fiocchi C. Soluble interleukin 2, CD8 and CD4 receptors in inflammatory bowel disease. A comparative study of peripheral blood

and intestinal mucosal levels. Gastroenterology. 1992;102:2006–14.

52. Murch SH, Lamkin VA, Savage MO, Walker-Smith JA, MacDonald TT. Serum concentrations of tumour necrosis factor a in childhood chronic inflammatory bowel disease. Gut. 1991;32:913–17.

53. Mahida YR, Ceska M, Effenberger F, Kurlak L, Lindley I, Hawkey CJ. Enhanced synthesis of neutrophil-activating peptide-I/interleukin-8 in active ulcerative colitis. Clin Sci. 1992;82:273–5.

54. Mahida YR, Kurlak L, Gallagher A, Hawkey CJ. High circulating levels of interleukin 6 in active Crohn's disease but not ulcerative colitis. Gut. 1991;32:1531–4.

55. Gross V, Andus T, Caesar I, Roth M, Scholmerich J. Evidence for continuous stimulation of interleukin-6 production in Crohn's disease. Gastroenterology. 1992;102:514–19.

56. Mosmann TR, Coffman RL. Th1 and Th2 cells: different patterns of lymphokine secretion lead to different functional properties. Ann Rev Immunol. 1989;7:145–73.

57. Mosmann TR, Moore KW. The role of IL-10 in crossregulation of Th1 and Th2 responses. Immunol Today. 1991;12:A49–53.

58. Heinzel FP, Sadick MD, Holoday BJ, Coffman RL LR. Reciprocal expression of interferon gamma or interleukin 4 during the resolution or progression of murine leishmaniasis: evidence for expansion of distinct helper T cell subsets. J Exp Med. 1989;169:59–72.

59. Wierenga EA, Snoek M, Jansen HM, Bos JD, Lier RAWV, Kapsenberg ML. Human atopen-specific types 1 and 2 T helper cell clones. J Immunol. 1991;147:2942–9.

60. Parronchi P, Macchia D, Piccinini M-P, Biswas P, Simonelli C, Maggi E, Ricci M, Ansari AA, Romagnani S. Allergen- and bacterial antigen-specific T-cell clones established from atopic donors show a different profile of cytokine production. Proc Natl Acad Sci USA. 1991;88:4538–42.

61. Salgame P, Abrams JS, Clayberger C, Goldstein H, Convit J, Modlin RL, Bloom BR. Differing lymphokine profiles of functional subsets of human CD4 and CD8 T cell clones. Science. 1991;254:279–82.

62. Akira S, Hirano T, Taga T, Kishimoto T. Biology of multifunctional cytokines: IL6 and related molecules (IL1 and TNF). FASEB J. 1990;4:2860–7.

63. Fernandex-Botran R. Soluble cytokine receptors: their role in immunoregulation. FASEB J. 1991;5:2567–74.

64. Dinarello CA, Thompson RC. Blocking IL-1: interleukin 1 receptor antagonist in vivo and in vitro. Immunol Today. 1991;12:404–10.

65. Cominelli F, Nast CC, Clark BD, Schindler R, Llerena R, Eysselein VE, Thompson RC, Dinarello CA. Interleukin 1 (IL-1) gene expression, synthesis, and effect of specific IL-1 receptor blockade in rabbit immune complex colitis. J Clin Invest. 1990;86:972–80.

66. Cominelli F, Fiocchi C, Eisenberg SP, Bortolami M. Imbalance of IL-1 and IL-1 receptor antagonist in the intestinal mucosa of Crohn's disease and ulcerative colitis patients. Gastroenterology. 1992;102:A609.

67. Sharon P, Ligumsky M, Rachmilewitz D, Zor U. Role of prostaglandins in ulcerative colitis, enhanced production during active disease and inhibition by sulfasalazine. Gastroenterology. 1978;75:638–40.

68. Rampton DS, Sladen GE. Prostaglandin synthesis inhibitors in ulcerative colitis: flurbiprofen compared with conventional treatment. Prostaglandins. 1981;21:417–25.

69. Sharon P, Stenson WF. Enhanced synthesis of leukotriene B4 by colonic mucosa in inflammatory bowel disease. Gastroenterology. 1984;86:453–60.

70. Eliakim R, Karmeli F, Razin E, Rachmilewitz D. Role of platelet-activating factor in ulcerative colitis. Gastroenterology. 1988;95:1167–72.

71. Stenson WF. Role of eicosanoids as mediators of inflammation in inflammatory bowel disease. Scand J Gastroenterol. 1990;25 (suppl 172):13–18.

72. Stenson WF, Cort D, Rodgers J, Bukaroff R, DeSchryver-Kecskemeti K, Gramlich TL, Beeken W. Dietary supplementation with fish oil in ulcerative colitis. Ann Intern Med. 1992;116:609–14.

73. Hawthorne AB, Daneshmend TK, Hawkey CJ, Belluzzi A, Everitt SJ, Holmes GKT, Malkinson C, Shaheen MZ, Willars JE. Treatment of ulcerative colitis with fish oil supplementation: a prospective 12 month randomised controlled trial. Gut. 1992;33:922–28.

74. O'Dorisio MS, Panerai A, editors. Neuropeptides and immunopeptides: messengers in a neuroimmune axis. New York: Ann NY Acad Sci. 1990; vol 594.

75. Bienenstock J, Perdue M, Stanisz A, Stead R. Neurohormonal regulation of gastrointestinal immunity. Gastroenterology. 1987;93:1431–4.
76. Eysselein VE, Reinshagen M, Cominelli F, Sternini C, Davis W, Patel A, Nast CC, Bernstein D, Anderson K, Khan H, Snape WJ. Calcitonin gene-related peptide and substance P decrease in the rabbit colon during colitis. Gastroenterology. 1991;101:1211–19.
77. Bishop AE, Polak JM, Bryant MG, Bloom SR, Hamilton S. Abnormalities of vasoactive intestinal polypeptide-containing nerves in Crohn's disease. Gastroenterology. 1980;79:853–60.
78. Kubota Y, Petras RE, Ottaway CA, Tubbs RR, Farmer RG, Fiocchi C. Colonic vasoactive intestinal peptide nerves in inflammatory bowel disease. A digitized morphometric immunohistochemical study. Gastroenterology. 1992;102:1242–51.
79. Mazumdar S, Das KM. Immunohistochemical localization of vasoactive intestinal peptide and substance P in the colon from normal subjects and patients with inflammatory bowel disease. Am J Gastroenterol. 1992;87:176–81.
80. Watanabe T, Kubota Y, Sawada T, Muto T. Distribution and quantification of somatostatin in inflammatory disease. Dis Colon Rectum. 1992;35:488–94.
81. Manyth PW, Catton MD, Boehmer CG, Welton ML, Passaro EP, Maggio JE, Vigna SR. Receptors for sensory neuropeptides in human inflammatory diseases: implications for the effector role of sensory neurons. Peptides. 1989;10:627–45.
82. Chiodini RJ, Kruiningen HJV, Thayer WR, Merkal RS, Coutu JA. Possible role of mycobacteria in inflammatory bowel disease. I. An unclassified *Mycobacterium* species isolated from patients with Crohn's disease. Dig Dis Sci. 1984;29:1073–9.
83. Chiodini RJ. Crohn's disease and the mycobacterioses: a review and comparison of two disease entities. Clin Microbiol Rev. 1989;2:90–117.
84. Butcher PD, McFadden JJ, Hermon-Taylor J. Investigation of mycobacteria in Crohn's disease tissue by Southern blotting and DNA hybridization with cloned mycobacterial genomic DNA probes from a Crohn's disease isolated mycobacteria. Gut. 1988;29:1222–8.
85. Sanderson JD, Moss MT, Tizard MLV, Hermon-Taylor J. *Mycobacterium paratuberculosis* DNA in Crohn's disease tissue. Gut. 1992;33:890–6.
86. Moss M, Sanderson J, Tizard M, Hermon-Taylor J, El-Zaatari F, Markesich D, Graham D. *Mycobacterium paratuberculosis* (*M. para*) in long term cultures of Crohn's disease tissue revealed by PCR amplification of IS900. Gastroenterology. 1991;100:A232.
87. Rosenberg WMC, Bell JI, Jewell DP. *Mycobacterium paratuberculosis* DNA cannot be detected in Crohn's disease tissues. Gastroenterology. 1991;100:A611.
88. Relman DA, Schmidt TM, MacDermott RP, Falkow S. Identification of the uncultured bacillus of Whipple's disease. N Engl J Med. 1992;327:293–301.
89. Kohn A, Prantera C, Mangiarotti R, Luzi C, Andreoli A. Antimycobacterial therapy and Crohn's disease: a randomized placebo controlled trial. Gastroenterology. 1992;102:A647.
90. Sartor RB, Cromartie WJ, Powell DW, Schwab JH. Granulomatous enterocolitis induced in rats by purified bacterial cell wall fragments. Gastroenterology. 1985;89:587–95.
91. Rutgeerts P, Goboes K, Peeters M, Hiele M, Penninckx F, Aerts R, Kerremans R, Vantrappen G. Effect of faecal stream diversion on recurrence of Crohn's disease in the neoterminal ileum. Lancet. 1991;2:771–4.
92. Wakefield AJ, Dhillon AP, Rowles PM, Sawyerr AM, Pittilo RM, Lewis AAM, Pounder RE. Pathogenesis of Crohn's disease: multifocal gastrointestinal infarction. Lancet. 1989;2:1057–62.
93. Wakefield AJ, Sankey EA, Dhillon AP, Sawyerr AM, L.More, Sim R, Pittilo RM, Rowles PM, Hudson M, Lewis AAM, Pounder RE. Granulomatous vasculitis in Crohn's disease. Gastroenterology. 1991;100:1279–87.
94. Wakefield AJ, Sawyerr AM, Hudson M, Dhillon AP, Pounder RE. Smoking, the oral contraceptive pill, and Crohn's disease. Dig Dis Sci. 1991;36:1147–50.
95. Lloyd AR, Hoppenheim JJ. Poly's lament: the neglected role of the polymorphonuclear neutrophil in the afferent limb of the immune response. Immunol Today. 1992;13:169–72.
96. Grisham MB, Volkmer C, Tso P, Yamada T. Metabolism of trinitrobenzene sulfonic acid by the rat colon produces reactive oxygen species. Gastroenterology. 1991;101:540–7.
97. Baker SS, Campbell CL. Rat enterocyte injury by oxygen-dependent processes. Gastroenterology. 1991;101:716–20.
98. Ma TY, Hollander D, Freeman D, Nguyen T, Krugliak P. Oxygen free radical injury of IEC-18 small intestinal epithelial cell monolayers. Gastroenterology. 1991;100:1533–43.

99. Keshavarzian A, Sedghi S, Kanofsky J, List T, Robinson C, Ibrahim C, Winship D. Excessive production of reactive oxygen metabolites in inflamed colon: analysis by chemiluminescence probe. Gastroenterology. 1992;103:177–85.

100. Simmonds NJ, Allen RE, Stevens TRJ, Niall R, Someren MV, Blake DR, Rampton DS. Chemiluminescence assay of mucosal reactive oxygen metabolites in inflammatory bowel disease. Gastroenterology. 1992;103:186–96.

101. Emerit J, Pelletier S, Tosoni-Verlignue D, Mollet M. Phase II trial of copper zinc superoxide dismutase (CuZnSOD) in treatment of Crohn's disease. Free Radical Biol Med. 1989;7:145–9.

102. Kolb H, Kolb-Bachofen V. Nitric oxide: a pathogenic factor in autoimmunity. Immunol Today. 1992;13:157–60.

103. Kubes P, Suzuki M, Granger DN. Nitric oxide – an endogenous modulator of leukocyte adhesion. Proc Natl Acad Sci USA. 1991;88:4651–5.

104. Snape WJ, Collins SM. Effects of immune cells and inflammation on smooth muscle and enteric nerves. Boca Raton: CRC Press; 1991.

105. Vermillion DE, Ernst PB, Collins SM. T-lymphocyte modulation of intestinal muscle function in the *Trichinella*-infected rat. Gastroenterology. 1991;101:31–8.

106. Adenis A, Colombel J-F, Lecouffe P, Wallaert B, Hecquet B, Marchandise X, Cortot A. Increased pulmonary and intestinal permeability in Crohn's disease. Gut. 1992;33:678–82.

107. Teahon K, Smethurst P, Levi AJ, Menzies IS, Bjarnason I. Intestinal permeability in patients with Crohn's disease and their first degree relatives. Gut. 1992;33:320–3.

108. Ruttenberg D, Young GO, Wright JP, Isaacs S. PEG-400 excretion in patients with Crohn's disease, their first-degree relatives, and healthy volunteers. Dig Dis Sci. 1992;37:705–8.

109. Gaginella TS, Walsh RE. Sulfasalazine. Multiplicity of action. Dig Dis Sci. 1992;37:801–12.

110. Hinterleitner TA, Powell DW. Immune system control of intestinal ion transport. Proc Soc Exp Biol Med. 1991;197:249–60.

111. Teahon K, Smethurst P, Pearson M, Levi AJ, Bjarnason I. The effect of elemental diet on intestinal permeability and inflammation in Crohn's disease. Gastroenterology. 1991;101:84–9.

112. Hillier K, Jewell R, Dorrell L, Smith CL. Incorporation of fatty acid from fish oil and olive oil into colonic mucosal lipids and effects upon eicosanoid synthesis in inflammatory bowel disease. Gut. 1991;32:1151–5.

113. Laursen LS, Naesdal J, Bukhave K, Lauritsen K, Rask-Madsen J. Selective 5-lipoxygenase inhibition in ulcerative colitis. Lancet. 1990;335:683–5.

114. Cominelli F, Nast CC, Duchini A, Lee M. Recombinant interleukin-1 receptor antagonist blocks the proinflammatory activity of endogenous interleukin-1 in rabbit immune colitis. Gastroenterology. 1992;103:65–71.

115. Feldmann M, June CH, McMichael A, Maini R, Simpson E, Woody JN. T-cell-targeted immunotherapy. Immunol Today. 1992;13:84–5.

116. Emmrich J, Seyfarth M, Fleig WE, Emmrich F. Treatment of inflammatory bowel disease with anti-CD4 monoclonal antibody. Lancet. 1991;1:570–1.

117. Deusch K, Reiter C, Mauthe B, Riethmuller G, Classen M. Chimeric monoclonal anti-CD4 antibody therapy proves effective for treating inflammatory bowel disease. Gastroenterology. 1992;102:A615.

118. Springer TA. Adhesion receptors of the immune system. Nature. 1990;346:425–34.

119. Adhesion molecules in diagnosis and treatment of inflammatory diseases. Lancet. 1990;336:1351–2.

120. Malizia G, Calabrese A, Cottone M, Raimondo M, Trejdosiewicz LK, Smart CJ, Oliva L, Pagliaro L. Expression of leukocyte adhesion molecules by mucosal mononuclear phagocytes in inflammatory bowel disease. Gastroenterology. 1991;100:150–9.

121. Koizumi M, King N, Lobb R, Benjamin C, Podolsky DK. Expression of vascular adhesion molecules in inflammatory bowel disease. Gastroenterology. 1992;102:A647.

122. Wallace JL, Higa A, McKnight GW, MacIntyre DE. Prevention and reversal of experimental colitis with a monoclonal antibody that inhibits leukocyte adherence. Gastroenterology. 1992;102:A710.

123. Bousvaros A, Stevens AC, Strom TB, Murphy JR, LaMont JT. Diphtheria toxin-interleukin-2 fusion protein (DAB-389 IL2) inhibits activated human blood and intestinal lymphocytes. Gastroenterology. 1992;102:A599.

124. Marx J. Testing of autoimmune therapy begins. Science. 1991;252:27–8.

Section VI
Implications of pathophysiology for diagnosis

26
Serological and mucosal markers of ulcerative colitis and Crohn's disease: implications of pathophysiology for diagnosis

S. R. TARGAN and L. K. MURPHY

INTRODUCTION

Biomedical research investigations have identified serological, genetic and mucosal markers that define distinct subgroups among the inflammatory bowel diseases. Systemic lupus erythematosus, primary sclerosing cholangitis and chronic active hepatitis are examples of chronic inflammatory disorders that demonstrate the clinical importance of such markers[1,2]. Recent discoveries regarding the interaction between disease-related autoantibodies and molecular and cell biology have generated a new perspective from which to consider the clinical implications of basic science findings[3]. In inflammatory bowel disease, antineutrophil cytoplasmic autoantibodies (ANCA) and MHC class II genes have been found in probands. ANCA has been also found in clinically unaffected family members of probands[4]. These data suggest a primarily determined, genetically distinct subgroup of disease and disease susceptibility. Expanded research has yielded specific markers at the mucosal level, for Crohn's disease[5]. A better definition of these markers and their relevance in linkage and natural history studies will be helpful in defining disease susceptibility.

EVIDENCE FOR DISEASE HETEROGENEITY

Evidence to suggest genetic predisposing factors in ulcerative colitis is based upon the percentage of concordance in monozygotic twins and dizygotic twins. In Crohn's disease, 67% of monozygotic twins are concordant, while only 8% of dizygotic twins are concordant[6]. Among twins with ulcerative colitis, 20% of monozygotic twins are concordant while few dizygotic twins were concordant[6]. The concordance among monozygotic twins, then, is greater than among dizygotic. There was no occurrence of mixed pairs. These data demonstrate that the well-recognized familial aggregation is genetic and complex.

Given the evidence of genetic predisposition, studies were begun in an attempt to demonstrate linkage. Linkage refers to the existence of two loci located so close together on chromosomes that they are inherited as a unit[6]. Recent genetic investigations have proposed an HLA linkage to the presence of IBD in families with multiple affected members[6]. The evidence points to forms of IBD that can be demonstrated to be linked to HLA, and forms of IBD in which no linkage can be determined. That 20 years of prior research have not yielded consistent findings regarding linkage is probably due to the likelihood that these diseases are genetically heterogeneous. A specific definition of disease subgroups will clarify the level of heterogeneity in these diseases and provide more homogeneous groups of patients to study the different immunopathogenic mechanisms related to each.

Studies of genetic associations using HLA class II genes delineated at the molecular level were performed using restriction fragment length polymorphism (RFLP) analysis and polymerase chain reaction (PCR)[7]. Forty-four per cent of subjects with ulcerative colitis expressed HLA-DR2 as compared to 21% of control subjects, and 22% of subjects with Crohn's disease. There was a negative association between ulcerative colitis and DR4 and DRw6, and no associations were observed between any DQ alleles and ulcerative colitis. Stratifying on DQ alleles reinforced the effect of DR2, arguing for a primary DR2 association with ulcerative colitis. In contrast, patients with Crohn's disease were found to have an increased frequency of both DR1, and DQw5. Stratifying independently on DR1 and DQw5 indicated that neither allele was independently associated with Crohn's disease alone, suggesting that the association was with the haplotype DR1-DQw5 rather than either of the individual alleles. These findings confirm the involvement of HLA-linked genes in the inflammatory bowel diseases, and illustrate that the genetic susceptibility provided by the HLA class II genes is not the same for ulcerative colitis as it is for Crohn's disease, thereby demonstrating heterogeneity of the genetic susceptibility to inflammatory bowel disease.

AUTOANTIBODIES

Antineutrophil cytoplasmic autoantibodies have been used to differentiate ulcerative colitis from Crohn's disease, and to separate ulcerative colitis into two subgroups. The antigen(s) to which ulcerative colitis-related ANCA react has yet to be identified. The ANCA associated with ulcerative colitisis found using the combination of a positive enzyme-linked immunosorbent assay with a perinuclear pattern on immunofluorescent staining. This method has proved to be a very specific and moderately sensitive test for the diagnosis of ulcerative colitis[8,9].

We were able to ascertain the frequency of ANCA positivity in unaffected relatives of patients with ulcerative colitis. The data were gathered from two centres: UCLA/Cedars–Sinai and Calgary, Canada. About 15–20% unaffected relatives were ANCA[+]. More importantly, when the family members of probands were divided into those that were ANCA[+] or those that were ANCA[−], a similar distribution was found. That is, ANCA[+] probands have relatives that were ANCA[+], and ANCA[−] probands had relatives that were ANCA[−] [4].

To provide further evidence of genetic heterogeneity, we investigated the association of ANCA positivity in ulcerative colitis to the DR2 association[10]. These findings led us to the hypothesis that the heterogeneity in ulcerative colitis may be further defined by this DR2 locus compared with controls. We found that the DR2 positivity within ulcerative colitis was only associated with ulcerative colitis patients that were ANCA[+], whereas the ulcerative colitis patients that were ANCA[−] had no increased association of the DR2 locus. These findings have allowed us to stratify further the population into ANCA[+]/DR2[+] and ANCA[−]/DR2[−] populations.

MUCOSAL MARKERS

Using ANCA as a precedent, Dr Jonathan Braun tested the hypothesis that additional B cell subsets exist which may define pathogenic mechanisms within ulcerative colitis. Dr Braun searched for such B cells within the mucosa of patients with ulcerative colitis and Crohn's disease. In a collaborative endoscopic project, 38 biopsy specimens from 20 individuals (six normal, seven ulcerative colitis, seven Crohn's disease) were analysed, using V gene specific oligonucleotides and polymerase chain reaction (PCR) technology. Several V genes were analysed including those clones generally constant (VH 4, 5, 6) and those developmentally regulated (VHe and Vκ134 and VκIIIa). Dr Braun found an over-abundance of VκIIIa and Vκ134 B cells in active Crohn's disease lesions (six of seven samples), but *not* in uninvolved Crohn's disease mucosa. Neither was there such an over-abundance in involved or uninvolved mucosa of patients with ulcerative colitis, nor in normals, supporting that this is a disease-specific phenomenon. These findings were not the result of migration of B cells from the blood, as peripheral blood B cells showed no increased expression[5]. Thus, as ANCA has been identified as a marker of ulcerative colitis, B cell markers within the mucosa of Crohn's disease lesions may well 'mark' the Crohn's disease-associated inflammatory response. These data, therefore, establish differing patterns of markers in Crohn's disease and ulcerative colitis (Table 1).

HETEROGENEOUS CLINICAL PROFILE

The notion that heterogeneous genetic and immunological markers reflect clinical and treatment subsets of patients is provocative and exciting. The likely response to medical therapy may be predicted within a subset of

Table 1 Markers associated with inflammatory bowel disease

	Marker type		
Disease	MHC	Autoantibody	Mucosal
Ulcerative colitis	DR2	ANCA$^+$	VκIIIa$^-$, Vκ134$^-$
Crohn's disease	DR1 DQw5	ANCA$^-$	VκIIIa$^+$, Vκ134$^+$

patients, as well as therapeutic compounds selected for treatment, and developed specifically to interact at certain parts of the inflammatory process. In the future the correlation of clinical subsets of inflammatory bowel disease patients with the distinct serological and molecular, peripheral and mucosal markers would allow selection of specific therapies, designed to modulate disease expression at the level of the earliest identified, preclinical lesion. Eventually these methods may be applied to inhibit expression of disease in relatives of patients with the highest likelihood of developing disease.

References

1. Smolen JS, Klippel JH, Penner E, Reichlin M, Steinberg AD, Chused TM, Scherak O, Graninger W, Hartter E, Zielinski CC, Wolf A, Davey RJ, Mann DL, Mayr WR. HLA-DR antigens in systemic lupus erythematosus: association with specificity of autoantibody responses to nuclear antigens. Ann Rheum Dis. 1987;46:457–62.
2. Farrant JM, Doherty DG, Donaldson PT, Vaughan RW, Hayllar KM, Welsh KI, Eddeleston ALWF, Williams R. Immunogenetic disease-severity markers in primary slcerosing cholangitis. Gastroenterology. 1992;102(4):A806.
3. Tan EM. Interactions between autoimmunity and molecular and cell biology. Bridges between clinical and basic sciences. J Clin Invest. 1989;84:1–6.
4. Shanahan F, Duerr RH, Rotter JI, Yang H, Sutherland LR, McElree C, Landers CJ, Targan SR. Neutrophil autoantibodies in ulcerative colitis: Familial aggregation and genetic heterogeneity. Gastroenterology. 1992;103(2):456–61.
5. Valles Y, Berberian LS, Targan SR, Braun J. Marker B cell clones in ulcerative colitis and Crohn's disease. Gastroenterology. 1992;102(4):A708.
6. Shohat T, Vadheim CM, Rotter JI. Genetics. In: Gitnick G, editor. Inflammatory bowel disease. New York: Igaku-Shoin; 1991:53–86.
7. Toyoda H, Wang S-J, Yang H-Y, Redford A, Magalong D, Tyan D, McElree CK, Pressman SR, Shanahan F, Targan SR, Rotter JI. Distinct associations of HLA class II genes with inflammatory bowel disease. Gastroenterology. 1992: in press.
8. Saxon A, Shanahan F, Landers C, Ganz T, Targan S: A subset of anti-neutrophil cytoplasmic antibodies associated with inflammatory bowel disease. J Allergy Clin Immunol. 1990;86(2):22022–10.
9. Duerr RH, Targan SR, Landers CJ, Sutherland LR, Shanahan F. Neutrophil autoantibodies in ulcerative colitis: comparison with other colitides and diarrheal disorders. Gastroenterology. 1991;100(6):1590–6.
10. Yang H, Rotter JI, Toyoda H, Wang S-J, McElree C, Landers CL, Shanahan F, Targan SR. Ulcerative colitis: a genetic heterogeneous group defined with genetic (DR2) and subclinical markers (ANCA). Gastroenterology. 1992;102(4):A716.

27

Cytokines in inflammatory bowel disease

Y. R. MAHIDA

Active inflammatory bowel disease (IBD) is characterized by infiltration of the intestinal mucosa with lymphocytes, macrophages and neutrophils. Granulomata are a characteristic feature of Crohn's disease, whereas neutrophils are prominent in ulcerative colitis, especially in the form of crypt abscesses. It is likely that cytokines play an important role in the migration of cells into the mucosa from the circulation (by acting as chemoattractants and by inducing expression of adhesion molecules on endothelial cells) and also the subsequent mediation of inflammatory and immunological responses. During relapse there is an acute-phase response as demonstrated by the rise in circulating levels of C-reactive protein, α_1 and glycoprotein, and fall in albumin levels. These parameters are commonly used to assess severity of disease as well as monitoring response to treatment, and have been shown to be secreted by hepatocytes in response to stimulation by cytokines such as interleukin 1 (IL-1), interleukin 6 (IL-6) and tumour necrosis factor alpha (TNF-α). Recent studies have examined the role of cytokines or their receptors in the assessment of intestinal inflammation in ulcerative colitis and Crohn's disease. The acute-phase response generally does not distinguish ulcerative colitis from Crohn's disease, but recent studies suggest that circulating cytokine levels may allow such distinctions to be made.

STUDIES ON IL-1

IL-1 is present in two forms, IL-1α and IL-1β, with the latter being the predominant secreted form which can be produced by a variety of cells, but mainly monocytes and macrophages. It mediates a wide range of effects which may play an important role in the pathogenesis of IBD. These activities include T lymphocyte activation, enhanced antibody synthesis and fibroblast proliferation. It also induces the expression of adhesion molecules on the surface of endothelial cells to facilitate migration of cells into the mucosa.

Mononuclear cells (lymphocytes and macrophages) isolated from the mucosa with active inflammatory bowel disease, when cultured *in vitro*, have been shown to produce significantly greater amounts of IL-1β compared to cells from the normal mucosa[1]. When the cells from normal mucosa were cultured in the presence of lipopolysaccharide (LPS; which is a very potent inducer of IL-1 synthesis by peripheral blood monocytes), there was no increase in the amount of IL-1β produced. However, mononuclear cells from inflammatory bowel disease musoca produced even more IL-1β when cultured in the presence of LPS. This suggests that the normal intestinal macrophages are down-regulated with respect to their capacity to produce IL-1, and that the increased mucosal production of the cytokine in IBD is due to recently recruited monocytes (from the circulation).

Studies on tissue homogenates confirmed that higher amounts of IL-1β are produced *in vivo* in the mucosa with active IBD[2,3]. The drug 5-aminosalicylic acid, at levels normally found in the colonic lumen of patients taking the compound, significantly inhibited production of IL-1β in organ cultures of inflamed colonic biopsies[2]. Peripheral blood mononuclear cells of patients with active Crohn's disease and ulcerative colitis have also been shown to produce higher amounts of IL-1 (compared to controls) when cultured *in vitro*, in the presence or absence of LPS[4]. Mucosal production of IL-1 is also enhanced in rabbit immune-complex colitis[5].

Although IL-1 may be responsible for some of the systemic effects such as pyrexia and the induction of an acute-phase response in IBD, there are no reported studies of the peptide in circulation, probably because it is difficult to measure it in plasma or serum.

TUMOUR NECROSIS FACTOR β

TNF-α shares many biological activities with IL-1. Animal studies suggest that it may also be important in the mediation of cachexia and tissue damage, and hence has been of interest in IBD. High serum levels of this cytokine have been reported in children with active colonic Crohn's disease and ulcerative colitis[6]. It has also been reported to be increased in stools of children with active IBD[7]. However, studies in adults have shown that isolated peripheral blood and intestinal mononuclear cells from patients with active inflammatory bowel disease produce similar amounts of TNF-α compared to normal controls[4,8,9]. Elevated plasma and serum levels are also only detected in occasional (adult) patients with active Crohn's disease (unpublished observations).

INTERLEUKIN 2 (IL-2) AND INTERLEUKIN 2 RECEPTOR (IL-2r)

IL-2 is a growth factor for T cells which is produced by lymphocytes upon stimulation with antigen or mitogen. Circulating levels of IL-2 have been detected in patients with active Crohn's disease, but in this study the levels did not correlate with the clinical index of disease activity[10].

High-affinity IL-2 receptors are made up of two polypeptides of molecular weight 55 000 (p55) and 75 000 (p75), which on their own have lower affinity. These peptides can be released from the cell surface and detected in circulation.

Activated T cells and macrophages bearing IL-2r are present in the mucosa with active IBD[11,12]. High circulating (plasma) levels of IL-2r (p55) have been demonstrated in patients with active Crohn's disease and ulcerative colitis[13-16]. Higher levels of the receptor in mesenteric veins draining diseased intestine (compared to peripheral circulation), suggest that a significant proportion of the circulating IL-2r in inflammatory bowel disease is derived from the inflamed mucosa. In Crohn's disease, circulating levels of the receptor have been shown to correlate with disease activity with levels falling only upon clinical response to treatment. It is possible that circulating IL-2r may reflect more sensitively (compared to the tests currently used) the intestinal inflammation in Crohn's disease, but further studies are required to confirm this.

It should be noted that high circulating IL-2r levels are not specific to IBD and occur in other diseases where there is chronic activation of the immune system such as in coeliac disease[17] and autoimmune diseases.

INTERLEUKIN 6 (IL-6)

IL-6 is a peptide with molecular weight of 25 000 which can be produced in a variety of cells, including macrophages, T cells, B cells, keratinocytes, endothelial cells and fibroblasts. Its biological functions include B cell differentiation and growth, induction of acute-phase protein synthesis by hepatocytes and T cell activation and differentiation[18].

As noted above, in active IBD there is T cell and macrophage activation and an acute-phase response, and therefore production of this cytokine has been studied[19]. IL-6 was detected (by ELISA) in plasma of 18 out of 21 patients with active Crohn's disease but only two (out of 20) with ulcerative colitis and two (out of 16) controls (Table 1). This somewhat surprising finding was not due to differences in disease activity between ulcerative colitis and Crohn's disease. Thus levels of C-reactive protein, α_1 acid glycoprotein, albumin, platelet count and ESR were similar in the two groups. IL-6 in plasma from peripheral and mesenteric vein (draining inflamed bowel) was

Table 1 Circulating (plasma) levels of interleukin-6 (pg/ml)

	Normal controls *(n = 16)*	*Active Crohn's disease* *(n = 21)*	*Active ulcerative colitis* *(n = 20)*
Median	<20	47	<20
Range	<20–30	<20–250	<20–80

Crohn's disease vs normal controls: $p < 0.001$
Crohn's disease vs ulcerative colitis: $p < 0.001$

detected in seven (out of eight) patients with Crohn's disease undergoing resection. In contrast, it was not detected in plasma samples from any of five patients with ulcerative colitis undergoing colectomy.

In the patients with Crohn's disease there was significant negative correlation between plasma IL-6 levels and the albumin level. There were no significant differences in IL-6 levels between patients with colonic and small intestinal disease, and steroid intake also appeared to have no effect. There were no significant correlations between plasma IL-6 levels and clinical disease activity, G-reactive protein or α_1 acid glycoprotein levels. Lack of direct relationship between IL-6 levels and the acute-phase proteins may be because there is a lag period between production of IL-6 and stimulation of hepatocytes to produce the proteins. Differences in circulating levels of IL-6 between active Crohn's disease and ulcerative colitis have also been demonstrated in two other, independently performed studies[20,21]. In the study of Gross *et al.* a bioassay was used to measure the concentration of IL-6 in serum[20].

Reasons for the differences in circulating IL-6 levels between ulcerative colitis and Crohn's disease are not clear. Further studies are required, and these may also give important clues about the pathogenesis of Crohn's disease.

INTERLEUKIN-8

IL-8 is a peptide which can be produced by a variety of cell types, but monocytes and macrophages are probably the major source. Its biological activities affect mainly the neutrophils for which it is a very potent chemoattractant (more potent than LTB4), induces expression of adhesion molecules and also release of stored enzymes[22]. Chemotactic activity for T cells has also been demonstrated.

In view of the predominant neutrophil infiltration of the mucosa in active ulcerative colitis, production of this cytokine in IBD has been studied[23]. Significantly higher tissue levels of the peptide have been found in mucosa with active ulcerative colitis compared to active Crohn's disease or normal controls (Table 2). However, circulating levels were detected only in occasional patients. When circulating anti-IL-8 antibodies (IgG) were studied, higher levels were found in patients with active ulcerative colitis when compared to active Crohn's disease or normal controls (Table 3). Plasma levels of the anti-IL-8 antibodies in ulcerative colitis in remission did not differ from controls.

Table 2 Levels of interleukin-8 in homogenates of mucosal tissue (pg/mg)

	Normal controls	Active ulcerative colitis	Active Crohn's disease
Median	10.4	74.5	10.4
Range	4–16.6	17.7–450.8	4–46.9

UC vs normal controls: $p < 0.002$
UC vs Crohn's disease: $p < 0.002$

Table 3 Circulating (plasma) levels of anti-IL-8 antibody (ng/ml)

	Normal controls	Active ulcerative colitis	Active Crohn's disease
Median	6.1	62.9	5.9
Range	3.2–15.8	3.4–239	2.1–18.1

UC vs normal controls: $p < 0.001$
UC vs Crohn's disease: $p < 0.001$

It can be postulated that the high mucosal levels of IL-8 (produced mainly by macrophages) may be responsible for the predominant neutrophil infiltration in ulcerative colitis. Since neutrophils have also been shown to be able to produce IL-8[24] it is also possible that the high mucosal levels of the peptide are secondary to the neutrophil infiltration. Circulating antibodies to IL-8 may protect against systemic effects of the peptide produced by the mucosa. The highly significant differences in plasma levels of anti-IL-8 antibodies may, like IL-6, allow active ulcerative colitis to be distinguished from active Crohn's disease.

References

1. Mahida YR, Wu KC, Jewell DP. Enhanced production of interleukin 1β by mononuclear cells isolated from mucosa with active ulcerative colitis or Crohn's disease. Gut. 1989;30:835–8.
2. Mahida YR, Lamming CED, Gallagher A, Hawthorne AB, Hawkey CJ. 5-Aminosalicylic acid is a potent inhibitor of IL1β production in organ culture of colonic biopsies from patients with inflammatory bowel disease. Gut. 1991;32:50–4.
3. Ligumsky M, Simon PL, Karmeli FC, Rachmilewitz D. Role of interleukin 1 in inflammatory bowel disease – enhanced production during active disease. Gut. 1990;31:686–9.
4. Mahida YR, Scott E, Kurlak L, Gallagher A, Hawkey CJ. Interleukin 1β, tumour necrosis factor α and interleukin 6 synthesis by circulating mononuclear cells isolated from patients with active ulcerative colitis and Crohn's disease. Eur J Gastroenterol Hepatol. 1992;4:501–7.
5. Cominelli F, Nast CC, Clark BD, Schindler R, Llerena R, Eyselein VE, Thompson RC, Dinarello CA. Interleukin-1 (IL-1) gene expression, synthesis and effect of specific receptor blockade in rabbit immune complex colitis. J Clin Invest. 1990;86:972–80.
6. Murch SH, Lamkin VA, Savage MO, Walker-Smith JA, MacDonald TT. Serum concentrations of tumour necrosis factor α in childhood chronic inflammatory bowel disease. Gut. 1991;32:913–17.
7. Braegger CP, Nicholls S, Murch SH, Stephens S, MacDonald TT. Tumour necrosis factor alpha in stool as a marker of intestinal inflammation. Lancet. 1992;339:89–91.
8. Mazlam MZ, Hodgson HJF. Peripheral blood monocyte cytokine production and acute phase response in inflammatory bowel disease. Gut. 1992;33:773–8.
9. Mahida YR, Wu K, Lamming CED, Jewell DP, Hawkey CJ. Human colonic tumour necrosis factor α production. Gastroenterology. 1989;96:A313.
10. Brynskov J, Tvede N. Plasma interleukin-2 and soluble/shed interleukin-2 receptor in serum of patients with Crohn's disease. Effect of cyclosporin. Gut. 1990;31:795–9.
11. Mahida YR, Wu K, Patel S, Jewell DP. Interleukin 2 receptor expression by macrophages in inflammatory bowel disease. Clin Immunol. 1988;74:382–6.
12. Choy MY, Walker-Smith JA, Williams CB, MacDonald TT. Differential expression of CD25 (interleukin 2 receptor) on lamina propria T cells and macrophages in the intestinal lesions in Crohn's disease and ulcerative colitis. Gut. 1990;31:1365–70.
13. Mahida YR, Gallagher A, Kurlac L, Hawkey CJ. Circulating and tissue interleukin 2 receptor levels in inflammatory bowel disease. Clin Exp Immunol. 1990;82:75–80.

14. Crabtree JE, Juby LD, Heatley RV, Lobo AJ, Bullimore DW, Axon ATR. Soluble interleukin-2 receptor in Crohn's disease: relation of serum concentrations to disease activity. Gut. 1990;31:1033-6.
15. Mueller Ch, Knoflach P, Zielinski CC. T-cell activtion in Crohn's disease. Gastroenterology. 1990;98:639-46.
16. Matsuura T, West GA, Klein JS, Ferraris L, Fiocchi C. Soluble interleukin 2 and CD8 and CD4 receptors in inflammatory bowel disease. Gastroenterology. 1992;102:2006-14.
17. Crabtree JE, Heatley RV, Juby LD, Howdle PD, Losowsky MS. Serum interleukin-2-receptor in coeliac disease: response to treatment and gluten challenge. Clin Exp Immunol. 1989;77:345-8.
18. Akira S, Hirano T, Taga T, Kishimoto T. Biology of multifunctional cytokines: IL-6 and related molecules (IL-1 and TNF). FASEB J. 1990;4:2860-7.
19. Mahida YR, Kurlak L, Gallagher A, Hawkey CJ. High circulating levels of interleukin 6 in active Crohn's disease but not ulcerative colitis. Gut. 1991;32:1531-4.
20. Gross V, Andus T, Caesar I, Roth M, Scholmerich J. Evidence for continuous stimulation of interleukin-6 production in Crohn's disease. Gastroenterology. 1992;102:514-19.
21. Lobo AJ, Jones SC, Evans SW, Banks R, Rathbone BJ, Axon ATR. Plasma interleukin-6 in inflammatory bowel disease. Gut. 1990;31:A1194.
22. Baggiolini M, Walz A, Kunkel SL. Neutrophil-activating peptide-1/interleukin 8, a novel cytokine that activates neutrophils. J Clin Invest. 1989;84:1045-9.
23. Mahida YR, Ceska M, Effenberger F, Kurlac L, Lindley I, Hawkey CJ. Enhanced synthesis of NAP1/IL8 in active ulcerative colitis. Clin Sci. 1992;82:273-5.
24. Bazzoni F, Cassatella MA, Rossi F, Ceska M, Dewald B, Baggiolini M. Phagocytosing neutrophils release high amounts of the neutrophil-activating peptide 1/interleukin 8. J Exp Med. 1991;173:771-4.

28
Prerequisites for treatment decisions – impact of pathophysiology on conservative or operative approaches

V. W. FAZIO and J. J. TJANDRA

INTRODUCTION

Chronic inflammatory bowel disease (IBD) includes Crohn's disease and ulcerative colitis. There are many overlapping features shared by the two conditions, such as sex, age of onset, geographical and social distribution, familial incidence, response to medical therapy and the need for surgery. However, there are also many differences in clinical, radiological and pathological features between them. Their causes remain obscure and the pathophysiology involves an interaction between host responses, immunological, genetic and environmental factors[1].

Over the past decade evidence continues to grow that in IBD there is a failure to dampen or down-regulate an active immune response[2]. It has also been hypothesized that intrinsic abnormalities in the mucosal barrier of the intestine may lead to the influx of both injurious antigens and molecules into the host[3]. Better understanding of the pathogenesis in IBD may lead to better medical control of undesirable elements of inflammation.

With our current knowledge[1], the causes of IBD still are not precisely known. As a result no consistently curative medical treatment exists, and the foundation of drug treatment remains empirical. Surgery is often necessary for refractory symptoms and/or to prevent or to treat complications. Nevertheless, there has been significant improvement in the understanding of the pathophysiology in IBD.

PATHOLOGY

Crohn's disease is a diffuse condition of the gastrointestinal tract with a high risk of relapse, often at the site of previous resection. Segmental or plurisegmental involvement of the intestinal tract with skip areas is common. Furthermore, microscopic changes of Crohn's disease may be present in a macroscopically normal-appearing bowel[4]. The initial lesion is usually in the lymphoid follicles and Peyer's patches of the mucous membrane, which undergo hyperplasia followed by ulceration. With time the inflammatory process in Crohn's disease tends to affect the full thickness of the wall, although not necessarily in all the areas involved. The bowel wall is thickened from a combination of oedema, lymphatic dilatation in the submucosa and fibrosis[5]. This mural thickening leads to narrowing of the lumen and rigidity. The mucosa may appear swollen and erythematous, but more severe changes of ulceration may occur, such as slit-like haemorrhagic erosions, aphthoid ulcers, linear guttering ulcers and large irregular serpiginous ulcers. Deep ulceration may extend into the bowel wall to cause fistulae or loculated abscesses. The absorptive function of the mucosa is grossly reduced by oedema and lymphatic stasis; as a result severe diarrhoea may occur.

By contrast, ulcerative colitis is confined to the mucosa and submucosa of the large bowel. The only exception is when transmural involvement produces toxic colitis and megacolon. There is a predilection for, and constant involvement of, the rectum with a variable proximal extension to the large bowel. Characteristically, the disease does not affect the ileum with the rare exception of 'backwash ileitis' resulting from non-specific inflammation of the terminal 2–3 cm of ileum because of its proximity to diffusely inflamed colon.

IMPACT OF BASIC RESEARCH IN PATHOPHYSIOLOGY ON CLINICAL THERAPY

There has been an overwhelming, complex and seemingly endless amount of data on possible pathogenesis and pathophysiology of IBD. However, little of the information generated so far has contributed to practical benefits in patient care. There is now a much greater therapeutic arsenal available than several decades ago. By the time medical or surgical therapy is instituted, the disease is usually already well established in the bowel. Earlier intervention in the course of the disease is not possible, as there are still no objective markers to indicate the presence of early subclinical disease.

Many of the current medications available share a common and non-specific anti-inflammatory activity, although this appears to be mediated at many different biochemical and immunological levels[6,7]. However, the action of many of these drugs is not really well understood. The best example of this is sulphasalazine, which displays a wide spectrum of *in vitro* activities ranging from modulation of arachidonic acid metabolism, inhibition of cytokine production, to modulation of antibody synthesis and cell-mediated cytotoxicity[6]. In practice, sulphasalazine has been mainly used for preventing relapses in ulcerative colitis. The oral aminosalicylate derivatives, a second generation of sulphasalazine that deliver mesalamine into the ileum, have been shown to be effective in preventing relapses in ulcerative colitis and Crohn's disease patients. When administered at high dosages they have also controlled mild attacks of both ulcerative colitis and Crohn's disease. In ulcerative colitis, mesalamine has not proven to be better than azulfidine[6]. Their primary indication, therefore, is for patients who cannot tolerate sulphasalazine.

Earlier studies have shown the utility of steroids for inducing remission of attacks of ulcerative colitis and for active Crohn's disease. Attacks of ulcerative colitis vary greatly in severity, and the medical treatment employed needs to be tailored accordingly; these have been discussed in depth previously[8]. Immunosuppressive agents such as azathioprine or 6-mercaptopurine have been used either in steroid-resistant patients or in those with refractory disease. The involvement of immunological mechanisms in the pathogenesis of inflammatory bowel disease is the rationale for their clinical use. A newer immunosuppressive agent with a relatively restricted and specific immune function similar to cyclosporin is now also under study[9]. The latency period of 4–8 weeks before traditional immunosuppressives show efficacy can be reduced by using cyclosporin.

Antibiotics, above all metronidazole, have shown efficacy in Crohn's disease, mainly with perianal involvement, and now tobramycin seems to have a role in active colitis. Topical medications such as steroids, mesalamine in enema or suppository form have also been used in distal colitis with excellent results[6].

New therapeutic options with variable scientific bases are constantly emerging. Our ignorance of the pathogenesis of IBD has contributed to this very confusing situation. Despite this, improved understanding of inflammatory intermediaries in IBD has been achieved recently[10]. A new exciting approach to therapy is the possibility of selective inhibition at different levels of the inflammatory cascade[10]. It is now known that several mediators such as prostaglandins, leukotrienes, cytokines and platelet-activating factors are involved in the inflammation of the bowel. Consequently future therapeutic approaches could include manipulation of these factors. In addition, the level of certain soluble mediators such as soluble interleukin-2 receptor is increased in IBD[11]. These may be useful indicators of activity early in the course of the illness.

INDICATIONS FOR SURGERY IN CROHN'S DISEASE

The indications for surgery in Crohn's disease are fundamentally different from those in ulcerative colitis. This is because patients with ulcerative colitis can be cured by proctocolectomy with or without intestinal restoration, whereas no such surgical cure can be guaranteed in Crohn's disease. The latter is potentially a panintestinal disease with a tendency to periodic exacerbation in any part of the gastrointestinal tract. The basis of surgical intervention in Crohn's disease is not to excise the whole of the disease but to treat only its complications. The anatomical pattern of the disease has an important bearing on the clinical course, indications for surgery, operative and recurrence rates[12].

ELECTIVE SURGERY IN SMALL BOWEL DISEASE

The decision for surgery is often a value judgement made collectively by the surgeon, the gastroenterologist and the patient, and is usually for obstructive symptoms refractory to medical therapy. It is uncertain whether the interval between diagnosis and surgery is related to the subsequent risk of recurrence, all other factors being equal. With current evidence[13], it would seem unreasonable to defer surgery in a symptomatic patient with a short history, merely because of the potential risk of earlier recurrence. Limited disease can usually be treated by resection and primary anastomosis. Extensive disease with skip lesions is best treated by strictureplasty, especially if the patient has had multiple prior resections (see below).

Extent of resection

The length of 'normal' bowel that should be included as resection margin has been a contentious issue, with a swing towards more conservative resection in recent years[13,14]. The main protagonists of radical resection have been the Scandinavians[15,16], but all studies have been retrospective. In these studies, overt disease often remained in the non-radical group. This would have exaggerated the 'recurrence' rate. Furthermore, the radical operations were often performed at a different institution from the non-radical or control operations. Other studies[17-19] have shown no difference in recurrence rates between patients with wide and narrow resection margins. Thus, it would be prudent to resect only the overtly diseased segment and to construct the anastomosis at the supple bowel ends. This conservative attitude will minimize the risk of short bowel syndrome.

Use of intraoperative frozen sections

Some centres[20,21] have advocated intraoperative frozen section examinations to ensure disease-free resection margins. However, microscopic changes are easily missed in frozen sections[22], and microscopic changes of Crohn's disease are often seen in areas remote from the macroscopically diseased area. Thus, the weight of evidence suggests that this is a waste of effort[14].

Strictureplasty

As an alternative to extensive repeat resections, Lee *et al.*, from Oxford[23], pioneered the technique of strictureplasty to relieve obstruction from strictures of the small bowel due to Crohn's disease. In subsequent studies[24-26] it has been shown to be safe and effective, and has the added advantage of bowel preservation. There has been no operative mortality related to the procedure and the incidence of enterocutaneous fistula or suture line dehiscence is similar to that seen with bowel resection[24]. In our experience[24] with 116 patients undergoing 452 strictureplasties in the small bowel, symptomatic restricture of the strictureplasty sites was around 3%, and most symptomatic recurrences were due to disease progression in a new site. Strictureplasty is most suitable for patients with diffuse symptomatic strictures, and in those who have had previous extensive resection(s) of small bowel[27]. It is to be avoided for phlegmonous or perforative disease. Multiple strictures within a short segment are also best resected for technical reasons. A serum albumin level $< 30\,g/l$ has been associated with an increased incidence of major septic complications.

ELECTIVE SURGERY IN LARGE BOWEL DISEASE

In general, few patients with extensive Crohn's colitis manage to secure long-term remission with medical treatment, and most require surgery. Common indications for surgery include chronic ill-health, troublesome bowel symptoms, colonic bleeding and gross perianal disease[28]. Bowel obstruction from stricture is another common indication. The need for surgery often becomes apparent gradually over a period of time with worsening bowel symptoms and large-dose steroid dependency or its side-effects. The probability of surgical treatment for primary Crohn's colitis has been estimated as $35 \pm 7\%$ at 5 years and $39 \pm 7\%$ at 10 years for recent-onset disease[29], rising to $72 \pm 6\%$ at 6 years from the first admission to hospital[30].

The commonest type of operation performed in our Department[31] was proctocolectomy (76%), followed by colectomy with or without anastomosis (21%). Much less commonly, ileostomy only, or bypass (3%), was performed.

PROCTOCOLECTOMY AND END ILEOSTOMY

This is the most appropriate operation for the treatment of extensive Crohn's colitis, especially if there is serious anorectal disease. This is associated with lower recurrence rates than other lesser colonic resections. It can be done either entirely in one stage or as a staged procedure after initial abdominal colectomy. Very rarely, initial diverting loop ileostomy followed later by proctocolectomy is performed in the presence of severe suppurative perineal disease, and in patients who are unwilling to have a permanent stoma at a particular time. The drawbacks of this operation are that, despite its extent, it does not eradicate the disease, and problems with persistent perineal sinus are not uncommon. Risk factors for poor perineal wound healing include severe rectal disease, active perianal disease, a high rectal fistula and faecal contamination at the time of operation[32]. In addition, subsequent reoperation for small bowel Crohn's disease is not uncommon, and was 23% after 10 years in one study[33].

Abdominal (subtotal) colectomy

This is considered when the rectum is free of disease, the anal function is adequate and there is a lack of perineal sepsis. None of these criteria is absolute. Experience and philosophy of an individual surgeon may favour a particular operation in an individual case. If possible the whole of the rectum is conserved, and the anastomosis made at the level of the sacral promontory. If the distal sigmoid is free of disease an ileosigmoid anastomosis is constructed instead. One-stage anastomosis is usually performed unless there is significant intra-abdominal sepsis, or if adverse factors to healing are present. Favourable results have been reported following ileorectal anastomosis even if a mild degree of Crohn's proctitis is present[34-36]. Complications related to the anastomosis are comparable whether the rectum is diseased or macroscopically normal. If in doubt, the anastomosis can be deferred and an initial ileostomy performed.

Some authors believe that, with diversion following abdominal colectomy, the diseased rectum will recover and may subsequently become suitable for ileorectal anastomosis[37]. This is not always possible, and in many cases the rectum has to be removed. In addition, cancer may occur insidiously in the rectal stump.

Ileorectal anastomosis has a higher incidence of recurrence than proctocolectomy. In our experience of 118 patients, 61% maintained a functioning ileorectal anastomosis after a mean of 9 years[36]. About one in three patients required regular medications with antidiarrhoeal agent and/or steroids. Although this procedure is associated with higher recurrence rates, it has a special place in young patients where the potential morbidity of pelvic dissection, a perineal wound and an abdominal stoma are avoided.

Segmental colectomy

Segmental disease occurred in about 6% of patients with Crohn's disease. While segmental ileocolic resection is well accepted for ileocolic disease, the role of segmental colectomy is less clear. A high rate of recurrence follows such procedure; up to 62% at 5.5 years has been reported[38]. Despite the high recurrence rate the procedure is safe, confers good function and delays the need for an ileostomy.

EMERGENCY OPERATION

Perforation/intra-abdominal abscess

Surgical management should include adequate drainage of the abscess and bacteriological study of the pus. Abscesses in Crohn's disease may form complex cavities, and may be difficult to define even with CT scan. In uniloculated abscess cavity, CT-guided drainage is useful. Even if a fistula develops, subsequent surgery may then be successfully confined to one stage. At the time of surgery a careful search for abscess ramifications and satellite cavities should be made.

Fistula

There are several varieties of entero-enteric fistulae. Most commonly they are from ileocaecal region to the sigmoid colon. The primary ileocolic lesion can be resected and the sigmoid opening trimmed and closed with interrupted absorbable sutures if sigmoid involvement is minimal macroscopically. However, phlegmonous changes are commonly present in the wall of the sigmoid colon and a double resection is often necessary[39]. Perioperative endoscopic examination of the sigmoid colon is helpful to evaluate the extent of disease.

Entero-enteric fistulae to the small bowel are often not detected before operation[40]. In themselves they do not necessarily constitute an indication for operation, but they are often associated with severe distal disease, luminal stenosis or abscess. These associated complications are generally the cause of symptoms rather than the fistula itself. Entero-enteric fistulae are usually treated by removal of the segment of diseased bowel from which they arise, and oversewing of the re-entry site in the non-diseased bowel. Any areas of distal stenosis may be widened by strictureplasty or resected.

Entero-enteric fistulae sometimes follow surgical resection of diseased bowel and are found to originate from areas with no macroscopic disease. The outcome is similar to a postoperative fistula in a patient without Crohn's disease. High-output fistulae that develop within 4–5 days of surgery usually indicate a major anastomotic dehiscence, and are probably best treated by further surgery, resection of fistula sites with or without a diverting stoma. Postoperative fistulae occurring later than the first week after operation are usually low-output, and can be managed by drainage of any associated sepsis, skin protection and parenteral nutrition. Provided there is no distal obstruction, most will heal with this treatment.

Fistulae that occur after abscess drainage usually do not heal with conservative treatment[40,41]. Preliminary drainage of abscess is useful to prepare the patient sufficiently to make definitive operation and anastomosis safe. Laparotomy is almost always needed. The affected bowel from which the fistula arises is resected together with any distal obstruction.

PERIANAL CROHN'S DISEASE

Perianal Crohn's disease occurs more commonly in association with colonic than with small bowel disease[42]. In 30% of patients, perianal disease may be the first manifestation of Crohn's disease[43]. These lesions include mucosal fissures, ulcerated oedematous piles and cavitating ulcers. Fissuring of the anal margin heals by fibrosis and may subsequently produce the anal stenosis commonly seen in these patients[44]. The majority of oedematous piles resolve to form anal skin tags, but it is the cavitating ulcers which progress to cause tissue destruction and spreading sepsis into the perirectal tissues. Perianal Crohn's disease can look alarming; however, the temptation to treat with aggressive surgery must be resisted to minimize the risk of incontinence by surgical intervention. They are often painless and generally 'benign', and are best managed conservatively because of the complicated nature of many fistulae and the risk of poor healing. There is evidence that perianal lesions may heal if active Crohn's disease elsewhere in the gut is successfully treated[45]. There are no prospective, controlled trials of drug therapy alone in perianal Crohn's disease; but azathioprine or 6-mercaptopurine[46] may be useful in healing perirectal fistulae. Unfortunately, prolonged drug therapy is often required with resultant side-effects. There is also mounting evidence that antibiotics such as metronidazole are effective in controlling perianal Crohn's disease[47]. The efficacy of metronidazole may be related to its antimicrobial action, effect on leucocyte chemotaxis and immunosuppressive effect[43].

The potential benefits of local surgical treatment must be carefully weighed against the possibility of spontaneous resolution of these complications. If pain develops, this usually indicates pus under tension, and requires simple incision and drainage. Short low anal strictures may respond to gentle dilatation. Low anal fistulae are often asymptomatic and may heal spontaneously. Few of these need surgical intervention. Coexisting haemorrhoids are not uncommon in patients with perianal Crohn's disease, and surgical treatment in the presence of active disease is not to be recommended and may eventuate in proctectomy because of failure to heal[48].

In retrovaginal fistulae, patients with minimal symptoms can be managed conservatively. Regular review is important to ensure that a carcinoma does not arise in the fistula track. Severe disabling symptoms will need surgical intervention by anorectal flap[49] if the rectum is minimally diseased, or by proctectomy if the rectum is contracted and severely diseased.

Advantages of anorectal flap technique include a reduction in the duration of healing, avoidance of damage to the anal sphincters, and no risk of deformity to the anal canal. This can be performed as a one-stage procedure without covering stoma in most cases[49,50]. The flap raised should include at least partial thickness of the rectal wall, but may include the full thickness of the rectum. The width of the proximally placed flap base should be at least twice as long as the width of the apex to ensure an adequate blood supply[50]. Curettage of the external portion of the track as opposed to fistulectomy or excision is regarded as being technically easier, with similar functional results[49,50].

Setons are useful in complex fistulae when the anatomical landmarks have been distorted, or if fistulotomy may render the patient incontinent. They may be used in several ways: applied loosely when used as drains, or as a stimulant to fibrosis around the track with the intention to cut slowly through the track, or as markers to enable better postoperative assessment by outlining the track. When used to promote fibrosis, setons act by holding the muscle ends together, thereby preventing separation of the anal sphincters when fistulotomy is performed.

FAECAL DIVERSION

Proximal diversion of the faecal stream to 'rest' inflamed intestine was first advocated by Brown[51], and was advocated by the Oxford group[52] for Crohn's colitis. Similar reduction of faecal stream can be achieved by elemental diet[53]. The mechanism by which faecal diversion produces disease remission is unknown. The faecal stream or one of its constituents may perpetuate the inflammatory process, and may be involved in disease pathogenesis. Microorganisms or their metabolic products, ingested materials or endogenous substances, such as digestive enzymes, might be provocative agents[54].

The overall results from many reports suggest that faecal diversion does seem to be effective in resting inflamed colon and facilitating healing of perianal disease, but the effect of restoring intestinal continuity is unpredicatable[55]. Even in patients obtaining early symptomatic relief, long-term results are unpredictable and relapse is common. In most cases faecal diversion is best regarded as a holding procedure to facilitate subsequent definitive surgical care[55]. Intestinal continuity has ultimately been restored in less than a third of patients with perianal disease[56], although it is useful in cases with gross perianal disease to facilitate subsequent proctocolectomy.

PERIOPERATIVE BLOOD TRANSFUSION

Blood transfusion has been shown to have an immunosuppressive effect on the recipient, which is thought to account for the improved survival of transplanted kidneys[57]. Immunological mechanisms and immune hyperactivity have been implicated in the pathophysiology of Crohn's disease[58] and a few studies have investigated the effect of blood transfusion on recurrence after surgery. In one study[59], the recurrence rate at 5 years after surgery for small bowel Crohn's disease in patients who had received a blood transfusion in the perioperative period was significantly lower than the recurrence rate in those who did not receive a transfusion (19% vs 59%). Similar findings were found by Peters et al.[60], although a third study did not confirm this[61]. Further study in this area is required before firm conclusions can be made.

DRUG TREATMENT AFTER RESECTION

Use of drug treatment after resection to prevent recurrence developing is an attractive concept. Several trials have evaluated steroids[62-64], sulphasalazine[63,64] and azathioprine[64] as prophylaxis against recurrence. In each case drug treatment was no better than placebo in preventing recurrence.

These studies illustrate the difficulties involved in therapeutic trials in Crohn's studies. All these studies had a small number of patients. Several hundred patients would be required to illustrate any significant benefit in either group. Many of the studies had a short follow-up of 2–3 years, and recurrent disease may develop many years after resection. However, potential side-effects of steroids or immunosuppressants would limit their long-term use.

ULCERATIVE COLITIS

The majority of patients with ulcerative colitis can be managed satisfactorily by medical means. The most common indication for an elective operation is to restore health in patients with chronic disease who are debilitated with weight loss and protein-losing enteropathy. Many of these patients are also taking high doses of steroids. In patients with chronic colitis with severe malnutrition, an initial course of nutritional support is advisable[8].

A further indication in long-standing ulcerative colitis is the risk of malignant change in the colon. The risk of cancer increases with increasing extent of disease, with increasing duration of disease and probably with increasing age at onset of symptoms[65]. In a retrospective study the cumulative risk in those with extensive ulcerative colitis was 0.6% at 10 years and 7.2% at 20 years from the onset of disease[66]. Thus the risk of developing colorectal carcinoma becomes a significant problem only after 10 years, and that risk increases with time[65]. The extent of disease is also an important risk factor. The incidence of malignancy in cases with extensive involvement was 7.2% compared with 1.3% for cases with left-sided disease[67].

Thus regular surveillance colonoscopy in patients with extensive colitis of more than 10 years' duration is recommended. The optimal frequency of examination is still not decided, but the presence of high-grade dysplasia or a mass lesion in association with ulcerative colitis is an indication for surgery[65,68]. An additional risk factor for colorectal cancer in ulcerative colitis is the presence of colonic stricture[68] in which there is a high incidence of carcinoma or dysplasia and may hinder adequate endoscopic surveillance of more proximal bowel.

Because a cure for ulcerative colitis can be offered by excising the colon and rectum, surgery is recommended more liberally. The range of surgical options includes:

Restorative proctocolectomy and ileoanal pouch
This involves a conventional total colectomy, rectal excision, construction of an ileal pouch and ileal pouch–anal anastomosis. This is viewed as the most recent development in the evolution of continence-preserving procedures for ulcerative colitis. It is preferable for the colitis to be inactive and a higher complication rate has been reported in patients on systemic steroids at the time of pouch construction[69]. A covering ileostomy is advisable in most cases, in view of the large number of suture or staple lines. Documented Crohn's disease, inadequate anal sphincter function, presence of advanced low-lying rectal cancer and serious co-morbid illness are contraindications to this procedure.

Techniques of restorative proctocolectomy have changed with improvement in stapling techniques and with increased understanding of the anal sphincter function[70]. In earlier experience, long rectal muscular cuff up to 10 cm was made in the belief that it would enhance continence. Instead, it was associated with increased intraoperative bleeding and higher septic complication rates. The current practice is to leave a shorter muscular cuff of no more than 1–2 cm above the levators if mucosectomy is performed. The functional results are comparable and there are less complications with the shorter cuff[71]. This suggests that receptors for sensation of defaecation do not lie predominantly in the rectal muscle.

The importance of sensory receptors in the anal transitional zone in the differentiation between faeces and flatus has recently been emphasized[71]. Vigorous anal manipulation and dilatation, associated with endoanal approaches to mucosectomy, is also now known to be harmful to nocturnal continence[70]. With the advent of modern circular staplers, we and others[71,72] have abandoned the routine practice of rectal mucosectomy, and the ileal pouch is stapled to the top of the anal canal. This led to improved continence, greater ease and speed of the operation and a safer anastomosis compared with the hand-sewn anastomosis associated with mucosectomy. Nevertheless, important questions remain concerning postoperative cancer risk and potential problems of persistent inflammation in the anal transitional zone.

Proctocolectomy and end ileostomy

This still has a place in patients who prefer a definitive procedure that is more consistent with their lifestyle, or who are not ideal candidates for restorative proctocolectomy, which is a more complex procedure. The morbidity, including sexual and bladder dysfunction, is higher than after restorative proctocolectomy.

Continent ileostomy of Kock

This procedure involves intricate construction and has a high rate of pouch and valvular dysfunction that requires frequent revisional surgery. There is also a recognized learning curve with the procedure, as in restorative proctocolectomy. It has a limited place in some patients in whom an ileal pouch has failed but are reluctant to have an end ileostomy.

Abdominal colectomy and ileorectal anastomosis

This procedure has always been controversial, and its role is even smaller with the advent of restorative proctocolectomy. It is a relatively simple procedure, preserves anal continence and avoids pelvic dissection. This is an acceptable compromise if there is a serious concern about Crohn's disease, if the rectum is minimally diseased and there is a good anal sphincter function. Other indications include patients who refuse to have an ileostomy and yet are not suitable candidates for restorative proctocolectomy or continent ileostomy. These include patients with gross obesity, significant portal hypertension, or advanced synchronous malignancy in whom life expectancy is limited. Careful surveillance of the rectum is important as there is a 5% risk at 20 years of carcinoma developing in the rectum. The carcinoma may arise without significant macroscopic changes in the mucosa, and can be advanced by the time it is diagnosed[73].

DYSPLASIA AND CANCER

The presence of dysplasia denotes increased risk of malignancy. The evaluation of dysplasia may be observer-dependent. Information on the time sequence of the transformation of dysplasia to carcinoma is sparse, and it is possible, in mild cases at least, that the dysplastic process can reverse. Furthermore, dysplasia and carcinoma can occur in flat mucosa[74]. To avoid blind monitoring, control endoscopic biopsies should ideally be taken by the same endoscopist, and a note should be made, each time, of the sites of biopsy.

In Crohn's disease also, dysplasia has been seen in surgical specimens containing cancer[75]. The evidence suggests that dysplasia in Crohn's disease is similar to that found in ulcerative colitis, in both appearance and timing[65]. However, owing to the relative rarity of cancers associated with Crohn's disease, it is not possible to state unequivocally that dysplasia represents a precancerous state. For Crohn's disease the risk of developing cancer in the first 10 years is virtually nil, as in ulcerative colitis; that risk then progressively rises[76]. There are difficulties with cancer prevention in Crohn's disease as the duration and extent of disease is often not clear; additional and currently unknown risk factors are likely to be present, and there is a lack of effective screening programmes as the cancer can arise in both small and large bowels.

Despite these considerations, dysplasia remains the most reliable marker of malignant transformation in ulcerative colitis. New indicators of premalignancy, such as DNA flow cytometry and proliferation kinetics of colonic epithelial cells, have shown interesting results, but further investigations are required[68].

TOXICITY

Severe colitis can occur with both ulcerative colitis and Crohn's disease. This can be initially treated with nutritional support, bowel rest and medical treatment until patients are fit for colectomy.

Toxic megacolon, refractory toxicity, perforation or massive haemorrhage is an absolute indication for urgent operation. The most satisfactory operation in this setting is an abdominal colectomy and end ileostomy. Depending on the state of the sigmoidorectal stump, it may be exteriorized, matured primarily as a mucous fistula or closed and anchored to the anterior abdominal wall. This removes most of the disease right away, and avoids a lengthy and hazardous pelvic dissection.

There is no evidence that hyperalimentation and bowel rest have any primary therapeutic effect in severe acute colitis[77]. Whether such treatment reduces the incidence of postoperative complications has not yet been proved. A patient with a temperature of $>38°C$ and a stool frequency of $>8/24\,h$ has an 80% chance of not responding to drug therapy and needing surgical intervention[78]. It has also been shown that continuing the conservative regimens for longer than 1 week does not significantly increase the number of patients entering a satisfactory remission, but mortality does rise[79].

INDETERMINATE COLITIS

In some patients the histological differentiation is not clear-cut, and falls within the domain of indeterminate colitis. In others an initial diagnosis of ulcerative colitis may later be revised to Crohn's disease if small bowel or perianal lesions appear. The differentiation of Crohn's disease from ulcerative colitis can be extremely difficult in toxic colitis even with full histological examination of the specimens. This is of particular importance with current interest in ileal pouch–anal anastomosis. Perianal lesions or any histological evidence suggestive of Crohn's disease in the rectum should be regarded with suspicion, and ileal reservoir surgery best avoided in these circumstances. If in doubt, it is prudent to preserve the rectum in the first instance.

The natural history of ileal pouch–anal anastomosis in indeterminate colitis is now better defined[70,80]. A number of patients will develop features of Crohn's disease with time. Outcome of patients in the short term, up to 4–5 years, is similar to patients with ulcerative colitis[80]. Late pouch complications appear to be related to the presence of preoperative features that are suggestive of Crohn's disease, such as perianal disease. If features of Crohn's disease develop only after pouch construction, one would still proceed to close the diverting ileostomy, after advising the patient of the possibility of future pouch excision.

GENERAL SUPPORT

Anaemia, fluid and electrolyte depletion must be rectified. Symptomatic relief of diarrhoea with codeine phosphate or loperamide may be appropriate in non-acute cases. Nutritional support in the form of elemental diet or parenteral nutrition seems to have a role as primary therapy in active Crohn's disease[81]. They also promote the replacement of protein body stores in both Crohn's disease and ulcerative colitis. In Crohn's disease complicated by short bowel syndrome, home parenteral nutrition results in improvement in nutritional status, quality of life and a decrease in the intensity of medical treatment[82]. However, it has no advantage with regard to the need for surgery or hospitalization.

References

1. Gibson PR. Etiology of inflammatory bowel disease. Curr Opinion Gastroenterol. 1991;7:642–8.
2. Mayer L. Immunology of inflammatory bowel disease. Curr Opinion Gastroenterol. 1990;6:556–60.
3. Hollander D, Vadheim CM, Bretholz E, Petersen M, Delahunty T, Rotter JI. Increased intestinal permeability in patients with Crohn's disease and their relatives. Ann Intern Med. 1986;105:883–5.
4. Dunne WT, Cooke WT, Allan RN. Enzymatic and morphometric evidence for Crohn's disease as a diffuse lesion of the gastrointestinal tract. Gut. 1977;18:290–4.
5. Cunningham IGE. Inflammatory bowel disease. In: Hughes ESR, Cuthbertson AM, Killingback MK, editors. Colorectal surgery. Edinburgh: Churchill Livingstone; 1983:265–88.
6. Campieri M, Brignola C, Miglioli M, Barbara L. Medical management of inflammatory bowel disease. Curr Opinion Gastroenterol. 1991;7:607–16.

7. Hawthorne AB, Hawkey CJ. Immunosuppressive drugs in inflammatory bowel disease. A review of their mechanisms of efficacy and place in therapy. Drugs. 1989;38:267–88.

8. Truelove SC. Medical management of ulcerative colitis and indications for colectomy. World J Surg. 1988;12:142–7.

9. Lichtiger S, Present DH. Preliminary report: cyclosporin in treatment of severe active ulcerative colitis. Lancet. 1990;336:16–19.

10. Fiocchi C. Immunology of inflammatory bowel disease. Curr Opinion Gastroenterol. 1991;7:654–61.

11. Mueller C, Knoflach P, Zielinski CC. T-cell activation in Crohn's disease: increased levels of soluble interleukin-2 receptor in serum and supernatants of stimulated peripheral blood mononuclear cells. Gastroenterology. 1990;98:639–46.

12. Farmer RG, Hawk WA, Turnbull RB. Clinical patterns in Crohn's disease: a statistical study of 615 cases. Gastroenterology. 1975;68:627–35.

13. Williams JG, Wong WD, Rothenberger DA, Goldberg SM. Recurrence of Crohn's disease after resection. Br J Surg. 1991;78:10–19.

14. Tjandra JJ, Fazio VW. The benefits of minimal surgery. Can J Gastroenterol. 1992: in press.

15. Bergman L, Krause U. Crohn's disease: a long-term study of the clinical course in 186 patients. Scand J Gastroenterol. 1977;12:937–44.

16. Krause U, Ejerblad S, Bergman L. Crohn's disease: a long-term study of the clinical course in 186 patients. Scand J Gastroenterol. 1985;20:516–24.

17. Kotanagi H, Kramer K, Fazio V, Petras R. Do microscopic abnormalities at resection margins correlate with increased anastomotic recurrence in Crohn's disease? Dis Colon Rectum. 1991;34:909–16.

18. Trynka YM, Glotzer DJ, Kasdon EJ et al. Long-term outcome of restorative operation in Crohn's disease. Ann Surg. 1982;196:345–55.

19. Speranza V, Simi M, Leardi S, Del Papa M. Recurrence of Crohn's disease: are there any risk factors? J Clin Gastroenterol. 1986;8:640–6.

20. Wolff BG, Beart RW Jr, Frydenberg HB, Weiland LH, Agrez MV, Ilstrup DM. The importance of disease-free margins in resection for Crohn's disease. Dis Colon Rectum. 1983;26:239–43.

21. Karesen R, Serch-Hanssen A, Thoresen BO, Hertzberg J. Crohn's disease: long-term results of surgical treatment. Scand J Gastroenterol. 1981;16:57–64.

22. Hamilton SR, Reese J, Pennington L et al. The role of resection margin frozen section in the surgical management of Crohn's disease. Surg Gynecol Obstet. 1985;160:57–62.

23. Lee ECG, Papaioannou N. Minimal surgery for chronic obstruction in patients with extensive or universal Crohn's disease. Ann R Coll Surg Engl. 1982;64:229–33.

24. Tjandra JJ, Fazio VW, Lavery IC, Church JM, Milsom JW, Oakley JR. Long-term follow up of strictureplasty in Crohn's disease. Dis Colon Rectum. 1992;35:P20.

25. Alexander-Williams J, Haynes IG. Up-to-date management of small bowel Crohn's disease. Adv Surg. 1987;20:245–64.

26. Dehn TCB, Kettlewell MGW, Mortensen NJMcC, Lee ECG, Jewell DP. Ten-year experience of strictureplasty for obstructive Crohn's disease. Br J Surg. 1989;76:339–41.

27. Tjandra JJ, Fazio VW, Lavery IC. Results of multiple ($\geqslant 4$) strictureplasties in Crohn's disease. Am J Surg. 1992: in press.

28. Tjandra JJ, Fazio VW. Surgery for Crohn's colitis. Int Surg. 1992;77:9–14.

29. Elliott PR, Ritchie JK, Lennard-Jones JE. Prognosis of colonic Crohn's disease. Br Med J. 1985;291:178.

30. Lennard-Jones JE, Ritchie JK, Zohrab WJ. Proctocolitis and Crohn's disease of the colon: a comparison of the clinical course. Gut. 1976;17:477–82.

31. Farmer RG, Hawk WA, Turnbull RB Jr. Indications for surgery in Crohn's disease: analysis of 500 cases. Gastroenterology. 1976;71:245–50.

32. Scammell BE, Keighley MRB. Delayed perianal wound healing after proctectomy for Crohn's colitis. Br J Surg. 1986;73:150–2.

33 Scammel BE, Andrews H, Allen RN et al. Results of proctocolectomy for Crohn's disease. Br J Surg. 1987;74:671–4.

34. Buchmann P, Weterman IT, Keighley MRB, Pena SA, Allan RN, Alexander-Williams J. The prognosis of ileorectal anastomosis in Crohn's disease. Br J Surg. 1981;68:7–10.

35. Lock MR, Fazio VW, Farmer RG, Jagelman DG, Lavery IC, Weakley FL. Proximal

recurrence and the fate of the rectum following excisional surgery for Crohn's disease of the large bowel. Ann Surg. 1981;194:754–60.

36. Longo WE, Oakley JR, Lavery IC, Fazio VW. Outcome of ileorectal anastomosis for Crohn's colitis. Dis Colon Rectum. 1991;34:23.

37. Morel P, Hawker PC, Allan RN, Dykes PW, Alexander-Williams J. Management of acute colitis in inflammatory bowel disease. World J Surg. 1986;10:814–19.

38. Longo WE, Ballantyne GH, Cahow E. Treatment of Crohn's colitis – segmental or total colectomy? Arch Surg. 1988;123:588–90.

39. Fazio VW, Wilk P, Turnbull RB Jr, Jagelman DG. The dilemma of Crohn's disease: ileosigmoidal fistula complicating Crohn's disease. Dis Colon Rectum. 1977;20:381–6.

40. Givel JC, Hawker PC, Allan RN et al. Enteroenteric fistula complicating Crohn's disease. J Clin Gastroenterol. 1983;5:321–3.

41. Givel JC, Hawker PC, Allan RN et al. Entero-vaginal fistulas associated with Crohn's disease. Surg Gynecol Obstet. 1982;155:494–6.

42. Heuman R, Bolin T, Sjodahl R, Tagesson C. The incidence and cause of perianal complications and arthralgia after intestinal resection with restoration of continuity for Crohn's disease. Br J Surg. 1981;68:528–30.

43. Allan A, Keighley MRB. Management of perianal Crohn's disease. World J Surg. 1988;12:198–202.

44. Hughes LE, Jones IRG. Perianal lesions in Crohn's disease. In: Allan RN, Keighley MRB, Hawkins C, Alexander-Williams A, editors. Inflammatory bowel disease. Edinburgh: Churchill-Livingstone; 1982:321–31.

45. Lockhart-Mummery HE, Morson BC. Crohn's disease of the large bowel. Gut. 1964;5:493–5.

46. Present DM, Korelitz BI, Wisch N, Glass JL, Sachar DB, Pasternack BS. Treatment of Crohn's disease with 6-mercaptopurine. N Engl J Med. 1980;302:981–7.

47. Ursing B, Alm T, Baramy F. A comparative study of metronidazole and sulfasalazine for active Crohn's disease. The cooperative Crohn's disease study in Sweden. II: Results. Gastroenterology. 1984;83:550–62.

48. Jeffrey PJ, Ritchie JK, Parks AG. Treatment of haemorrhoids in patients with inflammatory bowel disease. Lancet 1977;1:1084–5.

49. Jones IT, Fazio VW, Jagelman DG. The use of transanal rectal advancement flaps in the management of fistulas involving the anorectum. Dis Colon Rectum. 1987;30:919–23.

50. Stone JM, Goldberg SM. How I do it. The endorectal advancement flap procedure. Int J Colorect Dis. 1990;5:232–5.

51. Brown JY. The value of complete physiological rest of the large bowel in the treatment of certain ulcerative and obstructive lesions in this organ. Surg Gynecol Obstet. 1913;16:610–11.

52. Lee ECG. Split ileostomy in the treatment of Crohn's disease of the colon. Ann R Coll Surg Engl. 1975;56:94–7.

53. O'Morain C, Segal AW, Levi AJ. Elemental diet as a primary treatment of acute Crohn's disease: a controlled trial. Br Med J. 1984;288:1859–62.

54. Kivel RM, Taylor KB, Oberhelman H. Response to bypass ileostomy in ulcerative colitis and Crohn's disease of the colon. Lancet. 1967;2:632–4.

55. Goligher JC. Surgical treatment of Crohn's disease affecting mainly or entirely the large bowel. World J Surg. 1988;12:186–90.

56. Harper PH, Kettlewell MGW, Lee ECG. The effect of split ileostomy on perianal Crohn's disease. Br J Surg. 1982;69:608–12.

57. Opelz G, Graver B, Terasaki PI. Induction of high kidney graft survival by multiple transfusion. Lancet. 1981;1:1223–5.

58. Strober W, James SP. The immunologic basis of inflammatory bowel disease. J Clin Immunol. 1986;6:415–32.

59. Williams JG, Hughes LE. Effect of perioperative blood transfusion on recurrence of Crohn's disease. Lancet. 1989;2:131–3.

60. Peters WR, Fry RD, Fleshman JW, Kodner IJ. Multiple blood transfusions reduce the recurrence rate of Crohn's disease. Dis Colon Rectum. 1989;32:749–53.

61. Sutherland LR, Ramcharan S, Bryant H, Fick G. Effect of perioperative blood transfusion on recurrence of Crohn's disease. Lancet. 1989;2:1048.

62. Smith RC, Rhodes J, Heatley RV et al. Low dose steroids and clinical relapse in Crohn's disease: a controlled trial. Gut. 1978;19:606–10.

63. Bergman L, Krause U. Postoperative treatment with corticosteroids and salazosulphapyridine (Salazopyrin) after radical resection for Crohn's disease. Scand J Gastroenterol. 1976;11:651–6.
64. Summers RW, Switz DM, Sessions JT *et al*. National Cooperative Crohn's Disease Study: results of drug treatment. Gastroenterology. 1979;77:847–69.
65. Cola B. Inflammatory bowel disease and cancer. Int J Colorect Dis. 1989;4:128–33.
66. Gyde S, Prior P, Allan RN *et al*. Colorectal cancer in ulcerative colitis: a cohort study of primary referrals from three centers. Gut. 1988;29:206–17.
67. Edwards FC, Truelove SC. The course and prognosis of ulcerative colitis III. Complications. IV. Carcinoma of the colon. Gut. 1964;5:1–22.
68. Lashner BA. Cancer in inflammatory bowel disease. Curr Opinion Gastroenterol. 1991;7:622–7.
69. Nicholls RJ, Pescatori M, Motson RW, Pezim ME. Restorative proctocolectomy with a three loop ileal reservoir for ulcerative colitis and familial adenomatous polyposis. Ann Surg. 1984;199:383–8.
70. Tjandra JJ, Fazio VW. Indications for and results of ileal pouch. Curr Pract Surg. 1992: in press.
71. Fazio VW, Tjandra JJ, Lavery IC. Techniques in pouch construction. In: Bartolo D, Mortensen N, Nicholls RJ, editors. Techniques to restorative proctocolectomy. Oxford: Blackwell Scientific Publications; 1992: in press.
72. Wexner SD, Wong WD, Rothenberger DA, Goldberg SM. The ileoanal reservoir. Am J Surg. 1990;159:178–85.
73. Grunfest ST, Fazio VW, Weiss RA *et al*. The risk of cancer following colectomy and ileorectal anastomosis for extensive mucosal ulcerative colitis. Ann Surg. 1981;193:9–14.
74. Bozdech J, Petras R, Farmer R. Low-grade dysplasia in ulcerative colitis: its association with the development of carcinoma. Am J Gastroenterol. 1990;85:1272.
75. Craft CF, Mendelson G, Cooper HS, Yardley JH. Colonic 'precancer' in Crohn's disease. Gastroenterology. 1981;80: 578–84.
76. Shorter RG. Risk of intestinal cancer in Crohn's disease. Dis Colon Rectum. 1983;26:686–90.
77. Dickinson RJ, Ashon MG, Axon ATR *et al*. Controlled trial of intravenous hyperalimentation and total bowel rest as an adjunct to the routine therapy of acute colitis. Gastroenterology. 1980;79:1199–204.
78. Truelove SC, Willoughby CP, Lee FG *et al*. Further experience in the treatment of severe attacks of ulcerative colitis. Lancet. 1978;4:1086–8.
79. Oakley JR, Lavery IC, Fazio VW *et al*. The fate of the rectal stump after subtotal colectomy for ulcerative colitis. Dis Colon Rectum. 1985;28:394–6.
80. Hyman NH, Fazio VW, Tuckson WB, Lavery IC. The consequences of ileal pouch anal anastomosis for Crohn's colitis. Dis Colon Rectum. 1991;34:653–7.
81. Fazio VW, Harford F, Farmer RG. Total parenteral nutrition for Crohn's disease: a role as primary therapy. Ital J Gastroenterol. 1979;11:80–5.
82. Galandiuk S, O'Neill M, McDonald P, Fazio VW, Steiger E. A century of home parenteral nutrition for Crohn's disease. Am J Surg. 1990;159:540–5.

29

Prognostic factors in predicting the clinical course of inflammatory bowel disease

A. RAEDLER and S. SCHREIBER

Prognostic criteria have to fulfil two major expectations:

1. Forecasting the course of the disease in a defined population by providing data on the predictive relevance and incidence of complications and events in the natural course of disease.
2. Helping to determine the individual outlook of a single patient by giving the likelihood by which certain signs predict the development of defined events in the course of the disease (i.e. relapse).

Prognostic criteria have been searched for in a host of chronic disorders and have been regarded as particularly important to predict *mortality, morbidity,* and *complications* of the disease.

Mortality has been shown not to be increased in inflammatory bowel disease patients in comparison with the normal population. In contrast to earlier reports, in the past decade no significant excess mortality has been observed in Crohn's disease or ulcerative colitis. This development is probably due to an enhancement of surgical and conservative therapeutical strategies, in particular in the management of disease complications[1,2].

The prediction of disease *morbidity,* in particular of relapses, in patients with Crohn's disease has been of great interest in recent years. Brignola and co-workers[3] showed that a relapse in the near future was preceded by an increase in acid α_1-glycoprotein, α_2-globulin serum levels and ESR, whereas those patients remaining in remission maintained normal levels. Brignola and co-workers calculated a clinical prognostic score based on these three parameters, which they used to distinguish two groups of patients with a different clinical course of the disease regarding the development of an acute relapse[3]. In their patient population the authors could see only a small overlap between the groups. A similar score based on Crohn's disease activity index values, orosomucoid and α_1-antitrypsin serum concentrations has been proposed by Wright and co-workers[4] to predict relapse in Crohn's disease. De Boer Visser and co-workers investigated symptoms predictive of the patient's need of early hospitalization after the onset of acute Crohn's disease[5]. The authors reported that the presence of an abdominal mass, a raised body temperature, a pathological lymphocyte count, elevated serum urea levels and increased transferase activity were predictive of an adverse clinical course requiring earlier and longer hospital stays. Markowitz and co-workers evaluated rectal biopsies by pathohistological criteria, and found that the degree of inflammation seen would be of predictive significance for the clinical severity of the initial presentation of paediatric Crohn's disease[6]. Moreover, the presence of granulomas was reported to be associated with a poor clinical outcome[6]. The confirmation of this hypothesis, that certain laboratory parameters would be highly predictive for the occurrence of relapses, would be of great importance for treatment strategies, and requires further evaluation in a larger number of patients.

In ulcerative colitis the extent and development of disease activity can be assessed much more easily by endoscopy. Therefore, the development of prognostic scores to determine the clinical course of acute relapses is less important for the management of these patients. Of great interest, however, are the life habits probably inducing relapses and factors predicting the need for a colectomy. Leo and co-workers reported that a fibre-poor diet, frequent episodes of relapses and the presence of extraintestinal manifestations were associated with increased disease activity[7]. Most attempts to characterize a subgroup of patients by clinical parameters, which require colectomy at a later time, did fail[1,8].

Major *complications* in Crohn's disease are the development of abscesses, stenoses, episodes of acute colonic bleeding and fistulae. The occurrence of these complications is frequently the cause for surgical interventions. Kruis and co-workers showed that the presence of fistulae was associated to a high degree with malnutrition of the patient, high disease activity and certain localization of the disease[9]. A host of predictive parameters have been described, which are associated with the need for early surgical intervention. Markowiecz and co-workers divided their patient population into groups using haemoglobulin levels, serum albumin concentrations, height of the ESR and localization of the disease as discriminating criteria[10]. The authors reported that an early ileocolitis, together with anaemia, hypoalbuminaemia and an increased ESR, were associated with an aggressive course of the disease requiring early surgical intervention. Farmer and co-workers emphasized that Crohn's ileocolitis is compared to other localizations of the disease most frequently associated with an early need for abdominal surgery, in particular for lower gastrointestinal bleeding[11]. Factors predicting long intervals between surgical interventions are high age, a long interval between onset of symptoms and diagnosis, and an isolated localization of Crohn's disease in either colon or ileum[12]. Following surgical intervention, recurrence of inflammation is dependent on disease localization[13]. Griffiths and co-workers reported that Crohn's ileocolitis is the localization most frequently associated with a postoperative recurrence[13]. Moreover, Rutgeerts and co-workers convincingly demonstrated that colonoscopic lesions appearing early after resections are important predictors for a clinical relapse[14].

In ulcerative colitis, the extent of inflammation is correlated to the colectomy rate, which is highest in patients with pancolitis[15,16]. However, the extent of the disease is not associated with the likelihood of relapse after remission[15,16].

In contrast to the prediction of the course of the disease and the occurrence of complications in a study population, the forecast of complications and relapses in an individual patient is a great problem. No predictive parameters could be sufficiently established to justify prophylactic therapeutic interventions. Disease activity is poorly correlated to laboratory parameters, clinical indices and even to histological and endoscopic appearance[17,18]. State of health and, moreover, quality of life, is not dependent on the clinical activity of the disease as the sole determinant but is also influenced by coping capacity, psychological background, occurrence of stressful life events, and degree of social support. As long as no widely accepted definitions for clinical disease activity are available, and as long as our therapeutic approaches modulate symptoms rather than cure the cause of the disease, prognostic factors seem to be of limited value.

References

1. Hendriksen C, Binder V, Kreiner S. Long term prognosis in ulcerative colitis. Gut. 1985;26:158–63.
2. Binder V, Hendriksen C, Kreiner S. Prognosis in Crohn's disease. Gut. 1985;26:145–50.
3. Brignola C, Campieri M, Bazzochi G, Faruggia P, Tragnone A, Lanfranchi GA. A laboratory index for predicting relapse in asymptomatic patients with Crohn's disease. Gastroenterology. 1986;91:1490–4.
4. Wright JP, Young GO, Tygler-Wybrandi N. Predictors of acute relapse of Crohn's disease. Dig Dis Sci. 1987;32:164–70.
5. De Boer Visser N, Bryant HE, Hershfield NB. Predictors of hospitalization early in the course of Crohn's disease. Gastroenterology. 1990;99:380–5.
6. Markowitz J, Kahn E, Daum F. Prognostic significance of epithelial granulomas found in rectosigmoid biopsies at the initial presentation of pediatric Crohn's disease. J Pediatr Gastroenterol Nutr. 1989;9:182–6.
7. Leo S, Leandro G, Matteo GD, Caruso ML, Lorusso D. Ulcerative colitis in remission: is it possible to predict the risk of relapse? Digestion. 1989;44:217–21.
8. Leijonmarck CE, Persson PG, Hellers G. Factors affecting colectomy rate in ulcerative colitis: an epidemiologic study. Gut. 1990;31:329–33.
9. Kruis W, Scheuchenstein AM, Scheurlen C, Wenzierl M. Risikofaktoren für die Entstehung von Fisteln bei Morbus Crohn. Z Gastroenterol. 1989;6:313–16.
10. Markowiecz F, Starlinger M, Jenss H, Jehle E, Becker H-D. Prognostische Faktoren bei Morbus Crohn. Dtsch med Wochenschr. 1991;116:961–7.
11. Farmer RG. Lower gastrointestinal bleeding in inflammatory disease. Gastroenterol Jpn. 1991;26:93–100.
12. Basilisco G, Campanini M, Cesana B, Ranzi T, Bianchi P. Risk factors for first operation in Crohn's disease. Am J Gastroenterol. 1989;84:148–51.
13. Griffiths AM, Wesson DE, Shanding B, Corey M, Sherman PM. Factors influencing postoperative recurrence of Crohn's disease in childhood. Gut. 1991;32:491–5.

14. Rutgeerts P, Geboes K, VanTrappen G, Beyls J, Kerremans R, Hiele M. Predictability of the postoperative course of Crohn's disease. Gastroenterology. 1990;99:956–63.
15. Chawla LS, Chinna JS, Dilawari JB, Sood A. Course and prognosis of ulcerative colitis. J Indian Med Assoc. 1990;88:159–60.
16. Brostroem O. Prognosis in ulcerative colitis. Med Clin N Am. 1990;74:201–18.
17. Riley SA, Mani V, Goodman MJ, Dutt S, Herd ME. Microscopic activity in ulcerative colitis: what does it mean? Gut. 1991;32:174–8.
18. Mary JY, Modigliani R. Development and validation of an endoscopic index of the severity for Crohn's disease: a prospective multicentre study. Gut. 1989;30:983–9.

30
Inflammatory bowel disease: the diagnostic approach

B. LEMBCKE

In general, diagnosis may be defined as the sum of all relevant information concerning aetiology and actual course of a disease, its therapy, prognosis, complications, and prevention of recurrence. The diagnostic approach should thus allow sufficient characterization and understanding of the patient in his (her) disease. This is of particular importance in the case of chronic diseases, e.g. inflammatory bowel disease (IBD), with fluctuating inflammatory activity and a variety of complications resulting in diverse individual problems.

Ideally, Crohn's disease and ulcerative colitis have a clearly distinguished clinical presentation with diarrhoea, abdominal pain, weight loss, fatigue, bleeding, anorexia, fever, signs of inflammation and fistulae/perianal disease in Crohn's disease, and diarrhoea with blood and mucus, urgency, pain after defaecation, and anaemia in ulcerative colitis.

DIAGNOSTIC APPROACH IN ULCERATIVE COLITIS

Diagnostic activities in ulcerative colitis are aimed at establishing the diagnosis, extent of disease, its activity, and potential complications.

History plays an important role in this work-up and should include information on the patient's age; recent visits to foreign countries; potential infection with the human immunodeficiency virus (HIV); previous radiation; intake of prescribed (and non-prescribed) drugs, especially of antibiotics and NSAIDs; onset of symptoms and IBD among relatives.

In most instances, ischaemic colitis may be ruled out on the basis of age and known atherosclerosis, foregoing dialysis or a period of prostrated hypotension (e.g. in a case of myocardial infarction), a sharp onset of abdominal symptoms with subsequent quiescence (a period during which objective findings are very sparse but progressively deteriorating clinical status), segmental disease with a cutoff at the splenic flexure, painful barium enema, and characteristic 'thumbprints' either on plain abdominal films or after barium (Fig. 1).

Radiation colitis is mainly differentiated by the history of therapeutic radiation (which may have been more than 20 years ago!), and, at endoscopy, sometimes a bizarre branching of the mucosal vessels in addition to abnormal friability.

Pseudomembranous colitis will be recognized by the typical endoscopic

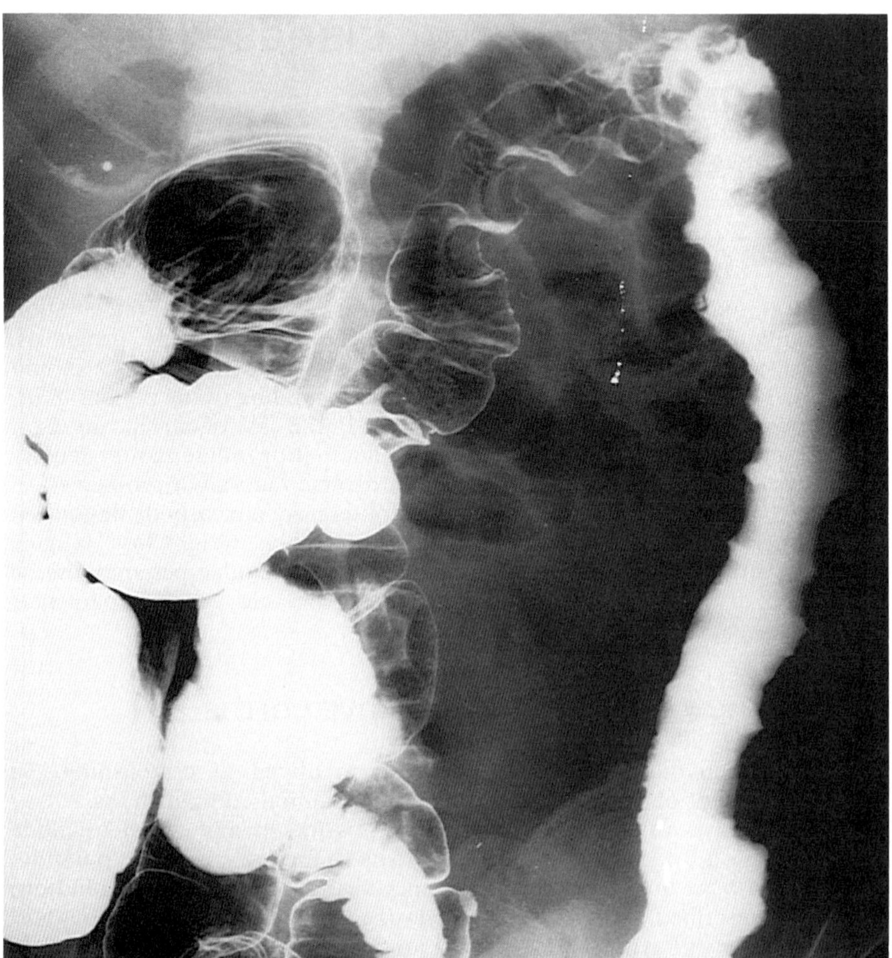

Fig. 1 Barium enema in ischaemic colitis. Thumbprints (intramural oedema and haematomas) narrowing the colonic lumen indicate ischaemia at the level of the inferior mesenteric artery. The patient improved without operation

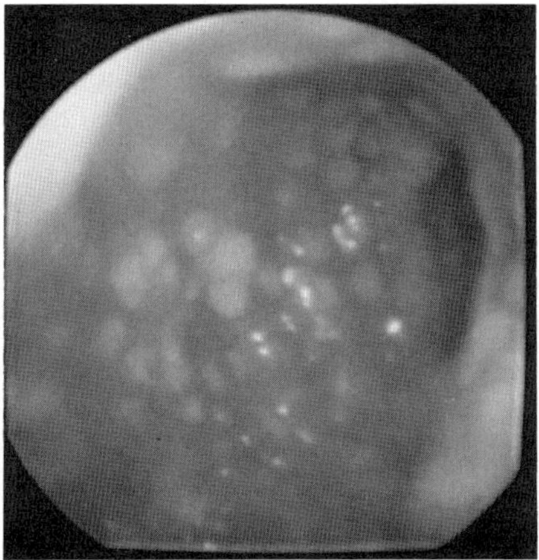

Fig. 2 Pseudomembranous colitis (cottage cheese-like pseudomembranes) due to *Clostridium difficile* toxin

aspect (Fig. 2) and the detection of *Clostridium difficile* in the stool by culture, or of one of their toxins (mostly toxin B) by means of a cytotoxin assay, while sigmoidal diverticulitis again will be demonstrable on endoscopy, colonic barium enema, or non-invasively during abdominal ultrasonography with a 5 MHz linear or curved-array transducer which allows detection of muscular hypertrophy, narrowing of the neck of the diverticulum, and of peridiverticular inflammation or abscess. Ultrasonography thereby enables distinguishing (peri-)diverticulitis from ulcerative colitis (Fig. 3a,b), which – in the case of severe inflammation – leads to a broadened mucosal layer with normal submucosal and muscular layers (Fig. 3b).

Sometimes endoscopy allows one to arrive at a presumptive diagnosis of intestinal infection with *Yersinia enterocolitica* (Fig. 4), but factors other than the mucosal aspect alone (e.g. in this particular patient the rather acute time-course of disease) will help to distinguish this from IBD. In the majority of cases, however, infectious colitis appears endoscopically indistinguishable from idiopathic IBD and stool and/or serological tests need to be repeated for potential pathogens including *Campylobacter* species, *Salmonella*, *Shigella* species, *Chlamydia*, giardiasis, *Yersinia enterocolitica* and pseudotuberculosis as well as the human immunodeficiency virus[1,2]. In special instances, e.g. after a stay in countries/areas with low standards of hygiene, additional aetiologies such as amoebiasis or ileocolonic tuberculosis must be considered. In difficult cases with atypical response to treatment, subtle cultures of mucosal biopsies are recommended for the detection of potential pathogens.

Basically, in ulcerative colitis the primary diagnostic work-up may be considered complete when the aforementioned infected aetiologies are appropriately excluded and characteristic findings of ulcerative colitis are obtained at procto-sigmoidoscopy (Table 1) or colonoscopy including biopsies for histology. Endoscopy is appropriate when the extent of disease can be clearly defined, not only by endoscopy but also by multiple biopsies obtained stepwise from both the endoscopically diseased and non-diseased

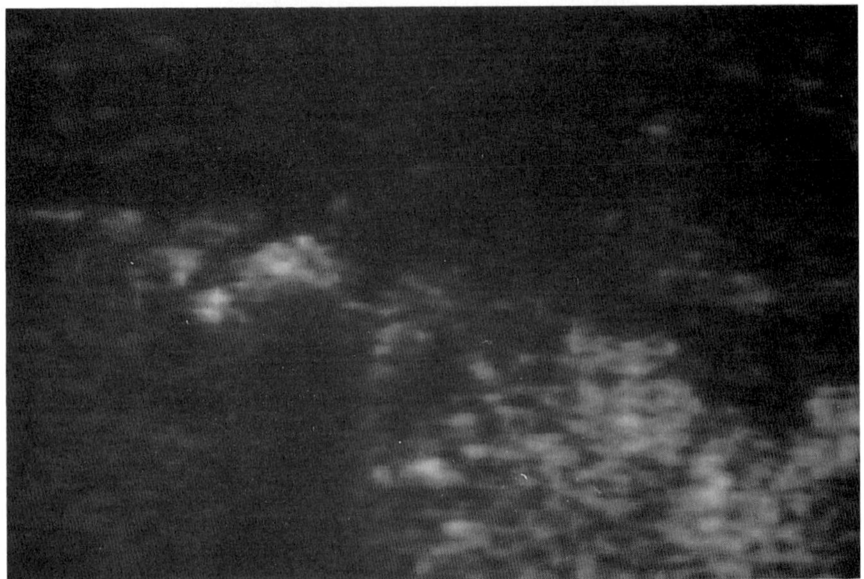

(a)

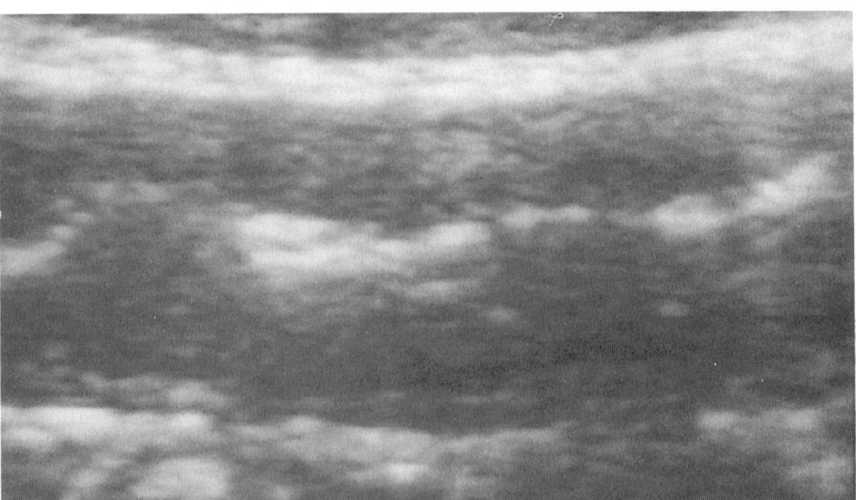

(b)

Fig. 3 (a) 5 MHz ultrasonography of diverticulitis complicating diverticular disease. The bright echo-cap is due to air in the diverticulum, showing an air-filled, narrow neck as a sequel to substantial hypertrophy of the muscular layer. The air-filled diverticulum (and another one at its right) are surrounded by a thin hypoechoic layer (inflamed mucosa) and a broad hyperechoic mesenteral structure. (b) Very severe form of ulcerative colitis: 5 MHz ultrasonographic image of the descending colon showing a wavy and broadened hypoechoic mucosal layer followed by a thin hyperechoic submucosa and a thin muscular layer. Regarding ultrasonographical morphology, Figs 3a and 3b cannot be confused

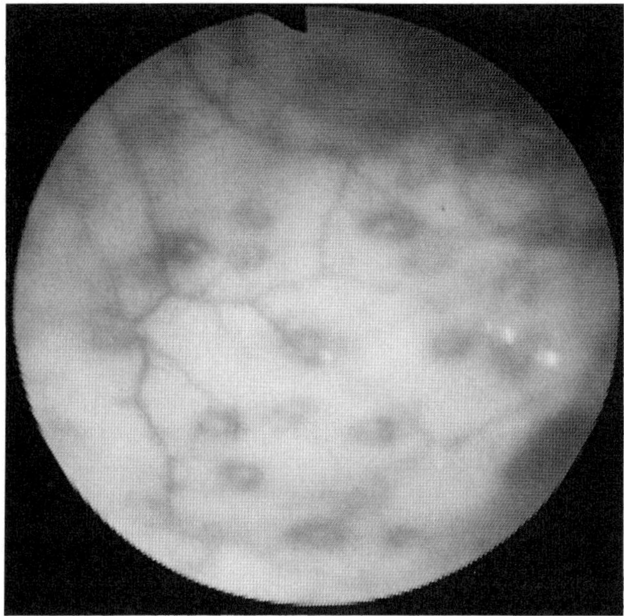

Fig. 4 Small superficial (aphthous) lesions with hyperaemic margins (so-called lymph follicle cockades) in *Yersinia* enterocolitis

mucosa. Thus proctosigmoidoscopy can be sufficient in cases with distal ulcerative colitis or proctitis only, and total colonoscopy is required if inflammation spreads beyond the splenic flexure.

For the diagnostic approach in ulcerative colitis, radiological examination is considered of lower priority than endoscopic methods because (a) the rectum is both easily and conveniently assessed by flexible proctosigmoidoscopy,

Table 1 Endoscopic differential diagnosis of ulcerative colitis and Crohn's disease

	Ulcerative colitis	*Crohn's disease*
Rectal involvement	+ + +	+
Continuous inflammation	+ + +	+
Symmetrical inflammation	+ + +	+
Friability	+ + +	+
Granularity	+ + +	+
Ileal ulcers	0	+ + + +
Aphthoid ulcers	0	+ + + +
Discrete ulcers	+	+ + +
Ulcers > 1 cm	+	+ + +
Linear ulcers	+	+ + +
Deep ulcers	+	+ +

0 = does not occur; + + + + = diagnostic feature
Adapted from Hogan *et al.*[3]

whereas sufficient radiological evaluation requires a subtle double-contrast technique; and (b) the earliest lesions detected by X-ray are discrete erosions with mucosal oedema corresponding to the endoscopic feature of granularity, but milder forms of inflammation (erythema, loss of vascular pattern) are not accessible to radiology. (c) Segmental disease with strictures and local complications requiring emphasis on topographical distribution of the lesions is atypical in ulcerative colitis compared to Crohn's disease.

Endoscopic features will usually help to distinguish ulcerative colitis from Crohn's disease (Table 1). However, it should be emphasized that about 10–20% of IBD patients initially cannot be classified as having either Crohn's disease or ulcerative colitis by history and physical findings, endoscopy with biopsy, radiology and bacteriological tests. This 'indeterminate' colitis may be further clarified with time.

Currently, there is also still no valid and convenient serological test for ulcerative colitis. A recently proposed assay of p-ANCA (antineutrophil cytoplasmic antibody with a perinuclear pattern) gave promising results in some (but not in all) patients if the experience of different groups is combined. Moreover, this is not yet a routine method for the clinical laboratory.

For assessing the extent of the disease, again endoscopic and radiological methods may be applied. If radiology instead of total ileocolonoscopy is considered necessary or preferential, a double-contrast barium enema technique is mandatory.

The more proximal parts of the colon are involved, the higher is the rate of an initially severe attack of ulcerative colitis (Table 2); however, frequency distribution shows that convenient proctoscopy or proctosigmoidoscopy will suffice in the majority of patients.

In very severe attacks it is wise to postpone total colonoscopy until some remission is achieved. The term 'severe attack' refers to the classification of Truelove and Witts[5] (see Table 3), which is based on stool frequency, the occurrence of blood, increased body temperature, pulse rate, haemoglobin and the 1 h ESR. Severity of activity, however, may also be assessed by means of endoscopy showing erythema, unsharp vessels (Fig. 5a), a velvet-like and friable mucosa, granularity, purulent exudation, and spontaneous petechiae or frank ulcerations and profuse bleeding (Fig. 5b).

Initial examination of the patient with suspected ulcerative colitis will be influenced by the clinical situation, since extensive and invasive diagnostic procedures may be useless on one hand and unfavourable or harmful on the other. Especially if initial presentation of ulcerative colitis occurs with

Table 2 Frequency of severe inflammatory attack in relation to the extent of disease at the time of initial diagnosis in patients with ulcerative colitis

Extent of disease	Percentage of patients	Incidence of severe attack (%)
Rectum	38	12.5
Left colon	40	37.3
Total colon	22	50.2

Adapted from Watts et al.[4]

Table 3 Criteria for assessment of disease activity in ulcerative colitis

Factor	Mild	Moderate	Severe
Bowel frequency	<4/day	4–6/day	⩾6/day
Blood in stool	±	+	+ +
Temperature	normal	intermediate	>37.7°C on 2 of 4 days
Pulse rate	normal	intermediate	>90/min
Haemoglobin	>10.5 g/dl (75%)	intermediate	⩽10.5 g/dl
ESR/1 h	⩽30/1 h		>30/1 h

Adapted from Truelove and Witts[5]

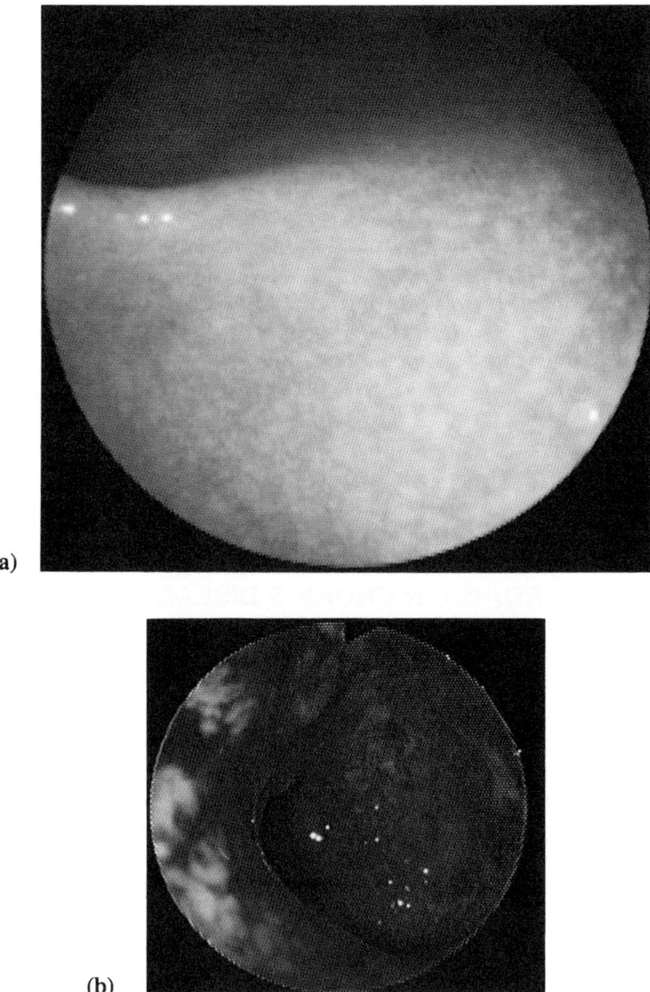

Fig. 5 (a) Velvet-like mucosal aspect of mild ulcerative proctitis. (b) Frank bleeding from the sigmoid colon in severe ulcerative colitis

Table 4 Characteristics of toxic megacolon

Radiographic distension of the transverse colon >5.5 cm; loss of normal haustral pattern

Tenderness/rebound tenderness at the colonic frame, diminished bowel sounds

In addition to

3 of 4 'inflammatory' signs $(+)$ve and	1 of 4 'toxicity' signs $(+)$ve
Fever $>38.6°$C	Dehydration
Pulse rate >120/min	Mental changes
Leucocytes $>10500/\mu$l	Electrolyte disturbance
Anaemia	Hypotension

Adapted from Jalan *et al.*[6]

developing or manifest toxic megacolon, reiterative sophisticated physical examination should be applied in close counselling with the surgeon, making use of plain abdominal X-ray and ultrasonography in addition to vital laboratory tests (haemoglobin, leucocytes, albumin, K^+, ESR), whereas enemas and intensive endoscopic investigations should be carefully avoided.

A toxic megacolon is characterized by air-filled, dilated loops of the colon (>5.5 cm at the transverse colon) with a loss of haustrae on plain abdominal X-ray, tenderness on abdominal palpation and quiescence during auscultation, and the presence of additional symptoms (given in Table 6).

Rarely, ulcerative colitis presents first with a typical associated complication, i.e. primary sclerosing cholangitis (PSC). These patients usually have a cholestasis syndrome. In about 80%, however, symptoms of ulcerative colitis precede those of the PSC. Overall, PSC complicates ulcerative colitis in 4–5.5%, accounting for 81% of cholestasis syndromes in ulcerative colitis[7]. Therefore, endoscopic cholangiography (ERCP) must be considered in any patient with IBD with a cholestasis syndrome while percutaneous liver biopsy is diagnostic in a minor proportion of patients only.

DIAGNOSTIC APPROACH IN CROHN'S DISEASE

Concerning Crohn's disease, diagnostic goals do not differ from those in ulcerative colitis. Similarly, having ruled out other conditions by laboratory tests for infectious diseases, a reliable diagnosis can usually be made by clinical criteria in conjunction with endoscopy or radiology. Sometimes, initial presentation includes primary operation, usually for appendicectomy. In contrast to a very conservative view, personal experience does not go against ileocaecectomy in this situation if substantial segmental inflammation or complications (e.g. narrowing) are present.

Laparotomy with biopsy or resection usually substantially improves pathological confirmation of the diagnosis. At present the Lennard-Jones criteria (Table 5), in conjunction with the exclusion of other aetiologies of IBD, are still the valid clinical mainstay to establish the diagnosis of Crohn's disease[8]. The presence of granulomas thus plays an important role, but it is well acknowledged that they are not specific for Crohn's disease and will be detected in some 40% or less of patients with Crohn's disease only.

Table 5 Criteria for Crohn's disease according to Lennard-Jones et al.[8]

A. Radiological, endoscopic or operative criteria
   1. Discontinuous disease
   2. Ileal involvement
   3. Deep mucosal fissures
B. Enterocutaneous involvement
   4. Enterocutaneous fistula
   5. Chronic anal disease
C. Histological findings
   6. Normal mucus content of goblet cells in inflamed mucosa
   7. Mucosal and submucosal lymphoid aggregates

Three positive criteria indicate Crohn's disease if other aetiologies are excluded, but one positive criterion is sufficient if a non-caseating granuloma is present

Differential diagnosis again will mainly rely on the exclusion of infectious and vascular diseases, as discussed above. Exclusion of Behçet's disease can be difficult[2], because other lesions (e.g. CMV ulcerations) may look very similar. Nowadays, in any case with clinically or endoscopically suspected IBD, immunoincompetence and HIV infection must be ruled out. Clinical presentation with a 'signum ab igne' or a palpable or even visible mass in the ileocaecal region, or the presence of either erythema nodosum or pyoderma gangrenosum, which occur mainly in patients with colonic disease, may give hints for localization or activity of Crohn's disease, but they have to be substantiated by other investigations such as ultrasonography, small bowel enteroclysis, colonic double-contrast examination or colonoscopy.

Initial work-up and diagnosis of Crohn's disease should include upper gastrointestinal endoscopy, a small bowel radiology series, and ileocolonoscopy with serial biopsies, both of inflamed and apparently normal mucosa. Upper gastrointestinal endoscopy detects Crohn's lesions in about 15% of patients (0.5% oesophagus, 6% stomach, 4.5% duodenum). Whether or not colonoscopy is replaced by radiological methods (double-contrast) is rather influenced by secondary criteria (availability of a careful and experienced endoscopist or, vice-versa, radiologist; patient's constraints) than a principal decision. Usually we undoubtedly prefer colonoscopy (allowing us to confirm the diagnosis by histology in addition to the visualization of mucosal damage), unless the question of fistulae or the dynamic significance of stenosing segments are of priority.

Typical radiological signs of advanced Crohn's disease of the small bowel include segmentation with asymmetry, narrowing ('string sign') and pseudosacculation[9] (Bodart's triad; Fig. 6) and a 'cobblestone' aspect in the terminal ileum. These correspond to the histological hallmark of Crohn's disease, e.g. transmural, segmental, and disproportionate inflammation. Since these criteria, as well as ileal involvement and deep mucosal fissures (group A criteria of Lennard-Jones 15 years ago), but also histological features such as lymphoid aggregates in the submucosa and external to the muscularis propria are well demonstrable by abdominal ultrasonography (if a 5 or 7.5 MHz linear or curved-array transducer is used and the examination is performed by a sonographically and clinically experienced physician), ultrasonography tends to become more and more important not only for

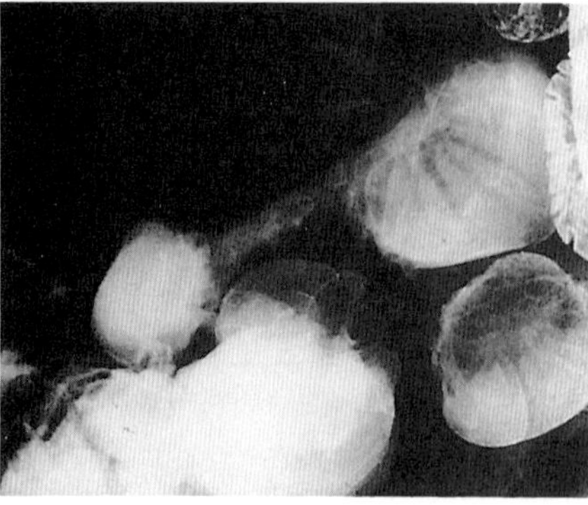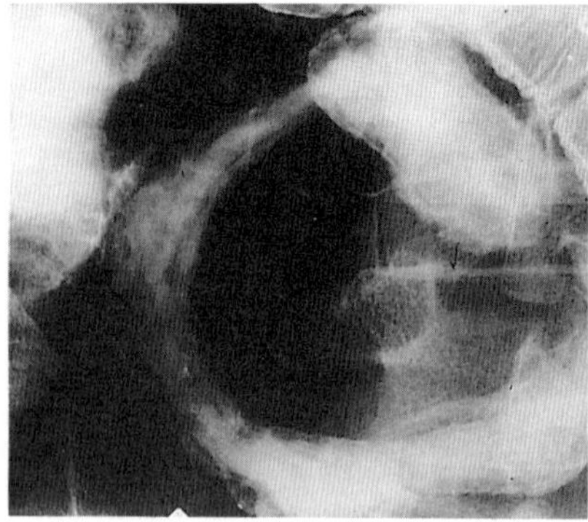

Fig. 6 Radiological aspect of chronic fibrotic small bowel Crohn's disease with a narrow segment and asymmetric pseudosacculations

surveillance of IBD but also for initial diagnosis[10]. This development has preferentially occurred in those countries where ultrasonography has achieved high quality and a high clinical impact, and thus is considered the 'second step of physical examination'.

Figure 7a shows a longitudinal section of the ileocaecal junction in chronic stenosing Crohn's disease (corresponding to the string sign), and Fig. 7b gives a transverse section of the caecum with broad, fibrotic submucosal 'pillows' corresponding to the radiological (luminal) aspect of cobblestones, covered by a thin and sharply delineated (non-inflammatory) mucosal layer.

The longitudinal extent of Crohn's disease may be investigated by testing specialized functions of the ileum (malabsorption of conjugated bile acids ($[^{14}C]$cholylglycine breath test, $[^{75}Se]$HCAT test) or diminished liberation of diaminoxidase activity (DAO) in response to heparin if the terminal ileum is inflamed, and malabsorption of $[^{57}Co]$cyanocobalamin (Schilling test with intrinsic factor) if $>100\,cm$ of the ileum are involved). However, this will rarely play a major role during initial diagnosis. Usually the extent of disease is estimated with reference to endoscopy (plus biopsy) or radiological methods. Among these, the double-contrast technique (Sellink) will give a more precise measure of small intestine involvement; however, advanced fibrotic shrinkage may lead to an underestimation of true functional impairment, and in these patients function tests may be of clinical significance.

Recent studies have demonstrated that ultrasonography is another valid method for assessing the extent of Crohn's disease correctly in 89–100%, but results are more favourable in ileocolonic, ileal and colonic disease than in patients with rectal or small intestinal involvement alone[11].

Ultrasonography, however, is the most useful tool for examination of the transverse section of the gut wall, and therefore represents a unique complementary parameter for either endoscopy or radiology (see Fig. 7a,b).

Characteristic features of Crohn's disease are the discontinuous, disproportional and transmural character of inflammation as opposed to the continuous, proportional and mucosal lesion in ulcerative colitis. Thus, apart

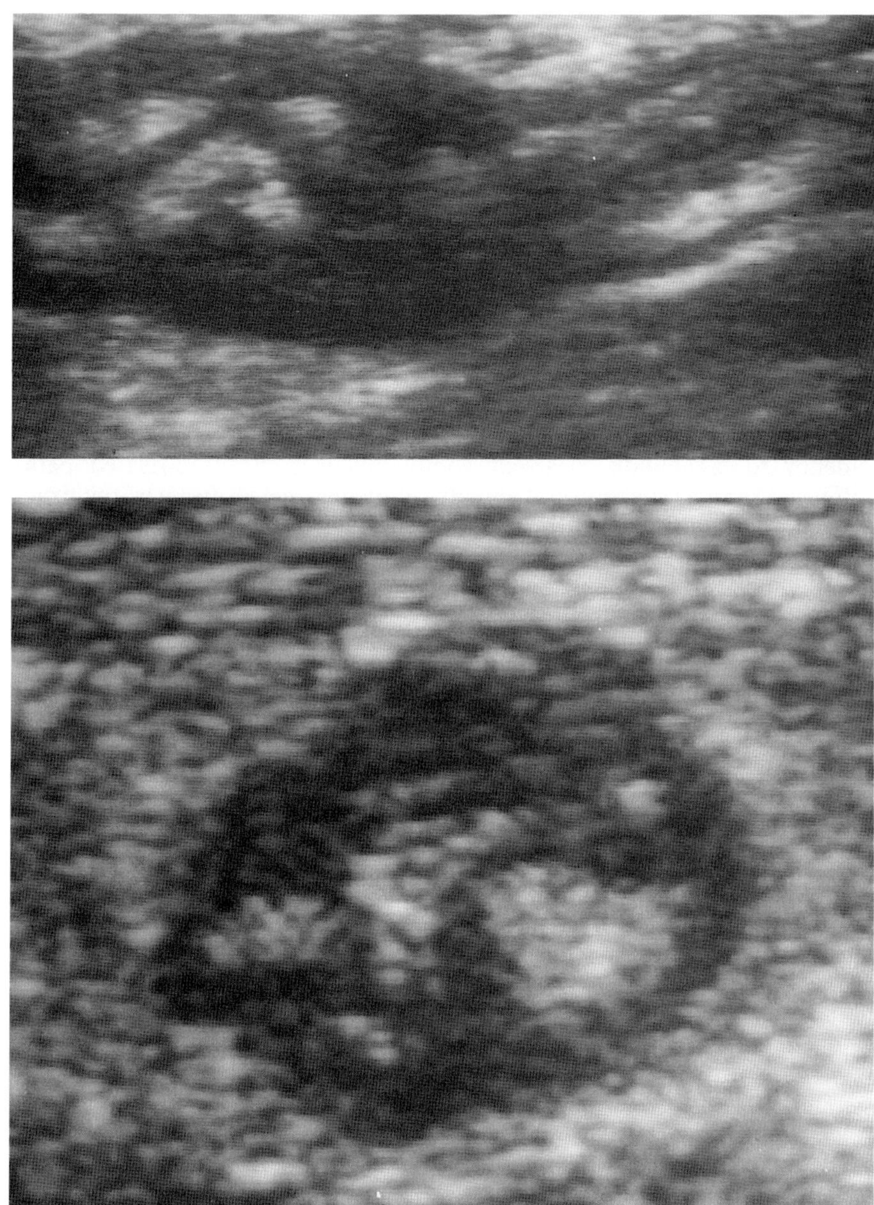

Fig. 7 (a) High-resolution ultrasonography of chronic fibrotic Crohn's disease. Longitudinal section of the shrunken ileocaecal region. There is only a narrow residual lumen surrounded by a thin but variable, well-delineated hypoechoic mucosal layer. Broadened hyperechoic submucosal layer, both in the terminal ileum (right) and the caecum (left). (b) Cross-section of the caecum with the pillow-like broadened asymmetric fibrosing submucosa, covered with a sharply delineated (non-inflammatory) mucosal layer

from imaging intestinal complications (fissures, fistulae (Fig. 8)), interenteric abscess, free peritoneal fluid accumulation, ileus, stenosis, inflammatory mass) and extraintestinal complications of Crohn's disease (nephrolithiasis, cholelithiasis, hydronephrosis, thrombosis of the iliac vein), ultrasonography may significantly and directly contribute to the understanding of the transverse aspect of inflammation and fibrotic healing with – in my experience – distinct patterns in inflamed and fibrotic segments. The series of ileal and colonic cross-sections in Fig. 9a,b and 9c–e reflects the different pattern of ultrasonography in different activity states of Crohn's disease.

Concerning activity of Crohn's disease, activity-dependent clinical symptoms such as gangrenous pyoderma, erythema nodosum, a variety of indices, laboratory parameters, excretion tests and imaging methods should be discussed.

In general, the well-known but less commonly used battery of activity indices (CDAI, van Hees, Harvey–Bradshaw and OMGE index, St Marks AI, SAI, prognostic index) are principally considered useful, although difficulties may arise from interobserver variability, practicability and a tendency to 'assimilate' clear-cut complaints (e.g. stricture-related pain) within a less precise score, not directly allowing one to discover the exact meaning of a high score to the patient and to the physician[12].

The most widely accepted indices are the Crohn's disease activity index (CDAI) and the more convenient Harvey–Bradshaw index (either as originally described or in the OMGE (Organisation Mondiale de Gastro-enterologie) modification) which requires a one-time evaluation of symptoms only (CDAI: 7 day-evaluation period)[13].

However, it should be recalled that these activity indices (as far as this has been investigated) do not correlate with endoscopic findings of activity in Crohn's disease or with faecal [^{111}In]leucocyte extrusion (which is related to both activity and extent of disease)[14–16].

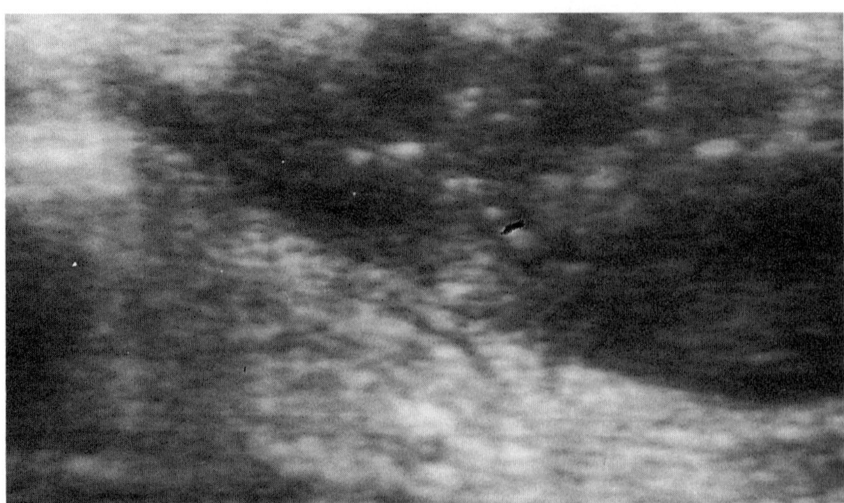

Fig. 8 Severe hypoechoic wall-thickening with apparent loss of layer differentiation, extramural effusions and a small interenteric fistula with bright air bubbles allowing easy fistula detection

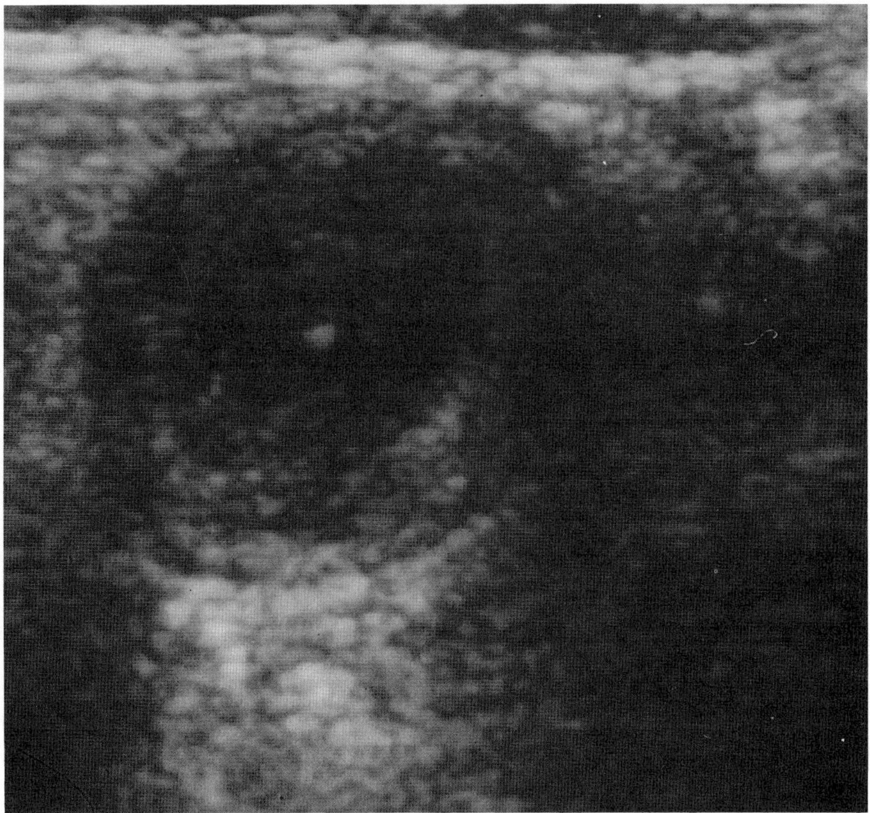

Fig. 9 (a) Cross-section of the ileum in a patient with 'hot Crohn'. The filiform residual lumen (bright reflex) is surrounded by a broad but unsharp hypoechoic mucosal layer which 'infiltrates' the submucosal layer. The muscular layer is attached to the bright (inflamed) mesenterium.

Laboratory parameters for Crohn's disease activity are affected in different ways and overall they reflect disease activity more or less well, but with some constancy in a given patient. ESR and CRP, together with serum orosomucoid, serum albumin, serum α_1- and α_2-globulins and cholinesterase activity are time-honoured, useful static laboratory parameters of Crohn's disease activity[17].

Among excretory tests, faecal α_1-antitrypsin appears to be the most valuable parameter for objectively assessing disease activity (and extent), provided the faecal α_1-antitrypsin *clearance* is measured, thereby correcting for the increase of acute-phase (α_1) proteins resulting from the inflammatory process[18]. Although faecal α_1-antitrypsin clearance is a recommendable parameter, its clinical role for assessing Crohn's disease activity is confined to difficult decisions in the management of individual patients or clinical studies, as it is also the case with ^{111}In-labelled or ^{99m}Tc-HMPAO-labelled leucocyte scintigraphy (Fig. 10).

Permeability tests, such as the double sugar ratio method using rhamnose

325

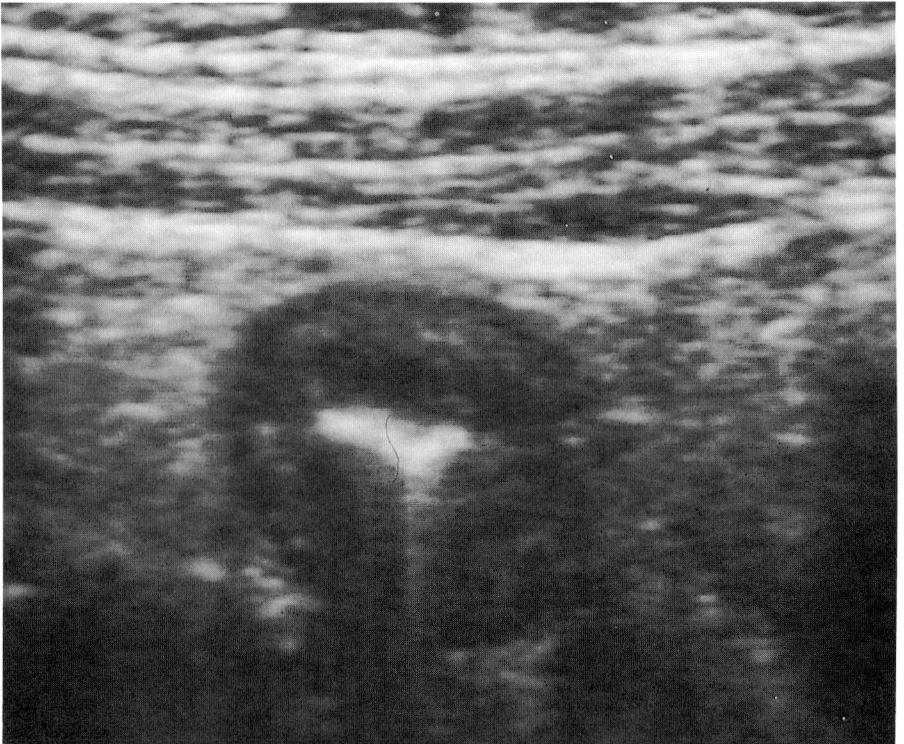

Fig. 9 (**b**) Very unsharp border zone of the ileal mucosa and submucosa; active Crohn's disease.

and lactulose as permeability markers which are recovered in the urine after oral administration, are clearly related to Crohn's disease activity, but not specific for Crohn's disease, and as a diagnostic parameter they are still premature.

Finally, endoscopy is frequently used to assess disease activity and the effect of therapy. In my opinion, however, endoscopy no longer has any justification for this purpose, since Modigliani *et al.*[15] have demonstrated virtually perfect disagreement of endoscopic and clinical scores for disease activity. Irrespectively, there are different patterns of active and suppurative (Fig. 11a), moderately active (Fig. 11b), and inactive, fibrotic Crohn's disease at endoscopy (Fig. 11c), and the findings of this Italian study group recall that our current therapy of Crohn's disease is symptomatic only. However, this study casts some doubt on the proposed anti-inflammatory action of steroid therapy in colonic Crohn's disease. This view is corroborated by Figs 9c–e, demonstrating progressive deterioration of the ileal wall at ultrasonography despite clinical remission (CDAI).

Metabolic disturbances (enteric hyperoxaluria with oxalate stones of the kidney, osteoporosis, zinc-depletion with acrodermatitis enteropathica),

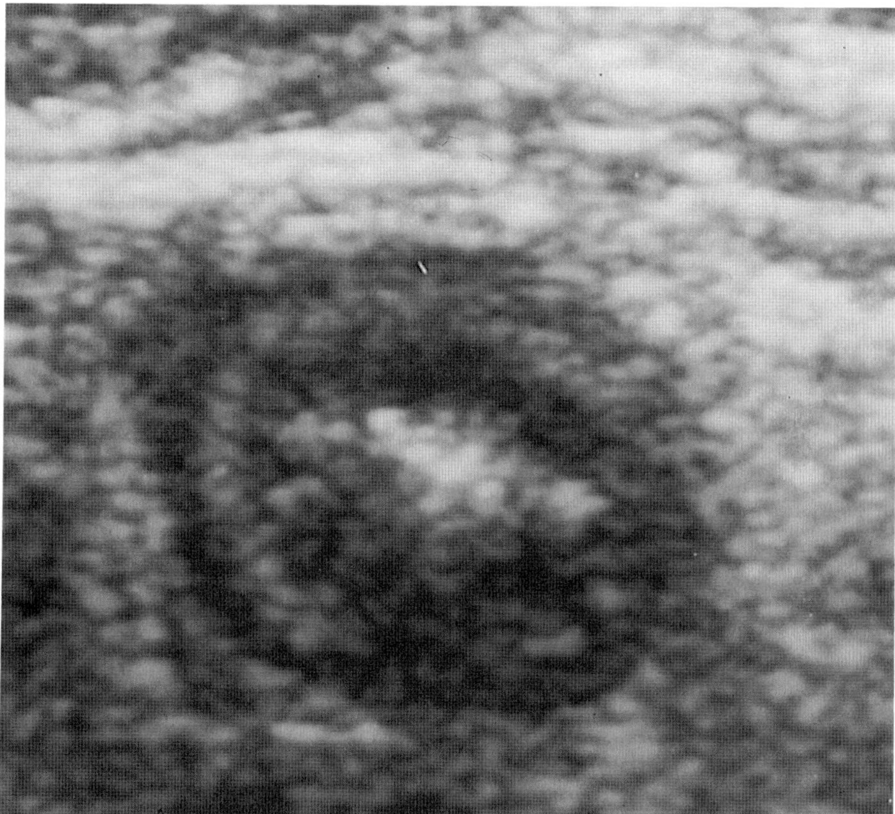

Fig. 9 (c) Active Crohn's disease of the ileum (unsharp border zone of the broadened mucosa and the submucosa) with (presumed) lymph follicular aggregation at the outside of the muscular layer (10 o'clock). Disproportionate inflammation.

various pathogenetic patterns of malabsorption (bacterial overgrowth syndrome, lactose intolerance, chologenic diarrhoea and decompensated bile acid malabsorption with steatorrhoea and diminished absorption of fat-soluble vitamins A, D, E and K, malabsorption of cyanocobalamin) and nutritional deficits (e.g. linoleic acid deficiency) may complicate Crohn's disease during the chronic intermittent course of the disease.

Since these complications usually develop slowly, and thus remain clinically silent for months and years, and since other aetiologies of disturbed bowel habits (e.g. superimposed giardiasis, recurrent inflammation) or other diseases may interfere with the clinical picture, specific and sensitive diagnostic tests are required to detect the presence and to quantitate the significance of these complications. The diagnostic approach to the patient with Crohn's disease thus is not complete, unless the physician can exclude or prove that respective symptoms are sequels to complications of Crohn's disease. However, it is neither useful nor necessary to assess all these functions in any patient with

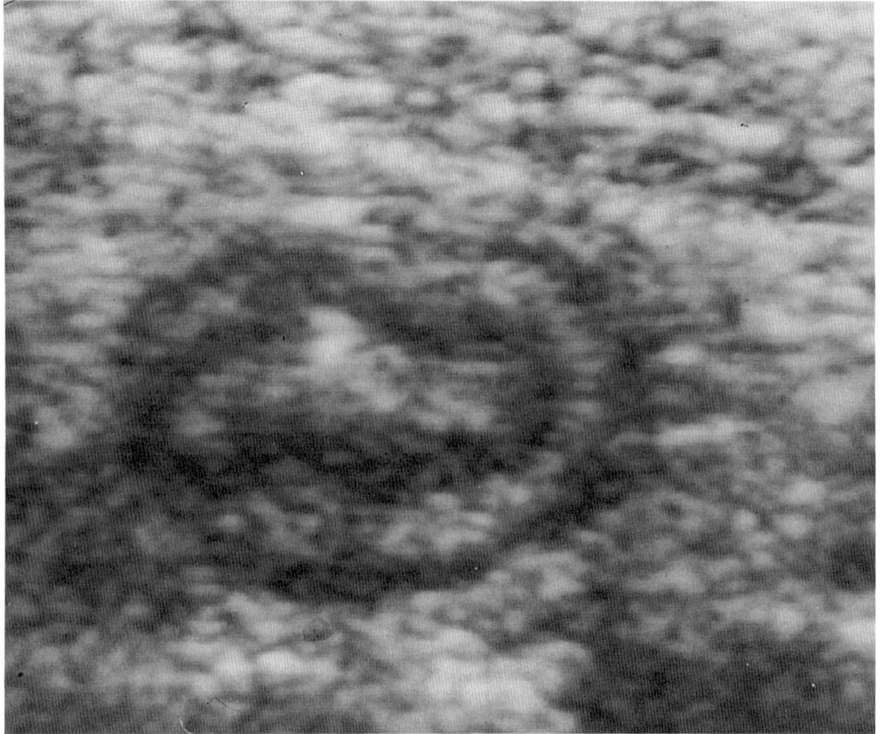

Fig. 9 **(d)** Same patient after achieving remission by steroids and elemental diet. Still disproportionate mucosal lesion, but better separation of the mucosa and submucosa.

Crohn's disease, since there are a number of risk factors indicating whether or not a patient is prone to one or other complication.

Chologenic diarrhoea (compensated bile acid malabsorption) is unlikely to occur unless >25 cm of the terminal ileum have lost their absorptive function for conjugated bile acids[19]. Diagnostic work-up includes a 72 h stool collection showing moderate diarrhoea (250–500 g/d), but no steatorrhoea, a therapeutic trial with cholestyramine (4–8 g/day) which will inevitably result in dramatic improvement of diarrhoea, and finally, as diagnostic confirmation, the demonstration of an abnormal $[^{75}Se]$HCAT- or $[^{14}C]$-cholylglycine-test. Decompensated bile acid malabsorption will occur if >50–100 cm of the ileum are involved, resulting in fatty acid malabsorption (steatorrhoea >7 g/day) which worsens during cholestyramine administration. In patients with such extensive impairment of ileal bile acid absorption, vitamin B_{12} malabsorption can almost regularly be demonstrated by means of the Schilling test (with intrinsic factor).

Ileal or extensive ileocaecal resections may aggravate the speed of developing bile acid malabsorption and its extent. Further, this is the 'classical' pathophysiological situation for developing enteric hyperoxaluria

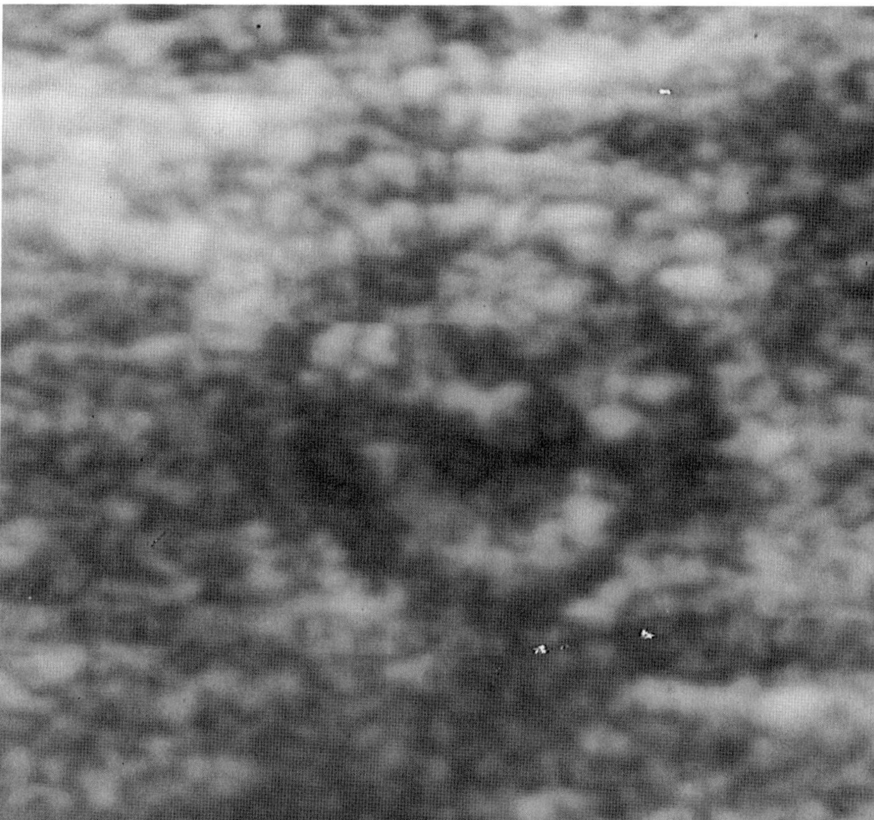

Fig. 9 **(e)** Same patient, 30 months after initial diagnosis (9c). Ultrasonography shows the progressive transmural destruction of the ileal wall with a cobblestone-like pattern of submucosal compartmentation and disproportionate broadening of the mucosa

(>35 mg/day), which is caused by the combination of increased colonic permeability for oxalic acid (effect of bile acid malabsorption) together with Ca^{2+} precipitation due to steatorrhoea (effect of fatty acid malabsorption). Thus, patients with ileocaecal disease and, more pronounced, with larger ileocaecal resections or the short bowel syndrome, are preferentially prone to develop enteric hyperoxaluria and oxalate stones of the kidneys (Table 6).

Patients developing zinc deficiency are primarily those with long-time parenteral zinc-deficient nutrition and/or extensive involvement of the small bowel and anorexia.

Lactose malabsorption rarely develops as a sequel of Crohn's disease but is present with the same prevalence as in the normal population (Germany: 10–20%). Patients with extensive resections, however, may malabsorb lactose at higher doses, whereas patients with strictures may develop a bacterial overgrowth syndrome not only resulting in diarrhoea and steatorrhoea but also causing falsely abnormal hydrogen breath tests after lactose administration.

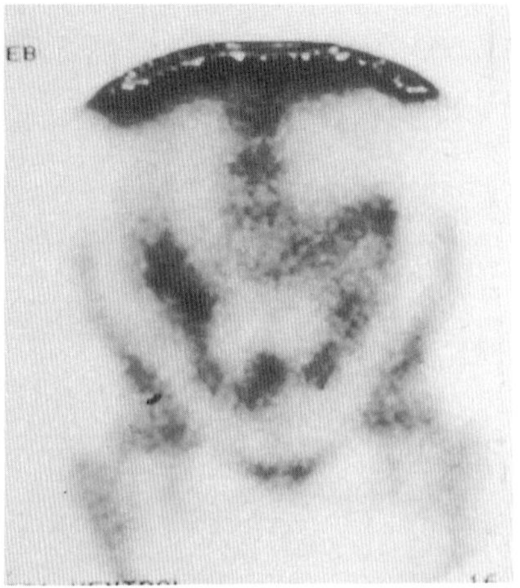
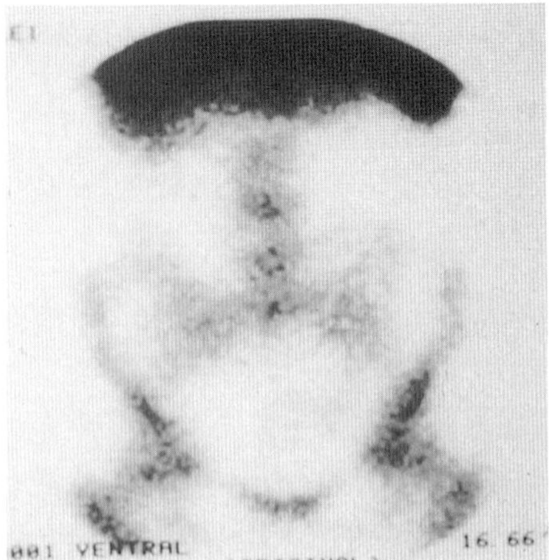

Fig. 10 ^{111}In-labelled autologous granulocytes visualize the area of inflammation in ileocolonic Crohn's disease 4 h after injection; 20 h later there is no residual ^{111}In activity in this area, indicating active Crohn's disease (sequestration of leucocytes due to active inflammation)

Since the [^{14}C]cholylglycine breath test does not differentiate bacterial overgrowth in Crohn's disease from ileal dysfunction, today the 75 g glucose H_2 breath test or the [^{13}C]D-xylose breath test are considered more appropriate.

Osteoporosis as a sequel of Crohn's disease has received increasing attention during recent years, and is now known to be a cause of considerable morbidity in these patients. Again, menopausal patients, those with long-standing steatorrhoea and malabsorption of vitamin D, with intolerance to milk (the most important nutritional source of calcium) and with continuous or frequent courses of steroid therapy and disease-related immobilization are thought to be at the highest risk of developing osteoporosis, although exact data on the respective significance of these factors are not yet available. Early diagnosis of osteoporosis in patients with Crohn's disease requires the reiterative use of highly sophisticated methods such as quantitative CT measures or radioisotope double- or triple-beam techniques, which allow detection of loss of bone mass 6–12 months after the first measurement obtained. These difficulties underscore the necessity for effective prevention of osteoporosis in Crohn's disease and, thereby, indirectly militate against unjustified dietary restriction such as avoiding milk or milk products. Similarly, except for children, nutritional deficiencies in patients with Crohn's disease hardly occur in our institution, unless peculiar dietary habits are involved.

Last, but by no means least, the physician diagnosing and treating patients with IBD should be aware of the psychological and social impact of chronic, disabling and little-understood diseases such as Crohn's disease and ulcerative colitis which may, additionally, become the cause of functional complaints and psychological complications.

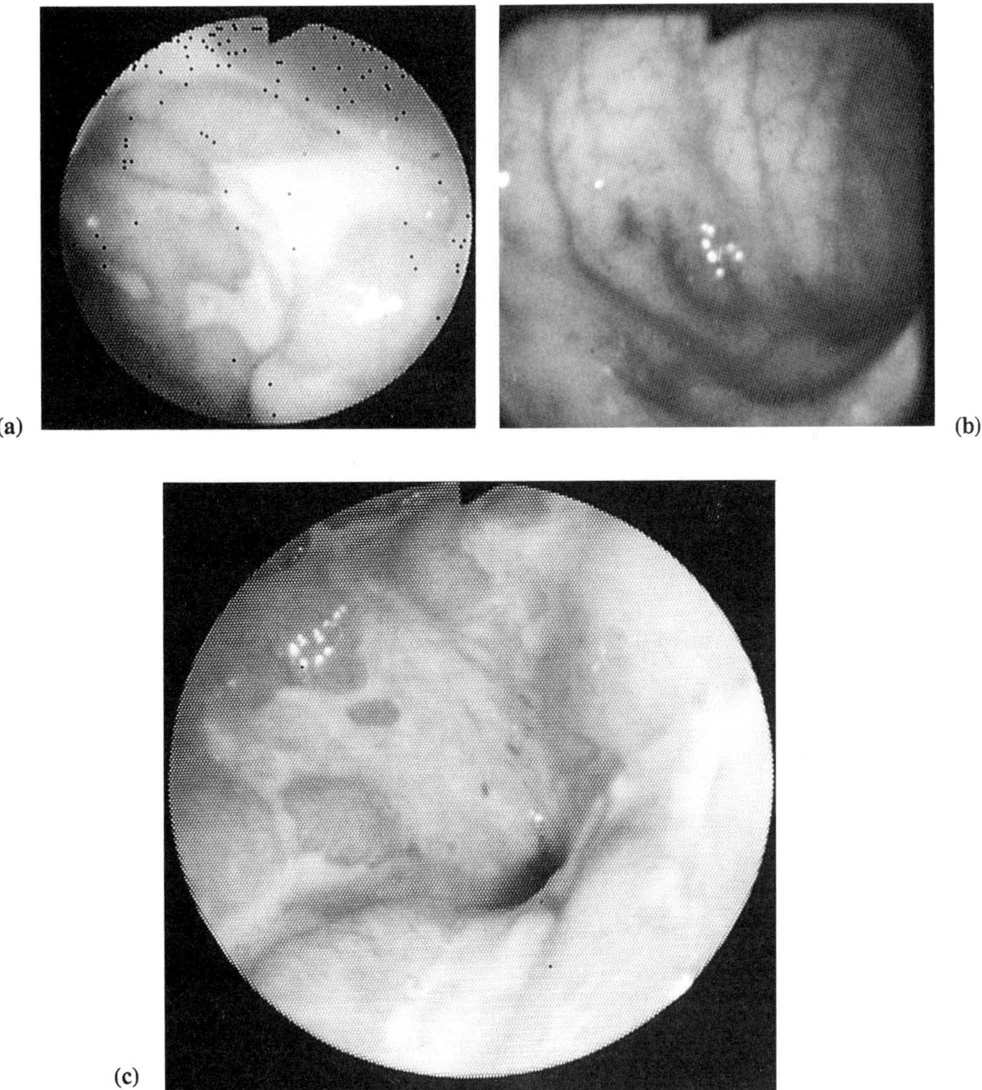

Fig. 11 (**a**) Colonoscopy in acute Crohn's disease with deep, purulent fissures and ulcerations among apparently normal mucosa. (**b**) Colonoscopy in acute Crohn's disease with snailtrack-like flat aphthous ulcerations among apparently normal mucosa. (**c**) Fibrous stenosis of the ileocolonic valve in a patient with inactive Crohn's disease

Table 6 Enteric hyperoxaluria in IBD (Division of Gastroenterology, Center of Internal Medicine, University Hospital, Frankfurt)

Patient group	No.	Urinary oxalate excretion [mg/24 h]	
1. Control	23	31.9 ± 2.2	
2. Ulcerative colitis	11	33.9 ± 4.2	
3. Crohn's disease			
Colon	11	34.5 ± 3.9	
Ileocaecal disease	42[a]	36.9 ± 2.7	
IC resection	16[b]	61.5 ± 8.1	$(p < 0.001)$
4. Short bowel syndrome	4	$87.7 - 114.0$	

[a] $n = 2$ with oxalate stones; [b] $n = 4$ with oxalate stones; all stone carriers had oxalate excretions of $65-90$ mg/day and a duration of Crohn's disease of $20-23$ years

References

1. Tedesco FJ, Hardin RD, Harper RN *et al*. Infectious colitis endoscopically simulating inflammatory bowel disease: a prospective evaluation. Gastrointest Endosc. 1983;29:195–7.
2. Höchter W, Kühner W, Ottenjann R. Rare forms of colitis. Hepato-gastroenterol. 1983;30:211–21.
3. Hogan WJ, Henshey GT, Geenen JE. Endoscopic evaluation of inflammatory bowel disease. Med Clin N Am. 1980;64:1083–102.
4. Watts J McK, deDombal FT *et al*. Early course of ulcerative colitis. Gut. 1966;7:16.
5. Truelove SS, Witts LJ. Cortisone in ulcerative colitis: final report on a therapeutic trial. Br Med J. 1955;2:1041–48.
6. Jalan KN, Sircus W, Card WI *et al*. An experience of ulcerative colitis: I. Toxic dilation in 55 cases. Gastroenterology. 1969;57:68.
7. Shepherd HA, Selby WS, Chapman RWG *et al*. Ulcerative colitis and persistent liver dysfunction. Q J Med. 1983;52:503–13.
8. Lennard-Jones JE, Ritchie JK, Zohrab WJ. Proctocolitis and Crohn's disease of the colon: a comparison of the clinical course. Gut. 1976;17:477.
9. Bodart P, Pringot J. Radiology of Crohn's disease. J Belge Radiol. 1977;60:83.
10. Lembcke B. Magen-Darm-Trakt. In: Lembcke B, ed., Clement TH, Cordes HJ. Die gastroenterologische Ultraschalluntersuchung. Einhorn-Presse Verlag, Reinbek; 1992:197–256.
11. Schwerk WB, Beckh K, Raith M. High resolution sonography in the diagnosis of inflammatory bowel disease. Gastroenterology. 1992;102:A693.
12. Camilleri M, Proano M. Advances in the assessment of disease activity in inflammatory bowel disease. Mayo Clin Proc. 1989;64:800–7.
13. Myren J, Bouchier IAD, Watkinson G *et al*. The O.M.G.E. multinational inflammatory bowel disease survey 1976–1982: a further report on 2,657 cases. Scand J Gastroenterol. 1984;Suppl. 95:1–27.
14. Gomes P, du Boulay C, Smith CL *et al*. Relationship between disease activity indices and colonoscopic findings in patients with colonic inflammatory bowel disease. Gut. 1986;27:92–5.
15. Modigliani R, Mary JY, Simon JF *et al*. Clinical, biological, and endoscopic picture of Crohn's disease: evolution on prednisolone. Gastroenterology. 1990;98:811–18.
16. Saverymuttu SH, Camilleri M, Rees H *et al*. Indium 111-granulocyte scanning in the assessment of disease extent and disease activity in inflammatory bowel disease: a comparison with colonoscopy, histology, and fecal indium 111-granulocyte excretion. Gastroenterology. 1986;90:1121–8.
17. Cooke WT, Prior P. Determining disease activity in inflammatory bowel disease. J Clin Gastroenterol. 1984;6:17–25.
18. Karbach U, Ewe K, Dehos H. Antiinflammatory treatment and intestinal alpha 1-antitrypsin clearance in active Crohn's disease. Dig Dis Sci. 1985;30:229–35.
19. Lembcke B. Ursachen und klinische Diagnostik der chologenen Diarrhoe. Z Gastroenterologie. 1989;27:279–84.

Section VII
Drugs – mechanisms and effects

31

Pharmacology of aminosalicylates: luminal and systemic availability

P. LAYER and H. GOEBELL

INTRODUCTION

Drug treatment with aminosalicylates is one of the main principles in the therapy of chronic inflammatory bowel disease. Their anti-inflammatory effects are mediated locally and probably dependent on their intraluminal concentration within the inflamed portion of the gastrointestinal tract. Consequently, because the distal segments of the small bowel and the colon are the sites most frequently affected by chronic inflammatory bowel disease, administration of aminosalicylates to the distal intestine has been a major aim in most established treatment concepts.

SALAZOSULPHAPYRIDINE

Oral *salazosulphapyridine* (SASP) is an effective treatment for colonic inflammatory bowel disease. Its local mechanism of action is explained by its pharmacochemical properties: the SASP molecule is composed of two components, *5-aminosalicylic acid* (5-ASA, mesalazine) and *sulphapyridine*, linked by a diazo bond. Only small quantities (10–20%) of intact SASP are absorbed by the human small intestinal mucosa, but after its passage into the distal gut the diazo bond is split by an azoreductase produced by the luminal bacterial flora present in the colon and (to a lesser extent) distal ileum. In consequence, large quantities of 5-ASA and sulphapyridine are delivered to, and released within, the proximal colonic lumen. Sulphapyridine is absorbed quantitatively by the colonic mucosa, and undergoes hepatic metabolism (acetylation, glucuronidation, hydroxylation) and subsequent renal excretion.

In contrast to earlier views, sulphapyridine has few or no therapeutic effects in colitis, while 5-ASA has been demonstrated to be the main active anti-inflammatory moiety[1]. On the other hand, the use of sulphapyridine as a carrier molecule to prevent proximal intestinal absorption of 5-ASA is disadvantageous, because the sulphapyridine component is responsible for most of the side-effects of SASP encountered in up to 20–25% of patients. These observations have stimulated efforts to eliminate or replace the sulphapyridine component from 5-ASA-containing compounds.

AMINOSALICYLATES: PHARMACOLOGICAL PROPERTIES AND CONCEPTS

The mechanism by which 5-ASA decreases inflammation within intestinal tissue is not fully elucidated but may be related to its effects on arachidonic acid metabolism and eicosanoid production (in particular its inhibition of leukotriene synthesis) and its action as a free radical scavenger[2–5]. The anti-inflammatory action of aminosalicylates is not dependent on the 5-amino configuration within the molecule. The 5-ASA isomer, 4-ASA, which has been used for decades under the name of para-aminosalicyclic acid (PAS) as an effective and safe antituberculotic drug, appears to have similar efficacy in decreasing inflammation in ulcerative colitis[6,7], but further studies are required to establish its role as an alternative treatment in chronic inflammatory bowel disease.

Pharmacokinetic properties and metabolism

Administration of 5-ASA as an uncoupled moiety into the proximal small intestine results in rapid and complete absorption and acetylation by the gastrointestinal mucosa with formation of the inactive metabolite acetyl-5-ASA (ac-5-ASA). As a consequence the major proportion ($>80\%$) of the absorbed amount is present in plasma as ac-5-ASA[8–10]. Another site of acetylation of 5-ASA is the liver. Systemic elimination occurs nearly exclusively as ac-5-ASA by renal excretion, while biliary excretion appears to play only a minor role. The plasma half-life of 5-ASA varies dose-dependently between 30 and 90 min, while that of ac-5-ASA is 6–10 h[5,11]. Upon direct administration of 5-ASA into the colon by means of enemas or oral slow-release galenics (see below), absorption and systemic availability is incomplete as estimated by cumulative renal elimination (20–30% of total dose) and the major proportion of the overall amount is excreted in faeces[11]. It is assumed that the absorption rate of 5-ASA is lower in the colon than in small bowel[12].

Galenic concepts

As a result of these pharmacokinetic properties (rapid absorption and inactivation in the proximal gastrointestinal tract), administration of pure 5-ASA to distal intestinal sites has been proved difficult. To achieve delivery of therapeutic amounts of 5-ASA into the ileum and the colon, several preparations have been developed in recent years with the aim of preventing or delaying release of free, absorbable 5-ASA into the gastric or small intestinal lumen. The different principal galenic or pharmacochemical approaches in these slow-release preparations included:

1. Tablets coated with Eudragit S (Asacol® or Eudragit L in combination with sodium bicarbonate/glycine buffering (Salofalk®, Claversal®); these acid-resistant preparations remain intact within the gastric lumen and disintegrate slowly in response to exposure to neutral pH (Eudragit S) or a milieu of pH $\geqslant$ 6.5 (Eudragit L) during duodenocaecal transit.
2. Microgranules coated with ethylcellulose (Pentasa®) within a tablet; the tablet releases the acid-stable microgranules within the stomach, which are then emptied into the duodenum. The ethylcellulose coating disintegrates gradually during small intestinal transit.
3. Replacement of sulphapyridine with other molecules for coupling with 5-ASA, e.g. coupling of two molecules of 5-ASA (olsalazine; Dipentum®). The resulting 5-ASA dimer is stable and unabsorbable within the proximal gastrointestinal lumen, and releases two molecules of free 5-ASA after bacterial cleavage of the compound in the colon.

While it has been demonstrated by indirect methods that delivery of 5-ASA into the colon is possible by means of these galenic measures, release and fate of 5-ASA within the small intestinal lumen has been unknown. However, availability of 5-ASA within different levels of the small bowel may be of interest because of its potential value in the treatment of Crohn's disease. We have determined luminal release and fate of 5-ASA from two preparations (Salofalk®, Pentasa®) by direct luminal measurements[13,14] in 12 healthy human volunteers who were intubated with an integrated multilumen oro-ileal tube which allowed marker perfusion, aspiration of luminal content from the duodenum, mid-jejunum and terminal ileum, and recording of intestinal motility[15,16]. This system permits measurement of intraluminal concentrations and flow rates of 5-ASA its main metabolite, acetyl-5-ASA (ac-5-ASA) within the duodenum, mid-jejunum, and terminal ileum. 5-ASA (either as Salofalk®, 500 mg, $n = 6$; or Pentasa®, 500 mg, $n = 6$) was administered as a single oral dose together with a standard meal (300 kcal). 5-ASA and ac-5-ASA were measured by HPLC prior to administration and for 7–10 h post-administration in duodenal, jejunal and ileal samples, as well as in plasma and urine (Prof. Dr U. Klotz, Dr Margarete Bosch Institute of Clinical Pharmacology, Stuttgart, Germany[11,17,18]). In addition, perfusion and meal markers were determined to calculate kinetic and cumulative luminal flow rates for each site[19,20].

INTRALUMINAL FATE OF 5-ASA SLOW-RELEASE PREPARATIONS

Eudragit L/bicarbonate-buffer tablets (Salofalk®)

Following administration of the slow-release preparation Salofalk®, gastric emptying of 5-ASA into the duodenum started 3 h after meal intake, at the time when gastric emptying of the meal was complete, i.e. after the end of the digestive period. This reflected the physiological emptying of resistant particles from the stomach which typically occurs in the interdigestive period. Mean small intestinal transit of 5-ASA lasted approximately 30 min on the duodenojejunal segment, and about 80 min between duodenum and ileum.

Cumulative delivery of free 5-ASA to the duodenum was less than 2% of the total dose. At the jejunal site approximately 6% were released; cumulative delivery to the ileum was 13%. In all samples and at all aspiration sites appearance of 5-ASA was accompanied by ac-5-ASA, with similar concentrations of both compounds in the proximal intestine and somewhat higher concentrations of ac-5-ASA compared with 5-ASA in the distal intestine. Thus, cumulative delivery of ac-5-ASA was between 1% and 2% in the duodenum, 12% in the jejunum and 18% in the ileum (Fig. 1). The simultaneous and approximately parallel appearance of 5-ASA and ac-5-ASA suggests mucosal generation and back-diffusion into the lumen rather than enterobiliary recirculation[21].

Intraluminal 5-ASA concentrations increased gradually on the passage from the proximal to the distal small intestine. In the duodenum, mean 5-ASA concentrations were 20–25 µg/ml for up to 2 h. Mean intrajejunal concentrations ranged between 35 and 70 µg/ml, and in the ileum usually exceeded 60 µg/ml and approached 100 µg/ml.

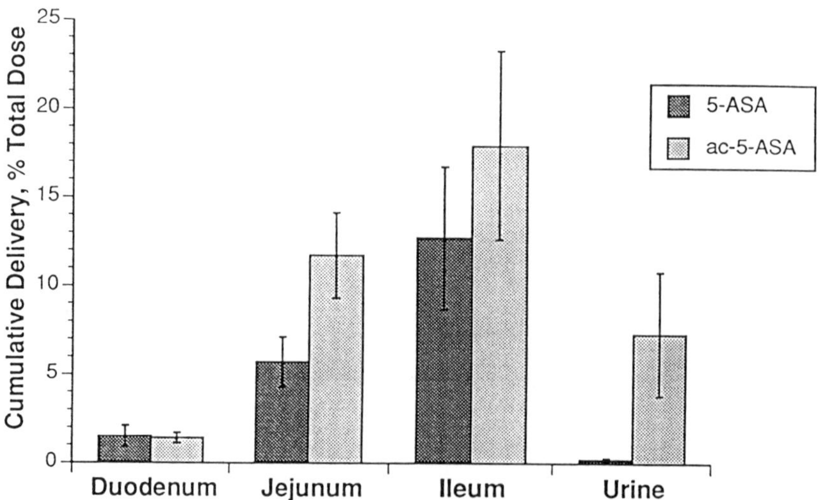

Fig. 1 Cumulative delivery (percentage of total dose) of free 5-ASA and ac-5-ASA to duodenum, jejunum and ileum, and cumulative urinary excretion, following ingestion of 500 mg of 5-ASA (Salofalk®) with a meal (modified from reference 13)

Early appearance of 5-ASA and ac-5-ASA in plasma coincided with their delivery to the proximal intestine. In the later phase plasma ac-5-ASA concentrations exceeded those of 5-ASA, which probably reflects intraintestinal acetylation and slower uptake and elimination of the metabolite[17,22]. Less than 0.5% of the total dose was excreted in the urine as 5-ASA; urinary excretion of ac-5-ASA over the 10 postprandial hours was about 7% of the administered dose.

Overall analysis of luminal, plasma and urinary data suggests that about 30% of the total dose was released (and partly acetylated) within the small intestine and reached the colon in solution, and another 60% reached the colon unreleased from tablets; less than 10% were absorbed.

Ethylcellulose-coated microspheres (Pentasa®)

Following administration of the 5-ASA microsphere preparation Pentasa®, 5-ASA appeared in the duodenum in the early postprandial phase (between 20 and 60 min) and was emptied roughly simultaneously with the meal, i.e. during the digestive period. Small intestinal transit times were similar to those following Salofalk®.

Cumulative delivery of free 5-ASA to each intestinal site was approximately 10% of the total dose, which reflects marked luminal pharmacokinetic differences compared with Salofalk®. Again, cumulative amounts of ac-5-ASA tended to be slightly greater at distal intestinal sites (Fig. 2).

In the duodenum, 5-ASA concentrations reached a persistent plateau of 50–60 μg/ml that was nearly as high as that produced in the distal intestine (60–70 μg/ml). In contrast to Salofalk®, plasma concentrations of 5-ASA were significantly lower than those of ac-5-ASA. Only traces of 5-ASA

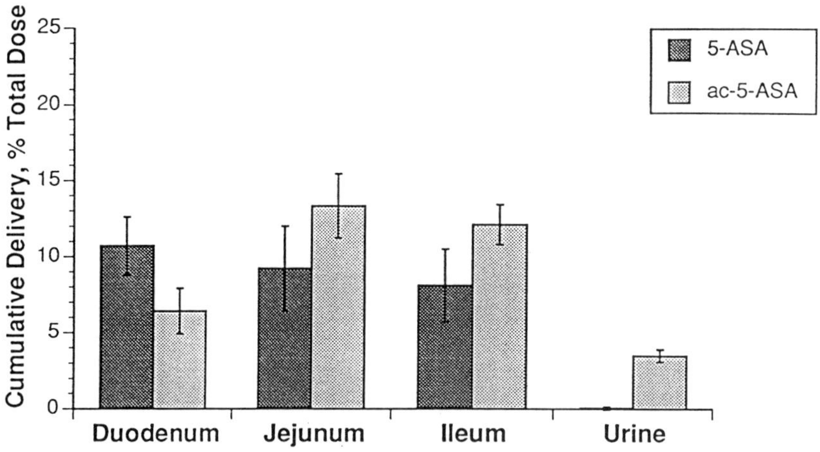

Fig. 2 Cumulative delivery (percentage of total dose) of free 5-ASA and ac-5-ASA to duodenum, jejunum and ileum, and cumulative urinary excretion, following ingestion of 500 mg of 5-ASA (Pentasa®) with a meal (modified from reference 14)

were present in urine; cumulative excretion of ac-5-ASA amounted to approximately 5% of the total dose.

Overall analysis suggests that about 20% of the total dose was released during small intestinal transit and reached the colon dissolved in luminal juice, and another 70% reached the colon unreleased as microspheres; about 5% were absorbed.

IMPLICATIONS

5-ASA has been shown to be the active anti-inflammatory moiety within SASP while sulphapyridine, the other component in SASP, is responsible for most of the side-effects. These observations have prompted the development of uncoupled 5-ASA preparations that remain, at least in part, unabsorbed during small intestinal transit and reach the ileocaecal region in sufficient quantities. Direct luminal measurements demonstrate that from enteric-coated slow-release forms, either tablets or microspheres, the major portion of 5-ASA is delivered into the colon, which explains the effectiveness of such preparations in ulcerative colitis[23,24].

However, there were marked differences in the patterns of gastric emptying and small intestinal transit between the two galenic preparations studied. Salofalk®, a coated, resilient tablet, was emptied after the meal in the subsequent interdigestive period. Upon its entrance into the small intestine, 5-ASA was released in increasing quantities as the tablet passed to the distal small bowel. Consequently, the highest luminal concentrations were observed in the terminal ileum. By contrast, 5-ASA from Pentasa® appeared in the duodenum in the early prandial period, and was emptied largely simultaneously with the meal, i.e. in the digestive period. These differences are due to the physiological gastric emptying mechanisms in humans: in the digestive period, gastric emptying of solid particles occurs together with meal nutrients only if their diameter does not exceed 1–2 mm. Larger particles are retained until the end of the digestive period and emptied in the subsequent interdigestive state.

Thus, Salofalk® tablets are emptied into the small bowel preferentially by interdigestive motility patterns. As the resilient coating disintegrates and its permeability increases gradually during small intestinal transit, increasing quantities of 5-ASA are released and maximal concentrations are produced in the ileal lumen. By contrast, Pentasa® micropellets are emptied into the duodenum essentially synchronously with the meal, and release of 5-ASA occurs relatively persistently throughout small intestinal transit, with similar intraluminal concentrations in duodenum, jejunum, and ileum.

5-ASA is acetylated (and thus inactivated) rapidly within the intestinal mucosa[25,26], but not by human intestinal juice. In addition, it has been shown that biliary re-secretion is no major source of intraluminal ac-5-ASA[21]. Therefore, the most likely pathway involves uptake of 5-ASA by the intestinal mucosa, acetylation and, in part, subsequent back-diffusion into the lumen. In consequence, because most of intramucosal 5-ASA is acetylated, the therapeutic effects of 5-ASA are probably mediated prior to its acetylation. Hence we suggest that the ac-5-ASA present in the lumen reflects the portion of total 5-ASA which already has exerted its anti-inflammatory effects within the intestinal tissue; conversely, free intraluminal 5-ASA has not yet penetrated into, and been active within, the mucosa. To assess the anti-inflammatory potential of luminal 5-ASA concentrations it may therefore be useful to consider intraluminal concentrations of both its free and acetylated forms.

With both preparations, considerable luminal concentrations are produced within the lumen of the small bowel, which suggests that they may also be effective in small intestinal Crohn's disease provided sufficient doses are administered. Their specific release patterns suggest that Salofalk® may have advantages in predominantly terminal ileal disease, while Pentasa® may be particularly effective in extensive (including proximal) small intestinal involvement.

References

1. Azad Khan AK, Piris J, Truelove SC. An experiment to determine the active therapeutic moiety of sulphasalazine. Lancet. 1977;1:892–5.
2. Ligumsky M, Karmeli F, Sharon P, Zor U, Cohen F, Rachmilewitz D. Enhanced thromboxane A2 and prostacyclin production by cultured rectal mucosa in ulcerative colitis and its inhibition by steroids and sulphasalazine. Gastroenterology. 1981;81:444–9.
3. Stenson WF, Lobos E. Sulfasalazine inhibits the synthesis of chemotactic lipids by neutrophils. J Clin Invest. 1982;69:494–7.
4. Nielsen OH, Ahnfelt-Ronne I. 4-Aminosalicylic acid has no effect on arachidonic acid metabolism in human neutrophils or on the free radical, 1.1-diphenyl-2-picrylhydrazyl. Pharmacol Toxicol. 1988;62:223–6.
5. Ireland A, Jewell DP. Mechanism of action of 5-aminosalicylic acid and its derivatives. Clin Sci. 1990;78:119–25.
6. Campieri M, Lanfranchi GA, Bertoni F, Brignola C, Bazzochi G, Minguzzi MR, Labo G. A double-blind clinical trial to compare the effects of 4-aminosaliylic acid in topical treatment of ulcerative colitis. Digestion. 1984;29:204–8.
7. Ginsberg AL, Davis ND, Nochomovitz E. Placebo-controlled trial of ulcerative colitis with oral 4-aminosalicylic acid. Gastroenterology. 1992;102:448–52.
8. Nielsen OH, Bondensen S. Kinetics of 5-aminosalicylic acid after jejunal instillation in man. Br J Clin Pharmacol. 1983;16:738–40.
9. Myers B, Evans DNW, Rhodes J, Evans BK, Hughes BR, Lee MG, Richens A, Richards D. Metabolism and urinary excretion of 5-aminosalicylic acid in healthy volunteers when given intravenously or released for absorption at different sites in the gastrointestinal tract. Gut. 1987;28:196–200.
10. Rijk MCM, van Schaik A, van Tongeren JHM. Disposition of 5-aminosalicylic acid by 5-aminosalicylic acid-delivering compounds. Scand J Gastroenterol. 1988;23:107–12.
11. Klotz U. Clinical pharmacokinetics of sulphasalazine, its metabolites and other products of 5-aminosalicylic acid. Clin Pharmacokinet. 1985;10:285–302.
12. Bondesen S, Bronnum-Schon J, Pedersen V, Rafiolsadat Z, Honoré Hansen S, Huidberg EF. Absorption of 5-aminosalicylic acid from colon and rectum. Br J Clin Pharmacol. 1988;25:269.
13. Goebell H, Layer P, Nehlsen B, Klotz U. Oro-ileal transit and intestinal delivery of 5-aminosalicylic acid in humans. Gastroenterology. 1990;98:A172.
14. Keller J, Layer P, Klotz U, Goebell H. Freisetzung von mikroverkapselter 5-Amino-salizylsäure (5-ASA; Pentasa®) im Dünndarmlumen des Menschen. Klin Wochenschr. 1992;69(Suppl 28):83.

15. Layer P, Chan ATH, Go VLW, DiMagno EP. Human pancreatic secretion during phase II antral motility of the interdigestive cycle. Am J Physiol. 1988;254:G249–53.
16. Layer P, Peschel S, Schlesinger T, Goebell H. Human pancreatic secretion and intestinal motility: effects of ileal nutrient perfusion. Am J Physiol. 1990;258(Gastrointest Liver Physiol. 21):G196–201.
17. Fischer C, Maier K, Klotz U. Simplified high-performance liquid chromatographic method for 5-aminosalicylic acid in plasma and urine. J Chromatogr. 1981;225:498–503.
18. Klotz U, Maier KE, Fischer C, Bauer KH. A new slow-release form of 5-aminosalicylic acid for the oral treatment of inflammatory bowel disease. Biopharmaceutical and clinical pharmacokinetic characteristics. Drug Res. 1985;35:636–9.
19. Layer P, Zinsmeister AR, DiMagno EP. Effects of decreasing intraluminal amylase activity on starch digestion and postprandial gastrointestinal function in humans. Gastroenterology. 1986;91:41–8.
20. Layer P, Jansen JBMJ, Cherian L, Lamers CBHW, Goebell H. Feedback regulation of human pancreatic secretion: Effects of protease inhibition on duodenal delivery and small intestinal transit of pancreatic enzymes. Gastroenterology. 1990;98:1311–19.
21. Fischer C, Maier K, Klotz U. Specific measurement of 5-aminosalicylic acid and its acetylated metabolite in human bile. Br J Clin Pharmacol. 1983;15:273–4.
22. Ireland A, Priddle JD, Jewell DP. A comparison of the uptake of 5-aminosalicylic acid (acetyl-mesalazine) and N-acetyl-aminosalicylic acid (Ac-ASA) into the isolated colonic epithelial cell. Gastroenterology. 1987;92:1447.
23. Riley SA, Mani V, Goodman MJ, Herd ME, Dutt S, Turnberg LA. Comparison of delayed-release 5-aminosalicylic acid (5-ASA) and sulfasalazine as maintenance treatment for patients with ulcerative colitis. Gastroenterology. 1988;94:1383–9.
24. Rachmelewitz D. On behalf of an international study group. Coated 5-ASA versus sulphasalazine in the treatment of active ulcerative colitis: A randomised trial. Br Med J. 1989;298:82–6.
25. Ireland A, Priddle JD, Jewell DP. Acetylation of 5-aminosalicylic acid by human colonic epithelial cells. Gastroenterology. 1986;90:1471.
26. Allgayer H, Ahnfelt NO, Kruis W, Klotz U, Frank-Holmberg K, Söderberg HNA, Paumgartner G. Colonic N-acetylation of 5-aminosalicylic acid in inflammatory bowel disease. Gastroenterology. 1989;97:38–41.

32

Topical use of steroids in gastroenterology

H. W. MÖLLMANN, G. HOCHHAUS, A. TROMM, J. BARTH,
C. BIGALKE, B. MAY, A. C. MÖLLMANN, U. SCHWEGLER,
H. DERENDORF, S. TUNN and M. KRIEG

Glucocorticoids are used most successfully as rapidly acting drugs in the treatment of acute or chronic inflammatory bowel disease (IBD)[1]. In controlled therapeutic trials they have been found to be effective in the treatment of both acute ulcerative colitis (UC) and active Crohn's disease (CD)[2-11]. Most clinical aspects of inflammatory bowel disease can be explained by the inflammatory and immunological mechanisms. Glucocorticoids inhibit many of these mechanisms, and this explains their considerable effectiveness.

Glucocorticoids induce their effects mainly via a receptor-mediated mechanism (Fig. 1)*. For this, the steroid molecule binds to an intracytoplasmatic receptor protein. This induces the activation of the receptor (dissociation from heat shock protein HSP90), upon which the receptor can induce its effect either directly, or upon transfer into the cell nucleus by modulating the expression of proteins. Although the mode of action is rather complex, the extent of the effect is solely determined by the degree of receptor occupancy. This depends on the affinity of the glucocorticoid to the receptor but also on the concentration of the glucocorticoid at the site of action.

Glucocorticoids differ in their glucocorticoid receptor affinity (Fig. 2); thus, for a glucocorticoid with lower affinity, higher concentrations at the receptor site are necessary to achieve the same therapeutic effects, as well as adverse glucocorticoid reactions. For glucocorticoid esters a clear distinction must be made: glucocorticoid-21-esters do not bind to the receptor, but represent prodrugs, which need to be activated to the corresponding free alcohols. On the other hand, esterification in 17α-position enhances glucocorticosteroid potency remarkably.

* Figures and Tables will be found between pages 346 and 347.

The use of glucocorticoids in high doses over a long period of time is linked to extensive systemic side-effects. Thus, the main therapeutic challenge in the treatment of chronic IBD is the realization of distinct local effects by preventing systemic adverse effects. Hence, a rational approach to glucocorticoid therapy is to find an optimal glucocorticoid profile for local anti-inflammatory and immunosuppressive therapy of IBD with high topical glucocorticoid potency and rather high metabolic stability in the bowel and rectum compartments which after systemic absorption show a rapid inactivation and elimination.

The choice of an optimal dosage form is limited by the localization of the inflammatory disorder and the size of the lesions (Fig. 3). If the disease area is accessible to local therapy the glucocorticoids should always be delivered directly to the target region using an enema or foam, because this form of administration results in the realization of high local steroid concentrations in the inflamed mucosa with a limited overall dose. As a consequence, the systemic spillover of the drug is relatively low, and systemic adverse effects, generally seen after systemic oral or i.v. administration of the same dose, are reduced.

Lee[12] reported the bioavailability of prednisolone after rectal enema administration to be only half of that after oral administration (Fig. 4).

Rectal delivery thus seems to be advantageous alone from the standpoint of reduced systemic bioavailability. This is, however, true only for the distal part of the colon, for if steroids pass the right flexura or in more proximal areas in IBD, they may show higher absorption rates (Fig. 5)[13].

The disease state changes membrane properties, and the absorption of rectally administered drugs to colitis patients might be different from those in healthy volunteers (Fig. 6). Usually a higher absorption rate was observed in patients with Crohn's disease[14,15] (Fig. 7), whereas in some cases lower systemic absorption was observed[16]. It was speculated that the increased systemic absorption of the glucocorticoid might be linked to the disease, and patients with acute symptoms might be at greater risk of developing corticoid side-effects. Under these conditions the drug would be systemically absorbed and might act upon systemic recirculation into the intestinal disease area.

Even if a local therapy can be applied, the selection of a glucocorticoid with a high benefit to risk ratio is of major importance. Therefore, not only pharmacodynamic but also pharmacokinetic characteristics should be considered. While pharmacodynamic activities describe the activity at the site of action, pharmacokinetic properties determine how fast the drug will be absorbed from the site of administration, and how fast it will be activated or eliminated from the systemic circulation. These properties consequently decide how much of a drug is available for induction of the pharmacodynamic effects. Among therapeutically employed glucocorticoids, there are essential differences which make it possible to modulate the time profiles of the glucocorticoid response.

In the following, rectally administered glucocorticoids will be discussed according to their classification as full agonists, lipophilic, or hydrophilic prodrugs (Table 1).

GLUCOCORTICOID AGONISTS

Table 2 classifies glucocorticoid agonists according to their use as topically employed drugs. Preferable topical glucocorticoids such as budesonide (BUD: RBA 935) or betamethasone valerate (BV: RBA 1600) show higher intrinsic activity than the mainly systemically employed steroids such as hydrocortisone (HC: RBA 9), prednisolone (P: RBA 16), methylprednisolone (MP: RBA 42), and betamethasone (B: RBA 58). These differences in intrinsic potency are of some impact in clinical practice, as budesonide has a 100-fold higher receptor binding activity than hydrocortisone. Budesonide may exert equipotent effects in a concentration 100 times lower (Fig. 8).

In addition to its pharmacodynamic properties, pharmacokinetic properties also need to be considered. HC, P, MP, B and the highly potent betamethasone-17-valerate, when given rectally, are likely to show more significant systemic side-effects because their fast absorption from colon leads to a high systemic bioavailability, which is often close to 50% compared to oral intake[12,17]. The same is also true for HC, which has a lower intrinsic activity, but after oral administration passes almost completely intact into the systemic circulation[18] and is able to induce steroid-relevant side-effects. Hence the esteration as acetate delays the release of HC.

In contrast, the 21-alcohol budesonide shows high topical activity, but also high metabolic inactivation. Its activity at the site of action is very high. It has a 9 times higher receptor binding affinity than dexamethasone (RBA: 100). It is efficiently metabolized in the systemic circulation with a half-life of less than 2 h, and the generated metabolites are pharmacologically inactive (Fig. 9). Approximately 90% of an oral or rectal dose of budesonide undergoes first-pass metabolism. The drug has a very high clearance. The rapid metabolism of budesonide is reflected in its plasma clearance which, at 0.9–1.4 l/min, is higher than that of most other glucocorticoids[19,20]. Due to its high liver first-pass effect, the oral bioavailability is very small (14.3%). Only 2% of budesonide in the body circulates in the blood; over 95% is tissue-bound (Figs 10 and 11)[21]. In addition, it has pronounced protein binding. All these facts argue for a low reduced systemic and systemic spill-over activity of budesonide, given rectally, quite in contrast to first-generation steroids. Indeed, after rectal application of budesonide, in comparison with equivalent doses of the 'classic' glucocorticoids, the systemic side-effects on therapeutic parameters were rather low (Fig. 12)[22].

A similar concept leads to the use of hydrocortisone thiopivalate (Table 3). This substance shows the same activity as hydrocortisone, but is metabolically converted to its inactive cortienic acid in blood and liver, and also in the intestinal wall. The partial inactivation in the target organ might however lead to a lower efficacy in the bowel wall. Its high first-pass metabolism leads to a rectal bioavailability of 10–20%[23]; thus, this drug needs to be given at very high doses to achieve clinically sufficient response. In humans an administration of 500–2000 mg tixocortol pivalate into the rectum did not markedly affect plasma or urinary cortisol levels[24]. On the other hand, the pronounced metabolic inactivation also ensures lack of any systemic side-effects. Thus, in therapy tixocortol pivalate has an improved profile for the selective glucocorticoid treatment of proctitis and left-sided colitis, but more studies are required to determine its therapeutic potency for that indication[25].

C21 ESTERS

Glucocorticoid-21-esters have been used widely for topical as well as systemic application. The 21-esters can be divided mainly into two classes: water-soluble prodrugs (phosphates, hemisuccinates, sulphobenzoates) and lipophilic esters, such as acetates and propionates.

Hydrophilic prodrugs

Hydrocortisone phosphate, prednisolone phosphate, methylprednisolone phosphate, betamethasone phosphate, hydrocortisone hemisuccinate, prednisolone hemisuccinate and methylprednisolone hemisuccinate represent examples of water-soluble C21-ester derivatives (Table 4). Hydrophilic esters dissolve very fast in the GI tract and are available for systemic absorption. As a result a high systemic bioavailability has been observed for glucocorticoids that have been applied as phosphate- and hemisuccinate-esters. Thus, the benefit of these water-soluble prodrugs is at least questionable. Additional clinical studies need to be performed in order to characterize the local component of the effects; especially whether intraluminal concentrations of active drug (cleaved prodrug), after rectal delivery of hydrophilic compounds, are comparable to those observed after systemic administration. Future studies should also investigate in far more detail the benefit/risk ratio after rectal delivery of phosphates and hemisuccinates, and should evaluate whether the currently employed dosage can be reduced to decrease systemic side-effects by retaining its local activity.

The clinical profiles of some other water-soluble prodrugs are promising. These prodrugs show very low rectal bioavailability, while local tissue levels are very high after rectal administration (Fig. 13)[26,27]. Thus sulphobenzoates might represent better water-soluble prodrugs for local delivery with a high benefit to risk ratio; but the mechanism for their optimal biopharmaceutical behaviour remains unclear (Table 5).

Lipophilic prodrugs

Another group of 21-esters are the lipophilic derivatives, such as the 21-acetates of hydrocortisone, methylprednisolone, or betamethasone-17,21-dipropionate esters (Table 6). These represent rather lipophilic glucocorticoid prodrugs and show a slow gastrointestinal release profile after local administration, in contrast to water soluble esters. They are prescribed

Glucocorticoids	C21 Agonists	C21 - ester (prodrugs) hydrophilic			C21 - ester (prodrugs) lipophilic		C16	C17
	- OH	- P	- HS	- SB	- AC	-PROP		
Hydrocortisone					foam			
Prednisolone				foam				
Methylprednisolone								
Betamethasone								
Betamethasonvalerate								
Budesonid								
Beclomethasondipropionate								
Beclomethasonmonpropionate								
Beclomethasone								
Fluticasone								THIO
Tixocortol	Thiopiv.							

Table 1   Synopsis of glucocorticoids for rectal administration

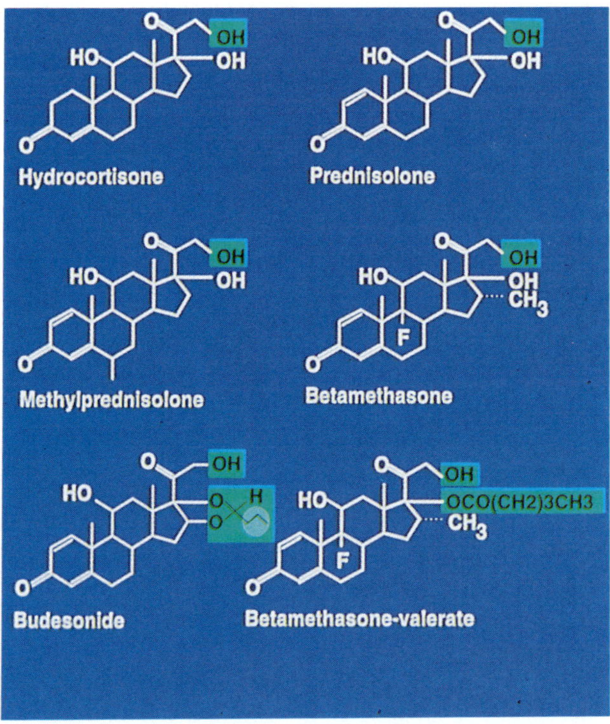

Table 2   Synopsis of chemical structures of agonists (C21-OH) glucocorticoids for topical treatment of IBD

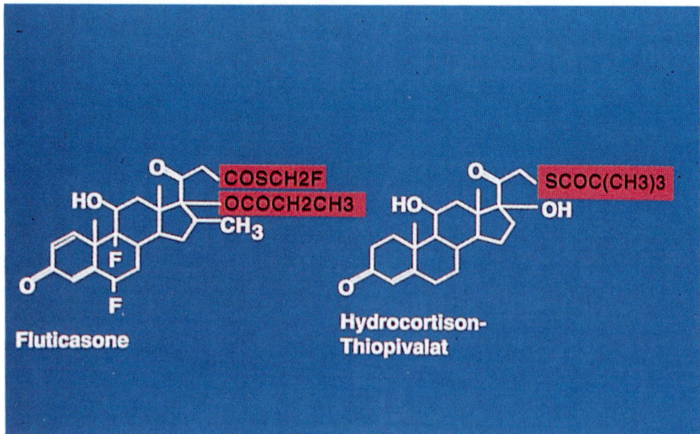

Table 3 Synopsis of chemical structures of agonists C21 thioester, which are rapidly transformed into metabolites with low glucocorticoid activity

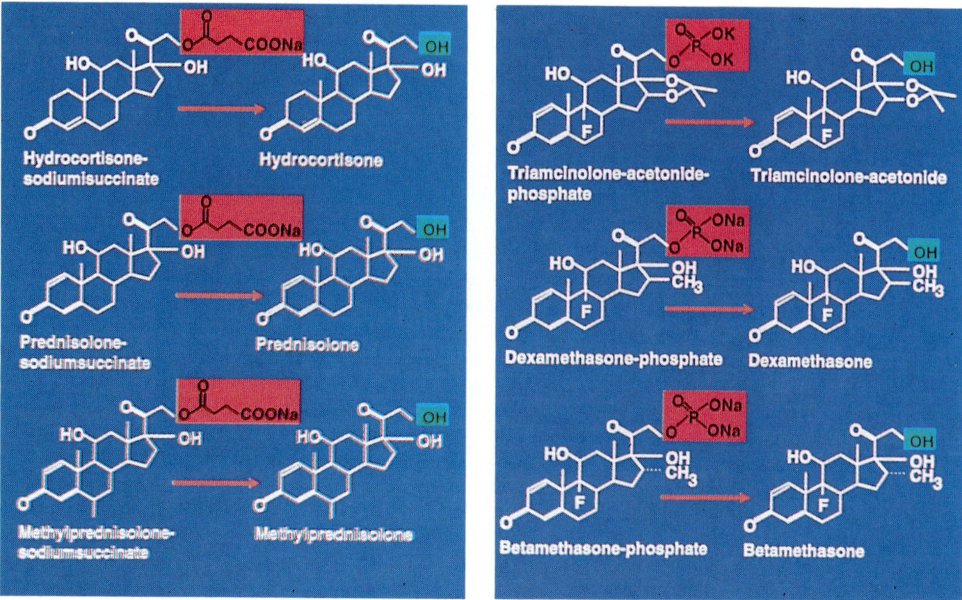

Table 4 Synopsis of chemical structures of hydrophilic C21-phosphates and sodium succinate ester (prodrugs), which need to be activated to the corresponding free C21-alcohols

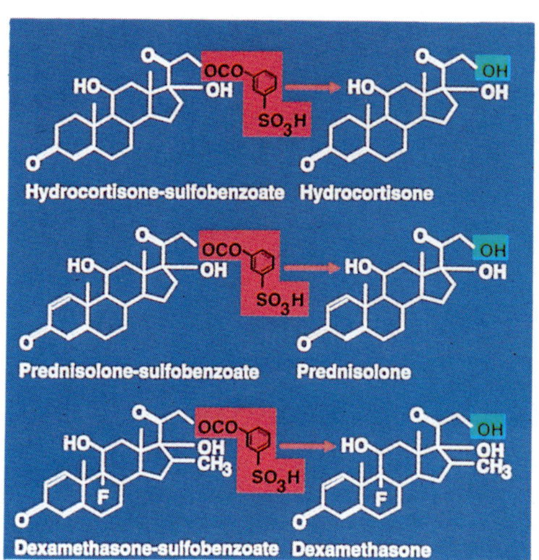

Table 5 Synopsis of chemical structures of hydrophilic C21-sulphobenzoate glucocorticoid ester (prodrugs), which need to be activated to the corresponding free C21-alcohols

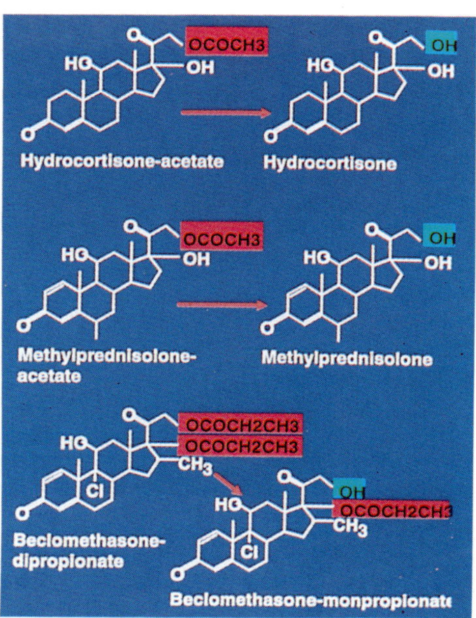

Table 6 Synopsis of chemical structures of lipophilic C21-acetate and propionate ester (prodrugs) which need to be activated to the corresponding free C21-alcohols

1 x 100 mg		Healthy volunteesrs Mean	S.D.	Patients Mean	S.D.
AUC	[ng / ml * h]	113,9	47,2	196,9	85,0
BA	[%]	2,2	0,9	3,8	1,6
Cmax	[ng / ml]	27,8	12,0	41,0	15,8
tmax	[h]	1,5	0,7	1,8	1,3

2 x 100 mg		Healthy volunteesrs Mean	S.D.	Patients Mean	S.D.
AUC	[ng / ml * h]	324,9	139,4	474,3	220,1
BA	[%]	3,1	1,3	4,6	2,1
Cmax 1	[ng / ml]	24,4	9,0	61,2	18,2
Cmax 2	[ng / ml]	39,9	12,0	65,2	26,9
tmax 1	[h]	1,4	0,2	2,5	0,9
tmax 2	[h]	1,5	0,7	2,9	1,3

3 x 100 mg		Healthy volunteesrs Mean	S.D.	Patients Mean	S.D.
AUC	[ng / ml * h]	426,8	132,6	589,6	381,6
BA	[%]	2,0	0,6	2,8	1,8
Cmax 1	[ng / ml]	19,3	8,8	38,8	21,0
Cmax 2	[ng / ml]	29,4	10,4	52,3	32,0
Cmax 3	[ng / ml]	38,4	14,2	61,4	37,3
Cmax 4	[ng / ml]	41,1	12,4	57,8	35,0
tmax 1	[h]	1,9	0,9	2,0	0,8
tmax 2	[h]	1,8	1,0	2,1	0,9
tmax 3	[h]	1,2	0,4	1,3	0,7
tmax 4	[h]	1,7	0,9	1,0	0,0

Table 7 Synopsis of the pharmacokinetic data of hydrocortisone after single and multiple rectal administration of hydrocorticoacetate foam in healthy volunteers and patients with inflammatory bowel disease

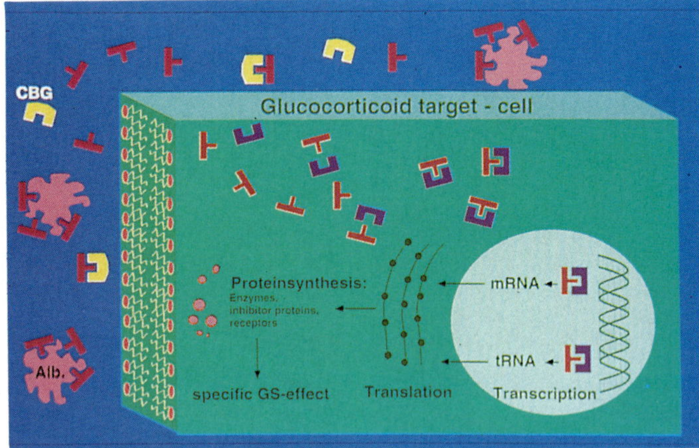

Fig. 1 Model for agonist interaction with the glucocorticoid receptor. Outline of receptor-mediated genomic mechanism of action of glucocorticoids. The diagram illustrates that transformed GR complexes are targeted to the nucleus, where they transcriptionally regulate a small set of primary target genes. Secondary hormone responses require *de novo* RNA and protein synthesis for the steroid effect

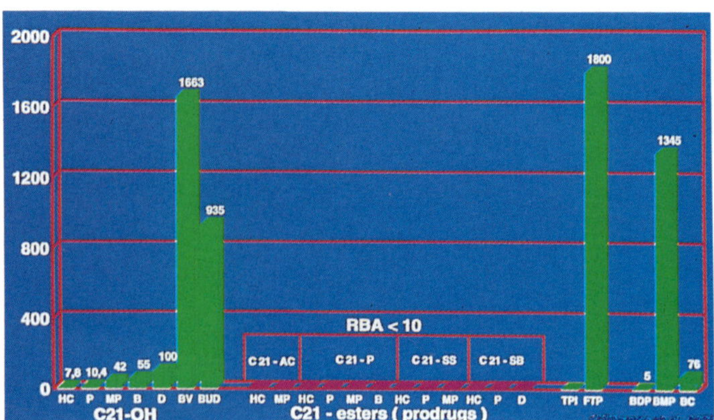

Fig. 2 Receptor binding affinities (RBA) to human tissue of different rectally administered glucocorticoids. HC = Hydrocortisone, P = Prednisolone, MP = Methylprednisolone, B = Betamethasone, D = Dexamethasone, BV = Beclomethasone valerate, BUD = Budesonide, HCP = Hydrocortisone phosphate, PP = Prednisolone phosphate, MPP = Methylprednisolone-phosphate, BP = Betamethasone, HCS = Hydrocortisone hemisuccinate, PHS = Prednisolone hemisuccinate, MPHS = Methylprednisolone hemisuccinate-sodiumaccinate, HCSB = Hydrocortisone sulphobenzoate, PSE = Prednisolone sulphobenzoate, DSP = Dexamethasone sulphobenzoate, TPI = Tixocortol pivalate, FTP = Fluticasone propionate, BDP = Beclomethasone dipropionate, BMP = Betamethasone monopropionate, BC = Beclomethasone

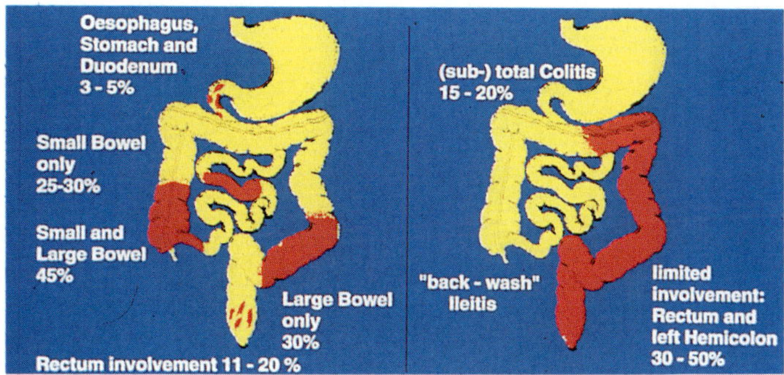

Fig. 3 Localization of Crohn's disease and ulcerative colitis in the gastrointestinal tract

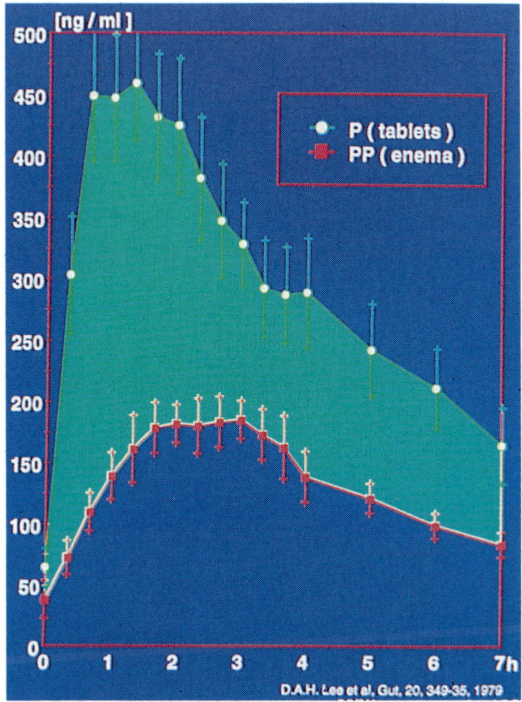

Fig. 4 Mean plasma prednisolone concentration–time profiles after administration of prednisolone-21-phosphate retention enema (20 mg) and oral prednisolone (20 mg) to healthy volunteers and to patients with idiopathic proctocolitis ($n = 10$) (rectal bioavailability 44.3%)[12]

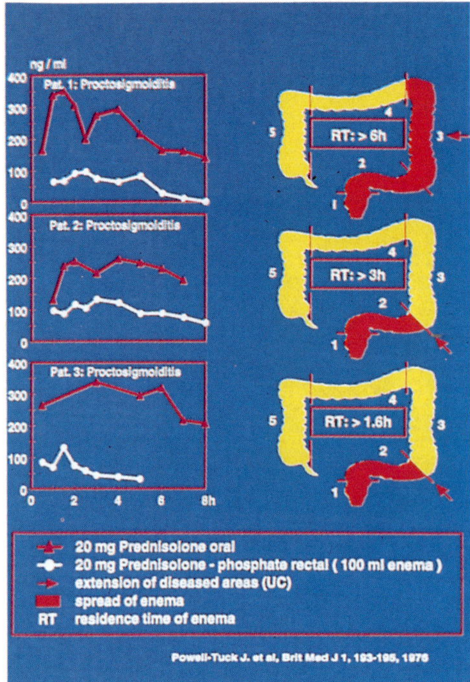

Fig. 5a

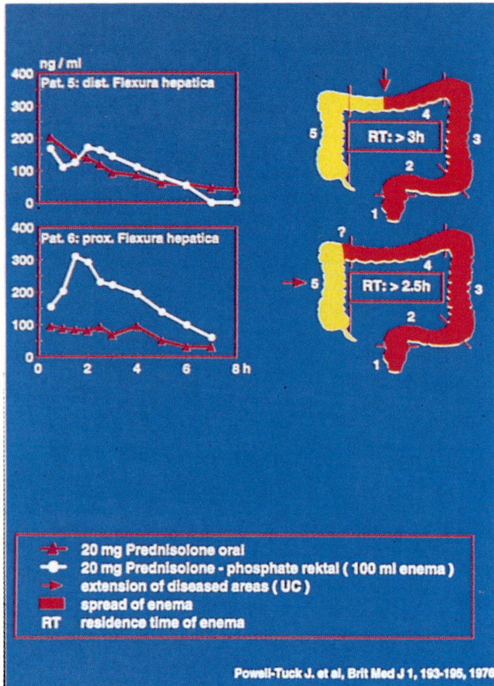

Fig. 5b

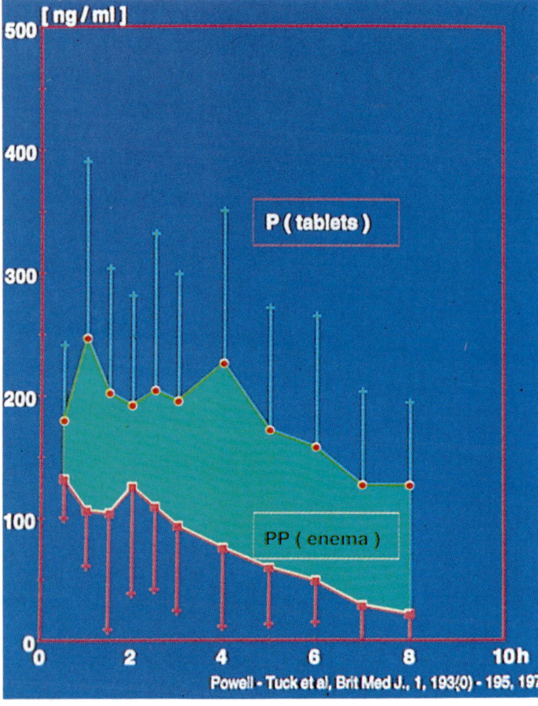

Figs 5 and 6 Prednisolone plasma concentration–time profiles in patients ($n = 5$) after intraindividual administration of 20 mg prednisolone oral in comparison to 20 mg prednisolone-21-phosphate rectal in dependence of the spread of the retention enema. In the individual patients the plasma levels achieved by enema were quite different from those achieved by mouth, but overall the levels by each mode of administration were of a similar order. The comparisons show that in two patients the plasma prednisolone levels were higher after rectal administration when the distance travelled by the enema to the distal and the hepatic flexura[13]

Fig. 6

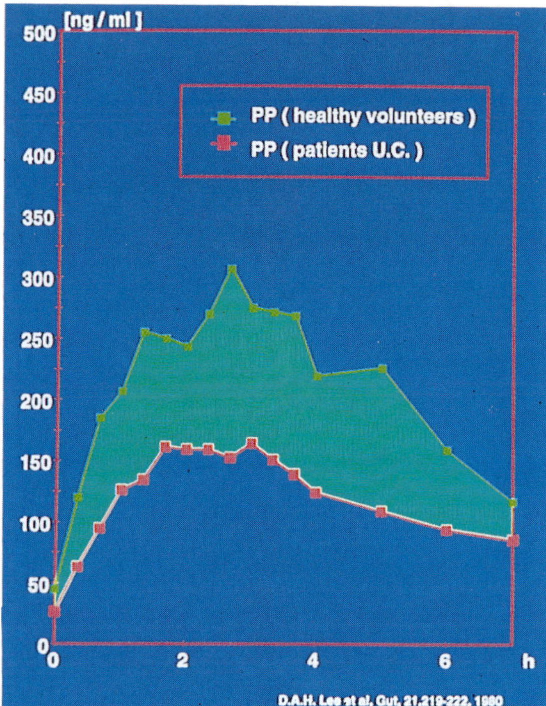

Fig. 7 Mean plasma prednisolone concentration–time profiles after administration of prednisolone-21-phosphate to healthy subjects ($n = 2$) and to patients ($n = 7$) with ulcerative colitis. Disease activity did not affect levels. The healthy subjects seem to achieve higher prednisolone-plasma concentration[14]

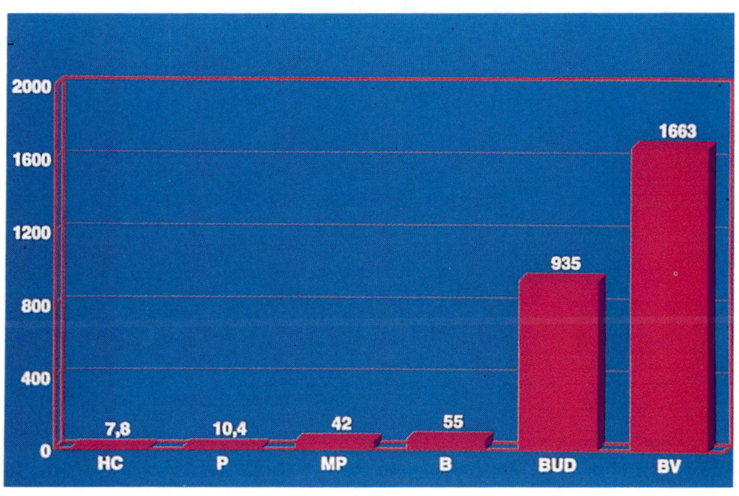

Fig. 8 Receptor binding affinities of glucocorticoid agonists to human tissue

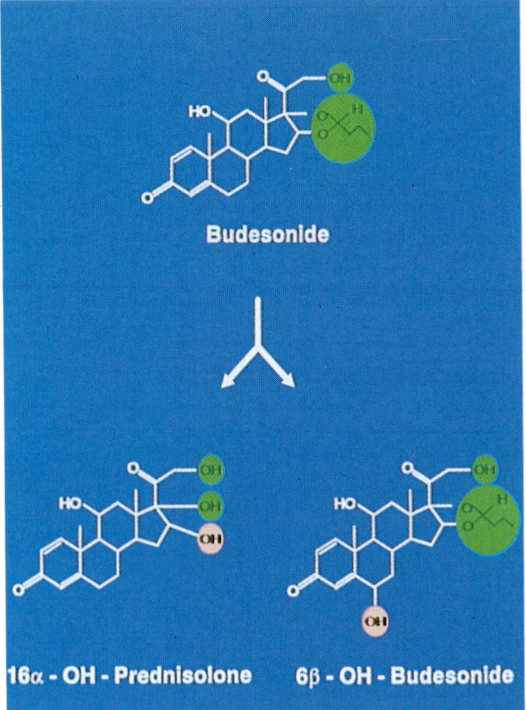

Fig. 9   Metabolic pathways of budesonide after rectal application in humans

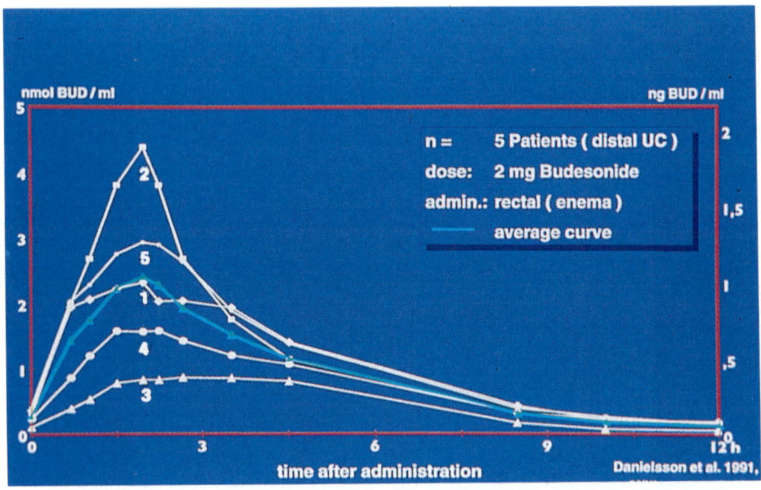

Fig. 10   Plasma concentration–time profiles of five patients after administration of 2 mg budesonide as retention enema[21]

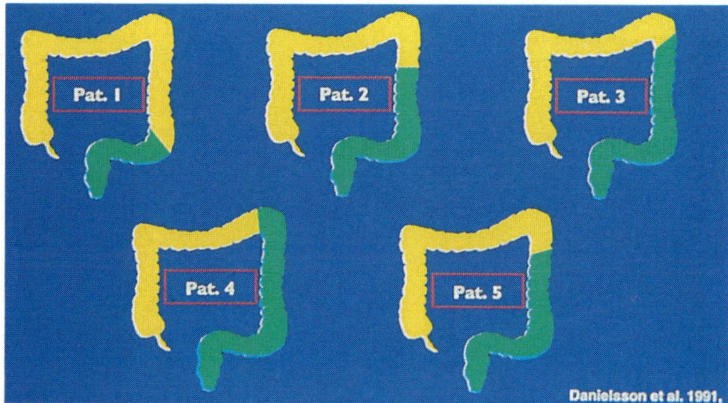

Fig. 11 The spread of budesonide enema in patients ($n = 5$) parallel to the plasma concentration–time profile

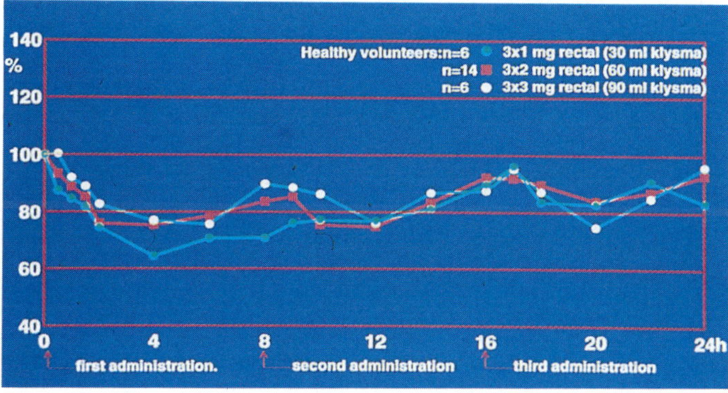

Fig. 12 Systemic pharmacodynamic effect after multiple rectal administered budesonide in different doses as retention enema

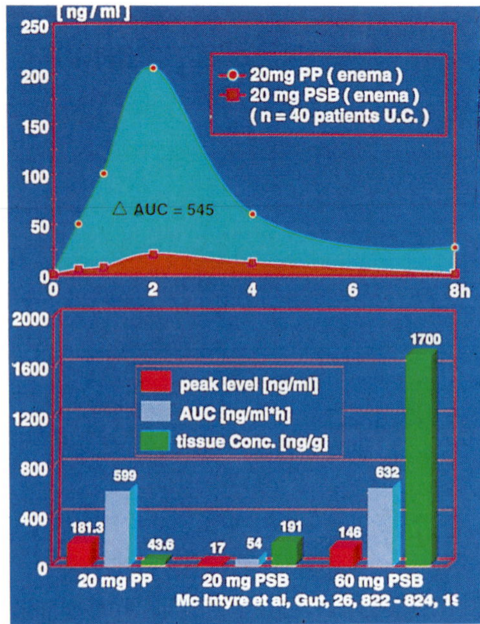

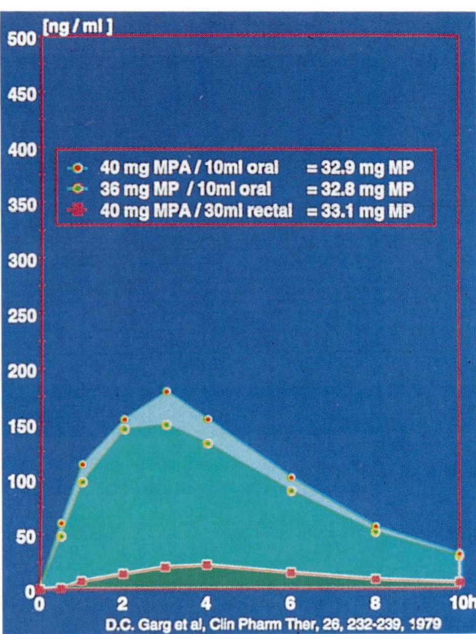

Fig. 13 Mean plasma prednisolone time-level profile and tissue concentration after administration of 20 mg prednisolone-21-phosphate sulphobenzoate retention enema to patients with distal ulcerative colitis ($n = 40$)

Fig. 14 Mean plasma methylprednisolone concentration–time profiles after administration of methylprednisolone acetate oral and retention enema (33 mg MP-equivalent) in a single-dose three-way crossover to normal male volunteers ($n = 12$) (BA:14.2%)[28]

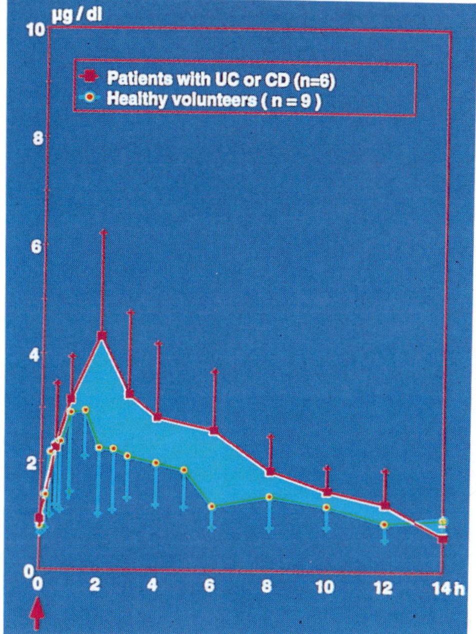

Fig. 15

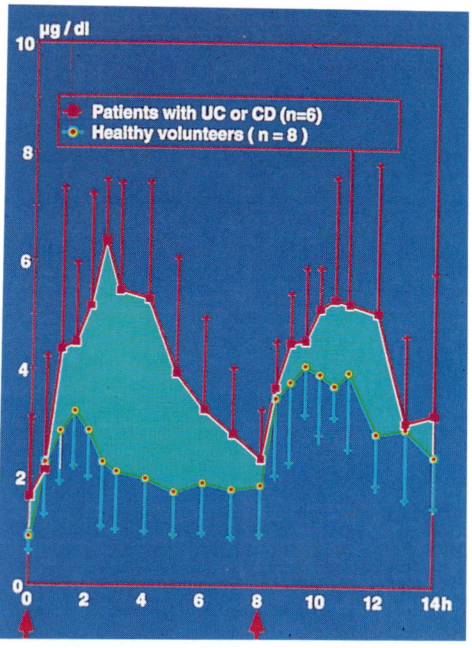

Fig. 16

Figs 15–17   Mean plasma HC-concentration–time profiles after 1 (Fig. 15); 2 (Fig. 16) and 4 (Fig. 17) times rectal administration of 100 mg HCA foam to healthy volunteers and patients with distal IBD after suppression of the endogenous HC production

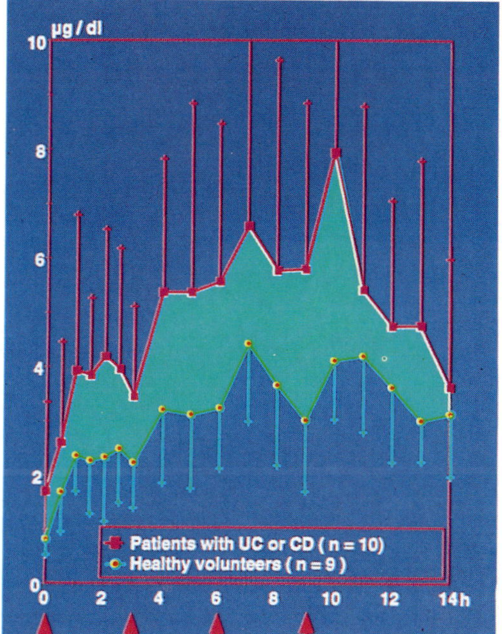

Fig. 17.

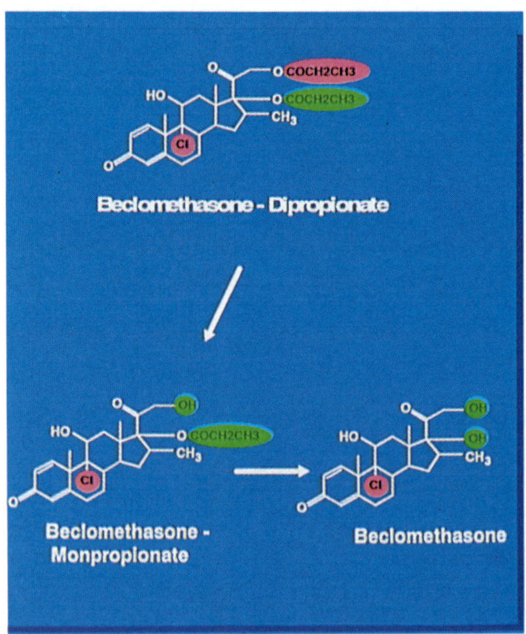

Fig. 18   Metabolic pathway of beclomethasone diprop-
rionate after rectal application in humans

because high local levels are achieved, while the slow systemic absorption is responsible for low systemic levels, and the lack of systemic side-effects. But it is necessary that the C21-esters are hydrolysed before they can be active.

Methylprednisolone acetate after rectal administration was intensively investigated by Garg *et al.*[28]. This group revealed a low rectal bioavailability of 14% and linked this observation in part to presystemic metabolism of MPAC (Fig. 14).

Möllmann *et al.*[22] have investigated the pharmacokinetic properties of hydrocortisone after administration of hydrocortisone acetate foam (HCAC). Studies were performed either in healthy volunteers or in patients with distal protocolitis. HCAC (100 mg), given as rectal foam, was applied once a day, twice every 8 h, or four times every 3 h. Hydrocortisone blood levels were compared to those after i.v. administration of 20 mg of hydrocortisone (Figs 15, 16, 17). The results showed that the bioavailability after single and multiple rectal administration in both healthy volunteers and patients with distal colitis, is very low in volunteers, (2.0–3.1%), and in patients (2.8–4.6%); these differences are not significant. Maximal plasma levels were observed in healthy subjects after 1.2–1.9 hours in the range 19.3–41.1 ng/ml, and in patients the C_{max} values of 38.8–65.6 ng/ml were found 1.0–2.9 hours after administration (Table 7). After administration of 2×100 mg HCA foam in an 8-hour interval, no accumulation of the drug was recorded, which is in agreement with the short half-life of hydrocortisone. Therefore, an 8-hour interval for the repeated administration should be recommended.

The rather low systemic level of hydrocortisone, observed in these and former studies, corresponds well to the low systemic side-effects reported after administration of hydrocortisone foam[29]. Thus, hydrocortisone acetate seems to have a much smaller systemic spillover than hemisuccinate and phsophate.

Easy application, good tolerance and high acceptance by patients in combination with a well documented efficacy are advantages of using HCA foam for the therapy of distal intestinal bowel disease.

Despite the success of ester derivatives, some research questions remain unanswered. Only a limited number of investigations suggest that lipophilic and hydrophilic prodrugs are cleaved locally, ensuring that active compounds are provided in the target tissue. Thus, it is not completely understood whether the necessary activation of these esters occurs locally, or upon absorption due to hepatic metabolism. The site of activation is, however, important. If glucocorticoid ester cleavage occurred after systemic absorption a topical effect could not be realized, and local delivery would not be of any advantage over systemic delivery. This problem is especially relevant for the use of beclomethasone dipropionate. BDP (RBA > 10) needs to be metabolized into BMP (RBA 1022), to become an active drug (Fig. 18). Previous studies have shown rather high oral bioavailability (70%) of BDP, when BDP, BMP, and beclomethasone (BC) derivatives were used for bioavailability calculations[30,31]. If BDP is not locally activated to BMP, a certain portion of the dose would not be available for the induction of topical effects, but for systemic side-effects. Additional clinical studies should elucidate the site of the activation processes for glucocorticoid prodrugs in more detail.

SUMMARY

The desired therapy goal, a high local activity with the lowest amount of systemic side-effects, can be realized by two methods:

1. Administration of lipophilic prodrugs of glucocorticoids with low intrinsic activity, e.g. hydrocortisone-acetate, provides a sustained release of active drug over time. Locally achievable drug concentrations are sufficiently high to realize the desired local effects, while systemically observed concentrations are negligible.
2. Highly active 21-alcohols, such as budesonide, with high systemic clearance and a high first-pass effect allow the use of relatively high doses without the induction of considerable systemic side-effects.

References

1. Lennard-Jones JE. Corticosteroids and immunosuppressive drugs. In: Inflammatory bowel disease. Chapman and Hall Medical, London. 1991;275–86.
2. Cooke W, Fielding J. Corticosteroid or corticotrophin therapy in Crohn's disease (regional enteritis). Gut. 1970;11:921–7.
3. Truelove S, Jewell D. Intensive intravenous regime for severe attacks of ulcerative colitis. Lancet. 1974;1:1067–70.
4. Schjonsby H, Heimann P, Kremer D et al. Intensive treatment in severe acute attacks of ulcerative colitis. Acta Med Scand. 1977;603(suppl.):43–6.
5. Truelove S, Lee E, Willoughby C. et al. Further experience in the treatment of severe attacks of ulcerative colitis. Lancet. 1978;2:1086–8.
6. Summers R, Switz D, Sessions J. Jr et al. National Cooperative Crohn's Disease Study: Results of a drug treatment. Gastroenterology. 1979;77:847–69.
7. Malchow H, Ewe K, Brandes J et al. European Cooperative Crohn's Disease Study: Results of a drug treatment. Gastroenterology. 1984;86:259–66.
8. Jarnerot G, Rolny P, Sandberg-Gertzen H. Intensive intravenous treatment of ulcerative colitis. Gastroenterology. 1985;89:1005–13.
9. Shepherd H, Barr G, Jewell D. Use of an intravenous steroid regimen in the treatment of acute Crohn's disease. J Clin Gastroenterol. 1986;8:154–9.
10. Powell-Tuck J, Bown R, Lennard-Jones JE. A Comparison of oral prednisolone as single or multiple daily doses for active procolitis. Scand J Gastroenterol. 1987;13:833–7.
11. Lennard-Jones JE. Corticosteroids and immunosuppressive drugs. In: Allan RN, Keighley MRB, Alexander-Williams J, Hawkins CF, editors. Inflammatory bowel disease. Churchill Livingstone, Edinburgh, London, Melborne and New York; 1990:373–89.
12. Lee DAH, Taylor GM, James VHT, Walker G. Plasma prednisolone levels and adrenocorticol responsiveness after administration of prednisolone-21-phosphate as a retention enema. Gut. 1979;20:349–50.
13. Powell-Tuck J, Lennard-Jones JE, May CS, Wilson CG, Paterson JW. Plasma prednisolone levels after administration of prednisolone-21-phosphate as a retention enema in colitis. Br Med J. 1976;1:193–5.
14. Lee DAH, Taylor GM, James VHT, Walker G. Rectally administered prednisolone-evidence for a predominantly local action. Gut. 1980;21:215–18.
15. Tanner AR, Halliday JW, Powell LW. Serum prednisolone levels in Crohn's disease or celiac disease following oral prednisolone administration. Digestion. 1981;21:310–15.
16. Shaffer JA. Absorption of prednisolone in patients with Crohn's disease. Gut. 1983;24:182–6.
17. Lennard-Jones JE. Betamethasone 17-valerate and prednisolone 21-phosphate retention enemata in proctocolitis. Br Med J. 1971;3:84–6.
18. Derendorf H, Möllmann HW, Barth J, Möllmann CR, Tunn S, Krieg M. Pharmacokinetics and oral bioavailability of hydrocortisone. J Clin Pharmacol. 1991;31:473–6.

19. Ryrefeldt A, Andersson P, Edsbäcker S, Tönnesson M, Davies D, Paulwels R. Pharmacokinetics and metabolism of budesonide, a selective glucocorticoid. Eur J Resp Dis. 1982;63(suppl. 122):86–95.
20. Edsbäcker S. Studies on the metabolic fate and human pharmacokinetics of budesonide. Thesis, Lund University, Sweden; 1990.
21. Danielsson A, Heller G, Lyrenäs E *et al.* A controlled trial of budesonide versus prednisolone retention enemas in active distal ulcerative colitis. Scand J Gastroenterol. 1987;22:987–92.
22. Möllmann HW, Derendorf H, Barth J, Möllmann CR, Tunn S, Krieg M. Biologische Verfügbarkeit von Hydrokortison nach rektaler Applikation von Hydrokortisonazctat-Foam. Med Welt. 1992;43:609–15.
23. Chanoine F. Tixocortol pivalate: pharmacokinetics and metabolism. In: Henry JF, editor. 1st Meeting 21-thiosteroids. Mediators of Inflammation: The Local Response. Montrouge: John Libbey Eurotext; 1988:71–82.
24. Larochelle P, Du Sowich P, Bolte E, Lelorier J, Goyer R. Tixocortol pivalate, a corticosteroid with no systemic glucocorticoid effect after oral, intrarectal and internasal applications. Clin Pharmacol Ther. 1983;33:343–50.
25. Brattsand R. Overview of newer glucocorticosteroid preparations for inflammatory bowel disease. Can J Gastroenterol. 1990;4:407–14.
26. McIntyre PB, Macrae FA, Berghouse F, English J, Lennard-Jones JE. Therapeutic benefits from poorly absorbed prednisolone enema in distal colitis. Gut. 1985;26:822–4.
27. Rodrigues C, Lennard-Jones JE, English J, Parsons DG. Systemic absorption from prednisolone rectal foam in ulcerative colitis. Lancet. 1987;27:1497.
28. Garg DC, Wagner JG, Sakmar E, Weidler DJ, Albert KS. Rectal and oral absorption of methylprednisolone acetate. Clin Pharm Ther. 1979;26:232–9.
29. Cann PA, Holdworth CD. Systemic absorption from hydrocortisone foam enema in ulcerative colitis. Lancet. 1987;1:922–3.
30. Martin EL, Tanner RJN, Clark TJ, Cochrane GM. Absorption and metabolism of orally administered beclomethasone dipropionate. Clin Pharmacol Ther. 1973;15:267–75.
31. Martin EL, Harrison C, Tanner RJN. Metabolism of beclomethasone dipropionate by animals and man. Postgrad Med J. 1975;51(suppl. 4):11–26.

33

Topical steroids in ileocolitis

C. J. J. MULDER, G. N. J. TYTGAT, P. FOCKENS and J. J. UIL

INTRODUCTION

Administration of corticosteroids is one of the mainstays in the treatment of immunologically mediated diseases. Topically applied newer corticosteroids have been shown to be very useful in a number of skin, eye, and joint diseases.

Topical use in inflammatory bowel disease (IBD) would therefore seem to be a logical application. Rectal instillation of steroids, alone or in combination with oral sulphasalazine, has been employed for the treatment of left-sided ulcerative colitis (UC) since the late 1950s, starting with the use of hydrocortisone by Truelove[1].

Topical treatment of an exacerbation of distal UC with corticosteroids containing enemas is well established[2-8]. However, prolonged treatment with enemas may produce suppression of the hypothalamic–pituitary–adrenal axis (HPA). The severity of side-effects and toxicity of rectally administered steroids varies with total dose, duration of administration, and extent of absorption. Short-term administration is rarely associated with serious side-effects, but prolonged therapy carries the same side-effects as prolonged oral or parenteral use. Therefore it would be preferable to treat distal colitis topically with corticosteroids which do not have systemic side-effects, or with steroids with a large first-pass metabolism, if at least the therapeutic efficacy is equivalent to the standard steroid enemas.

The purpose of this analysis is to give a review of topical steroid therapy in ileocolitis.

HYDROCORTISONE

Observations such as those reported by Truelove, and by Watkinson[1,9], leave little doubt as to the immediate beneficial effect of hydrocortisone, locally applied to the rectal mucosa[1,2,9-11]. With local application of hydrocortisone in alcohol to the rectal mucosa, a striking scopic improvement occurred in all patients who went into clinical remission, but the histological appearance of biopsy specimens did not show a marked favourable response. The alcohol vehicle was responsible for this[1]. The histological response was better when hydrocortisone hemisuccinate sodium was used, a water-soluble corticosteroid[10]. However, HPA suppression and side-effects, including fluid retention and acne, are associated with the use of hydrocortisone hemisuccinate sodium solutions and hydrocortisone-acetate foams[12-14].

PREDNISOLONE-21-PHOSPHATE

Prednisolone-21-phosphate (PP) is one of the most commonly used therapeutic agents in ulcerative colitis[2,6]. Slow intrarectal drip of a prednisolone solution has been shown to be effective in distal disease[3,15]. However, prolonged use of PP enemas in the treatment of UC produces profound suppression of the HPA[16,17]. In comparison to monotherapy with 5-ASA enemas, monotherapy with PP enema is cheap and at least of equal anti-inflammatory efficacy[5,6]. Whether combination of 5-ASA and PP is superior to single-agent therapy has not been investigated[8].

Prednisone, which is given orally, requires activation in the liver (i.e. 11-keto to 11-hydroxy conversion) to become active. It is therefore inactive topically and cannot be used in enemas.

BETAMETHASONE

Betamethasone enemas are frequently used in France. In a dose-range study improvement occurred with betamethasone phosphate in 100% of patients at a dose of at least 5 mg, which is considered to be the minimum effective dose. However, 5 mg or more per day produces side-effects in almost all subjects[18].

In a later study, a 5 mg betamethasone 17-valerate enema was shown to be as effective as a 20 mg PP enema. The betamethasone 17-valerate enema produced less HPA suppression compared to PP. The difference in absorption and HPA suppression may be due to the fact that the valerate is less readily absorbed than the phosphate[4].

However, substantial absorption was found to occur when 5 mg of betamethasone was compared to 250 mg tixocortol pivalate. Reduction in plasma cortisol occurred in 9% of patients on tixocortol pivalate compared to 67% of patients on betamethasone (unpublished data, G. Friedman, New York).

STEROIDS FOR TOPICAL TREATMENT

A steroid for local treatment of IBD should have a high intrinsic glucocorticoid activity, be readily absorbed into the target organ, and be rapidly inactivated. A few years ago prednisolone metasulphobenzoate, tixocortol pivalate, fluticasone propionate, beclomethasone dipropionate, and budesonide were supposed to fulfil these requirements.

PREDNISOLONE METASULPHOBENZOATE

Prednisolone metasulphobenzoate (PMSB) is a drug with minor absorption compared with prednisolone-21-phosphate. The larger molecule probably gives a slower release of prednisolone[15,19]. PMSB has been shown to give higher rectal tissue levels than rapidly absorbed systemic steroids in patients with ulcerative colitis[19].

Rectal administration is quite commonly used in England[19,20]. A foam preparation of PMSB has been introduced but, unexpectedly, this appeared to be absorbed as well as prednisolone-21-phosphate. HPA suppression can be demonstrated[20]. Raw material is available for low prices (outside the USA). Recently a preliminary study of an oral Eudragit-coated preparation in ulcerative colitis has been published. It was minimally absorbed and, in an open study, it induced remission in the majority of patients[21].

TIXOCORTOL PIVALATE

Tixocortol pivalate (TP) is a steroid molecule derived from cortisol. Its anti-inflammatory activity was considered its only steroid-related property. All information on TP in IBD has been published in abstract form and in reviews[22]. The local anti-inflammatory activity is equivalent to, or greater than, that of hydrocortisone[23,24]. No changes in plasma cortisol, leucocyte count, blood glucose, or 24-h excretion of sodium or potassium have been found[23]. A multicentre trial in the USA compared the effect and safety of rectally instilled TP (250 mg/100 ml) with the effect of hydrocortisone (100 mg/60 ml). This study, not yet published, suggests that TP is an effective local anti-inflammatory steroid comparable in efficacy to hydrocortisone and without undesirable systemic activity[25]. In another trial 250 mg TP in a 100 ml retention enema was compared with 100 mg hydrocortisone in a 100 ml retention enema in left-sided ulcerative colitis. The treatments were equally effective[24]. Promising results were obtained with a nightly rectal suspension of 250 or 500 mg TP[26]. A co-worker of Draco suggested that its very low topical potency excludes its use in slow-release formulations[27]. However, until now it is the only topical steroid commercially available as enema (250 mg/100 ml; Rectovalone®: Jouveinal France) in several countries in Europe.

FLUTICASONE PROPIONATE

Fluticasone propionate (FP) is a new steroid which is more potent than beclomethasone dipropionate (BDP) and which induces minimal systemic activity after oral dosing[28]. Its topical potency is double that of BDP[29].

Application of equal doses of both FP and BDP improves pulmonary function in patients with severe asthma; no significant changes in HPA function occurred[28]. However, after 10 days of administration of either FP or BPD, a comparable transient fall of urinary cortisol excretion (24-h) has been found[30]. In oral studies an adrenal suppression in a minority of the patients was suggested[31]. Until 1989 FP seemed a very promising drug for ileocolitis. One study with promising results with this drug in Crohn's disease has been published as an abstract with 20 mg pure substance[32]. Several other trials in England were undertaken: however, because of disappointing results Glaxo stopped development for ileocolitis (Anonymous, SCRIP, 1990;1521:11). In our opinion enema studies, and especially slow-release tablets, might still be of interest because of the high topical potency and extensive first-pass metabolism. FP seemed worthy of further assessment in coeliac disease[31]. This suggests that it might be effective in ileitis.

BECLOMETHASONE DIPROPIONATE

Beclomethasone dipropionate (BDP) is a corticosteroid which has a topical anti-inflammatory activity. This drug is effective in asthma and allergic rhinitis, reducing oral steroid requirements in many of these patients[33,34]. Under these conditions 24-h cortisol excretion remains within normal ranges[35].

BDP has been used in distal ulcerative colitis, in enema therapy[16,36-39]. The usually rapid improvement seen with PP (30 mg enema), can also be seen with BDP enemas, if given in adequate doses (2 or 3 mg)[16,38]. Also, compared with betamethasone phosphate (5 mg/100 ml), BDP (0.5 mg/100 ml) exhibits an equal anti-inflammatory action[39]. The lack of interference of BDP enemas with HPA function in these trials indicates that the absorption of this drug is insignificant, or that first-pass metabolism to metabolism is very rapid[40]. Daily doses of up to 4 mg BDP taken orally or by inhalation have been shown not to interfere with the HPA axis, possibly by converting the absorbed BDP, to pharmacologically inactive metabolites[40]. One of these metabolites is beclomethasone, which retains gluococorticosteroid activity in a tissue model[41]. ACTH, plasma cortisol and synacthen tests are not influenced by enema therapy. Only in a dosage of 6 mg is there an influence on 24-h urinary cortisol excretion[42].

Enema administration of BDP in dosages up to 2 or 3 mg, rarely 6 mg, permitted us to decrease and later to discontinue oral and topical prednisone therapy in patients with left-sided colitis (author's observation). Enema studies are under way in The Netherlands and Italy (Campieri). BDP might be of interest in aphthous oral ulceration[43].

Dose–response studies with doses of up to 10 mg/24 h are needed, including detailed HPA studies, to appreciate the full potential and the full range of safety of this drug in enema and slow-release oral formulations. A major disadvantage for trials with BDP is that Glaxo has no interest in developing the drug for ileocolitis, Gist-Brocades and Henning-Berlin have been involved in further development of BDP since 1989. Raw material is available for low prices (outside the USA).

BUDESONIDE

High-dose budesonide (BUD) treatment has shown an improvement in patients with severe steroid-dependent asthma, without causing systemic side-effects[44,45]. BUD is rapidly eliminated by a very rapid biotransformation in the liver (first-pass metabolism). The systemic activity is 2–4 times less than that of BDP[46]. Because of this it seemed suitable for the treatment of IBD.

Trials are supported by Draco/Astra, Lund, Sweden. In a first controlled randomized trial of BUD (2 mg/100 ml) versus PP (31.25 mg/100 ml), both used as retention enemas in the treatment of distal UC, BUD was found to be superior[17]. The patients receiving PP showed a significant depression of endogenous cortisol levels during the treatment period, in contrast with the patients receiving BUD[17]. The effect of budesonide, 1, 2 and 4 mg/100 ml in enemas, on distal UC, was compared with PP, 25 mg/100 ml, in a Danish Study group[47]. One milligram was less effective than the 2 or 4 mg, BUD may be an attractive alternative to PP. Two other trials have been published in abstract form[48,49]. Two milligrams of BUD showed good results compared to placebo in enema therapy[48]. Two milligrams of BUD proved to be effective and safe as 4 g/60 ml 5-ASA (Salofalk)[49].

After 4 and 8 weeks a small and stable decrease in plasma cortisol levels was seen in another study; however, it was significantly lower than with the use of 20 mg methyl prednisolone[50].

Budesonide 0.5 mg suppositories seem to be effective in pouchitis, when used three times daily[51]. All 10 patients in this study were in remission after 4 weeks, but six relapsed within 4 weeks after the drug was stopped.

Probably the most exciting field for the use of topical corticosteroids in IBD, is the development of oral slow-release formulations. With these formulations also other localizations of IBD can possibly be treated, for instance terminal ileitis and extensive colitis. One case of oral untreated BUD treatment has been published in Crohn's disease[52]. The BUD slow-release tablet consists of a central sugar core, a second layer of budesonide in combination with ethylcellulose and an outer coating of Eudragit-L. Two different release profiles have been developed, one for the ileum (controlled ileum release CIR) and one for the colon (controlled colon release CCR). The 9 mg CIR formulation is currently being investigated for Crohn's disease against 25 mg of prednisolone in a large multicentre controlled trial. Results of a small uncontrolled trial in nine patients are promising, for efficacy as well as for side-effects[53]. Although baseline cortisol was suppressed in five out of six patients after 6 weeks use of 9 mg budesonide, response to cortisol releasing factor (CRF) was preserved in all patients except one. The results of the large controlled trials are eagerly awaited. The release pattern of CIR is probably quite similar to Claversal/Salofalk; the need for a CCR formulation is therefore doubtful.

Data concerning ACTH, synacthen test and urinary coristol excretions are mandatory to discuss its systemic side-effects. The drug is running out of patent in 1 year and only slow-release formulations are patented. Raw material will be available for low prices.

ENEMA PREPARATIONS WITH CORTICOSTEROIDS

Commercially available steroid enemas are known for prednisone, beta-methasone phosphate and tixocortol pivalate. In most countries in Europe prescriptions according to the Formularies of the National Pharmacists are available. Prescriptions for BDP have been used and developed[54]:

BDP	1–6 mg
Ethanol 96%	0.2–0.3 ml
Methyloxybenzoate 15% w/v in propylene glycol	0.2 ml
Carbomer water gel 0.7%	10–25 gr
Distilled water	ad 40–100 gr

The stability of this formula, even in combination with 5-ASA, has been proven to be good and can be prepared in every pharmacy.

The BUD enema consists of a BUD tablet and an enema vehicle, prepared by combining the components before administration. Because of its excellent water-solubility enema prescription will be simple[27]. Exact formulations have not been published.

The effect of glycyrrhetinic acid and potentiation of corticosteroid activity in enema solutions should be investigated, as was recently suggested for the skin[55]. The retrograde spread of therapeutic enemas in IBD is in general good, and makes them suitable for treatment of left-sided colitis[56].

DISCUSSION

The beneficial effect of steroid enemas in the treatment of distal colitis has been established[1-6]. Trials with topical steroids in enema form, compared to systemically active steroids, have been reported. Studies with BUD and BDP show no clear suppression of the HPA function after 4 weeks of enema therapy. However, no adequate therapeutic and endocrinological data are available following longer periods of administration. Enema studies are at least promising. Slow-release formulations are needed for ileocolitis.

Oral administration of BDP capsules coated with cellulose acetate phthalate allows topical delivery of adequate concentrations of the drug to the terminal ileum[57]. Slow-release formulations for BDP and PMSB have been developed[21,57] BUD as CIR tablet is in progress for a multicentre trial.

We hope that the supposed reduced risk of serious adverse risks makes protracted therapeutic treatment possible. The next few years will show whether one or more of these drugs will be commercially available.

ACKNOWLEDGEMENTS

We thank Karin Dhaenens for her fine secretarial work.

References

1. Truelove SC. Treatment of ulcerative colitis with local hydrocortisone. Br Med J. 1956;2:1267–72.
2. MacDouglas I. Treatment of ulcerative colitis with rectal steroids. Lancet. 1963;1:826–7.
3. Matts SGF. Intrarectal treatment of 100 cases of ulcerative colitis with prednisolone 21-phosphate retention enemata. Br Med J. 1961;1:165.
4. Lennard-Jones JE. Betamethasone 17-valerate and prednisolone 21-phosphate retention enemata. Br Med J. 1971;3:84–6.
5. Campieri M, Lanfranchi GA, Bazzocchi G et al. Treatment of ulcerative colitis with high dose 5-aminosalicylic acid enemas. Lancet. 1981;2:270–1.
6. Mulder CJJ, Tytgat GNJ, Wiltink EHH, Houthoff HJ. Comparison of 5-aminosalicylic acid (3 g) and prednisolone phosphate sodium enemas (30 mg) in the treatment of distal ulcerative colitis. Scand J Gastroenterol. 1988;23:1005–8.
7. Jewel DP. Corticosteroids for management of ulcerative colitis and Crohn's disease. Gastroenterol Clin N Am. 1989;18:21–34.
8. Mulder CJJ, Rondas AALM, Wiltink EHH, Tytgat GNJ. Topical corticosteroids in inflammatory bowel disease. Neth J Med. 1989;35:S27–34.
9. Watkinson G. Treatment of ulcerative colitis with topical hydrocortisone hemissuccinate sodium; a controlled trial employing restricted sequential analysis. Br Med J. 1958;2:1077–82.
10. Truelove SC. Treatment of ulcerative colitis with local hydrocortisone. Br Med J. 1957;1:1437–43.
11. Truelove SC. Treatment of ulcerative colitis with local hydrocortisone hemisuccina sodium; a report on a controlled therapeutic trial. Br Med J. 1958;2:1072–7.
12. Spencer JA, Kirsner JB. Experience with short and longterm courses of local adrenal steroid therapy for ulcerative colitis. Gastroenterology. 1962;6:669–77.
13. Farmer RG, Schumacher OP. Treatment of ulcerative colitis with hydrocortisone enemas; relationship of hydrocortisone absorption, adrenal suppression and clinical response. Dis Colon Rectum. 1970;13:355–61.
14. Cann PA, Holdsworth CD. Systemic absorption from hydrocortisone foam enema in ulcerative colitis. Lancet. 1987;1:922–30.
15. Lee DAH, Taylor M, James VTH, Walker G. Rectally administered prednisolone evidence for a predominantly local action. Gut. 1980;21:215–18.
16. Van der Heide H, Van den Brandt-Grädel V, Tytgat GNJ et al. Comparison of beclomethasone dipropionate and prednisolone 21-phosphate enemas in the treatment of ulcerative proctitis. J Clin Gastroenterol. 1988;10:169–72.
17. Danielsson A, Hellers G, Lyrenäs E et al. A controlled trial of budesonide versus prednisolone retention enemas in active distal ulcerative colitis. Scand J Gastroenterol. 1987;22:987–92.
18. Matts SGF. Betamethasone enemata in ulcerative colitis. Gut. 1962;3:312–14.
19. McIntyre PB, Macrea FA, Berghouse L, English J, Lennard-Jones JE. Therapeutic benefits from a poorly absorbed prednisolone enema in distal colitis. Gut. 1985;26:822–4.
20. Rodrigues C, Lennard-Jones JE, English J, Parsons DG. Systemic absorption from prednisolone rectal foam in ulcerative colitis. Lancet. 1987;1:1497.
21. Ford GA, Oliver PS, Shephard NA, Wilkinson SP. An eudragit-coated prednisolone preparation for UC: pharmacokinetics and preliminary therapeutic use. Aliment Pharmacol Ther. 1992;6:31–40.
22. Hanauer SB. Clinical experience with tixocortol pivalate. Can J Gastroenterol. 1988;2:156–8.
23. Larochelle P, Du Souich P, Bolte E, Lelorier J, Goyer R. Tixocortol pivalate, a corticosteroid with no systemic glucocorticoid effect after oral, intrarectal, and intranasal application. Clin Pharmacol Ther. 1983;3:343–50.
24. Hanauer SB, Kirsner JB and Barrett WE. The treatment of left-sided ulcerative colitis with tixocortol pivalate. Gastroenterology. 1986;90:1449A.
25. Levinsson P. Tixocortol pivalate versus hydrocortisone enemas in ulcerative colitis: a multicenter comparative clinical trial. IBD symposium, 12 April 1985, Phoenix AZ, USA.
26. Friedman G. Treatment of refractory proctosigmoiditis and left sided colitis with a rectally instilled non-mineralocorticoid. Gastroenterology. 1985;88:1388A.
27. Brattsand R. Overview of newer glucocorticosteroid preparations for inflammatory bowel disease. Can J Gastroenterol. 1990;4:407–14.

28. Bauer K, Bamtje TA, Sips AP *et al*. The effect of inhaled fluticasone propionate, a new potent corticosteroid in severe asthma. Eur Resp J. 1988;2:201A.
29. Harding S. Human pharmacology of fluticasone. XIV congress of the European Academy of Allergology and Clinical Immunology. Berlin, 17–22 September 1989, AS 04.04.
30. Harding SM, Felstaed S. A comparison of the tolerance and systemic effects of fluticasone propionate and beclomethasone dipropionate in healthy volunteers. Eur Resp J. 1988;2:196A.
31. Carpani de Kaski M, Peter AM, Lavender JP, Hodgson HJF. Fluticasone propionate in coeliac disease. Gut. 1991;32:657–61.
32. Carpani de Kaski M, Peter AM, Lavender JP, Hodgson HJF. Oral fluticasone propionate in active Crohn's disease. Gut. 1989;30:A1480.
33. Williams MH. Diagnosis and treatment-drugs five years later: beclomathasone dipropionate. Ann Intern Med. 1981;95:464–7.
34. Brogden RN, Heel RC, Speight TM, Avery GS. Beclomethasone dipropionate: a reappraisal of its pharmacodynamic properties and therapeutic efficacy after a decade of use in asthma and rhinitis. Drugs. 1984;29:99–126.
35. Smith MJ, Hodgson ME. Effects of long term inhaled high dose beclomethasone dipropionate on adrenal function. Thorax. 1983;38:676–81.
36. Kumana CR, Seaton T, Meghji M, Casteli M, Benson R, Sivakumaran T. Beclomethasone dipropionate enemas for treating inflammatory bowel disease without producing Cushing's syndrome or hypothalamic–pituitary–adrenal suppression. Lancet. 1982;1:579–83.
37. Levine DS, Rubin CE. Topical beclomethasone dipropionate enemas improve distal ulcerative colitis and idiopathic proctitis without systemic toxicity. Gastroenterology. 1985;88:1473A.
38. Mulder CJJ, Endert E, van der Heyde H, Tytgat GNJ, Wiltink EHH, Wiersinga W, Houthoff HJ. Comparison of beclomethasone dipropionate (2 and 3 mg) and prednisolone-sodium phosphate enemas (30 mg) in the treatment of distal ulcerative colitis. Neth J Med. 1989;35:18–24.
39. Bansky G, Buhler H, Stamm B, Häcki WH, Buchmann P. Treatment of distal ulcerative colitis with beclomethasone enemas: high therapeutic efficacy without endocrine side effects. Dis Colon Rectum. 1987;30:288–92.
40. Martin L, Harrison C, Tanner RJN. Metabolism of beclomethasone dipropionate by animals and man. Postgrad Med J. 1975;51(Suppl. 14):11–20.
41. Axelsson B, Brattsand R, Anderson PH, Ryrfeldt A, Thalén A. Relationship between glucocorticosteroid effects of beclomethasone 17α,21-dipropionate, beclomethasone 17α-propionate and beclomethasone as studies in human, mouse and rat tissue. Respiration. 1984;46(Suppl. 4):11–20.
42. Mulder CJJ, Kneppelhout JC, Verschoor L, Willekens FLA. Beclomethasone dipropionate enema (6 mg). Sydney World Congress, abstr. PD 566.
43. Thompson AC, Nolan A, Laney PJ. Minor aphthous oral ulceration: a double-blind cross-over study of beclomethasone dipropionate aerosol spray. Scott Med J. 1989;34:531–2.
44. Tukianen P, Lahdensuo A. Effect of inhaled budesonide on severe steroiddependent asthma. Eur J Respir Dis 1987;70:239–44.
45. Clissold SP, Heel RC. Budesonide. A preliminary review of its pharmacodynamic properties and therapeutic efficacy in asthma and rhinitis. Drugs. 1984;28:485–518.
46. Johansson SA, Andersson KE, Brattscand R, Gruvstad E, Hedner P. Topical and systemic glucocorticoid potencies of Budesonide and Beclomethasone dipropionate in man. Eur J Clin Pharmacol. 1982;22:523–9.
47. Matzen P. Budesonide enema in distal ulcerative colitis. A randomized dose–response trial with prednisolone enema as positive control. Scand J Gastroenterol. 1991;26:1225–30.
48. Danielson Å, Loftberg R, Salde L, Schöler R, Suhr O, Willén R. A new steroid enema without systemic side-effects for treatment of proctitis and distal ulcerative colitis. Scand J Gastroenterol. 1989;245:88A.
49. Lamers C, Meijer J, Engels L *et al*. Comparative study of the topically acting glucocorticosteroid budesonide and 5-aminosalicylic acid enema therapy of proctitis and proctosigmoiditis. Gastroenterology. 1991;100:5;A223.
50. Bianchi Porro G, Campieri M, Bianchi P *et al*. Comparative trial of budesonide and methylprednisolone enemas in the treatment of ulcerative colitis. Gastroenterology. 1992;102:A595.

51. Beluzzi A, Campieri M, Miglioli M *et al*. Evaluation of phlogistic pattern in "pouchitis" before and after the treatment with budesonide. Gastroenterology. 1992;102:A593.
52. Wolman SL. Use of oral budesonide in a patient with small bowel Crohn's disease and previous pseudotumour cerebri secundary to steroids. Scand J Gastroenterol. 1989;24:S158: 146–7.
53. Roth M, Ueberschaer K, Ewe K, Gross V, Scholmerich J. Oral slow release budesonide induces remission in active Crohn's disease with little effect on adrenal function. Gastroenterology. 1992;102:A688.
54. Stolk LML, Gerrits M, Wiltink EHH, Mulder CJJ, Tytgat GNJ. Formulation and stability of a beclomethasone dipropionate enema. Pharm Weekbl (Sci). 1989;11:20–2.
55. Teelucksingh S, Mackie ADR, Burt D, McIntyre MA, Brett L. Potentiation of hydrocortisone activity in skin by glycerrhetinic acid. Lancet. 1990;335:1060–3.
56. van Buul MMC, Mulder CJJ, Wiltink EHH, van Ryen EA, Tytgat GNJ. Retrograde spread of therapeutic enemas in patients with IBD. Hepatogastroenterology. 1989;36:199–201.
57. Levine DS, Raisys VA, Ainardi V. Coating of oral beclomethasone dipropionate capsules with cellulose acetate phtalate enhances delivery of topically active antiinflammatory drug to the terminal ileum. Gastroenterology. 1987;92:1037–44.

34
Immunosuppressive therapy for refractory inflammatory bowel disease

R. A. KOZAREK

INTRODUCTION

The use of immunosuppressive agents to treat refractory inflammatory bowel disease (IBD) remains an art form as opposed to a science. Not only is there debate about which particular patient requires treatment, but even which disease process. To that end, most clinicians have a greater comfort level utilizing these drugs in Crohn's disease (CD) as opposed to chronic ulcerative colitis (CUC), a disease that is not only surgically curable, but also has a much higher incidence of superimposed colorectal carcinoma. Once such therapy is considered, however, a plethora of secondary questions arise: What are the clinical goals? Which drug should be used? and For how long?

6-MERCAPTOPURINE/AZATHIOPRINE (6-MP/AZ)

An analogue of the purine bases hypoxanthine and adenine, 6-MP ultimately inhibits purine ribonucleotide synthesis[1,2]. AZ, in turn, is an S-substituted 6-MP, converted into its parent compound within the liver. Both drugs suppress natural killer lymphocyte activity and affect humoral responsiveness[3,4]. Whether such effects account for the drugs' anti-inflammatory capabilities remains uncertain, although recent data suggest that clinical response in IBD appears to be contingent upon development of leukopenia[5,6].

Crohn's disease

A large number of uncontrolled trials have been published using 6-MP or AZ for CD with variable results[2]. A recent study by O'Brien *et al.* reported 78 patients treated with AZ for a mean of 1.6 years[7]. At a median treatment time of 3 months, 70 patients responded clinically, achieving such predefined goals as steroid reduction (76%), control of refractory disease (73%), and improvement of fistulae (63%). Side-effects severe enough to require medication withdrawal occurred in 10% and included serious infections in three patients and pancreatitis in a fourth. Mendelsohn *et al.*, in turn, used 6-MP for at least 6 months in 162 of 230 CD patients, effecting such therapeutic goals as steroid elimination (66%), fistula or abscess healing (66%) and a reduction in disease activity (78%)[8]. Additional studies by Markowitz *et al.* demonstrated improvement in fistulous disease, decrease in steroid requirement and reduction in disease activity in 36 adolescents treated for at least 6 months with 6-MP, whereas Korelitz and Present have confirmed a favourable effect of the latter drug in fistulous CD[10].

In addition to the uncontrolled data cited above there have been two large, randomized, prospective trials using 6-MP or AZ for CD[11]. In the National Cooperative Crohn's Disease Study, patients with active disease were randomized into 17-week treatment arms and received placebo, prednisone, sulphasalazine, or 25 mg/kg of AZ. Although sulphasalazine- and prednisone-treated patients had significant clinical improvement, AZ and placebo treated patients did not. In addition, the significant incidence of AZ-induced pancreatitis ultimately led to its withdrawal from the trial. In contrast, Present *et al.* studied 83 patients with refractory CD, randomizing them to either placebo therapy or 6-MP for 1 year[12]. Only 8% of the patients receiving placebo responded in contrast to two-thirds of 6-MP-treated patients.

Chronic ulcerative colitis

In addition to efficacy in CD, 6-MP/AZ may play a role in CUC despite concerns that prolonged treatment may result in an increased risk of colorectal neoplasia. For instance, Present *et al.* have reported in abstract form that 43% of 56 steroid-resistant CUC patients experienced full remission, and an additional 30% partial remission with long term 6-MP therapy[13]. Adler and Korelitz, in turn, used 6-MP in 81 patients who underwent 91 courses of therapy for a minimum of 6 months[14]. Mean treatment was 1.8 years. Sixty three per cent of patients ultimately responded, and corticosteroids were eliminated in approximately one-half. Mean time to relapse after discontinuation of the drug was 21 months. In contrast to the above studies, Lobo *et al.* describe AZ use in 47 patients with intractable or steroid-dependent disease[15]. Forty-six per cent (13/28) of patients with resistant disease achieved initial remission, 11 of 13 maintaining this remission for approximately 2 years. Fifteen of the patients with refractory disease underwent colectomy acutely or during the follow up period. In the steroid-dependent group, 63% of patients had either steroid reduction or withdrawal of corticosteroids.

Complications

In the Lobo study noted above, 26% of patients had side-effects necessitating medication withdrawal[15]. These included haematological effects in six, gastrointestinal problems in two and miscellaneous complications in an additional two patients. This complication rate is significantly higher than that reported in the 396 IBD patients reported by Present *et al.*[16]. The latter included pancreatitis (3.3%), marrow suppression (2%), allergic-type reactions (2%), drug-induced hepatitis (1%) and possible medication-related neoplasia (0.3%).

METHOTREXATE (MTX)

A folic acid antagonist, MTX has both immunosuppressant and anti-inflammatory effects[17-21]. From the latter perspective the drug has been widely used for various forms of arthritis as well as psoriasis[22-27] and it is currently undergoing investigation in asthma[28,29], primary biliary cirrhosis[30], and sclerosing cholangitis[31]. We postulated in 1987 that it may have similar anti-inflammatory capabilities in IBD, and subsequently utilized a 12-week parenteral and subsequent oral course to treat refractory CUC and CD patients. Using a modified disease activity index and steroid requirements to define efficacy, approximately three-quarters of 21 previously refractory IBD patients had significant clinical response, including 11 of 14 patients with CD and five of seven with CUC[32] (Tables 1 and 2). Moreover, five patients with Crohn's colitis had endoscopic healing, four of whom had normal histology at 12 weeks. Side-effects were generally minor, including transient leukopenia or minor elevations in liver function tests, nausea, and diarrhoea exacerbation for 24 h following an injection.

Additional data from our group have noted that 16 of 20 IBD patients who had proved refractory to at least 6 months of 6-MP or AZ therapy, or who had developed toxicity necessitating discontinuation of these drugs, subsequently responded to parenteral MTX[33]. At a mean follow-up of 72 weeks, two-thirds of the initial respondees maintained a clinical remission on subsequent oral MTX. Five patients, comprising three with CUC and two with obstructive CD, ultimately required surgery. Such data suggest that failure to respond to 6-MP/AZ does not preclude subsequent response to MTX, and further suggest that there are differences either in medication potency or mechanism of action.

Prolonged follow-up of IBD patients treated with MTX suggests that there is a significant discordance between CUC and CD patients[34]. Whereas two-thirds of the latter remained in remission at a mean follow-up of 69 weeks, only 40% of CUC patients continued therapay at $1\frac{1}{2}$ years and fully 50% required or elected colectomy ultimately. The latter results are sobering, and suggest that additional anti-inflammatory or immunosuppressive drugs should supplant or supplement MTX in CUC patients undergoing prolonged therapy.

Table 1 Methotrexate administration in CUC†

Patients	Disease extent	F/U (weeks)	Response	Prednisone (mg) onset/ 12 weeks	Activity index onset/ 12 weeks	Ongoing MTX
1	Pancolitis	12	No	30/30	13/12	No
2	Pancolitis	34	Yes	60/10	15/7	Yes
3	Left colon	12	No	30/10	11/10	Yes
4	Pancolitis	20	Yes	15/0	15/2	Yes
5	Pancolitis	20	Yes	60/10	15/4	Yes
6	Left colon	20	Yes → R*	35/15	15/7	No
7	Left colon	24	Yes → R*	40/15	9/2	No
		$\bar{x} = 20.3$		$\bar{x}(SEM) =$ 38.6(6.35)/ 12.9(3.4), $p = 0.01$	$\bar{x}(SEM) =$ 13.3(0.9)/ 6.3(1.5), $p = 0.007$	

R* = relapse; $\bar{x}$ = mean; SEM = standard error of mean; p determined by paired t-test
† Adapted from ref. 32

Table 2 Methotrexate administration in Crohn's disease†

Patients	Disease site	F/U (weeks)	Response	Prednisone (mg) onset/ 12 weeks	Activity index onset/ 12 weeks	Ongoing MTX
1	Colon	40	Yes	20/0	15/5	Yes
2	Colon	30	Yes	0/0	10/2	Yes
3	Small bowel	36	Yes	20/0	15/6	Yes
4	Colon	22	Yes	15/10	15/2	No
5	Colon	22	Yes	10/2.5	7/2	Yes
6	Colon	12	No	40/15	14/9	No
7	Small bowel	12	No	0/0	15/15	No
8	Small bowel	9	Yes	60/0	15/7	Yes
9	Small bowel/ Colon	18	Yes → R*	0/0	15/7	Yes
10	Small bowel	12	Yes	15/15	13/6	Yes
11	Small bowel	20	Yes	60/20	15/3	Yes
12	Colon	32	Yes	20/0	11/1	Yes
13	Small bowel/ Colon	12	No	40/15	12/10	No
14	Small bowel/ Colon	26	Yes	0/0	4/0	Yes
		$\bar{x} = 22.5$		$\bar{x}(SEM) =$ 21.4(5.6/ 5.5(2.0), $p = 0.006$	$\bar{x}(SEM) =$ 13.3(0.9)/ 6.3(1.5), $p = 0.0001$	

R* = relapse; $\bar{x}$ = mean; SEM = standard error of mean; p determined by paired t-test
† Adapted from ref. 32

Toxicity

The lack of controlled trials, as well as concern about long-term toxicity, have limited the use of MTX at many medical centres. Based upon our anecdotal experience demonstrating dramatic clinical and, at times, endoscopic improvement in previously refractory IBD patients, we no longer consider this an investigational drug at our institution. We are concerned about toxicity issues, however, and do not recommend its use without a thorough informed consent detailing potential complications with the drug and alternative treatment modalities to include surgery. Side-effect liability in our patients has generally included post-injection nausea, diarrhoea, or stomatitis, minor degrees of leukopenia or transaminase elevation, brittle nails or accentuated hair loss[32]. There are three toxicities that deserve special mention. Hypersensitivity pneumonitis is a rare, allergic response to MTX which can cause non-productive cough, progressive shortness of breath and variable pulmonary infiltrates in an interstitial pattern[35]. Treated with medication withdrawal and high-dose steroids, deaths have been reported, and accordingly, patients with ongoing pulmonary complaints should be instructed to hold their weekly medication prior to physician evaluation. We have seen a single case. Hepatic histological abnormalities have been noted to occur in up to one-quarter of patients treated with long-term MTX[36]. Such abnormalities appear to be more common in obesity, with concomitant alcohol use, and with higher total cumulative MTX dose. Accordingly, our group not only interdicts alcohol but recommends liver biopsy at cumulative doses of 1.5, 3.0, and 5.0 cumulative grams of MTX. No histological abnormalities have been noted to date[37]. Finally, methotrexate has the capability of inducing fetal abnormalities, and should not be taken in fertile individuals of either sex without adequate instruction and contraceptive control. A single small series suggests that patients taking MTX for rheumatological purposes may have a higher incidence of spontaneous abortion, but did not deliver infants with congenital defects[38]. Such data are comparable to those recently reported in patients undergoing conception while on AZ therapy[39].

CYCLOSPORIN A (CyA)

Derived from the fermentation broth of soil fungi, CyA selectively interferes with interleukin-2 release and/or synthesis and inhibits helper T-lymphocyte function[40,41].

Crohn's disease

In a placebo-controlled, randomized trial, Brynskov et al. demonstrated a statistically significant improvement (50% vs 32%, $p = 0.032$) in 71 CD patients randomized to receive either 5–7.5 mg/kg per day of CyA or placebo[42]. There was also a significant, albeit mild, improvement in the Crohn's Disease Activity Index (CDAI) and orosomucoid levels. In contrast, only 19% of the patients in this study remained moderately or substantially improved 6 months after tapering and discontinuing the active medication, suggesting that long-term efficacy may require chronic therapy[43]. In an attempt to address the latter question, Lobo *et al.* utilized 5 mg/kg per day in 14 patients with CD, reducing the dose by 1 mg/kg per day every 2 months until a maintenance dose of 2 mg/kg per day was reached[44]. Twelve of 14 (86%) of patients in remission ultimately relapsed, suggesting that, in the doses utilized, CyA was not effective in maintaining remission.

Additional studies suggesting either acute or chronic efficacy in Crohn's disease have been published by Allison and Pounders[45], and Fukushima *et al.*[46], whereas Archambault *et al.*[47] and Baker and Jewel[48] have reported negative or equivocal results. Some of this discrepancy may be related to dosing and blood level of CyA, patient selection criteria, and drug toxicity necessitating medication discontinuation or decrease.

Ulcerative colitis

CyA has been utilized sparingly in CUC. Baker and Jewell reported its use in 12 patients with severe CUC, treating patients with 15 mg/kg per day in conjunction with ongoing corticosteroid therapy[48]. These authors noted no benefit when compared with hospital controls. Lichtiger and Present, in turn, treated 15 patients with refractory CUC with constant infusion CyA, demonstrating a response in 11 (73%)[49]. Nine of the 11 had prolonged remission after 6 months of subsequent oral therapy in doses ranging from 6 to 8 mg/kg per day. Additional studies have been reported by Gupta *et al.*[50], Porro *et al.*[51], and Hyams and Treem[52], with variable results. Finally, two studies have looked at use of rectal CyA for distal proctosigmoiditis[53,54]. While there was rapid improvement in the majority of treated patients, approximately one-half relapsed immediately after the drug's cessation.

Toxicity

CyA is not only an expensive medication, it is also one with a high side-effect profile[40,41] (Table 3). It is this latter problem, particularly the acute nephrotoxicity, that will probably limit widespread usage of this medication

Table 3 Cyclosporin side-effects (autoimmune disease use) (percentages)

Nephrotoxicity	19
Hypertension	11
Tremor	13
Paraesthesias	48
Hypertrichosis	46
Gingival hyperplasia	35
Nausea/vomiting	39
Seizures*	?

* Modified from ref. 41

in IBD patients. Moreover, particular care must be exercised in the acutely and chronically ill patient with very low serum cholesterol levels, as CyA application in this setting can induce seizures in a significant subset.

MISCELLANEOUS DRUGS

Immunosuppressive activity is an element of efficacy not only with corticosteroids, but also variably used drugs to include metronidazole, anti-malarial medications, and possibly sulphasalazine[55-57]. T-lymphocyte apheresis, while not classically defined as a medication, has also been used in CD and might be considered the ultimate form of immunosuppression[59]. Used anecdotally in 65 patients with refractory disease, Bicks et al. have reported signficiant clinical response in a subset of such patients[60]. Finally, Deusch et al. have recently reported the use of monoclonal antibodies to the CD4 lymphocyte for patients with otherwise refractory inflammatory bowel disease[61]. Preliminary results have been encouraging.

CONCLUSIONS AND FUTURE

Having undergone prolonged scrutiny over a several-decade period, 6-MP/AZ currently remain the immunosuppressive agents of choice in patients with refractory IBD. Both MTX and CyA appear promising, particularly in the setting of CD, but additional data to include efficacy and long-term medication-related toxicity are required before widespread utilization of either.

The future includes application of the above-mentioned drugs both in different vehicles (e.g. topical) and the development or application of additional immunosuppressive agents with greater efficacy or less toxicity than current ones. To that end, a number of centres are utilizing the recently developed immunosuppressive agent, FK-506, for refractory IBD, although, as of this writing, there have been no reports of clinical results.

Recently, oncological research has discovered that drug-induced induction of P-170 glycoprotein is associated with the development of resistance to multiple unrelated chemotherapeutic agents[62-64]. Researchers have further been able to block such induction with verapamil, quinidine, tamoxifen, CyA, and monoclonal antibodies, postulating that such blockage may prove to be clinically important in overcoming development of multiple drug resistance[65]. These developments probably have application in a number of gastroen-terological disorders as development of drug resistance or tolerance is common, particularly in refractory inflammatory bowel disease.

Finally, the future may allow better selection of combinations of immunosuppressive and anti-inflammatory agents, each attacking one particular aspect of the inflammatory or immunological cascade. After disease control is effected, individual agents can then be withdrawn, leaving a single medication to maintain disease control. This 'reverse-pyramid' concept of drug therapy is already being widely applied in oncology, and is currently being evaluated by other medical disciplines.

References

1. Elion GB. Biochemistry and pharmacology of purine analogues. Fed Proc. 1967;26:898–904.
2. Adler DJ, Korelitz BI. 6-mercaptopurine and azathioprine. In: Gitnick G, editor. Inflammatory bowel disease. Diagnosis and treatment. New York: Igaku-Shoin; 1991:323–46.
3. Brogan M, Stevens R, Histerodt J *et al.* Effects of 6-MP on the impaired in vivo humoral responsiveness in Crohn's disease. Gastroenterology. 1984;86:1035A.
4. Brogan M, Histerodt J, Stevens R *et al.* The effects of 6-mercaptopurine on the natural killer cell activities in Crohn's disease. J Clin Immunol. 1985;5:204.
5. Burke DA, Dixon MF, Axon ATR. Ulcerative colitis. Prolonged remission following azathioprine-induced pancytopenia. J Clin Gastroenterol. 1989;11:327–30.
6. Colonna T, Korelitz BI. The role of leukopenia in the 6-mercaptopurine induced remission of Crohn's disease. Am J Gastroenterol. 1991;86:1345A.
7. O'Brien JJ, Bayless TM, Bayuless JA. Use of azathioprine or 6-mercaptopurine in the treatment of Crohn's disease. Gastroenterology. 1991;101:39–46.
8. Mendelsohn RA, Adler DJ, Korelitz BI. The long term efficacy of 6-mercaptopurine in the treatment of Crohn's disease; an update. Am J Gastroenterol. 1991;86:1347A.
9. Markowitz J, Rosa J, Grancher K *et al.* Long term 6-mercaptopurine treatment in adolescents with Crohn's disease. Gastroenterology. 1990;99:1347–51.
10. Korelitz BI, Present DH. Favorable effect of 6-mercaptopurine on fistulae of Crohn's disease. Dig Dis Sci. 1985;30:58–64.
11. Summers RW, Switz DM, Sessions JT Jr *et al.* National Cooperative Crohn's Disease Study: results of drug treatment. Gastroenterology. 1979;77:847–69.
12. Present DH, Korelitz BI, Wisch N *et al.* Treatment of Crohn's disease with 6-mercaptopurine. A long term, randomized, double blind study. N Engl J Med. 1980;302:981–7.
13. Present DH, Chapman ML, Rubin PH. Efficacy of 6-mercaptopurine in refractory ulcerative colitis. Gastroenterology. 1988;94:359A.
14. Adler DJ, Korelitz BI. The therapeutic efficacy of 6-mercaptopurine in refractory ulcerative colitis. Am J Gastroenterol. 1990;85:717–22.
15. Lobo AJ, Foster PN, Burke DA *et al.* The role of azathioprine in the management of ulcerative colitis. Dis Colon Rectum. 1990;33:374–7.
16. Present DH, Meltzer SJ, Krumholz MP. 6-Mercaptopurine in the management of inflammatory bowel disease: short- and long-term toxicity. Ann Inter Med. 1989;111:641–9.
17. Bleyer WA. The clinical pharmacology of methotrexate. New applcations of an old drug. Cancer. 1978;41:36–51.
18. Calabrese LH, Taylor JV, Wilke WS *et al.* Response of immunoregulatory lymphocyte subsets to methotrexate in rheumatoid arthritis. Cleve Clin J Med. 1990;57:232–41.
19. Miller LC, Cohen SE, Orencole SF *et al.* Interleukin-1 is structurally related to dihydrofolate reductase: effect of methotrexate on IL-1. Lymphokine Res. 1988;7:272A.
20. Mitchell LC, Turk JL. Effect of the immune modulating agents cyclophosphamide, methotrexate, hydrocortisone, and cyclosporin A on an animal model of granulomatous bowel disease. Gut. 1990;31:674–8.
21. Olsen NJ, Murray LM. Antiproliferative effects of methotrexate on peripheral blood mononuclear cells. Arthritis Rheum. 1989;32:378–85.
22. Weinblatt ME, Coblyn JS, Fox DA, Fraser PA. Efficacy of low-dose methotrexate in rheumatoid arthritis. N Engl J Med. 1985;312:818–22.
23. Lanse SB, Arnold GL, Gowans JDC, Kaplan MM. Low incidence of hepatotoxicity associated with long-term, low-dose oral methotrexate in treatment of refractory psoriasis, psoriatic arthritis, and rheumatoid arthritis. An acceptable risk/benefit ratio. Dig Dis Sci. 1985;30:104–9.
24. Healey LA. The current status in methotrexate use in rheumatoid diseases. Bull Rheum Dis. 1986;36:1–10.
25. Williams HJ, Willkens RF, Samuelson CO Jr *et al.* Comparison of low-dose oral pulse methotrexate and placebo in the treatment of rheumatoid arthritis. A controlled clinical trial. Arthritis Rheum. 1985;28:721–30.
26. Andersen PA, West SG, O'Dell JR *et al.* Weekly pulse methotrexate in rheumatoid arthritis. Clinical and immunlogic effects in a randomized, double-blind study. Ann Intern Med. 1985;103:489–96.

27. Lally EV, Ho G Jr. A review of methotrexate therapy in Reiter syndrome. Semin Arthritis Rheum. 1985;15:139–45.
28. Mullarkey MF, Webb DR, Pardee NE. Methotrexate in the treatment of steroid-dependent asthma. Ann Allergy. 1986;56:347–50.
29. Mullarkey MF, Blumenstein BA, Andrade WP et al. Methotrexate in the treatment of corticosteroid-dependent asthma. A double-blind cross-over study. N Engl J Med. 1988;318:603–7.
30. Kaplan MM, Knox TA, Arora S. Primary biliary cirrhosis treated with low-dose oral pulse methotrexate. Ann Intern Med. 1988;109:429–31.
31. Knox TA, Kaplan MM. Treatment of primary sclerosing cholangitis with oral methotrexate. Am J Gastroenterol. 1991;86(5):546–52.
32. Kozarek RA, Patterson DJ, Gelfand MD et al. Methotrexate induces clinical and histologic remission in patients with refaractory inflammatory bowel disease. Ann Intern Med. 1989;110:353–6.
33. Kozarek RA, Patterson DJ, Botoman VA et al. Methotrexate use in inflammatory bowel disease patients who have failed azathioprine or 6-mercaptopurine. Gastroenterology. 1991;100:222A.
34. Kozarek RA, Patterson DJ, Gelfand MD et al. Long-term use of methotrexate in inflammatory bowel disease. Gastroenterology. 1992;102:648A.
35. Searles G, McKendry RJR. Methotrexate pneumonitis in rheumatoid arthritis: potential risk factors. Four case reports and a review of the literature. J Rheumatol. 1987;14:1164–71.
36. Whiting-O'Keefe QE, Fye KH, Sack KD. Methotrexate and histologic abnormalities: a meta-analysis. Am J Med. 1990;90:711–16.
37. Kozarek RA, Bredfeldt JE, Rosoff LE et al. Does chronic methotrexate cause liver toxicity when used for refractory inflammatory bowel disease? Gastroenterology. 1991;100:221A.
38. Kozlowski RD, Steinbrunner JV, MacKenzie AH et al. Outcome of first-trimester exposure to low-dose methotrexate in eight patients with rheumatic disease. Am J Med. 1990;88:589–92.
39. Alstead EM, Ritchie JK, Lennard-Jones JE et al. Safety of azathioprine in pregnancy in inflammatory bowel disease. Gastroenterology. 1990;90:443–6.
40. Hodgson HJF. Cyclosporin in inflammatory bowel disease. Aliment Pharmacol Ther. 1991;5:343–50.
41. Lowes JR, Jewell DP. Cyclosporin A in inflammatory bowel disease. In: Gitnick G, editor. Inflammatory bowel disease. Diagnosis and treatment. New York: Igaku-Shoin; 1991:359–64.
42. Brynskov J, Freund L, Rasmussen SN et al. A placebo-controlled, double-blind, randomized trial of cyclosporine therapy in active Crohn's disease. N Engl J Med. 1989;321:845–50.
43. Brynskov J, Freund L, Rasmussen SN et al. Final report on a placebo-controlled, double-blind, randomized, mutlicenter trial of cyclosporin treatment in active Crohn's disease. Scand J Gastroenterol. 1991;26:689–95.
44. Lobo AJ, Juby LD, Rothwell J. Long term treatment of Crohn's disease with cyclosporine; the effect of a very low dose on maintenance of remission. J Clin Gastroenterol. 1991;13:42–5.
45. Allison MC, Pounder E. Cyclosporin for Crohn's disease. Aliment Pharmacol Ther. 1987;1:39–43.
46. Fukushima T, Sugita A, Musuzawa S et al. Effects of cyclosporin A on active Crohn's disease. Gastroenterol Jpn. 1989;24:12–15.
47. Archambault A, Feagan B, Fedorak R et al. The Canadian Crohn's relapse prevention trial (CCRPT). Gastroenterology. 1992;102:591A.
48. Baker K, Jewell DP. Cyclosporin for the treatment of severe inflammatory bowel disease. Aliment Pharmacol Ther. 1989;3:143–9.
49. Lichtiger S, Present DH. Preliminary report: cyclosporin in treatment of severe active ulcerative colitis. Lancet. 1990;36:16–19.
50. Gupta S, Keshavarzian A, Hodgson HJF. Cyclosporin in ulcerative colitis. Lancet. 1989;1:1277–8.
51. Porro BG, Panza E, Petrillo M. Cyclosporin A in acute ulcerative colitis. Ital J Gastroenterol. 1987;19:40–41.
52. Hyams JS, Treem WR. Cyclosporine treatment of fulminant colitis. J Pediatr Gastroenterol Nutr. 1989;9:383–7.
53. Brynskov J, Freund L, Thomsen OO et al. Treatment of refractory ulcerative colitis with cyclosporin enemas. Lancet. 1989;1:721–2.

54. Ranzi T, Campanini MC, Velio P *et al*. Treatment of chronic proctosigmoiditis with cyclosporin enemas. Lancet. 1989;1:97.
55. Hawthorne AB, Hawkey CJ. Immunosuppressive drugs in inflammatory bowel disease. A review of their mechanisms of efficacy and place in therapy. Drugs. 1989;38:267–88.
56. Hanauer SB, Stathopoulos G. Risk–benefit assessment of drugs used in the treatment of inflammatory bowel disease. Drug Saf. 1991;6:192–19.
57. Freeman HJ. Immunosuppressive drug therapy of inflammatory bowel disease. Endosc Rev. 1991;8:26–31.
58. Aparico-Pagies MN, Verspaget HW, Hafkenscheid JC *et al*. Inhibition of cell mediated cytotoxicity by sulphasalazine: effect of *in vivo* treatment with 5-aminosalicylic acid and sulphasalazine on *in vitro* natural killer cell activity. Gut. 1990;31(9):1030–2.
59. Bicks RO, Groshart KD. The current status of TM-lymphocyte apheresis (TLA) treatment of Crohn's disease. J Clin Gastroenterol. 1989;11(2):136–8.
60. Bicks RO, Groshart KD. T-lymphocyte apheresis. In: Gitnick G, editor. Inflammatory bowel disease. Diagnosis and treatment. Nerw York: Igaku-Shoin; 1991:377–95.
61. Deusch K, Reiter C, Mauthe B *et al*. Chimeric monoclonal anti-CD4 antibody therapy proves effective for treating inflammatory bowel disease. Gastroenterology. 1992;102:615A.
62. Chabner BA, Wilson W. Editorial: reversal of multidrug resistance. J Clin Oncol. 1991;9:4–6.
63. Goldstein LJ, Ozols RF. Blocking P-glycoprotein action. Contemp Oncol. 1991(May/June):38–47.
64. Pastan I, Willingham MC, Gottesman M. Molecular manipulations of the multidrug transporter: a new role for transgenic mice. FASEB J. 1991;5(11):2523–8.
65. Lehnert M, Dalton WS, Roe D *et al*. Synergistic inhibition by verapamil and quinine of *p*-glycoprotein-mediated multidrug resistance in a human myeloma cell line model. Blood. 1991;77:348–54.

35
Mechanism of action of salicylates

H. ALLGAYER

Sulphasalazine (SAZ) and, more recently, the newer aminosalicylate preparations, are the drugs of choice in the treatment of mild to moderate attacks and relapse prevention of inflammatory bowel disease (IBD). Almost a decade and a half ago the 5-aminosalicylic acid (5-ASA) component of the SAZ molecule was recognized as the therapeutic moiety acting locally at the inflamed ileal and colonic mucosa[1-3]. Despite their successful use the precise mechanisms of the anti-inflammatory action in IBD are still poorly understood. In view of the complex pattern of actions found in experimental and clinical studies, and the still unknown aetiology of IBD, it is difficult to define a clear picture. This chapter will focus on those effects which contribute to clinically relevant therapeutic actions.

Currently there are three major groups of action which need to be considered (Table 1). These include: (i) the inhibition of early steps of the intestinal inflammatory response most likely at the level of immune cell activation involving cytokines and other factors; (ii) suppression of neutrophil functions, particularly the production and action of inflammatory mediators and toxic oxygen compounds including the inhibition of lipid peroxidation; and (iii) inhibition of enzymes, metabolism and function of the intestinal epithelial cell. In addition a structure–activity relationship of the aminosalicylate molecule with regard to certain defined anti-inflammatory actions can be demonstrated.

Table 1 Mechanisms of action of aminosalicylates

Inhibition of immune activation and antibody secretion

Suppression of neutrophil functions, inflammatory mediators, oxygen metabolites, lipid peroxidation

Inhibition of metabolism and function of epithelial cells

As previously suggested, the intestinal inflammatory response of IBD most likely evolves over three distinct stages, each of which includes specific cellular and biochemical events[4-7]. The first stage is characterized by an activation of macrophages, lymphoid and monocytic cells of the GALT/MALT system within the intestinal wall (GALT/MALT, gut/mucosa-associated lymphatic tissue) triggered by (an) as yet undefined stimulus. These processes include elevated production and levels of immunoregulators, e.g. different interleukins, soluble IL-2 receptors, HLA expression, tumour necrosis factors (TNF), interferons and other compounds[8-12]. The second phase is determined by an amplification of this initial response with increased production and concentrations of potent inflammatory mediators including complement binding factors[13], platelet-activating factor (PAF)[14] and arachidonic acid metabolites, particularly leukotrienes[7,15-19]. The third phase is characterized by cytotoxic interactions of activated inflammatory cells, particularly neutrophils, with the intestinal epithelium leading to a loss of function (e.g. disturbed water and electrolyte movements) and tissue damage (erosions and ulcers). Toxic oxygen metabolites and proteases are believed to be the main mediators of these effects[20-23]. In the absence of a defined aetiology pharmacological intervention at one or more levels by drugs, particularly aminosalicylates, is a desirable goal of the symptomatic treatment of IBD.

ACTIONS OF AMINOSALICYLATES IN PHASE I

Elevated local and systemic levels of interleukin 1 (IL-1), interleukin 2 (IL-2), interleukin 6 (IL-6), TNF-α and others increasingly are believed to play an important role in the permanent 'up-regulation' of the intestinal immune system in IBD[24-33]. IL-1, IL-2 receptors, and IL-6 were found to be correlated with disease activity[26-28]. In addition, receptors of formyl-methionyl-leucyl-phenylalanine (FMLP), a proinflammatory bacterial oligopeptide on neutrophils, have been shown to be increased in Crohn's disease, most likely as a further sign of general cellular activation[34]. SAZ and, to a lesser degree 5-ASA, are able to block FMLP receptors dose-dependently[35]. Corticosteroids and 5-ASA have recently been demonstrated to inhibit the production of IL-1β in cells cultured from mucosal specimens of IBD patients[29]. Increased cell surface expression of activation markers on lamina propria mononuclear cells (LPMC) such as adhesion molecules, IL-2 and transferrin receptors, were found to be suppressed by 5-ASA at concentrations normally found in the colonic lumen of IBD patients on SAZ or 5-ASA maintenance treatment[32]. This inhibition was further corroborated by observations showing that the biosynthesis of cytokines can be blocked at the m-RNA level by 5-ASA but not by cyclosporin[28]. TNF-α synthesis in peripheral blood cells from patients with Crohn's disease is dose-dependently inhibited by cortico-steroids[26-28], suppressing effects of aminosalicylates are possible, but have not yet been studied. A recent investigation showed that SAZ, but not 5-ASA, inhibits TNF-α receptors on human neutrophils[33]. The actions of other aminosalicylates on the different cytokines or their receptors have not yet been formally evaluated, but presently are being investigated in our and other laboratories. An altered secretion pattern of immunoglobulins with potential cytotoxicity by monocytic cells derived from peripheral blood or intestinal lamina propria cells of IBD patients has been reported[24,25]. It was shown that 5-ASA was able to suppress this antibody secretion dose-dependently without cell damage, whereas other compounds including SAZ were found to inhibit this action only unspecifically with major cytotoxicity[30].

Deactivation of natural killer (NK) cells and lymphocyte proliferation was observed with SAZ, but not consistently with 5-ASA, leaving the significance of these findings still unclear[36].

Taken together the presently available data suggest that suppression or modification of the early 'up-regulation' of the intestinal immune response at the levels of cytokines, FMLP receptor or antibody production may be a new and clinically important aspect of anti-inflammatory action of aminosalicylates.

ACTIONS OF AMINOSALICYLATES IN PHASE II

The second phase of the intestinal inflammatory response is characterized by increased production and levels of soluble mediators produced in and secreted from activated blood cells, mainly neutrophils, migrated from the peripheral compartment into the inflamed colonic or ileal sites[37]. These include C5a[13], PAF[14], histamine[38] and the products of the arachidonic acid cascade: prostanoids and leukotrienes[39–44]. Most of these mediators, especially the leukotrienes, have pronounced proinflammatory properties contributing to the amplification of the initial response (Table 2). Particularly leukotriene B_4 (LTB$_4$) has potent chemokinetic and chemotactic capabilities[7,39]. SAZ and 5-ASA were found to inhibit LTB$_4$ and 5-hydroxytetraenoic acid (5-HETE), the LTB$_4$ precursor of the 5-lipoxygenase reaction of arachidonic acid, in neutrophils dose-dependently with an IC_{50} of 1–6 mmol/l[42,44]. Although this inhibition is regarded as a non-specific action, lipoxygenase inhibition by aminosalicylates and, more recently, specific inhibitors, is considered a major mechanism of action in IBD[7,40–46]. This view is supported by the following observation: the concentrations necessary to inhibit lipoxygenase *in vitro* have been found to be in the same range as those present intraluminally in IBD patients taking SAZ or 5-ASA[45]. A second argument

Table 2 Biological effects of leukotrienes

5-HETE	Water and electrolyte disturbances
LTB$_4$	Chemokinesis, chemotaxis, adherence, degranulation, superoxide production, pain threshold decrease
LTC$_4$	Vasoconstriction
LTD$_4$	Capillary permeability
LTE$_4$	Smooth muscle contraction

5-HETE, 5-hydroxytetraenoic acid; LTB$_4$, leukotriene B$_4$; LTC$_4$, leukotriene C$_4$; LTE$_4$, leukotriene E$_4$

derives from different animal models showing a significant decrease of colonic inflammation as assessed macroscopically, histologically and by the myeloperoxidase (MPO) assay as a measure of infiltration with inflammatory neutrophils following pre and/or post-treatment with 5-ASA and more specific inhibitors such as Revlon 5901, BW 755 C or others[43,44,46] (Figs 1 and 2). Colonic 5-HETE and LTB_4 production was concomitantly decreased after treatment. First data from a study using zileuton, one of the newly developed more specific lipoxygenase inhibitors[47], in 30 patients with ulcerative colitis of mild to moderate disease activity showed that treatment led to a significantly decreased inflammation and an improvement of the clinical score, together with decreased colonic levels of 5-HETE and LTB_4[47]. The last argument is the observation that modification of leukotrienes to less potent derivatives, e.g. LTB_5, by $\omega-3$ fatty acids (fish oil) leads to diminished inflammation in animals and humans[48]. The presently available data strongly suggest that the extent of leukotriene suppression is almost linearly correlated with the degree of reduction of colonic inflammation; a complete reduction, however, cannot be achieved even if LTB_4 is suppressed by $>95\%$[43]. This supports the view that lipoxygenase inhibition by aminosalicylates is an important pharmacological action in the symptomatic

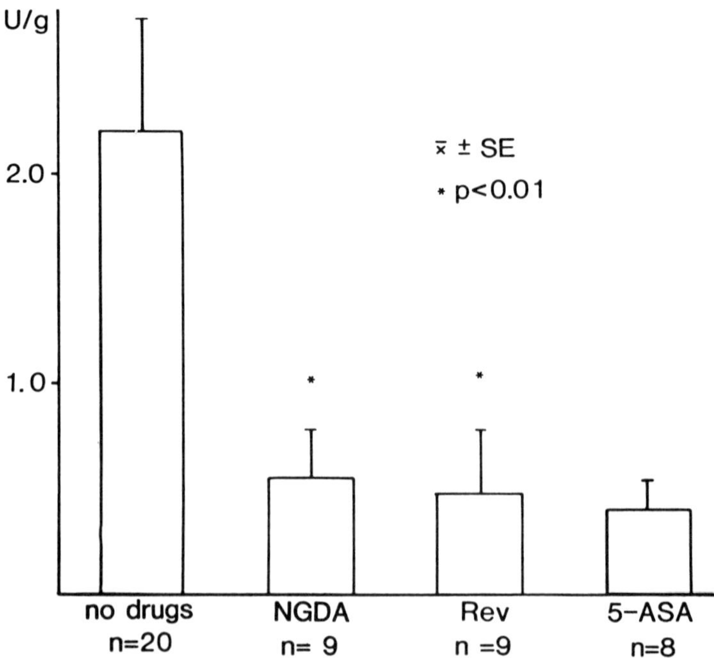

Fig. 1 Effects of treatment with lipoxygenase inhibitors: nordihydroguaretic acid (NGDA) (0.12 mg/kg), Revlon 5901 (0.12 mg/kg) and 5-ASA (4.8 mg/kg) on colonic myeloperoxidase activity (U/g) in trinitrobenzene sulphonic acid (80 mg/kg) induced colitis in rats. $\bar{X} \pm$ SEM; $n =$ number of animals in each group

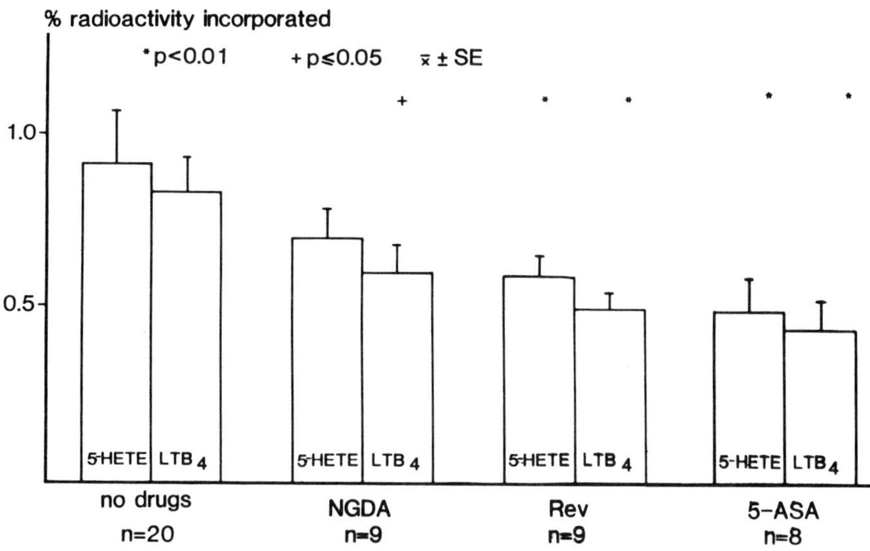

Fig. 2 Effects of treatment with nordihydroguaretic acid (NGDA) (0.12 mg/kg), Revlon 5901 (0.12 mg/kg) and 5 ASA (4.8 mg/kg) on colonic production of LTB_4 and 5-HETE in trinitrobenzene sulphonic acid (80 mg/kg) induced colitis in rats. Production is expressed as percentage of radioactivity incorporated from exogenous ^{14}C-arachidonic acid. $\bar{X} \pm$ SEM; $n =$ number of rats in each group

treatment of IBD, but that other factors also have to be considered. From observations in animal models leukotriene synthesis and MPO activity follow a certain time-course with most activity within the first 2 weeks after induction of the colitis and a rapid decline thereafter[43]. The time of administration of lipoxygenase inhibitors, including aminosalicylates, therefore, may be critical. Inhibition of leukotrienes at the receptor level by specific antagonists may also be a new attractive approach: Studies with aminosalicylates, however, are not yet available.

A structure–effect relationship is likely to exist with regard to the lipoxygenase inhibition. Thus, an intact aminophenolic structure with a free aminogroup at postion 5 seems to be necessary as salicylates alone (no amino group) or substitution of the amino group (*N*-acetylation) have been found to be either without effects or with only weak actions on lipoxygenases from different sources[49–52]. 4-ASA is unlikely to inhibit the lipoxygenase in human neutrophils[53]; the results of the studies, however, are inconsistent[54]. The precise molecular mechanism by which 5-ASA acts on lipoxygenase remains speculative. According to our present knowledge the lipoxygenase reaction is a multi-step process, the first involving the abstraction of a hydrogen atom at position 11L very close to the cyclooxygenase reaction leading to intermediate fatty acid radicals, as evidenced by ESR spectroscopy in our and other laboratories[55,56]. The subsequent steps include different cyclization reactions involving molecular oxygen[52]. From our ESR studies showing that

5-ASA does not directly react with intermediate fatty acid radicals[56] we speculate that aminosalicylates may interfere with one or more of the oxygen-dependent cyclization steps following the generation of fatty acid radicals. In addition, 5-ASA was demonstrated to form intermediate N-oximes non-enzymatically with LTB_4 precursors[57].

Platelet-activating factor (PAF), also a potent inflammatory mediator, was found to be increased in acute phases of IBD[14,58]. Aminosalicylates were shown to inhibit increased production and levels in animal models and human disease, suggesting that PAF suppression may have a therapeutic role[14,58].

Suppression of prostaglandin and thromboxane A_2 synthesis, and histamine release from anti-IgE stimulated mast cells, was described[38,59]; the clinical relevance of these findings, however, remains doubtful, as more specific inhibition of prostaglandins with indomethacin, naproxen or other NSAIDs was without any therapeutic effects in IBD[60,61]. Specific histamine suppression, e.g. by cromoglycate, was also ineffective[62]. Clinical trials with thromboxane inhibitors are in progress; results, however, are not yet available.

ACTIONS OF AMINOSALICYLATES IN PHASE III

Tissue damage as a result of cytotoxic interactions between activated inflammatory cells, particularly neutrophils, and the intestinal epithelium is a main feature of this stage. These effects are believed to be mainly mediated by toxic oxygen metabolites such as superoxide (O_2^-), hydroxyl ($OH^{\cdot}$) radicals, hydrogen peroxide, hypochlorous acid (OCl^-), chlorinated organic compounds and proteases produced in and released from stimulated neutrophils[63-70]. SAZ and aminosalicylates, including olsalazine, a newly introduced double molecule consisting of two 5-ASA, and benzalazine, another newly developed aminosalicylate derivative, are able to directly scavenge these molecular species. Thus, one of the most important extracellular actions of 5-ASA is its direct reaction (scavenging)[65-70] with O_2^-, $OH^{\cdot}$ and OCl^-. In addition, 5-ASA was found to inhibit the production of superoxide in neutrophils, following different stimuli of the respiratory burst, thus further contributing to the attenuation of tissue damage[71]. Superoxide, although only moderately toxic by itself, further leads to more reactive species including $OH^{\cdot}$, OCl^- and H_2O_2. The iron-dependent Haber–Weiss reaction yields $OH^{\cdot}$ and the myeloperoxidase (MPO) reaction the highly cytotoxic hypochlorite[63,64]. This reaction was found to be inhibited by 5-ASA and 4-ASA[75]. Olsalazine, benzalazine, or other derivatives have not yet been formally tested. Figure 3 summarizes the present view of the different actions of aminosalicylates on oxygen metabolites. According to our present knowledge an intact aminophenolic group seems to be necessary with respect to superoxide scavenging, as recently suggested by a comparative ESR study[56]. Presently there are three major arguments for a role of oxygen radicals in IBD and their pharmacological manipulation by drugs, including aminosalicylates as an important therapeutic modality in the symptomatic treatment of IBD:

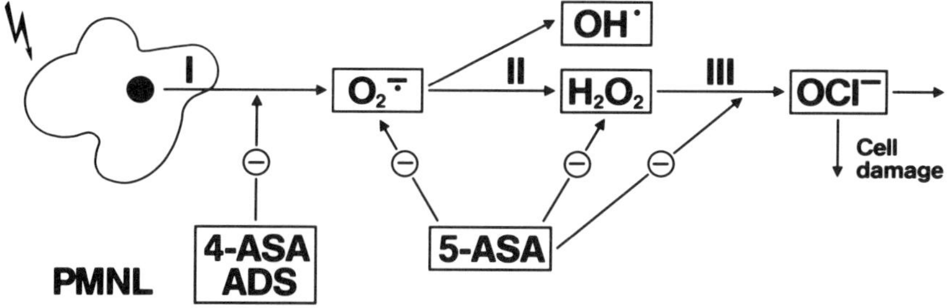

PMNL : Polymorphonuclear leukocytes
⚡ : activating steps
I : NADP-dependent oxidases: respiratory burst
II : Haber-Weiss reaction
III : Myeloperoxidase reaction

Fig. 3 Inhibition of oxygen species by aminosalicylates at different cellular and extracellular levels: 4-ASA, 4-aminosalicylic acid; 5-ASA, 5-aminosalicylic acid; ADS, azodisalicylte (olsalazine)

1. Inflamed colonic tissue from animal models and human disease contains increased levels of MPO[22] and hypochlorite[66,69].
2. Biopsy specimens from diseased areas produce a significantly higher chemoluminescence (an indirect measure of oxygen metabolites, especially OCl^-)[69,70] following appropriate incubation conditions compared to normal mucosa.
3. Treatment with specific scavengers leads to decreased inflammation in animal models[72].

A clinical argument is the recent study with 30 patients with steroid refractory Crohn's disease showing that treatment with superoxide dismutase, an enzyme which inactivates O_2^-, for 4 weeks, was associated with clinical and histological improvement[73]. One of the major destructive effects of radicals is lipid peroxidation[76]. Sulphasalazine and 5-ASA, but not sulphapyridine, have recently been shown to prevent lipid peroxidation in red cell membranes[76]. It is therefore likely that those effects may contribute significantly to the anti-inflammatory action.

While the inhibition (scavenging) of superoxide radicals, H_2O_2 and hypochlorite in IBD by aminosalicylates is increasingly appreciated as a potential therapeutic action, the role of OH· inhibition remains controversial[74]. Although 5-ASA was shown to scavenge OH·, most likely due to its iron chelating properties preventing the Haber–Weiss reaction[75], the clinical significance of this observation remains unclear, as treatment with more specific OH scavengers in animal models was found to be ineffective in decreasing inflammation[72]. In addition, 4-ASA, the *p*-analogue of 5-ASA, was recently shown to lack iron-chelating (unpublished) and OH·-scavenging properties[56], but was demonstrated to be clinically effective in the treatment of mild to moderate ulcerative colitis[77], suggesting that OH· may not be directly involved in the pathogenesis of IBD.

INHIBITION OF ENZYMES, METABOLISM AND FUNCTIONS IN EPITHELIAL CELLS BY AMINOSALICYLATES

The third group of actions of aminosalicylates comprises the inhibition of enzymes, metabolism and function in epithelial cells, including the suppression of the β-oxidation of fatty acids[78], DNA synthesis[79], bacterial growth[74], water and electrolyte movements across the intestinal barrier[79] and important membrane enzymes, such as the colonic $(Na^+ + K^+)$-ATPase[80]. Whereas the latter potentially may be clinically relevant with regard to potential side-effects of the aminosalicylate therapy, e.g. diarrhoea, the significance of the other observations remains unclear.

In summary, aminosalicylates inhibit the intestinal inflammatory response at multiple levels. The most prominent feature of the anti-inflammatory action is the inhibition of cytokines, antibody secretion, FMLP receptors, arachidonic acid metabolites, toxic oxygen species and lipid peroxidation. The present view is that not a single action, but rather the combination of these effects, may contribute to the therapeutic action in IBD.

ACKNOWLEDGEMENT

The author thanks Mrs T. Gerach for expert secretarial help.

References

1. Azad Khan AK, Piris J, Truelove SC. An experiment to determine the active moiety of sulphasalazine. Lancet. 1977;1:892–5.
2. van Hees AM, Bakker JH, van Tongeren. Effect of sulphapyridine, 5-aminosalicylic acid and placebo in patients with idiopathic proctitis: a study to determine the active therapeutic moiety of sulphasalazine. Gut. 1980;21:632–5.
3. Klotz U, Maier K, Fischer C, Heinkel K. Therapeutic efficacy of sulfasalazine and its metabolites in patients with ulcerative colitis and Crohn's disease. N Engl J Med. 1980;303:1499–1506.
4. Gibson PR. Current concepts in the pathogenesis of Crohn's disease and ulcerative colitis. Gastroenterol Hepatol. 1991;5:44–65.
5. Auer IO. Der Dünndarm als Immunorgan. Fortschr Med. 1990;108:292–6.
6. Allgayer H, Kruis W. New aspects of the pathophysiology of inflammation in Crohn's disease and ulcerative colitis: Z Gastroenterol. 1990;28:117–20.
7. Stenson WF. Leukotriene B_4 in inflammatory bowel disease. In: Goebell H, Peskar BM, Malchow H, editors. Inflammatory bowel diseases. Lancaster: MTP Press; 1988:143–52.
8. Dinarello JH. Interleukin 1. Dig Dis Sci. 1988;33:255–355.
9. Ligumsky M, Simon PL, Karmeli F, Rachmilewitz D. Role of interleukin 1 in inflammatory bowel disease- enhanced production during active disease. Gut. 1990;31:686–9.
10. Schreiber S, Raedler A, Conn AR, Rombeau IL, MacDermott RP. Increased in vitro release of soluble interleukin 2 receptor by colonic lamina propria mononuclear cells in inflammatory disease. Gut. 1992;33:236–41.
11. Brynskov J, Tvede N, Andersen CB, Vilien M. Increased concentrations of interleukin 1β, interleukin 2 and soluble interleukin-2 receptor in endoscopical mucosal biopsy specimens with active inflammatory bowel disease. Gut. 1992;33:55–8.

12. Crotty B, Hoang P, Dalton HR, Jewell DP. Salicylates used in inflammatory bowel disease and colchicine impair interferon-γ induced HLA- DR expression. Gut. 1992;33:59–64.
13. Weissmann G, Smolen JE, Korchak HM. Release of inflammatory mediators from stimulated neutrophils. N Engl J Med. 1980;303:27–34.
14. Eliakim R, Karmeli F, Razin E, Rachmilewitz D. Role of platelet-activating factor in ulcerative colitis. Gastroenterology. 1987;95:1167–72.
15. Boughton-Smith NK, Whittle BJR. The role of eicosanoids in animal models of inflammatory bowel disease. In Goebell H, Peskar BM, Malchow H, editors. Inflammatory bowel disease. Lancaster: MTP Press; 1988:175–9.
16. Lauritsen K, Laursen LS, Bukhave K, Rask-Madsen J. Effects of topical 5-aminosalicylic acid and prednisone on prostaglandin E_2 and leukotriene B_4 levels determined by equilibrium in vivo dialysis of rectum in relapsing ulcerative colitis. Gastroenterology. 1986;91:837–44.
17. Sharon P, Stenson WF. Enhanced synthesis of leukotriene B_4 by colonic mucosa in inflammatory bowel disease. Gastroenterology. 1984;86:453–60.
18. Zipser RD, Patterson JD, Le Duc E. Chemotactic peptide stimulation of leukotrienes from healthy and inflamed rabbit colon. J Pharmacol Exp Ther. 1987;241:218–22.
19. Peskar BM, Coersmann C. Effect of antiinflammatory drugs on human colonic leukotriene formation. In: Goebell H, Peskar BM, Malchow H, editors. Inflammatory bowel diseases. Lancaster: MTP Press; 1988:153–61.
20. Koningsberger JC, Marx M, van Hattum J. Free radicals in gastroenterology – a review. Scand J Gastroenterol. 1988;23(suppl.):30–40.
21. Williams JG, Hallett MB. The reaction of 5-aminosalicylic acid with hypochlorite. Implications for its mode of action in inflammatory bowel disease. Biochem Pharmacol. 1989;38:149–54.
22. Allgayer H. Clinical relevance of oxygen radicals in inflammatory bowel disease – facts or fashion. Klin Wochenschr. 1991;69:1001–3.
23. Tamura K, Manabe T, Imanishi K, Nonaka A et al. Effect of synthetic protease inhibitors on superoxide (O_2), hydrogen peroxide (H_2O_2) and hydroxyl radical production by human polymorphonuclear leukocytes. Hepatogastroenterology. 1992;39:59–61.
24. MacDermott RP, Nash GS, Bertovitch MJ, Seiden MV, Bragdon MJ, Beale MG. Alterations of IgM, IgG and IgA synthesis and secretion by peripheral blood and intestinal mononuclear cells from patients with ulcerative colitis and Crohn's disease. Gastroenterology. 1981;81:844–52.
25. MacDermott RP, Nash GS, Bertovitch MJ et al. Altered pattern of secretion of monomeric IgA and IgA subclasses from intestinal mononuclear cells in inflammatory bowel disease. Gastroenterology. 1986;91:379–85.
26. Groß V, Andus T, Leser HG, Roth M, Schölmerich J. Inflammatory mediators in chronic inflammatory bowel disease. Klin Wochenschr. 1991;69:981–7.
27. Hodgson HJF, Mazlam MZ. Cytokines – are they different in ulcerative colitis and Crohn's disease? In: Goebell H, Ewe K, Malchow H, Koelbel C, editors. Inflammatory bowel diseases: progress in basic research and clinical implications. Dordrecht: Kluwer; 1991:161–9.
28. James SP, Mullin GE. Lymphokine production by mucosal T cells in inflammatory bowel disease. In: Goebell H, Ewe K, Malchow H, Koelbel C, editors. Inflammatory bowel diseases: progress in basic research and clinical implications. Dordrecht: Kluwer; 1991:71–83.
29. Mahida JR, Lamming CED, Gallagher A, Hawthorne AB, Hawkey CJ. 5-Aminosalicylic acid is a potent inhibitor of interleukin-1β production in organ cultures of colonic biopsy specimens from patients with inflammatory bowel disease. Gut. 1991;32:50–4.
30. MacDermott RP, Schloemann SR, Bertovitch MJ, Nash GS, Peters M, Stenson WF. Inhibition of antibody secretion by 5-aminosalicylic acid. Gastroenterology. 1989;96:442–8.
31. Molin L, Stendahl O. The effect of sulfasalazine and its active components on human polymorphonuclear leukocyte function in relation to ulcerative colitis. Acta Med Scand. 1979;206:451–7.
32. Schreiber S, MacDermott RP, Raedler A, Pinnau K, Bertovitch MJ, Nash GS. Increased activation of isolated intestinal lamina propria mononuclear cells in inflammatory bowel disease. Gastroenterology. 1991;101:1020–30.
33. Shanahan F, Niederlehner A, Caramanzana N, Anton P. Sulfasalazine inhibits the binding of TNF a to its receptors. Immunopharmacology. 1990;20:217–24.
34. Anton P, Targan SR, Shanahan F. Increased neutrophil receptors for and response to the proinflammatory bacterial peptide formyl–methionyl–leucyl–phenylalanine in Crohn's

disease. Gastroenterology. 1989;97:20–8.

35. Stenson WF, Mehta J, Spilberg J. Sulfasalazine inhibition of binding of *N*-formyl–methionyl–leucyl–phenylalanine (FMLP) to its receptors on human neutrophils. Biochem Pharmacol. 1984;33:407–12.

36. Gibson PR, Jewell DP. Sulphasalazine and derivatives: natural killer activity and ulcerative colitis. Clin Sci. 1985;69:177–84.

37. Saverymuttu SH, Camilleri M, Rees H, Lavender JP, Hodgson HJF, Chadwick VS. Indium 111-granulocyte scanning in the assessment of disease extent and disease activity in inflammatory bowel disease. Gastroenterology. 1986;90:1121–8.

38. Fox C, Moore C, Lichtenstein LM. Modulation of mediator release from human intestinal mast cells by sulfasalazine and 5-aminosalicylic acid. Dig Dis Sci. 1991;36:179–84.

39. Bray A, Ford-Hutchinson AW, Smith MJH. Leukotriene B_4, an inflammatory mediator *in vivo*. Prostaglandins. 1981;22:213–22.

40. Stenson WF, Lobos E. Sulfasalazine inhibits the synthesis of chemotactic lipids by neutrophils. J Clin Invest. 1982;659:494–7.

41. Peskar BM, Dreyling KW, May B, Schaarschmidt K, Goebell H. Possible mode of action of 5-aminosalicylic acid. Dig Dis Sci. 1987;32:519–69.

42. Allgayer H, Stenson WF. Comparison of effects of sulfasalazine and its metabolites on the metabolism of endogenous vs. exogenous arachidonic acid. Immunopharmacology. 1988;15:39–46.

43. Wallace JL. Strategies for therapeutic modulation of colitis. In: Goebell H, Ewe K, Malchow H, Koelbel C, editors. Inflammatory bowel diseases. Progress in basic research and clinical implications. Dordrecht: Kluwer; 1991:179–89.

44. Peskar BM. Eicosanoids in inflammatory bowel disease and their pharmacological modulation. In: Goebell H, Ewe K, Malchow H, Koelbel C, editors. Inflammatory bowel diseases. Progress in basic research and clinical implications. Dordrecht: Kluwer; 1991:169–78.

45. Lauritsen K, Laursen S, Bukhave K, Rask-Madsen J. Use of colonic eicosanoid concentrations as predictors of relapse in ulcerative colitis: double blind placebo-controlled study on sulfasalazine maintenance treatment. Gut. 1988;29:1316–21.

46. Allgayer H, Stenson WF. Role of lipoxygenase products in an animal model of colitis. Gastroenterology. 1988;95(5):A6.

47. Stenson WF, Lauritsen K, Laursen LS, Rask-Madsen J *et al*. A clinical trial of zileuton, a specific inhibitor of 5-lipoxygenase, in ulcerative colitis. Gastroenterology. 1991;100(5):A253.

48. Stenson WF, Cort D, Deschryver-Kecskemeti K, Rodgers J, Burakoff W, Beeken W. A trial of fish oil supplemented diet in inflammatory bowel disease. Gastroenterology. 1991;100(5):A252.

49. Gombar V, Kapoor VK, Singh H. Quantitative structure–activity relationships: antiinflammatory activity of salicylic acid and derivatives. Arzneim Forsch/Drug Res. 1983;33:1226–30.

50. Ligumsky M, Hansen DG, Kauffman L. Salicylic acid blocks indomethacin- and aspirin-induced cyclo-oxygenase inhibition in rat gastric mucosa. Gastroenterology. 1982;83:1043–6.

51. Duniec Z, Robak J, Gryglewski R. Antoxidant properties of some chemicals vs their influence on cyclo-oxygenase and lipoxidase activities. Biochem Pharmacol. 1983;32:2283–6.

52. Mason RP, Chignell CF. Free radicals in pharmacology and toxicology – selected topics. Pharmacol Rev. 1982;33:189–211.

53. Nielson OH, Ahnfelt-Ronne I. 4-Aminosalicylic acid has no effect on arachidonic acid metabolism in human neutrophils or on the free radical 1.1 diphenyl-2-picrylhydrazyl. Pharmacol Toxicol. 1988;62:223–6.

54. Allgayer H, Stenson WF. *N*-acetylaminosalicylic acid and 4-(*p*)-aminosalicylic acid inhibit 5-HETE and leukotriene B_4 formation from endogenous arachidonic acid in ionophore stimulated human neutrophils. Gastroenterology. 1986;90(5):1324 (abstr.).

55. De Groot JJMC, Garssen GJ, Vliegenhart JFG, Boldingh J. The detection of linoleic acid radicals in the anaerobic reaction of lipoxygenase. Biochim Biophys Acta. 1973;326:274–84.

56. Allgayer H, Höfer P, Böhne P, Schmidt M, Kruis W, Gugler R. Superoxide, hydroxyl and fatty acid radical scavenging by aminosalicylates: direct evaluation with electron spin resonance spectroscopy. Biochem Pharmacol. 1992;43:259–63.

57. Stenson WF. A molecular mechanism for the inhibition of the synthesis of leukotriene B_4 (LTB$_4$) by 5-aminosalicylic acid (5-ASA). Gastroenterology. 1986;90(5):1648.

58. Rachmilewitz D, Eliakim R, Simon P, Ligumski M, Karmeli F. Role of cytokines and platelet activating factor in the pathogenesis of inflammatory bowel disease. In Goebell H, Ewe K, Malchow H, Koelbel C, editors. Inflammatory bowel diseases. Progress in basic research and clinical implications. Dordrecht: Kluwer; 1991:153–9.
59. Stenson WF, Lobos E. Inhibition of platelet thromboxane synthetase by sulfasalazine. Biochem Pharmacol. 1983;32:2205–9.
60. Rampton DS, Sladen GE. Prostaglandin synthesis inhibitors in ulcerative colitis. Flurbiprofen compared with conventional treatment. Prostaglandins. 1981;21:417–25.
61. Hawkey CJ, Rampton DS. Prostaglandin and the gastrointestinal mucosa: are they important in its function, disease or treatment? Gastroenterology. 1985;84:1162–88.
62. Buckell NA, Gould SR, Day DW, Lennard-Jones E, Edwards AM. Controlled trial of disodium chromoglycate in chronic persistent ulcerative colitis. Gut. 1978;19:1140–3.
63. Weiis SJ. Tissue destruction by neutrophils. N Engl J Med. 1989;320:3654–76.
64. Grisham MB, Granger DN. Neutrophil-mediated mucosal injury: role of reactive oxygen metabolites. Dig Dis Sci. 1988;33(suppl.):6S–15S.
65. Dull BJ, Salata K, Langenhove AV, Goldman P. 5-Aminosalicylate: oxidation by activated leukocytes and protection of cultured cells from oxidative damage. Biochem Pharmacol. 1987;36:2467–72.
66. Ahnfelt-Ronne I, Nielsen OH, Christensen A, Langholz E, Binder V, Riis P. Clinical evidence supporting the radical scavenger mechanism of 5-aminosalicylic acid. Gastroenterology. 1990;98:1162–8.
67. Arouma OI, Wasil M, Halliwell B. Hoey BM, Butler J. The scavenging of oxidants by sulfasalazine and its metabolites. Biochem Pharmacol. 1987;36:3739–42.
68. Grisham MB, Volkmer C, Tso P, Yamada T. Metabolism of trinitrobenzene sulfonic acid by rat colon produces reactive oxygen species. Gastroenterology. 1991;101:540–7.
69. Simmons NJ, Allen RE, Stevens J, van Someren RNM, Blake DR, Rampton DS. Colorectal mucosa in inflammatory bowel disease produces reactive oxygen metabolites, principally hypochlorite. Gut. 1991;32:A589.
70. Gionchetti P, Guarnieri C, Campieri M *et al.* Scavenger effects of sulfasalazine (SASP), 5-aminosalicylic acid (5-ASA) and olsalazine (OAZ). Gut. 1990;312:730–1.
71. Allgayer H, Rang S, Klotz U, Retey J, Kruis W, Gugler R. Superoxide inhibition following different stimuli of the respiratory burst and metabolism of aminosalicylates in neutrophils. Dig Dis Sci. 1992 (submitted).
72. Keshavarzian A, Morgan G, Sedghi S, Gordon H, Doria M. Role of reactive oxygen metabolites in experimental colitis. Gut. 1990;31:786–90.
73. Emerit J, Pelletier S, Tosoni-Verlignue D, Mollet M. Phase II trial of copper zinc superoxide dismutase (CuZnSOD) in treatment of Crohn's disease. Free Radical Biol Med. 1987;7:145–49.
74. Halliwell B. Free radical scavengers and inflammatory bowel disease. Gastroenterology. 1991;1012:872 (letter).
75. Grisham MB. Effect of 5-aminosalicylic acid in ferrous-sulfate-mediated damage to deoxyribose. Biochem Pharmacol. 1990;39:2060–3.
76. Greenfield SM, Punchard NA, Thompson PH. Inhibition of red cell membrane lipid peroxidation by sulphasalazine and 5-aminosalicylic acid. Gut. 1991;32:1156–9.
77. Ginsberg AL, Davis D, Nochomovitz LE. Placebo-controlled trial of ulcerative colitis with oral 4-aminosalicylic acid. Gastroenterology. 1992;102:448–2.
78. Roediger W, Schapel G, Lawson M, Radcliff B, Nunce S. Effect of 5-aminosalicylic acid (5-ASA) and other salicylates on short chain fat metabolism in the colonic mucosa. Biochem Pharmacol. 1986;35:331–5.
79. Ireland A, Jewell DP. Mechanisms of action of 5-aminosalicylates and its derivatives. Clin Sci. 1990;78:283–9.
80. Scheurlen C, Allgayer H, Kruis W. Inhibition of human ileal and colonic Na^+-pump activities by olsalazine and mesalazine: is it clinically relevant? Klin Wochenschr. (submitted).

Section VIII
Controversies in surgical treatment

36
Recurrent Crohn – impact of surgical strategy

H. J. BUHR, F. KALLINOWSKI, S. POST and Ch. HERFARTH

INTRODUCTION

At present, Crohn's disease can be cured by neither conservative nor surgical management. Therefore, the time of remission or the disease-free period are highly relevant for the effectiveness of a certain treatment regimen. In this respect it should be noted that recent publications report high recurrence rates within the first year after treatment. Are these recurrent clinical manifestations true recurrences or are we simply confronted with a recrudescence of the disease? Can specific surgical strategies influence the rate or timing of recurrences?

DEFINITION OF RECURRENT CROHN'S DISEASE

A recurrence can be defined as the occurrence of the disease in a bowel segment previously known to be free of disease. Crohn's disease is particularly well known for asymptomatic granulomas to occur along the full length of the gastrointestinal tract. Thus, simple progression of a microscopically manifest but asymptomatic disease could mimic a true clinical recurrence. Recurrent disease can further be defined by clinical symptoms, e.g. gastrointestinal cramps or fever, or by objective methods including laboratory measures. A likely recurrence can be detected by the radiologist or localized with certainty on endoscopy. The histological examination of tissue biopsies can confirm the clinical suspicion. Symptomatic disease which requires surgery in previously uninvolved bowel segments can certainly be called a recurrence. Recurrence rates vary widely depending on the means of diagnosis. Recurrence rates defined by repeated surgical interventions are lowest. High rates are obtained if only clinical symptoms are considered[1]. Compiling data of 487 patients from five groups[2-6], recurrence rates defined as a need for surgical intervention were at least one-third lower than those derived from clinical investigations including radiology, endoscopy and histology (Fig. 1). More detailed data were obtained by systematic endoscopic follow-up of 89 patients treated by ileal resection for Crohn's disease[7]. Five years after surgical treatment the recurrence rates were above 80% on endoscopy, between 30% and 40% by laboratory investigation or clinical evaluation and below 20% considering only surgical reoperations. These data indicate that the need for a surgical intervention may be taken as a 'gold standard' regarding recurrent Crohn's disease.

INFLUENCES ON RECURRENCE RATES OF CROHN'S DISEASE

Possible influences include age at the onset of disease, age at first resection, duration of Crohn's disease before resection, site of involvement in the bowel, previous resection, extent of resection performed, involvement of disease at the resection margin and drug treatment after resection. A universally accepted, surgically relevant predisposing factor for the relapse of Crohn's disease has so far not been reported (for an extensive review see ref. 1).

The surgical management of Crohn's disease follows well-defined guidelines[8]. Different strategies are based on the various clinical presentations of the disease. Greenstein et al.[9] differentiated a perforating and a non-perforating clinical manifestation of Crohn's disease and claimed that relapses followed the pattern of the first manifestation (Fig. 2, left panel). These authors based their classification on intraoperative findings rather than on indications for surgery. McDonald et al.[10] classified their patients related to the indication for surgery and could not confirm this claim (Fig. 2, right panel). In a

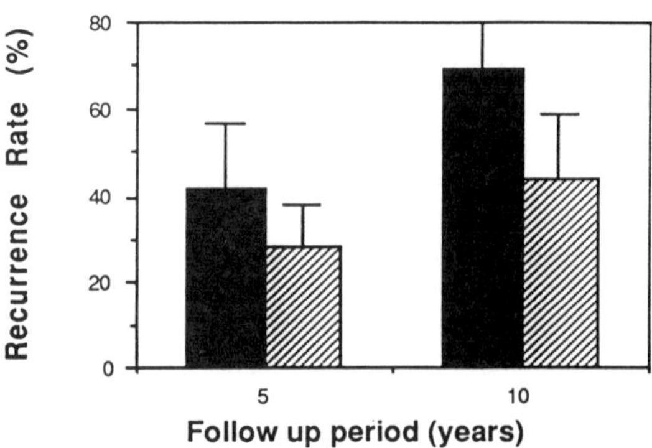

Fig. 1 Recurrence rates of 487 patients investigated by five groups[2-6], based on clinical data (black bars) and the need for surgical reintervention (shaded bars), after follow-up periods of 5 and 10 years

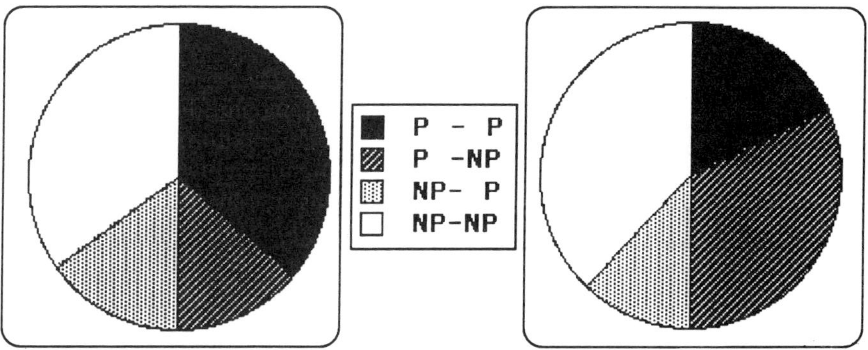

Fig. 2 Type of recurrence after surgery for perforating (P) and non-perforating (NP) disease. Data according to Greenstein *et al.*[9] (left circle) and McDonald *et al.*[10] (right circle)

multicentre trial including 232 patients, followed for 3 years postoperatively, recurrence rates increased after more radical resections[11]. In this study prophylactic adminstration of sulphasalazine reduced postoperative recurrence rates. However, an immunosuppression as expressed by reduced recurrence rates was not obvious after perioperative blood transfusions[12]. Thus, it can be concluded that a patient suffering from Crohn's disease does not benefit from an extended resection, that the involvement of diseased resection margins does not increase the risk for recurrence and that the type of recurrence cannot be predicted.

Our own data, published by Post *et al.*[13], demonstrated the risk of intestinal anastomoses to be independent of a possible involvement of the resection margins. On 843 patients, operated on between 1982 and 1992 at the Department of Surgery, University of Heidelberg, Germany, a more extended analysis was performed. A total of 325 males and 518 females with a mean age of 33 years (range 13–80 years) were included into the study. On average the patients suffered for 8.8 ± 6.0 years from Crohn's disease. The disease was limited to small bowel in 29.5% and to large bowel in 27.5% of the cases. A combined involvement of small and large bowel was noted in 36.0% of the patients. The indications for surgery, complemented by the intraoperative findings, are given in Table 1. Only 5% of the patients were treated on an emergency basis, rendering most patients subject to an adequate preoperative preparation. In the majority of patients, bowel resections were performed, the extent of which was limited to relief of the urgent symptomatology only. A total of 1082 anastomoses were performed. Postoperative complications were classified as slight (e.g. wound infections) and severe (e.g. abscesses, fistulae, anastomotic dehiscence). The complication rates as given in Table 2 were unrelated to the localization or the number of anastomoses or to the involvement of the resection margins (Figs 3–5). It can be concluded that complication rates were not elevated by multiple anastomoses or by diseased resection margins.

A common complication in Crohn's disease are short strictures, particularly in the small bowel. Within the last 10 years, stricturoplasties have become

Table 1 Preoperative indications and intraoperative findings in 843 patients operated on for Crohn's disease at the Department of Surgery, University of Heidelberg, Germany, between 1982 and 1992. Multiple listing is possible

Chronic ileus or stenosis	464
Internal fistulae	384
Septic complications	134
Perianal fistulae	158
Colitis unresponsive to therapy	66
Closure of stoma	61
Perforation	13
Bleeding	13
Blind loop syndrome	12
Toxic megacolon	5

Table 2 Postoperative complication rates in 843 patients operated on for Crohn's disease at the Department of Surgery, University of Heidelberg, Germany, between 1982 and 1992 (percentages)

	First surgery	Recurrent surgery
Without complications	91	93
Wound infection	3	4
Relaparotomy for		
abscess/ileus	3	1
dehiscence	2	1
Lethality	1	1

increasingly popular as a bowel-sparing surgical technique. We performed 148 stricturoplasties in 54 patients including six stricturoplasties in the duodenum without any anastomotic complications. Dehn et al.[14] performed 86 stricturoplasties and 15 resections in 24 patients. Within the follow-up period of 40 months no anastomotic dehiscence or fistulae were seen.

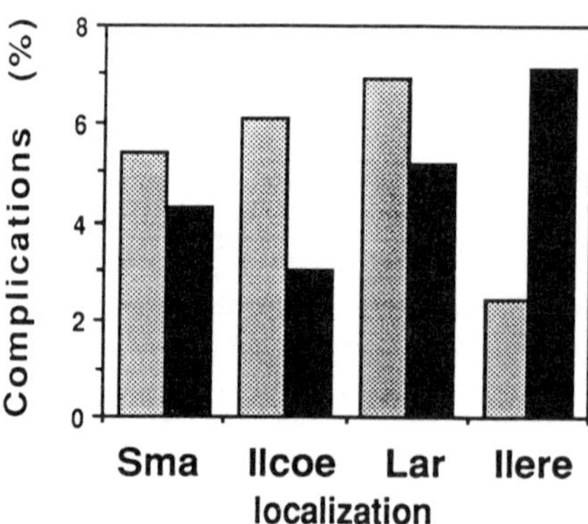

Fig. 3 Complication rates after anastomosis of the small bowel (sma), after the ileocaecal resection (ilcoe), after anastomosis of the large bowel (lar) and after ileorectostomy. Minor complications are indicated by the shaded bars, major complications by the black bars

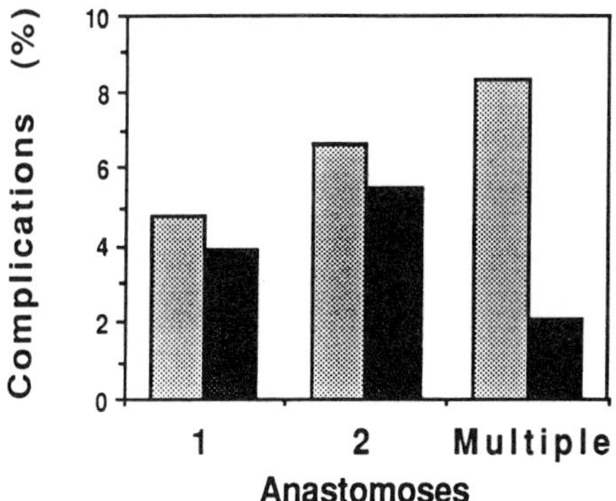

Fig. 4 Complication rates after one, two or multiple anastomoses in the same patient. Minor complications are indicated by the shaded bars, major complications by the black bars

Postoperatively, the patients experienced a mean weight gain of 4 kg. In five patients an additional 13 stricturoplasties were necessary within 12 and 36 months after the first operation. In one patient a recurrence was noted at a stricturoplasty. Sayfan *et al.*[15] reported the experiences from Birmingham: 41 patients with 93 resections solely and another 41 patients with 149 stricturoplasties and 81 small bowel resections. The patients were followed for 60 months. The recurrence rate was assessed for the area of the primary operation only. As expected, the recurrence rate increased with longer observation periods and reached 25% approximately 60 months after surgery. However, a significant difference between the treatment with resection alone and combined with stricturoplasty was not obvious.

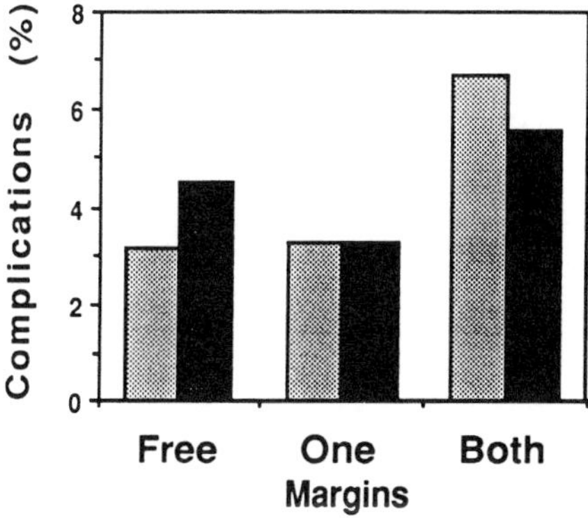

Fig. 5 Complication rates after anastomosis with free margins and with one or both margins involved in the disease process. Minor complications are indicated by the shaded bars, major complications by the black bars

CONCLUSION

The recurrence rate of Crohn's disease is independent from the extent of the surgical therapy. In particular, the involvement of the resection margin does not alter the recurrence rate. A radical surgical treatment cannot expand the time period of clinical remission. Complication rates after multiple anastomoses, even in diseased bowel segments, are not elevated. Surgical treatment should relieve clinical complications preserving as much bowel as possible. The use of stricturoplasties contributes towards this important goal.

References

1. Williams JG, Wong WD, Rothenberger DA, Goldberg SM. Recurrence of Crohn's disease after resection. Br J Surg. 1991;78:10–19.
2. Lennard-Jones JE, Stalder GA. Prognosis after resection of chronic regional ileitis. Gut. 1971;8:332–6.
3. Greenstein AJ, Sachar DB, Paternack BS, Janowitz HD. Reoperation and recurrence in Crohn's colitis and ileocolitis. N Engl J Med. 1975;293:685–90.
4. Nygaard K, Fausa O. Crohn's disease: recurrence after surgical treatment. Scand J Gastroenterol. 1977;12:577–84.
5. Trnka YM, Glotzer DJ, Kasdon EJ et al. Long-term outcome of restorative operation in Crohn's disease. Ann Surg. 1982;196:345–55.
6. Heen LO, Nygaard K, Bergan A. Crohn's disease: results of excisional surgery in 133 patients. Scand J Gastroenterol. 1984;19:747–54.
7. Rutgeerts P, Geboes K, Vantrappen G, Beyls J, Kerremans R, Hiele M. Predictability of the postoperative course of Crohn's disease. Gastroenterology. 1990;99:956–63.
8. Betzler M, Schürmann G, Herfarth C. Chirurgisches Vorgehen bei Morbus Crohn. Chirurg. 1992;63:13–19.
9. Greenstein AJ, Lachman P, Sachar DB et al. Perforating and non-perforating indications for repeated operations in Crohn's disease: evidence for two clinical forms. Gut. 1988;29:588–92.
10. McDonald PJ, Fazio VW, Farmer RG et al. Perforating and non-perforating Crohn's disease. Dis Colon Rectum. 1989;32:117–20.
11. Post S, Betzler M, Ditfurth B, Schürman G, Küppers P, Herfarth C. Risk of intestinal anastomoses in Crohn's disease. Ann Surg. 1991;213:37–42.
12. Ewe K, Herfarth C, Malchow H, Jeschinsky HJ. Postoperative recurrence of Crohn's disease in relation to radicality of operation and sulfasalazine prophylaxis: a multicenter trial. Digestion. 1989;42:224–32.
13. Post S, Kunhardt M, Sido B, Schürmann G, Herfarth C. Der Einfluß von Bluttransfusionen auf die Rezidivrate bei Morbus Crohn. Chirurg. 1992;63:35–8.
14. Dehn TCB, Kettlewell MGW, Mortensen NJ, Lee ECG, Jewell DP. Ten-year experience of stricturoplasty for obstructive Crohn's disease. Br J Surg. 1989;76:339–41.
15. Sayfan J, Wilson DAL, Allan A, Andrews H, Alexander-Williams J. Recurrence after stricturoplasty or resection for Crohn's disease. Br J Surg. 1989;76:335–8.

37
Postoperative treatment: impact on relapse rates

L. R. SUTHERLAND

INTRODUCTION

Most patients with Crohn's disease will eventually require surgery for either complications associated with their disease or failure to respond to medical therapy. The issue of when to perform surgery is made even more difficult by the reality that Crohn's disease is a chronic disease which will eventually recur. The definition of recurrence varies. Lennard-Jones[1] offered three definitions of recurrence: (1) recurrent symptoms, (2) recurrent symptoms with radiological or surgical evidence of recurrent disease or (3) need for further resection. The use of any of these definitions has become more difficult. Postoperative symptoms may not be related to recurrence disease and many patients are unwilling to undergo repeat investigations. With the increasing emphasis on conservative surgery including stricturoplasty it will be difficult to determine whether the need for a second operation represents a recurrence or simply worsening of disease which was left behind.

If endoscopy is used to define recurrence, then evidence of new disease occurs promptly following surgery. The studies of Rutgeerts and associates suggest that the endoscopic lesions of Crohn's disease appear in the neoterminal ileum within 6 months following surgery[2]. The type of endoscopic recurrence may predict how quickly patients will have a clinical recurrence.

Physicians and patients are naturally interested in any intervention which might alter the relentless progression of the disease. Given the prompt recurrence of disease, interventions within the first few months following resection may be important. This paper will focus on the postoperative period, reviewing risk factors for recurrence, models to predict recurrence and finally pharmacotherapy to maintain remission.

ARE THERE RISK FACTORS FOR RECURRENCE?

Greenstein and associates[3] have noted that patients can be divided into two groups: those with 'perforating' indications and those with 'non-perforating' indications for initial surgery. They report that patients tend to have their second operation for the same indication as the first, and suggest that this may be evidence that there are at least two types of Crohn's disease.

Within the epidemiology community there appears to be consensus that cigarette smoking is a risk factor for the development of Crohn's disease[4]. The risk would appear to be 2–3 times that of the non-smoking population. If smoking is a risk factor for development of Crohn's disease, it would be of interest to determine if smoking is a factor for continued disease activity. To date the evidence to support a positive association between smoking and recurrence has been retrospective. Holdstock noted that patients with Crohn's disease who smoked reported more relapses which tended to be characterized as severe as compared to non-smokers[5]. In a review of 174 patients who underwent their first resection for Crohn's disease at our institution, 70% of smokers required a second resection over the next 10 years compared to 41% of non-smokers[6]. A Belgian group[7] also reported that smokers were more likely to have surgery than non-smokers. It is important to point out that another interpretation of smoking as a *risk factor* for ongoing disease activity is the hypothesis that smoking is a *risk marker* for severe disease. In this scenario smoking is seen as a relaxant which suppresses appetite and offers psychological relief to patients.

Another lifestyle issue which has been assessed is the association between oral contraceptive use and Crohn's disease. Rhodes *et al.* were the first to review their patients with Crohn's disease and report an increased use of oral contraceptives amongst women with colonic Crohn's disease[8]. A variety of case–control studies have been performed, one of which is positive[9], others are equivocal (confidence intervals include unity)[10–12]. In our retrospective follow-up of women who had undergone resection for Crohn's disease we were unable to detect any difference in recurrence rates for users as compared to non-users. There was no evidence for an interaction between smoking and oral contraceptive users[13].

There are no studies to date which specifically examine the role of diet in maintaining surgically induced remission. The use of an unrefined carbohydrate, fibre-rich diet in a large group of patients with either inactive or mildly active Crohn's disease was not superior to a regular diet[14]. Alun Jones and associates claimed that elimination diets which establish which foodstuffs are associated with symptoms, are effective in maintaining remission, but this work has not been replicated[15]. The recent work by Rutgeerts and associates[16] demonstrating that diversion of the faecal stream protects against the development of endoscopic lesions could be consistent with the hypotheses that dietary factors influence recurrence rates.

CAN WE PREDICT RECURRENCE?

Not every patient will have a relapse in a particular year, and it would be advantageous to be able to identify patients at higher risk of recurrence, offering them pharmacotherapy. There have been numerous attempts to produce models of recurrence. One problem is that most models are developed on small data sets and generate self-fulfilling prophecies. At this time there is no single blood test that is a reliable predictor of recurrence[17], although recent reports that measurements of post-heparin plasma diamine oxidase[18] predict recurrence are encouraging. As this test requires an infusion of heparin prior to blood sampling it may not be readily acceptable.

Italian workers have developed a model using simple blood tests to predict recurrence, and have used it to test the efficacy of prednisone in preventing recurrence. In a pilot study of patients predicted to be at high risk of recurrence, fewer corticosteroid-treated patients relapsed compared to placebo-treated patients[19].

PHARMACOTHERAPY FOR MAINTENANCE OF REMISSION

Pharmacotherapy to maintain patients in remission has been assessed on a variety of occasions. The early trials (1970s) which did not demonstrate efficacy can be characterized as having a variety of deficiencies including insufficient numbers of patients and thus having insufficient statistical power[20] to detect significant differences. The patient groups also tended to be heterogeneous by disease location, adding additional complexity to the analysis which was already limited by the small sample. In the last 5 years, new studies suggest there may be effective therapy for maintaining remission.

5-AMINOSALICYLATES

Sulphasalazine has been demonstrated to be effective in active Crohn's disease[21] and pure 5-ASA, if at least 3 g/day is given, has also demonstrated efficacy[22,23]. There are several trials involving larger numbers of patients assessing a variety of 5-ASA compounds for maintaining remission (Table 1, Fig. 1). They include studies using Asacol®[24], Claversal®/Mesasal®/Salofalk®[25], Pentasa®[26-28], and sulphasalazine[29]. The majority of studies have demonstrated efficacy in maintaining remission – if not in the entire patient sample, then in a subgroup of patients. Various studies suggest that patients who enter remission surgically, or who begin treatment soon after remission is induced, are excellent candidates for maintenance therapy.

Many issues remain, including what is the effective dose required. For many gastroenterologists, maintenance therapy refers to the practice of giving half of the active dose to maintain healing of peptic ulcers. For maintenance therapy in Crohn's disease it may be more appropriate to refer to 'continuous' therapy, by which a full dose of medication is simply continued after remission is induced.

Table 1 Trials of 5-ASA therapy for maintenance of remission

First author	Drug and dose	No. of patients	Comments
Ewe[29]	Sulphasalazine: 3.0 g daily	232	Sulphasalazine-treated patients had significantly fewer recurrences during the first 2 years following surgery.
Thomson[25]	Claversal®, Mesasal®, Salofalk®; 1.5 g daily	206	Treated patients had significantly fewer recurrences; best effect for patients with ileal disease or previous resection.
Gendre[26]	Pentasa®; 2.0 g daily	161	Efficacy if given within 3 months of either surgically or medically induced remission.
Pallone[24]	Asacol®; 2.4 g daily	125	Relapse rate significantly lower at 12 months for 5-ASA-treated patients
Bondeson[27]	Pentasa®; 3.0 g daily	202	Equal relapse rates; suggestion that patients who entered within 6 months of surgery did better.
Brignola[28]	Pentasa®; 2.0 g daily	44	No difference overall; suggestion that patients with ileal disease had a better response.

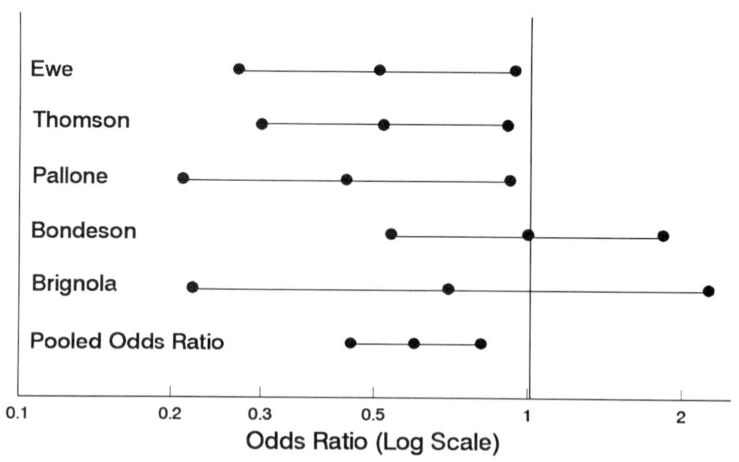

Fig. 1 Odds ratio (with 95% confidence intervals) for having a recurrence of Crohn's disease while taking 5-ASA. The pooled odds ratio represents a summary statistic for all trials combined. A value less than unity represents a protective effect for 5-ASA in maintaining remission

CORTICOSTEROIDS

There are only a few studies which have examined the use of prednisone or prednisolone in maintaining remission. Past reports were not promising[30]. The National Cooperative Crohn's Disease Study (NCCDS) failed to demonstrate any effect of corticosteroids in maintaining either a medically or surgically induced remission[21]. The European Cooperative Crohn's Disease Study (ECCDS) suggested that continuous low-dose prednisolone therapy offered a modest benefit for patients who entered the study with active disease, but provided no benefit to patients who had already entered remission[31]. Current studies with budesonide, a corticosteroid with high first-pass metabolism, already demonstrated in pilot trials to have efficacy in Crohn's disease[32], could offer another opportunity to assess the role of corticosteroids.

IMMUNOSUPPRESSIVES

The use of the immunosuppressants, azathioprine and 6-mercaptopurine (6-MP), for the treatment of active Crohn's disease remains controversial, with the NCCDS reporting no effect[21] and the Mount Sinai group demonstrating effectiveness[33]. The use of either azathioprine or 6-MP to maintain remission has only been examined in a few studies involving a sufficient number of patients. The NCCDS found no benefit with azathioprine therapy in maintaining remission. An interesting study by O'Donoghue et al.[34] reported the results of a placebo-controlled withdrawal of azathioprine therapy from patients who had previously entered remission using azathioprine. Over the next year 41% of patients randomized to placebo relapsed, compared to 5% of patients who continued taking azathioprine.

To date only one randomized placebo controlled study has demonstrated efficacy for cyclosporin A in the treatment of active Crohn's disease[35]. The Canadian Crohn's Relapse Prevention Trial (CCRPT) failed to demonstrate any protective effect in terms of maintenance of remission, and in fact suggested that the use of cyclosporin might be associated with increased disease activity[36].

Pilot, uncontrolled studies from Seattle suggest that methotrexate may be of benefit in the treatment of active disease[37] and in maintenance of remission for those who responded to acute therapy[38]. Randomized, controlled trials will be required before the use of methotrexate can be recommended.

METRONIDAZOLE

Metronidazole is effective in the treatment of active Crohn's disease[39,40]. Recently Rutgeerts and colleagues[41] reported a placebo-controlled trial of metronidazole (2 g daily) for the prevention of endoscopic recurrence in the neoterminal ileum of recently resected patients. Although the use of metronidazole did not prevent the development of endoscopic recurrence, it appeared to protect against the development of the more severe lesions.

CONCLUSIONS

Patients should be counselled to stop smoking following surgery. There is no convincing evidence that dietary manipulation has a role to play. In this time of increasing concerns regarding health care expenditures, it will become increasingly important to target therapy for patients who are at a higher risk of recurrence, rather than simply give medication to all patients regardless of risk. Attempts to develop models which predict those at risk of recurrence and who might benefit from therapy are ongoing. Preliminary studies suggest it may be possible to identify patients at risk and change the natural history of relapse following surgery.

References

1. Lennard-Jones JE, Stadler GA. Prognosis after resection of chronic regional ileitis. Gut. 1967;8:332–6.
2. Rutgeerts P, Geboes K, Vantrappen G, Beyls J, Kerremans R, Hiele M. Predictability of the postoperative course of Crohn's disease. Gastroenterology. 1990;99:956–63.
3. Greenstein AJ, Lachman P, Sachar DB et al. Perforating and non-perforating indications for repeated operations in Crohn's disease: evidence for two clinical forms. Gut. 1988;29:588–92.
4. Calkins BM. A meta-analysis of the role of smoking in inflammatory bowel disease. Dig Dis Sci. 1989;34:1841–54.
5. Hodstock G, Savage D, Harman M, Wright R. Should patients with inflammatory bowel disease smoke? Br Med J. 1984;288:362.
6. Sutherland LR, Ramcharan S, Bryant H, Fick G. Effect of cigarette smoking on recurrence of Crohn's disease. Gastroenterology. 1990;98:1123–8.
7. BACD. Effect of cigarette smoking on the prognosis of Crohn's disease. Gastroenterology. 1990;98:A209 (abstr.).
8. Rhodes JM, Cickel R, Allan RN, Hawker PC, Dawson J, Elias E. Colonic Crohn's disease and use of oral contraception. Br Med J. 1984;288:595–6.
9. Lesko SM, Kaufman DW, Rosenberg L et al. Evidence for an increased risk of Crohn's disease in oral contraceptive users. Gastroenterology. 1985;89:1046–9.
10. Calkins BM, Mendeloff AI, Garland C. Inflammatory bowel disease in oral contraceptive users. Gastroenterology. 1986;91:523–4.
11. Lashner BA, Kane SV, Hanauer SB. Lack of association between oral contraceptive use and Crohn's disease. Gastroenterology. 1989;97:1442–7.
12. Wurzelmann JL, Sandler RS, McDonnell CW. Oral contraceptive use and the risk of inflammatory bowel disease. Gastroenterology. 1991;100:A263 (abstr.).
13. Sutherland LR, Ramcharan S, Bryant H, Fick G. Effect of oral contraceptive use on reoperation following surgery for Crohn's disease. Dig Dis Sci. 1992: in press.
14. Ritchie JK, Wadsworth J, Lennard-Jones JE, Rogers E. Controlled multicentre therapeutic trial of an unrefined carbohydrate, fibre rich diet in Crohn's disease. Br Med J. 1987;295:517–20.
15. Alun Jones V, Dickinson RJ, Workman E, Wilson AJ, Freeman AH, Hunter JO. Crohn's disease: maintenance of remission by diet. Lancet. 1985;2:177–80.
16. Rutgeerts P, Goboes K, Peeters M et al. Effect of faecal stream diversion on recurrence of Crohn's disease in the neoterminal ileum. Lancet. 1991;338:771–4.
17. Wright JP, Alp MN, Young GO, Tigler-Wybrandi N. Predictors of acute relapse of Crohn's disease. A laboratory and clinical study. Dig Dis Sci. 1987;32(2):164–70.
18. D'Agostino L, Pignata S, Daniele B et al. Prediction of relapses in patients with Crohn's disease by postheparin plasma diamine oxidase. Gastroenterology. 1991;100:A205 (abstr.).

19. Brignola C, Campieri M, Farruggia P *et al*. The possible utility of steroids in the prevention of relapses of Crohn's disease in remission. A preliminary study. J Clin Gastroenterol. 1988;10:631–4.
20. Sutherland LR. Editorial: 5-aminosalicylates for prevention of recurrence in patients with Crohn's disease: time for a reappraisal? J Clin Gastroenterol. 1991;13:5–7.
21. Summers RW, Switz DM, Sessions JT Jr *et al*. National Co-operative Crohn's Disease Study: results of drug treatment. Gastroenterology. 1979;77:847–69.
22. Martin F, Sutherland LR, Beck IT *et al*. Oral 5-ASA versus prednisone in short term treatment of Crohn's disease: a multicentre controlled trial. Can J Gastroenterol. 1990;4:452–7.
23. Hanauer SB, Belker ME, Gitnick G *et al*. Multi-centre, placebo-controlled, dose-ranging study of oral pentasa (controlled release mesalamine) for active Crohn's disease: preliminary results. Gastroenterology. 1990;98:A173 (abstr.).
24. Pallone F, Prantera C, Cottone M, Brunetti G, Miglioli M, Italian Study Group. Maintenance treatment of Crohn's disease with oral 5-ASA (ASACOL). Results of a multicentre controlled trial. Gastroenterology. 1991;100:A237 (abstr.).
25. International Mesalazine Study Group. Coated oral 5-aminosalicylic acid versus placebo in maintaining remission of inactive Crohn's disease. Aliment Pharmacol Ther. 1990;4:55–64.
26. Gendre JP, Mary JY, Florent C *et al*. Does Pentasa prevent relapses in quiescent Crohn's disease (QCD)? A multicentre placebo-controlled trial. Gastroenterology. 1990;98:A171 (abstr.).
27. Bondesen S, Danish 5-ASA Group. Mesalazine (Pentasa) as prophylaxis in Crohn's disease. A multicenter, controlled trial. Scand J Gastroenterol. 1991;26, Supplement 183:68 (abstr.).
28. Brignola C, Iannone P, Pasquali S *et al*. Placebo-controlled trial of oral 5-ASA in relapse prevention of Crohn's disease. Dig Dis Sci. 1992;37:29–32.
29. Ewe K, Herfarth C, Malchow H, Jesdinsky HJ. Postoperative recurrence of Crohn's disease in relation to radicality of operation and sulfasalazine prophylaxis: a multicentre trial. Digestion. 1989;42:224–32.
30. Jewell DP. Corticosteroids for the management of ulcerative colitis and Crohn's disease. Gastroenterol Clin N Am. 1989;18(1):21–34.
31. Malchow H, Ewe K, Brandes JW *et al*. European Cooperative Crohn's Disease Study (ECCDS): results of drug treatment. Gastroenterology. 1984;86:249–66.
32. Loftberg R, Danielsson A, Salde L. Oral budesonide in active ileocecal Crohn's disease – a pilot trial with a topically acting steroid. Gastroenterology. 1991;100:A226 (abstr.).
33. Present DH, Korelitz BI, Wisch N, Glass JL, Sachar DB, Pasternack BS. Treatment of Crohn's disease with 6-mercaptopurine (6-MP) a long-term, randomized, double blind study. N Engl J Med. 1980;302:981–7.
34. O'Donoghue DP, Dawson AM, Powell-Tuck J, Bown RL, Lennard-Jones JE. Double-blind withdrawal trial of azathioprine as maintenance treatment for Crohn's disease. Lancet. 1978;2:955–7.
35. Brynskov J, Freund L, Rasmussen SN *et al*. A placebo-controlled, double-blind, randomized trial of cyclosporine therapy in active chronic Crohn's disease. N Engl J Med. 1989;321:845–50.
36. Archambault A, Feagan B, Fedorak R *et al*. The Canadian Crohn's Relapse Prevention Trial (CCRPT). Gastroenterology. 1992;102:A591 (abstr).
37. Kozarek RA, Patterson DJ, Felfand MD, Botoman VA, Ball TJ, Wilske KR. Methotrexate induces clinical and histologic remission in patients with refractory inflammatory bowel disease. Ann Intern Med. 1989;110(5):353–6.
38. Kozarek RA, Patterson DJ, Botoman VA, Ball TJ, Gelfand MD. Methotrexate: the long and the short of it. Gastroenterology. 1990;98:A183 (abstr.).
39. Ursing B, Alm T, Barany F *et al*. A comparative study of metronidazole and sulfasalazine for active Crohn's disease: the Cooperative Crohn's Disease Study in Sweden. II. Result. Gastroenterology. 1982;83:550–62.
40. Sutherland L, Singleton J, Sessions J *et al*. Double blind, placebo controlled trial of metronidazole in Crohn's disease. Gut. 1991;32:1071–5.
41. Rutgeerts P, Peeters M, Hiele M *et al*. A placebo controlled trial of metronidazole for recurrence prevention of Crohn's disease after resection of the terminal ileum. Gastroenterology. 1992;102:A688 (abstr.).

38

Fistulae in Crohn's disease: wait or operate?

K. W. ECKER

INTRODUCTION

Fistulae are one of the characteristic features of Crohn's disease[1]. Although the aetiology and pathogenesis of the underlying inflammatory disease are still largely unknown, there are plausible theories to explain the pathogenesis of the complicating fistulae[2]. These may aid in the decision to use curative surgical approaches for the treatment of such complicating manifestations of Crohn's disease, while the primary underlying disorder remains incurable, whether by medical or by surgical treatment[34].

The development of therapeutic concepts is made more difficult by the fact that the individual morbidity of the different types of fistulae is variable, and that both asymptomatic courses and spontaneous closures have been reported[5,6]. The questions as to the general possibilities of surgery, the best time for surgery, and the further prognosis both with respect to the fistula itself and to the underlying disorder, remain.

PATIENTS AND METHODS

In this chapter a distinction is made between intestinal and perianal fistulae. It was therefore necessary to carry out two different prospective studies.

In the first study the primary indication for carrying out abdominal surgery was defined preoperatively in 241 patients. It was also documented in the case report forms whether there were secondary indications for surgery, and whether there were any intraoperative findings which had not been known preoperatively, but would generally be considered part of the range of indications for surgery in Crohn's disease. The origins and target organs of intestinal fistulae were documented. This was to further elucidate the significance of intestinal fistulae for the morbidity of Crohn's patients, and for making decisions with regard to the indications for surgical treatment.

A second, independent study was carried out in 459 patients with Crohn's disease to determine the incidence and severity of complicating perianal fistulae and abscesses over a follow-up period of up to 9 years. During this time all acute infectious anal complications were relieved by a sphincter-sparing drainage operation, while the intestinal Crohn's disease itself was treated medically or, in the presence of abdominal complications or resistance to conservative therapy, surgically. The rate of spontaneous fistula closure at the end of the observation period, the need for re-drainage or stoma formation, and the possibility of safely carrying out classical fistula surgery, were all investigated. The findings were analysed in relation to the intestinal localization of the Crohn's disease and the treatment thus required. The aim was to assess the influence of the natural history of the disease and the effect of active surgical intervention.

RESULTS

Intestinal fistulae – surgical indications and clinical significance

Intestinal fistulae (Table 1) were of primary importance in determining the need for surgery in only 18% ($n = 43$) of the 241 patients. However, intestinal fistulae were also present in a further 17% ($n = 41$) of patients. Thus the actual prevalence of intestinal fistulae at the time of surgery was twice as high as their frequency as indications for surgery. Interestingly, not a single intestinal fistula – independent of its importance as an indication for surgery – constituted the sole reason for surgery. There were always additional features meriting operation, principally stenoses, abscesses, penetrations and perforations. It was the combination of different complications, rather than the presence of a fistula itself, that determined the patients' overall morbidity.

Table 1 Indications for abdominal surgery in 241 patients suffering from Crohn's disease (1982–1988).

	A		B
Stenosis	120		46
Abdominal mass			92
Fistula	*43*	*(18%)*	*41*
Abscess	11		34
Penetration/perforation	8		22
Chronic course	44		
Fulminant course	15		
	241		235

A = Indication leading to operation; B = additional finding at operation

Types of intestinal fistulae and special indications for surgery

Predominant among the fistulae of primary importance as indications for surgery were enterocutaneous fistulae, while the commonest 'incidental' type were interenteric (Table 2). A striking finding in this context was that the majority of patients with enterocutaneous fistulae had a history of previous surgery. The morbidity associated with these fistulae was related to high fistula output or to phlegmonous subcutaneous infections. The clinical relevance of interenteric fistulae was rarely related to quantitative faecal shunting, but rather to aggravation of the symptoms caused by other complications, in the context of conglomerate tumours. Enterovesical fistulae were less common overall. They were diagnosed in 10 cases, and in the presence of urinary tract infections or urosepsis constituted an absolute indication for surgery. Only three female patients had enterogenital fistulae, extending from the rectum to the vagina. These always represented absolute indications for surgery, due to the extraordinary distress implied. Retroperitoneal fistulae were not evaluated in this context, since they were always treated as an indication for urgent abscess removal.

Incidence and severity of perianal fistulae

During the follow-up period of up to 9 years and after a mean duration of the disease of 10.4 ± 7.8 years, a total of 190 out of 459 patients (41%) were found to have suffered infectious or septic anal complications (Table 3). In the final evaluation no distinction was drawn between fistulae and abscesses, since both complications were observed either simultaneously or successively in all patients affected, either from the outset or later during the course of their disease. There was an almost linear increase in the frequency and severity of perianal sepsis with more distal disease localization – from 8% in ileitis to 88% in proctitis.

Table 2 Differentiation of the 84 intestinal fistulae in Crohn's disease (1982–1988)

	A		B	
Enterocutaneous	22		3	
Spontaneous		3		2
Postoperative		9		1
Peristomal		10		
Interenteric	12		34	
Ileal origin		8		25
Colonic origin		4		9
Enterovesical	6		4	
Enterogenital	3			
	43		41	

A = Fistulae leading to operation; B = fistulae found at operation in addition to A

Table 3 Incidence (crude rates) of perianal fistulae and abscesses in Crohn's disease and proportion of perianal sepsis (1982–1990)

	Patients (n)	Fistulae/abscesses		Perianal sepsis	
Ileitis	140	11	(8%)		
Segmental (ileo-)colitis	96	34	(35%)	5	(5%)
Total (ileo-)colitis	206	130	(63%)	90	(44%)
Proctitis	17	15	(88%)	8	(47%)
	459	190	(41%)		

Outcome following initial drainage of acute manifestations

Following a sphincter-sparing drainage operation as an initial procedure in the presence of acute septic anal complications, the final outcome in ileitis and segmental colitis bore no relation to whether the intestinal inflammation had responded to drug treatment by the end of the observation period, or whether intestinal resection had been required (Table 4). In the end, 62% of the 45 patients had shown spontaneous closure, 20% had undergone re-drainage, and 18% had required classical fistulotomy because of continuing suppuration, despite remission of the intestinal disease. In patients with pancolitis and proctitis this continence-preserving regime was successful only as long as the intestinal Crohn's disease continued to respond to treatment. By the end of the observation period, 79 patients still showed adequate continence, though the proportion of patients requiring re-drainage had risen to 64% at the expense of the proportion showing uncomplicated healing. In 66 patients, resistance of the intestinal disease to treatment had necessitated laparotomy. Due to concomitant severe fistulous disease accompanied by anorectal destruction, these operations involved creation of a permanent stoma.

DISCUSSION

Pathogenesis of fistula formation

Intestinal fistulae are to be distinguished from perianal fistulae[3]. Nevertheless, they have some pathogenetic factors in common. Among the intestinal fistulae, a further differentiation between spontaneous and postoperative fistulae is necessary. Spontaneous fistula formation originating from the intestine is the end-result of the transmural inflammatory process characteristic of Crohn's disease. The presence of stenoses is thought to be a predisposing factor for fistula formation[2]. Postoperative fistulae often form following appendicectomy, or as a consequence of suture defects at the site of anastomosis. In addition, fistulae often form in the vicinity of enterostomies. This observation explains why fistulae connecting to the body surface are usually seen in patients who have undergone previous surgery, while spontaneous fistulae are more likely to connect intra-abdominally with some other hollow viscus[1]. Since intestinal fistulae become contaminated with the

Table 4 Follow-up after local drainage of 190 perianal fistulae and abscesses

Intestinal					
Inflammation	Treatment	n	Spontaneous closure	Re-drainage	Fistulotomy, fistulectomy
Ileitis Segmental colitis	Conservative Operation	45	28 (62%)	9 (20%)	8 (18%)
Total colitis	Conservative	79	22 (28%)	51 (64%)	6 (8%)
Proctitis	Operation	66 190		Stoma creation	

The table represents the endpoint of observation after 9 years at maximum (crude rates)

bacterial bowel flora, they are often associated with simultaneous or subsequent abscess formation[7].

There are parallels between the pathogenesis of spontaneous intestinal fistulae and that of perianal fistulae: the former arise from penetration of Crohn's lesions through the mucosa anywhere in the intestinal tract, while the latter are thought to have their origin in primary Crohn's lesions of the anal canal[8]. Both types of fistulae are also associated with abscesses, an association that is even more pronounced in the case of perianal fistulae[9]. With respect to perianal fistulae, cryptogenic infections are increasingly being discussed as a possible causative mechanism[10]. According to both these pathogenetic theories, there is a clear correlation between the frequency and severity of perianal fistulae on the one hand, and impairment of colorectal function (and hence the intestinal localization of Crohn's disease) on the other[11,12]. Severe infections and septic anal complications are thus a pathognomonic manifestation of Crohn's proctocolitis[13,14].

Fistula-related morbidity

The clinical significance of a fistula in Crohn's disease is related not so much to its presence as such, as to the context in which it arises and to its sequelae[1,6,15]. Intestinal fistulae are often found in the context of additional abdominal complications, including mainly stenoses and abscesses related to the presence of conglomerate tumours[2]. With perianal fistulae the context is essentially one of irreversibly impaired colorectal function followed by treatment-resistant diarrhoea[11].

The acute consequences of fistula formation result from the infectious and septic potential of the fistulae; in the long term, functional disturbances become more prominent. With intestinal fistulae, abdominal and in particular retroperitoneal sepsis acquires prognostic significance, but urinary tract infections can also lead to dangerous urosepsis[1,3]. Functional disturbances due to fistulae affect the digestive tract only if significant faecal shunting occurs. In such cases a syndrome due to bacterial contamination of the upper small bowel leads to further impairment of absorption, particularly if the fistula arises from a stenosis[6,16]. The development of necrotizing fasciitis has been described as a severe acute septic complication of perianal fistulae (citation from ref. 12). A more common complication, however, is the gradual destruction of the anal continence mechanism by the chronic infectious process, which may ultimately lead to incontinence[14].

Apart from these severe consequences of the disease that can be assessed objectively, the morbidity associated with fistulae always involves a variable degree of subjective distress as well, particularly if there is involvement of the genital region in the disease process.

Implications for the therapeutic concept

Treatment of fistulae will usually represent only one part, albeit an essential part, of the overall therapeutic strategy for Crohn's disease. Our considerations must therefore take into account the natural history of Crohn's disease itself, and that of the complicating fistulae. We must verify whether our intended therapeutic approach is merely symptomatic in nature, or curative. From this point of view, the surgical treatment of intestinal fistulae must be evaluated differently from that of perianal fistulae[1].

Intestinal fistulae, together with other abdominal complications, are usually responsible for making the patient's clinical condition untreatable by conservative means[17,18]. Surgical treatment, consisting of resection of the diseased, fistula-bearing intestinal segment and excision of fistulous tracks into otherwise healthy organs, not only eliminates the fistula with no fear of recurrence, but also prevents all its complications[1,2,19]. This justifies the indication for surgery. The only differentiation necessary relates to the urgency of the procedure, which depends on septic risk, functional impairment, and subjective symptoms. This provides the rationale for the differentiation between absolute and relative indications[2,20]. Experience shows that all relative indications sooner or later become absolute ones.

The morbidity associated with perianal fistulae ultimately is a function of the degree of activity of the intestinal inflammation[11,20]. This means that when treating the acute manifestations, treatment should simultaneously aim at both the underlying disease and the complication[20]. From a surgical point of view the procedure indicated for treating infectious perianal complications is the simplest way of achieving adequate drainage of pus[9]. Indications for abdominal surgery can only relate to the requirements posed by intestinal Crohn's disease[1]. Local surgery in this context can never be anything else but symptomatic. Nonetheless, permanent closure of a fistula is by no means an exceptional occurrence, provided stable intestinal remission can be achieved[20,21]. The natural history of the underlying disorder is a more powerful determinant of future prognosis than surgery. Hence it is advisable to abstain from curative treatment attempts unless an unequivocal cryptogenic infection can be demonstrated, usually with a deep fistula track[10]. In severe cases of perianal sepsis, faecal diversion combined with local drainage is an appropriate means of keeping infection under control[1]. Subsequent restoration of continence, however, is only rarely possible, implying that a definitive stoma, usually created in the context of a two-stage proctocolectomy, represents the final solution for most patients with severe perianal infection[13,22,23].

References

1. Herfarth C. Fisteln beim Morbus Crohn – Konservative versus operative Behandlung. Chirugischer Standpunkt. Z Gastroenterologie. 1985;23:34–7.
2. Alexander-Williams J. Surgical aspects of inflammatory bowel disease. Scand J Gastroenterol. 1990;25(Suppl 172):39–42.
3. Betzler M, Schürmann G, Herfarth C. Chirurgisches Vorgehen bei M. Crohn. Chirurg. 1992;63:13–19.
4. Domschke W. Morbus Crohn: I. Möglichkeiten und Grenzen der konservativen Therapie. Langenbeck's Arch Chir. 1984;364:413–17.
5. Buchmann P, Keighley RMB, Allan RN, Thompson H, Alexander-Williams J. Natural history of perianal Crohn's disease. Am J Surg. 1980;140:642–44.

6. Broe PJ, Bayless TM, Cameron JL. Crohn's disease: are enteroenteral fistulas an indication for surgery? Surgery. 1982;91:249–53.
7. Hill GL, Bourchier RG, Witney GB. Surgical and metabolic management of patients with external fistulas of the small intestine associated with Crohn's disease. World J Surg. 1988;12:191–7.
8. Hughes LE. Surgical pathology and management of anorectal Crohn's disease. J Roy Soc Med. 1978;71:644–51.
9. Pritehard TJ, Schoetz PJ Jr, Roberts PL, Murray JJ, Coller JA, Veidenheimer MC. Perirectal abscess in Crohn's disease: drainage and outcome. Dis Colon Rectum. 1990;33:933–7.
10. Hancke, E. Perianale Infektionen bei M. Crohn. Med Klin. 1992;87:305–9.
11. Hellers G, Bergstand O, Ewerth S, Holmström B. Occurrence and outcome after primary treatment of anal fistulas in Crohn's disease. Gut. 1980;21:525–7.
12. Keighley MRB, Allan RN. Current status and influence of operation on perianal Crohn's disease. Int J Colorect Dis. 1986;1:104–7.
13. Scammell BE, Andrews H, Allan RN, Alexander-Williams J, Keighley MRB. Results of proctocolectomy for Crohn's disease. Br J Surg. 1987;74:671–4.
14. Williams JG, Hughes LE. Abdominoperineal resection for severe Crohn's disease. Dis Colon Rectum. 1990;33:402–7.
15. Broe PJ, Cameron JL. Surgical management of ileosigmoid fistulas in Crohn's disease. Am J Surg. 1982;143:611–13.
16. Goebell H. Pathophysiologische Grundlagen des Malabscryptionssyndroms. Chirurg. 1974;45:1–6.
17. Block GE, Schraut WH. The operative treatment of Crohn's enteritis complicated by ileosigmoid fistula. Ann Surg. 1982;196:356–60.
18. Thiele H, Lorenz D. Ileocoecaler Crohn mit Sigmabeteiligung. Chirurg. 1985;56:798–802.
19. Hultén L. Frühoperation beim M. Crohn, ja oder nein? Internist. 1979;20:171–5.
20. Allan A, Keighley MRB. Management of perianal Crohn's disease. World J Surg. 1988;12:198–202.
21. Herfarth C, Buidewald H. Perianale Erkrankung beim M. Crohn. Chirurg. 1986;57:304–8.
22. Grant DR, Cohen Z, McLeod RS. Loop-ileostomy for anorectal Crohn's disease. Can J Surg. 1986;29:32–7.
23. Harper PH, Fazio VW, Lovery IC, Jagelman DG, Weakley FL, Farmer RG, Easley KA. The long-term outcome in Crohn's disease. Dis Colon Rectum. 1987;30:174–9.

39

Early surgery – a reappraisal: a discussion paper based on the Malmö experience

T. LINDHAGEN, M. STARCK and G. EKELUND

ULCERATIVE COLITIS

The timing of surgery in inflammatory bowel disease has been different over the years.

In ulcerative colitis we are aware of the risk for cancer and therefore more or less prophylactic colectomy was earlier often advocated after some 10 years disease duration[1]. Today to a great extent we rely on colonoscopic surveillance with multiple biopsies from various parts of the colon. This in spite of the fact that we have no real hard data relating to how this influences the rate of malignancy. There still is an ongoing debate concerning the magnitude of the cancer risk. There are reports indicating that the risk is much lower than earlier believed, especially if the patient's age is taken into consideration[2]. In ulcerative colitis we need further studies on the risk of cancer and on the effect of surveillance before firm conclusion can be drawn. This is especially important as there have probably been some changes in the indications for colectomy, as an opportunity now exists for sphincter-saving coloproctectomy, using the pouch operation. For these reasons ulcerative colitis will not be discussed further here.

CROHN'S DISEASE

In Crohn's disease the timing of surgery has fluctuated over the past 60 years and also from hospital to hospital. The reason for this is that we still do not know the aetiology and that we have no curative therapy[3].

Well-conducted controlled studies concerning the effect of medical treatment have been reported[4,5] but so far not so much concerning surgical therapy. Most studies are reports on results and experiences at various centres. Thus we are only able, in broad terms, to get some idea of the results from different management policies. Of course we would know much more if we had controlled studies to evaluate. To perform such studies, however, requires multicentre – maybe multinational – studies in order to have a sufficient number of patients in the various subgroups for randomization and statistical analysis. Furthermore long-term follow-up is necessary[6].

Today, at many centres, patients with Crohn's disease are primarily treated conservatively[7]. Such treatment may often lead to remission, but with a risk of adverse effects[8,9].

From many reports it is obvious that most patients will sooner or later have to undergo surgery due to the complications of the disease, but, as mentioned above, the timing varies. If surgery is delayed until it is unavoidable, many patients seem to develop complicated disease. In some centres, especially in Scandinavia, a policy of earlier surgery appears to prevail, while in the USA the policy seems to be towards prolonged primary conservative treatment[10–14].

Two US centres, for example, which have an outstanding experience in Crohn's disease (i.e. Mount Sinai Hospital in New York and the Cleveland Clinic in Ohio) report a higher frequency of preoperative complications than we have in Malmö. We have earlier reported our results compared to results from these centres[3,6]. The major indication for surgery at Mount Sinai Hospital was obstruction or abscess/fistula in 45% and 34% respectively[11].

The indications for surgery reported from the Cleveland Clinic are given in Table 1. It is obvious that most patients had advanced disease when operated on. In another report from the Cleveland Clinic it was stated that 'Crohn's disease is not a benign disease', as patients followed up for a minimum of 15 years showed a relentless progression of the disease with a high incidence of complications[15].

First Malmö study

In contrast to the above, we reported that the policy at our department was relatively early resection. Thus 8% of those operated on had at the most

Table 1 Indications for original surgery in relation to clinical pattern at the Cleveland Clinic[12] (percentages)

Indication	Small intestine pattern	Ileocolic pattern	Colonic or anorectal pattern
Obstruction	61	48	22
Toxic megacolon	2	5	27
Perianal disease	16	32	38
Fistula/abscess	38	48	31

minor symptoms. In total, during a 17-year period, 94% of all patients with Crohn's disease within the population of Malmö were operated on[16].

In an analysis of 133 cases in which the diagnosis of Crohn's disease was established preoperatively, and where referred patients from other areas were excluded, 11% had minor symptoms while only 4% had intra-abdominal abscesses or fistulae. One motive for this policy of early surgery was an attempt to forestall serious progress of the disease[12].

A comprison of rates on preoperative complications is difficult, as the length of the preoperative period is not always given, and series are not quite comparable for other reasons.

Figure 1 shows the reported mean time (median time seldom reported) between onset of symptoms and time of operation in three series from the UK, one from Malmö and in one early series from the Cleveland Clinic[12,17–20]. A later report from the latter clinic states only that the mean duration of symptoms until operation was 2 years[21]. From Figure 1 it is evident that most patients, especially those with large bowel disease, were generally operated on after several years duration. The results indicate a relatively more aggressive surgical policy in Leeds in the UK, and in Malmö in Sweden[6].

Given these figures it is possible to compare the rate of preoperative complications, i.e. indications for surgery in the different series. In Figure 2 and Figure 3 the rates between Malmö and the Cleveland Clinic for cases with predominantly small and large bowel disease respectively are compared. The figures show that the rates are lower for all preoperative complications in Malmö. It must, however, be considered that the Malmö series consists of unselected primary cases, whereas the figures from the USA represent both primary and referred cases, i.e. probably relatively more advanced cases. The data nevertheless indicate the inherent dangers of advanced and complicated disease[6,7,12].

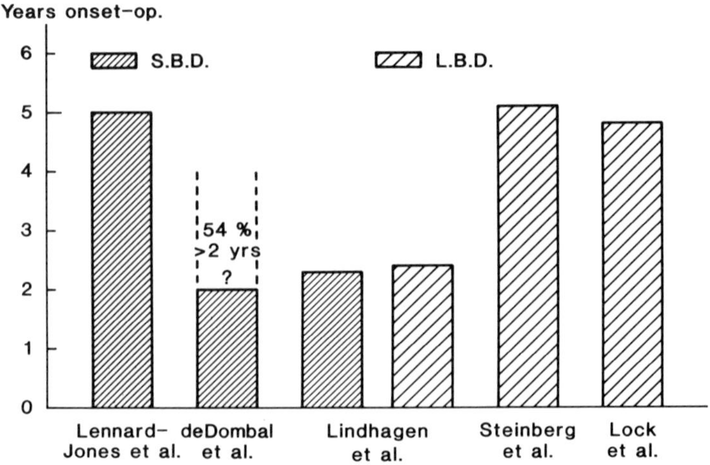

Fig. 1 Duration of symptoms from onset to first operation according to various series (from ref. 3)

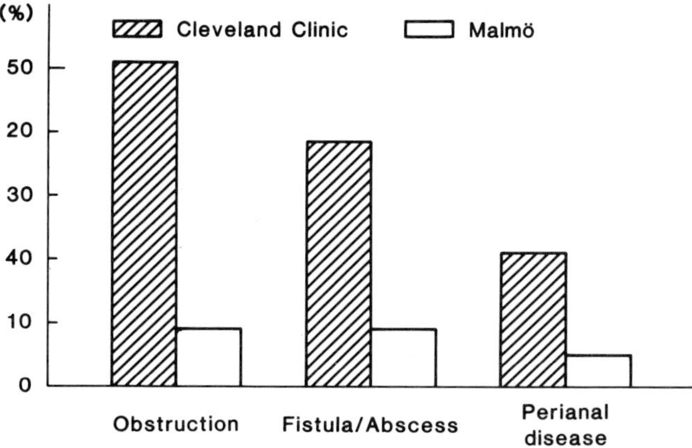

Fig. 2 Main indications for surgery in a series from Cleveland and one from Malmö (predominantly small bowel disease) (from ref. 3)

Another motive for early surgery is to prevent preoperative and postoperative complications. In the Malmö series of patients diagnosed as having Crohn's disease preoperatively the postoperative mortality rate was 1.5% as the late related mortality was 2.3% compared to 7.3% in the Cleveland Clinic series[12,22].

In Malmö none of the patients not operated on died, while this was the case for 2.6% of the Cleveland Clinic patients. Several reports indicate that preoperative septic complications increase the risk of postoperative complications. This was the case in both the compared series[12,21].

From Mount Sinai Hospital, New York, it has been reported that almost all patients will get recurrent disease if followed for a sufficient time. In the Malmö series, however, this recurrence rate, crude as well as actuarial, was close to 50% during the first 15 years[23]. Thus the recurrence risk is not

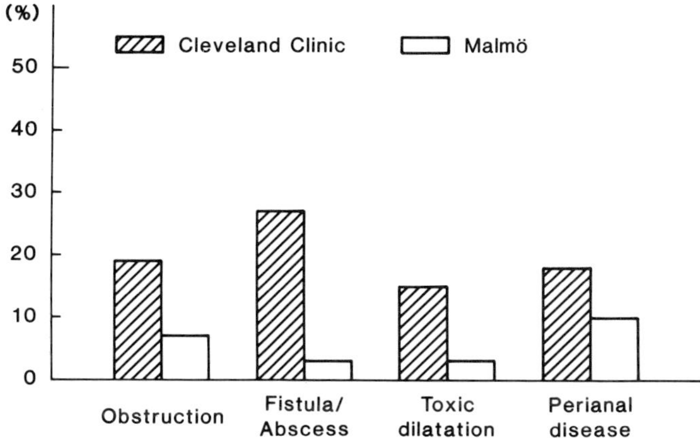

Fig. 3 Main indications for surgery in a series from Cleveland and one from Malmö (predominantly large bowel disease) (from ref. 3)

necessarily an argument against early surgery, especially as all patients without surgery have demonstrable disease.

Second Malmö study

It may be argued that the results from this Malmö study, reported 10 years ago, as well as those from other older studies, are invalid today when so much has improved lately in overall medical care. We therefore analysed the results from the following 10-year period, 1975–1984, with a mean observation period (from diagnosis) of 58 months (3 months–15 years).

During this study period there were 184 new patients with Crohn's disease in the city of Malmö, 78 (42%) of which had predominantly small bowel disease, 102 (55%) had predominantly large bowel disease while four had merely Crohn's disease of the appendix. The results are given in Tables 2–4. The diagnosis was established preoperatively in 88 cases. These are of special interest since there was a choice concerning timing of surgery.

Table 2 Crohn's disease in Malmö, 1975–84 (excluding four patients with Crohn's disease of the appendix)

	SBD	LBD	Total
Number of patients	78	102	180
Conservative treatment	11%	39%	27%
Operated on	89%	61%	73%
Recurrence rate (percentage of operations	35%	37%	35%
Related mortality			1.6%

Table 3 Diagnosis of Crohn's disease established preoperatively, Malmö, 1975–84

	SBD	LBD
Number of patients	44	44
Time diagnosis until operation (median, months)	2	5
Recurrence rate	32%	39%

Table 4 Diagnosis of Crohn's disease established preoperatively: main indications for surgery, Malmö, 1975–84 (percentages)

	SBD	LBD
Pain, diarrhoea, malnutrition	46	79
Minor symptoms	32	7
Fistulae	13	5
Obstruction	9	—
Anal disease	—	9

Comparison between the two series from Malmö shows that the frequency of operations is lower, and especially for patients with predominantly large bowel disease, in the later series; also the rates for preoperative complications were somewhat higher. This is so without any change in official policy. Admitting that the series are not quite comparable, as the observation time is different, the results suggest that, in spite of our policy we have been influenced by a widespread opinion that patients should be treated conservatively to a greater extent. So far we do not have complete data showing the quality of life for those under conservative treatment as compared to those operated on. However, of those 40 not operated on, 12 are doing well without any treatment, 18 are doing well on drug treatment while five on treatment are doing less well. In patients with predominantly small bowel disease it is apparent that we to a greater extent have adhered to our policy.

Experience from Birmingham and Gothenburg

In a report on 139 patients during 19 years from Birmingham, UK, concerning management of distal ileal disease it was shown that the outcome for primary and referred patients was similar even if there was a high proportion of referred patients in their group of patients with delayed surgery[24]. In their policy they prescribed no treatment for asymptomatic patients and a short course of sulphasalazine or 5-aminosalicylates for patients with mild symptoms. For symptomatic patients with active disease short courses with steroids were prescribed. When the authors compared their groups according to various lengths of delay in surgical treatment they found that such delay did not reduce reoperation rates for recurrent disease. They also found that 'the excess mortality previously associated with Crohn's disease has now been largely eliminated', and concluded that 'in experienced hands surgical intervention is an effective and rapid method of restoring patients to good health and is usually a good alternative to prolonged medical treatment during which the patient is improved but often remains unwell'[24].

The risk of creating short bowel syndrome by early surgical resection seems to be overestimated, as it has been shown by Hultén and co-workers in Gothenburg that the activity of the disease is a more important cause of malnutrition than is the loss of diseased bowel. They therefore concluded that only rarely should surgery be withheld from malnourished patients with Crohn's disease[25].

CONCLUDING REFLECTIONS

When all these experiences are considered together it is apparent that there are still reasons for early surgery. The key question then is what 'early' means. The answer is that surgery should be performed before serious complications of the disease occur, and when patients are unwell on medical treatment[6]. The report from Birmingham was a joint venture by medical and surgical gastroenterologists who apparently shared their policy[24]. In other places where cooperation between gastroenterologists and surgeons is not that well established it may turn out differently. If one part is more interested, or more active, than the other part, the treatment offered might be either surgical or medical. This might be an unfavourable situation, but on the other hand if gastroenterologists and surgeons start to discuss management in a positive and polite way there may be a risk that they start to negotiate, and it may then still be an unfavourable situation, if for the sake of peace, they end up with something in between. Probably the most optimal situation exists if gastroenterologists and surgeons work integrated, and see each others' patients regularly. Doing so it will be more obvious which patients should be operated on and when this should be performed.

In summary, when surgical treatment is indicated, due to symptoms or as prophylaxis against serious complications, it should not be delayed. Early surgery thus still plays an important role in the treatment of patients with Crohn's disease.

References

1. Kewenter J, Ahlman H, Hultén L. Cancer risk in extensive ulcerative colitis. Ann Surg. 1978;188:824–28.
2. Broström O, Löfberg R, Öst Å, Reichard H. Cancer surveillance of patients with longstanding ulcerative colitis: a clinical, endoscopical, and histological study. Gut. 1986;27:1408–13.
3. Ekelund G, Lindhagen T, Lindström C, Stewenius J. Surgical treatment of inflammatory bowel disease. Jpn J Surg. 1987;17:413.
4. Summers RW, Switz DM, Sessions JT Jr, Becktel JM, Best WR, Kern F Jr, Singleton JW. National Cooperative Crohn's Disease Study: results of drug treatment. Gastroenterology. 1979;77:847–69.
5. Rosén A, Ursing B, Alm T, Bárány F, Bergelin I, Ganrot-Norlin K, Hoevels J, Huitfeldt B, Järnerot G, Krause U, Krook A, Lindström B, Nordle Ö. A comparative study of metronidazole and sulfasalazine for active Crohn's disease: the Cooperative Crohn's Disease Study in Sweden. Gastroenterology. 1982;83:541–9.
6. Ekelund G, Lindhagen T. Controversies in the surgical management of Crohn's disease. Perspect Colon Rectal Surg. 1989;2:1–18.
7. Farmer RG, Hawk WA, Turnbull RB Jr. Indications for surgery in Crohn's disease. Gastroenterology. 1976;71:245–50.
8. Nyman M, Hansson I, Eriksson S. Long-term immunosuppressive treatment in Crohn's disease. Scand J Gastroenterol. 1985;20:1197–203.
9. McManus JM. Comment on 6-mercaptopurine in Crohn's fistulas. Gastroenterology. 1985;89:223–4.
10. Farmer RG, Whelan G, Fazio VW. Long-term follow-up of patients with Crohn's disease. Gastroenterology. 1985;88:1818–25.
11. Heimann TM, Greenstein AJ, Medchanic L, Aufses AH Jr. Early complications following surgical treatment for Crohn's disease. Ann Surg. 1985;201:494–8.
12. Lindhagen T, Ekelund G, Leandoer L, Hildell J, Lindström C, Wenckert A. Pre- and post-operative complications in Crohn's disease with special reference to duration of preoperative disease history. Scand J Gastroenterol. 1984;19:194–203.
13. Krause U. Early or late operation in the treatment of Crohn's disease. Scand J Gastroenterol. 1971;6:479–81.
14. Fasth S, Hellberg R, Hultén L, Magnusson O. Early complications after surgical treatment for Crohn's disease with particular reference to factors affecting their development. Acta Chir Scand. 1980;146:519–26.
15. Harper PH, Fazio VW, Lavery IC, Jagelman DG, Weakley FL, Farmer RG, Easley KA. The long-term outcome in Crohn's disease. Dis Colon Rectum. 1987;30:174.

16. Lindhagen T. Crohn's disease in a defined population. Results of surgical treatment. Academic thesis, Malmö, 1982.
17. Lennard-Jones JE, Stalder GA. Prognosis after resection of chronic regional ileitis. Gut. 1967;8:332.
18. deDombal FT, Burton I, Goligher JC. Recurrence of Crohn's disease after primary excisional surgery. Gut. 1971;12:519.
19. Steinberg DM, Allan RN, Thompson H, Brooke BN, Alexander-Williams J, Cooke WT. Excisional surgery with ileostomy for Crohn's colitis with particular reference to factors affecting recurrence. Gut. 1974;15:845–51.
20. Lock R, Farmer RG, Fazio VW, Jagelman DG, Lavery IC, Weakley FL. Recurrence and reoperation for Crohn's disease. N Engl J Med. 1981;304:1586–8.
21. Farmer RG, Whelan G, Fazio VW. Long-term follow-up of patients with Crohn's disease. Gastroenterology. 1985;88:1818–1825.
22. Fazio VW. Regional enteritis (Crohn's disease): indications for surgery and operative strategy. Surg Clin N Am. 1983;63(1):27–48.
23. Greenstein AJ, Sachar DB, Pasternack BS, Janowitz HD. Reoperation and recurrence in Crohn's colitis and ileocolitis. N Engl J Med. 1975;293:685–90.
24. Andrews HA, Keighley MRB, Alexander-Williams J, Allan RN. Strategy for mangement of distal ileal Crohn's disease. Br J Surg. 1991;78:679–82.
25. Hellberg R, Hultén L, Lindstedt G, Björn-Rasmussen E. The nutritional and haematological status before and after primary and subsequent resectional procedures for classical Crohn's disease and Crohn's colitis. Acta Chir Scand. 1982;148:453–60.

40

Aims of surgical treatment: which patient will benefit?

R. G. FARMER

During the course of inflammatory bowel disease (IBD), the majority of patients will either have, or be considered for, an operation. The decision is often a complicated one, frequently involving several physicians as well as the patient and family. While some decisions are obvious, many are not, and there may be conflicting opinions. Thus, assessment of the results of the operation is not only important to that patient, it can also be beneficial to subsequent patients in similar situations. Therefore, careful attention to assessment of the indications as well as the benefits of surgery constitutes valuable, but difficult, clinical research.

At the Cleveland Clinic for more than 25 years we have had the opportunity to follow patients with IBD and to evaluate both the indications for and the results of surgery. This has enabled us to determine the benefits derived from operations performed under various circumstances and for various reasons for patients with either ulcerative colitis or Crohn's disease.

CROHN'S DISEASE

In the mid-1960s at the Cleveland Clinic we developed a registry of 615 consecutive patients newly diagnosed with Crohn's disease. After following these patients for 10 years the thesis was proposed that the initial anatomical involvement in Crohn's disease was a major determinant in prognosis[1]. Approximately 96% of these patients were then followed for an additional 10 years[2]. Analysis of the cases revealed the occurrence of clinical patterns of the disease process that were dependent on initial location of disease. Clinical patterns were established for the following anatomical locations of disease: ileocolic (involvement of right colon and distal ileum), 252 patients (41%); small intestine (without colon involvement), 176 patients (28.6%);

colon (without small intestine involvement), 166 patients (27%); and anorectal (without other demonstrable involvement initially), 21 patients (3.4%). A small number of patients had gastroduodenal involvement.

Statistically significant symptoms ($p < 0.001$) were rectal bleeding with colon involvement and rectal fistulae with ileocolic or colon involvement. Among statistically significant complications ($p < 0.001$) were: perianal fistulae, internal fistulae and intestinal obstruction with ileocolic pattern; perianal fistulae, toxic megacolon and arthritis with the colon pattern; and intestinal obstruction with the small intestine pattern. Surgery was required for 73% of patients with the ileocolic clinical pattern and for 51% of patients with each of the small intestine and colon patterns. Subsequently, others adopted a similar approach, and Table 1 illustrates the results of this type of study from four other institutions besides our own[3-6].

Indications for surgery

Among these 615 patients, 316 had primary operations performed at the Cleveland Clinic between 1966 and 1969. In addition, in 1972 and 1973 there were 184 patients for whom the primary decision for surgery was made at the Cleveland Clinic, and the operation then performed. Thus, in the 6-year period (1966–1969 and 1972–1973) there were 500 patients who had indications for surgery[7]. The indications for surgery for these patients, in tabular form, are described in Table 2.

Of the 225 patients with the ileocolic pattern, 91% had specific surgical indications as follows: internal fistula and abscess, 44%; intestinal obstruction, 35%; and perianal disease, 12%. Among the 130 patients with the small intestine pattern, two indications made up 87% of the surgical indications: intestinal obstruction, 55% and internal fistula with abscess, 32%. Of the 127 patients with the colon pattern, a greater variety of surgical indications was observed. These included poor response to medical therapy (26%), internal fistula and abscess (23%), toxic megacolon (20%), perianal disease (19%) and intestinal obstruction (12%). For the patients with the anorectal patterns in whom colonic disease developed, indications for surgery were either the perianal disease itself or poor response to therapy.

Comparison was made of the three major patterns, and the statistical significance of each surgical indication was defined. There were highly significant statistical differences in indications for surgery based on anatomical location of Crohn's disease (Table 3).

Table 1 Crohn's disease: initial location of disease (percentages)

Series	Ileocolic	Small intestine	Colon	Other
Cleveland Clinic	41	29	27	3
NCCDS	55	30	14	1
Stockholm	41	41	17	1
Oxford	42	30	26	2
European	49	30	21	0

Table 2   Indications for surgery in Crohn's disease

Ileocolic pattern
    Intestinal obstruction
    Internal fistula and abscess
    Perianal disease, severe

Small-bowel pattern
    Intestinal obstruction
    Internal fistula and abscess

Colonic pattern
    Toxic megacolon
    Internal fistula
    Stricture with obstruction
    Perianal disease, severe
    Poor response to medical therapy and chronic disability, malnutrition

Anorectal pattern
    Severe perianal disease

Other
    Hydronephrosis (ileal)
    Pyoderma (colon), severe
    Arthritis (colon), severe
    Eye manifestations (colon), severe
    Growth retardation (colon)
    Massive haemorrhage (rare)

Recurrence and reoperation

In the 1981 study of recurrences and reoperation for patients with Crohn's disease, it was found that recurrence after surgery in Crohn's disease could be correlated with the original location of disease[8]. In this study 361 patients were followed for a mean of 11.5 years following the first operation for Crohn's disease. Among these patients 40% had ileocolic location of disease, 30% small intestine disease and 30% large intestine disease. There were 123 patients (34%) who had a recurrence requiring operation. The incidence of recurrence was lowest in patients with disease of the large bowel (24%) or small bowel (28.5%); the recurrence rate was highest for patients with ileocolic disease (44%).

These data showed that for the first 8 years there was a 3.9% per year risk of recurrence requiring resection, and after 8 years the risk declined to

Table 3   Statistical differences in indications for surgery in Crohn's disease

	Clinical pattern		
Indications for surgery	*Ileocolic*	*Small intestine*	*Colon*
Perianal disease	+	0	+
Intestinal obstruction	+	+	0
Internal fistula and abscess	+	+	0
Toxic megacolon	0	0	+
Poor response to medical therapy	0	0	+

about 1.4% per year. The cumulative risk was about 42% at 15 years. However, 85% of all recurrences had occurred within the first 8 years following the initial operation, and the risk did not appear to increase as time elapsed. Further analysis of the data revealed that the initial surgical indication of intestinal fistula with abscess, particularly when associated with ileocolic location of disease, was associated with the highest risk of recurrence requiring further operation[9].

Long-term prognosis

As the mean follow-up of the original cohort of patients approached 15 years it became quite apparent that the majority of patients had required an operation (Table 4)[2]. Evaluation was made of quality of life as assessed by 502 patients with a mean 15-year follow-up[2]. Questions directed to the patients related to their ability to function generally in comparison with their peers socially and economically; to the frequency and type of symptoms; to the frequency and type of medication used; and to the need for hospitalization. Quality of life was considered good if the patient had normal or nearly normal function, in comparison to peer group, and had few, if any, symptoms and no regular use of medications; the patient was rated as fair if there was suboptimal overall functioning with symptoms or use of medications, or both, on a sporadic basis; and quality of life was considered poor if there was impaired function with need for hospitalization or regular use of medications, or both (Table 5).

Many patients were found to function on a suboptimal basis. Patients who fared best were those who had undergone one operation and who had no recurrence and those who had not required surgery. There was also a relationship between disease location and prognosis: patients who had the most favourable prognosis, with both fewer complications and better quality of life, were those with localized ileal disease or segmental colonic involvement. Among 50 patients with segmental colonic disease, 33 (66%) described their quality of life as good, whether or not they had undergone an operation. Of the 123 patients with ileal disease location, 57 (46%) described their quality of life as good, regardless of whether or not a resection had been necessary[2].

In the most recent study at the Cleveland Clinic the long-term outcome of Crohn's disease was reviewed in 139 patients who were treated and followed

Table 4 Crohn's disease study from the Cleveland Clinic

Clinical pattern	Original diagnosis – 1966–1969	Follow-up*		Patients with operations	
Ileocolic	252	246	(41.5%)	225	(91.5%)
Small intestine	176	165	(28%)	108	(65.5%)
Colon/anorectal	187	181	(30.5%)	105	(58%)
Total	615	592	(96.3%)	438	(74%)

*Mean duration exceeded 13 years; minimum 7 years (adapted from Farmer RG, Whelan G and Fazio VW. Gastroenterology 1985;88:1818)

Table 5 Quality of life for patients with Crohn's disease

Status	Operated		Non-operated	
Quality of life				
Good	149	(40%)	69	(53%)
Fair	185	(50%)	57	(44%)
Poor	37	(10%)	5	(3%)
Total	371		131	

Good = normal or nearly normal functioning, with comparison to peer group: (1) few if any symptoms and (2) no regular use of medications. Fair = suboptimal overall functioning with symptoms or use of medications, or both, on a sporadic basis. Poor = impaired functioning, with need for hospitalization or regular use of medications, or both

for a minimum of 15 years with a mean of 23 years (Table 6)[10]. At the time of diagnosis, 27%, 28% and 43% of patients had small bowel, large bowel and ileocolic disease, respectively. A total of 122 patients (88%) underwent at least one definitive operation for the disease. As can be noted, the long-term complications include both renal and biliary calculi as well as, of course, the risk of a short bowel syndrome, usually associated with multiple operation (Table 6).

Prognostic indicators

Despite continued efforts to find predictive factors indicating prognostic variability in Crohn's disease, many aspects of the 'natural course' of the disease remain unpredictable, although some generalizations can be made. Using the anatomical classifications as the primary clinical characteristic of Crohn's disease, a temporal relationship can be established, as well as a disease behavioural characteristic. The complications of the disease are usually associated with a clinical event, such as need for operation. Table 7 attempts to illustrate these events on a temporal basis, also correlated with disease behaviour and disease location. Disease which is diffuse has more of a 'systemic' effect than does disease which is localized. In the experience at the Cleveland Clinic[1,2,7-9] the indicators of a poor prognosis include sepsis, malnutrition, megacolon and abscess; the indicators of a good prognosis include localized disease, particularly to the ileum or the colon.

Table 6 Crohn's disease: long-term complications*

Indications	Small bowel disease (n = 38)		Large bowel disease (n = 39)		Ileocolic disease (n = 62)		Total (n = 139)	
Ureteric calculi	8	(21%)	3	(8%)	12	(19%)	23	(17%)
Gallstones	6	(16%)	3	(8%)	10	(16%)	19	(14%)
Short bowel syndrome	4	(11%)	1	(3%)	2	(3%)	7	(5%)
Death	6	(16%)	2	(5%)	2	(3%)	10	(7%)

*Mean follow-up 23 years

Table 7 Crohn's disease complications

Early (less than 2 years)
  Perianal disease
Early to mid course (0–5 years) ('aggressive')
  Fistula/abscess
  Megacolon
  Extraintestinal
Late in course (more than 5 years) ('indolent')
  Obstruction
  Renal and gallstones
  'Chronic illness'
  Cancer

Surgical intervention in Crohn's disease may not be preventable but may be predictable, which may help the physician communicate to the patient a realistic view of prognosis. Certainly the presence of disease itself is not an indication for surgery. Likewise, when surgical resection is indicated, extensive resections are usually not advisable because of recurrence[2,4,5,9]. A recent study by Greenstein et al.[11], indicated that one could correlate disease activity based on 'perforating and non-perforating indications' for operation, and that this could be correlated with aggressive or indolent disease, but appeared to be independent of anatomical distribution. However, in concordance with Cleveland Clinic studies, the indications for second operation were closely dependent on the indication for primary resection, thus emphasizing the value of disease classification. This concept has been expressed recently by Sachar[12], noting that Crohn's disease may follow at least two different patterns: 'aggressive' disease characterized primarily by fistulae and abscesses, early requirement for surgery, and relatively rapid fistulizing-type recurrence; versus 'indolent' disease characterized mostly by fibrotic stenosis and strictures, late requirement for surgery, and relatively slower obstructive type recurrence. However, as has been emphasized[13], prevention of death and significant morbidity remain the primary concern of the clinician dealing with a patient who has Crohn's disease over a long period of time. This has been confirmed in a recent study by Andrews et al.[14], who correlated mortality in Crohn's disease with anatomical location and other factors, the most common causes of death being sepsis, digestive disease, cancer, pulmonary embolism and metabolic disorders; these occurred particularly after emergency surgical treatment.

Comment

Based on our long-term studies at the Cleveland Clinic[1,2], the following observations can be made: the anatomical location of disease (clinical pattern) is a major determinant of clinical course, complications and reasons for operation in patients with Crohn's disease; although long-term mortality is similar among the three clinical patterns, morbidity is greater with ileocolic location of disease, particularly in terms of need for operation. Crohn's disease is associated with specific complications; particularly obstruction with small intestine location, fistula/abscess with ileocolic location and megacolon with colonic location of disease. The most frequent complication overall is perianal disease, which is an early manifestation and is associated more with colonic and ileocolic patterns than with small intestine location of disease. The most favourable long-term prognosis is for patients with segmental colonic or localized ileal disease.

ULCERATIVE COLITIS

Long-term prognosis

The long-term prognosis for patients who have ulcerative colitis has been the subject of a number of studies over the years[15-20], and is dependent on four factors: location (extent) of disease, activity (severity), duration and impact on the patient.

1. *Location of disease.* Ulcerative colitis affects only the colon and does not extend proximally, except for an occasional instance of 'backwash ileitis'. On the other hand, ulcerative colitis may involve only certain segments or the entire colon.
2. *Activity of disease.* Activity may vary from (a) acute and severe or even fulminating to (b) chronic and recurrent to (c) chronic continuous; even inactive disease may have implications for the potential development of colonic carcinoma.
3. *Duration of disease.* This relates to the length of time the various patterns of disease have been present, and their nutritional and other systemic effects on the patient. Furthermore, the duration of disease may influence the effectiveness of therapy, side-effects of therapy and therapeutic response. In addition, duration of disease may be an important factor in determining the need for operation. Finally, duration of disease is an important factor in concern over development of dysplasia and/or colonic carcinoma.
4. *The overall impact of the disease on the patient.* This includes the ability of the patient to function normally in social, economic, and cultural situations. Included here are the 'psychological' factors that are sometimes considered important for patients with ulcerative colitis. Additional factors that can be considered under this heading include the family history, the effect on the patient and family, the general ability of the patient to adapt to the disease, and the overall quality of life experienced by the patient.

Ritchie and co-workers[21] described four questions that patients may ask regarding the prognosis in ulcerative colitis:

> 'Is my condition dangerous?'
> 'Will the inflammation spread?'
> 'Will I need an operation?'
> 'Will I develop cancer?'

Variations on these four questions have been reviewed from a number of centres and economic factors have been included, as well as problems associated with medications, surgery, and nutrition[22]. A Scandinavian study[23] indicated a mortality rate of 1.3% among 322 patients with ulcerative colitis followed for 1 year and noted that, in the short term, the mortality rate was related to the severity of the illness and the need for operation. In another study of mortality[24], the risk was 1.7 times that of the general population, particularly during the first year after diagnosis in the first year after surgery.

Interest in the 'natural history' of ulcerative colitis has focused on changes in the patterns of disease which have occurred recently. This was addressed by Softley *et al.*[25] in a review of 2657 cases registered by the World Organization of Gastroenterology (OMGE). It was observed that the mortality rate from ulcerative colitis is now 4% in 10 years, and similar to that of Crohn's disease and much less than that recorded in early years. Factors relating to this lower mortality include the fact that the frequency of severe attacks is now less than 10%, which likely relates to the disease location. However, two recent surveys from Sweden[26,27] have emphasized that there is still 'an appreciable excess mortality in the first year after diagnosis which relates to presence of severe attacks, total colitis and relatively high age at time of diagnosis'[26]. In the long-term prognosis, liver disease (sclerosing cholangitis) and the development of colon cancer account for the major part of colitis-related deaths. In another Swedish study looking at colectomy rates for 1586 patients with ulcerative colitis seen in Stockholm[27], the major factor affecting colectomy rate was extent of disease at diagnosis. Patients showed a cumulative colectomy rate of 32% at 5 years and 65% at 25 years. In the Cleveland Clinic survey of 1116 cases, factors affecting the prognosis adversely, and thus relating to colectomy[28], included the following: severe attacks of colitis, disease extent at diagnosis, presence of arthritis or arthralgia as a significant symptom, age at diagnosis (older) and presence of severe bleeding.

In the long term, several additional factors are also important. These include (a) the age of onset, and thus the duration of the disease; (b) the need for follow-up; (c) the importance of appropriate and cost-effective surveillance; and (d) the need for attention to psychological and nutritional factors.

The long-term prognosis is good for 90% or more of patients with proctitis or proctosigmoiditis[21,29-34]. These patients exhibit no progression, do not need continuous therapy, and have few, if any, symptoms. In the other 10% the inflammation extends[29-35] and may involve the entire colon, and the prognosis becomes similar to that of patients with total colon disease. This has recently been emphasized by the Cleveland Clinic experience[28] in which patients whose disease began as distal colon inflammation had a much higher progression rate if: (a) symptoms were severe, (b) joint symptoms were present, (c) there was severe bleeding early in the course of disease, and (d) the condition was diagnosed at a relatively young age. An adjusted odds ratio was developed, which also indicated an increased risk of colectomy, comparable to the Swedish study[27]. In a recent study from England[35] the relative frequency of episodes and the duration of the first attack, as well as the development of a recurrence, were also factors indicating progression of disease and a poor overall prognosis. With regard to morbidity, for patients with proctitis or proctosigmoiditis the disease generally resolves completely for about 75% of patients, with approximately 15% having multiple recurrences but without progression[30].

There is less likelihood of extension of disease after a given period of time – approximately 5 years after onset of disease. However, as has been demonstrated in a number of recent studies[27,28,35], while the frequency of distal colon ulcerative colitis, both proctitis and proctosigmoiditis, has appeared to increase in recent years, the long-term prognosis relates directly to the initial extent and severity of disease present.

The long-term prognosis for patients with childhood onset of ulcerative colitis includes features that are related to the age of onset and vulnerability to factors adversely affecting growth and development. Michener et al.[36] reported on 316 patients with childhood-onset ulcerative colitis for whom there was a follow-up of greater than 10 years. Subsequently, Michener et al.[37] have continued to follow up for as long as 30 years with these patients. Colectomy was required in 37%, 12% had only the single episode, 20% had an intermittent course, 52% had a chronic course and were incapacitated, 5.4% died, and 3% developed cancer. Edwards and Truelove[18] also reported that most patients have a relapsing–remitting course with intervals of variable duration in which the patient may have relatively few or no symptoms.

In a review of long-term prognosis for patients with ulcerative colitis, Sales and Kirsner[38] analysed actuarially the cumulative colectomy rates from several centres and from series recorded in the medical literature. They found that the cumulative colectomy rates ranged from 4% to 9% after 1 year of the disease, from 6% to 27% after 5 years, and from 14% to 50% after 10 years of ulcerative colitis. The recent review by Leijonmarck et al.[27], as well as Cleveland Clinic data[28], continues to confirm, generally, these rates. It has been noted that the major risk of colectomy occurs within the first few years of disease[26,27], and that the most important prognostic factors correlating directly with need for surgery and also with mortality are the severity of the initial attack and the extent of the disease. Most of the deaths that occur in ulcerative colitis do so within the first 2 years of illness. Subsequently, survival curves approximately parallel those of the general population. This 'early' mortality is due to severe onset of ulcerative colitis with increased risk of life-threatening complications such as massive haemorrhage, toxic dilatation of the colon, and perforation[24–27].

Another subset of patients with an unfavourable prognosis are those with onset of disease after the age of 50[19,23,39]. Decreased survival results not only from increased mortality during the first attack of colitis, but also from debility from the acute disease and higher surgical mortality related to associated illness.

It has been shown that the initial episode of colitis was often more protracted with a shorter remission in onset recurring after the age of 50, and that the inflammation is often relatively refractory to treatment. However, many patients with late-onset disease have distal colon involvement, which improves the prognosis[39].

Several comparative studies have been performed on patients who have ulcerative colitis and those having Crohn's colitis. Noteworthy is the study by Lennard-Jones and colleagues[40], in which ulcerative colitis was found to be 'an illness with an acute and potentially dangerous onset but which appears to become less severe after survival for one year'. This is in contrast with Crohn's disease, which 'tends to be a more chronic and progressive illness over several years with greater need for surgical treatment'. This study indicated that ulcerative colitis was often acute and that more patients required an operation within the first year of onset of illness than did those who had Crohn's disease. However, if patients were followed for 6 years or longer, the possibility of operation among patients who had Crohn's colitis was 72% compared with 44% for patients who had ulcerative colitis. This study is in very close agreement with our results[38]. In a Danish study of 709 patients having inflammatory bowel disease, a survival rate of about 94% was found in the first year of observation compared with an expected survival rate in the general population of 99.5%, matched for sex and age[41]. After 12 years the survival rate was about 77% for patients with both ulcerative colitis and Crohn's disease, which was about 2 or 3 times less than that in the matched population.

There has been a considerable amount of recent work attempting to explain why patients with ulcerative colitis have relapses[42]. A survey study addressed infections, compliance with therapy, new drug treatment, dietary changes, life stresses, anxiety and depression, and previous relapses. Factors of significance included number of previous relapses (i.e. relapses tended to perpetuate themselves) and occurred most frequently between August and January. However, there was no relationship of respiratory tract symptoms, antibiotic ingestion, analgesic intake and stressful life events. Other recent work has associated the presence of various infections with relapse or exacerbation of ulcerative colitis, including presence of *Clostridium difficile*, bacterial enteric pathogen and enteroviruses. In addition, use of antibiotics and possibly even sulphapyridine may be associated with relapses[43]. Another study attempted to correlate clinical features with histological characteristics[44]; factors of significance were an insidious onset of diarrhoeal symptoms (as contrasted with an acute episode in patients with non-relapsing colitis), and distorted crypt architecture and basal plasmacytosis on biopsies.

Studies have compared the postoperative course of patients having ulcerative colitis and Crohn's colitis (following colectomy) with particular concern over recurrences[45-47]. For patients having ulcerative colitis the main problem was need for ileostomy revision, but this occurred in only a small number of cases; after the first 2 years the risk of having an ileostomy revision was low. In an English study[48] a comparison of the course following colectomy of 73 patients with Crohn's colitis and 442 patients with ulcerative colitis showed a difference in the immediate mortality of Crohn's disease (4%) and ulcerative colitis (10%). The difference was primarily because of the higher proportion of emergency operations in the latter group. The late mortality in both groups was 10%, mainly because of recurrence in Crohn's disease and the sequelae of colonic malignancy in ulcerative colitis. The hospital readmission rate was twice as high for Crohn's disease patients, as was the need for ileostomy reconstruction. Furthermore, Crohn's disease required another operation because of recurrences. Nugent and Haggitt[49] followed patients on a long-term basis and graded the clinical status as excellent or good in 70% of those with Crohn's disease compared with 95% with ulcerative colitis, thus re-emphasizing the long-term favourable prognosis following total colectomy for patients with ulcerative colitis. Fawaz et al.[45] studied a group of patients of similar make-up who had total colectomy, and found that the postoperative recurrence rate for patients with Crohn's disease was 38%, whereas there were no recurrences in those with ulcerative colitis. The only problems encountered among the patients having ulcerative colitis were those related either to sepsis at the time of surgery (often related to the severity of illness or to the emergency circumstances under which the operation was performed) or to repair or revision of ileostomy.

The results of these studies reiterate and emphasize the comments made earlier regarding questions which patients ask about the overall long-term prognosis. The maximum impact of ulcerative colitis on the patient generally appears to occur earlier in the course of disease than in Crohn's colitis, and mortality is related to the severity of the disease at the time of onset, to associated sepsis, to the need for operation, and to postoperative problems.

Quality of life

Edwards and Truelove[18] found that 69% of 101 survivors of ulcerative colitis led an entirely normal life, with another 19% having an essentially normal lifestyle except for frequent outpatient hospital visits. A more recent study from the Cleveland Clinic determined the quality of life in 308 patients with onset of ulcerative colitis in childhood and adolescence[37]. Of these patients, 21% considered their health good (normal or nearly normal functioning in comparison with their peer group; no medications on a regular basis); 72% rated their quality of life as fair (suboptimal functioning in comparison with their peer group; occasional symptoms, occasional use of medications, occasional impairment of function because of illness); and only 7% considered their health to be poor (inability to function satisfactorily, continuous use of medications, and frequent need for hospitalization).

Whether owing to improved therapeutic regimens; better understanding of the disease by physicians, patients, and their families; improved nutritional status; better surgical techniques; or improved preoperative and postoperative care, the prognosis for patients with ulcerative colitis does appear to be improving. Hendricksen and Binder[50] compared the 'social prognosis' for 122 randomly selected patients with ulcerative colitis with a similar group of age- and sex-matched controls. The two groups were found to be similar in many respects, including marital status, sexual problems, leisure activities, physical functioning, and economic earning capacity. They concluded that the majority of patients with ulcerative colitis 'seem to adapt themselves well to their condition and suffer few social or professional disabilities'.

In recent years there has been an attempt to try and quantify various aspects of health-related quality of life in patients with inflammatory bowel disease. Drossman *et al.*[51] used a standardized measure, the Sickness Impact Profile, as well as their own questionnaire relating specifically to worries of patients with inflammatory bowel disease. Their data indicated that patients do indeed experience 'moderate functional impairment, more in the social and psychological than in the physical dimensions', that these problems are greater in patients with Crohn's disease than ulcerative colitis, that patients have their greatest concerns about the need for operation, degree of energy and body image issues. In an attempt to amplify and find a means of quantification of quality of life in patients with inflammatory bowel disease, we[52] compared our own instrument with that of the Sickness Impact Profile, and found the one we had developed to be much easier to use, requiring much less time, and that it could be administered by non-professionals verbally. We assessed four basic categories of activity: functional and economic; social and recreational; affect, attitudes and life in general; and medical symptoms. Statistical analyses were carried out, and it was found that patients with ulcerative colitis had better quality of life than those with Crohn's disease, and that patients without surgery had better quality of life than those with surgery. The implication of the latter finding is often that patients who have experienced an improved quality of life after time, fail to comply with, for example, surveillance systems for cancer detection. In general, however, results of our study were encouraging regarding the overall long-term prognosis for patients with ulcerative colitis.

In addition to these more general assessments of quality of life in patients with long-standing ulcerative colitis, recent emphasis has likewise been on relatively specific aspects of the disease. Of particular interest was a survey for patients who had liver transplantation for sclerosing cholangitis[53]. The data demonstrated that the symptoms of ulcerative colitis improved and that the quality of life of the patients who had undergone liver transplantation for sclerosing cholangitis was substantially improved by the procedure, as well as the immunosuppression with cyclosporin and prednisone.

Two other recent studies have looked at the quality of life of patients before and after surgery, particularly in light of the recent emphasis on surgery which avoids a permanent ileostomy, both the Koch pouch and the ileal pouch–anal anastomosis. The first of these[54] showed no significant differences regarding the type of operation which had been performed, but that there was significant improvement in quality of life for patients who had undergone operation. The other study[55] assessed various categories of social life, recreation, work and family, and found results similar among the various groups, except that the presence of a stoma with faecal incontinence impaired the quality of life after proctocolectomy. Their study emphasized that ileal pouch–anal anastomosis, which avoids both stoma and incontinence, offers the best quality of life among the three operations available to patients.

Emphasis on the long-term prognosis for patients with ulcerative colitis must take into account the extent and severity of disease, as noted, the frequency of relapses, the need for medications and the side-effects which may result, the need for proctocolectomy or not, the potential risk of cancer, and the need for long-term therapy. Attempts to quantify the quality of life have improved the ability to perform assessments of the prognosis which are more objective than was possible previously, and this illustrates the value of continued long-term clinical research and surveillance of such patients.

References

1. Farmer RG, Hawk WA, Turnbull RB. Clinical patterns in Crohn's disease. A statistical study of 615 cases. Gastroenterology. 1975;70:369–70.
2. Farmer RG, Whelan G, Fazio VW. Long term follow up of patients with Crohn's disease: relationship between the clinical pattern and prognosis. Gastroenterology. 1985;88:1818–25.
3. Mekhijian HS et al. Clinical features and natural history of Crohn's disease. Gastroenterology. 1979;77:898–906.
4. Hellers G. Crohn's disease in Stockholm County, 1955–1974. A study of epidemiology, results of surgical treatment and long term prognosis. Acta Chir Scand. (S) 1979;490:1–84.
5. Truelove SC, Pena AS. Course and prognosis of Crohn's disease. Gut. 1976;17:192–201.
6. Steinhardt HJ, Loeschke K, Kasper H et al. European cooperative Crohn's disease study (ECCDS): clinical features and natural history. Digestion. 1985;31:97–108.
7. Farmer RG, Hawk WA, Turnbull RB. Indications for surgery in Crohn's disease. An analysis of 500 cases. Gastroenterology. 1976;71:245–50.
8. Lock MR, Farmer RG, Fazio VW et al. Recurrence and reoperation for Crohn's disease: the role of disease location in prognosis. N Engl J Med. 1981;304:1585–8.
9. Whelan G, Farmer RG, Fazio VW, Goormastic M. Recurrence after surgery in Crohn's disease – relationship to location of disease (clinical pattern) and surgical indication. Gastroenterology. 1985;88:1826–33.
10. Harper PH, Fazio VW, Lavery IC et al. The long term outcome in Crohn's disease. Dis Colon Rectum. 1987;30:174–9.
11. Greenstein AJ, Lachman P, Sachar DB et al. Perforating and non-perforating indications for repeated operations in Crohn's disease: evidence for two clinical forms. Gut. 1988;29:588–92.
12. Sachar DB. The problem of postoperative recurrence of Crohn's disease. Med Clin N Am. 1990;74:183–8.
13. Sachar DB. Crohn's disease in Cleveland: a matter of life and death. Gastroenterology. 1985;88:1996–7.
14. Andrews HA, Lewis P, Allan RN. Mortality in Crohn's disease – a clinical analysis. Q J Med. 1989;71:399–405.
15. Bargen JA, Jackman RJ, Kerr JG. Studies on the life histories of patients with chronic ulcerative colitis (thrombo-ulcerative colitis) with some suggestions for treatment. Ann Intern Med. 1938;12:339.
16. Bockus HL, Roth JLA, Buckman E et al. Life history of non-specific ulcerative colitis: Relation of prognosis of anatomical and clinical varieties. Gastroenterologia. 1956;86:549.
17. Banks BM, Korelitz BI, Zetzel L. The course of nonspecific ulcerative colitis. Review of twenty years' experience and late results. Gastroenterology. 1957;32:983.
18. Edwards FC, Truelove SC. The course and prognosis of ulcerative colitis. Part II. Long-term prognosis. Gut. 1963;4:309.
19. Watts JMcK, deDombal FT, Watkinson G et al. Long-term prognosis of ulcerative colitis. Br Med J. 1966;1:1447.
20. Jalan KN, Prescott RJ, Sircus W et al. An experience of ulcerative colitis. III. Long-term outcome. Gastroenterology. 1970;59:598.
21. Ritchie JK, Powell-Tuck J, Lennard-Jones JE. Clinical outcome of the first ten years of ulcerative colitis and proctitis. Lancet. 1978;1:1140–3.
22. Prior P, Gyde P, Allan RN. Mortality in ulcerative colitis: Methods of analysis. Gastroenterology. 1982;83:524–5.
23. Bonnevie O, Binder V, Anthonisen P, Riis P. The prognosis of ulcerative colitis. Scand J Gastroenterol. 1974;9:81–91.
24. Gyde S, Prior P, Dow JM. Mortality in ulcerative colitis. Gastroenterology. 1982;83:36–43.

25. Softley A, Clamp SE, Watkinson G, Bouchier IA, Myren J *et al*. The natural history of inflammatory bowel disease: has there been a change in the last 20 years? Scand J Gastroenterol. (Suppl.) 1988;144:20–3.
26. Brostrom O. Prognosis in ulcerative colitis. Med Clin N Am. 1990;74:201–18.
27. Leijonmarck CE, Persson PG, Hellers G. Factors affecting colectomy rate in ulcerative colitis: an epidemiologic study. Gut. 1990;31:329–33.
28. Farmer RG, Easley KA, Rankin GB. Clinical patterns in ulcerative colitis: disease location, progression and prognosis. Gastroenterology. 1992 (in press).
29. Farmer RG, Brown CH. Ulcerative proctitis: course and prognosis. Gastroenterology. 1966;51:219–23.
30. Farmer RG. Long-term prognosis for patients with ulcerative proctosigmoiditis (ulcerative colitis confined to the rectum and sigmoid colon). J Clin Gastroenterol. 1979;1:47–50.
31. Lennard-Jones JE, Cooper GW, Newell AC *et al*. Observations on idiopathic proctitis. Gut. 1962;3:201–6.
32. Nugent FW, Veidenheimer MC, Zuberi S *et al*. Clinical course of ulcerative proctosigmoiditis. Am J Dig Dis. 1970;15:321–6.
33. Powell-Tuck J, Ritchie JK, Lennard-Jones JE. Prognosis of idiopathic proctitis. Scand J Gastroenterol. 1977;12:727–32.
34. Farmer RG. Evolution of the concept of proctosigmoiditis: clinical observation. Med Clin N Am. 1990;74:91–102.
35. Juby LD, Long DE, Dixon MF *et al*. Prognostic indicators and clinical course in proctosigmoiditis. Colorectal Dis. 1990;5:177–80.
36. Michener WM, Farmer RG, Mortimer EA. Long-term prognosis of ulcerative colitis with onset in childhood or adolescence. J Clin Gastroleterol. 1979;1:301–5.
37. Michener WM, Caulfield M, Wyllie R *et al*. Management of inflammatory bowel disease: 30 years of observation. Cleveland Clin J Med. 1990;57:685–91.
38. Sales DJ, Kirsner JB. The prognosis of inflammatory bowel disease. Arch Intern Med. 1983;143:585–90.
39. Zimmerman J, Gavish D, Rachmielwitz D. Early and late onset ulcerative colitis: distinct clinical features. J Clin Gastroenterol. 1985;7:492–8.
40. Lennard-Jones JE, Ritchie JK, Zohrab WJ. Proctocolitis and Crohn's disease of the colon. A comparison of the clinical course. Gut. 1976;17:477–82.
41. Storgaard L, Bischorr N, Hendriksen C *et al*. Survival rate in Crohn's disease and ulcerative colitis. Scand J Gastroenterol. 1979;14:225–30.
42. Riley SA, Mani V, Goodman MJ, Lucas S. Why do patients with ulcerative colitis relapse? Gut. 1990;31:179–83.
43. Hermens DJ, Miner PB Jr. Exacerbation of ulcerative colitis. Gastroenterology. 1991;101:254–62.
44. Schumacher G, Sandstedt B, Mollby R *et al*. Clinical and histologic features differentiating non-relapsing colitis from first attacks of inflammatory bowel disease. Scand J Gastroenterol. 1991;26:151–61.
45. Fawaz KA, Glotzer DJ, Goldman M *et al*. Ulcerative colitis and Crohn's disease of the colon – a comparison of the long-term post-operative courses. Gastroenterology. 1976;71:372–8.
46. Vender RJ, Rickert RR, Spiro HM. The outlook after total colectomy in patients with Crohn's colitis and ulcerative colitis. J Clin Gastroenterol. 1979;1:209–17.
47. Watts JM, Hughes ESR. Ulcerative colitis and Crohn's disease: Results after colectomy and ileorectal anastomosis. Br J Surg. 1977;64:77–83.
48. Steinberg DM, Allan RN, Brooke BN *et al*. Sequelae of colectomy and ileostomy: comparison between Crohn's colitis and ulcerative colitis. Gastroenterology. 1973;68:33–9.
49. Nugent FW, Haggitt RC. Long-term follow up including cancer surveillance for patients with ulcerative colitis. Clin Gastroenterol. 1980;9:459–68.
50. Hendricksen C, Binder V. Social prognosis in patients with ulcerative colitis. Br Med J. 1980;2:581–7.
51. Drossman DA, Patrick DL, Mitchell CM *et al*. Health-related quality of life in inflammatory bowel disease. Dig Dis Sci. 1989;34:1379–86.
52. Farmer RG, Easley KA, Farmer JM. Assessing quality of life for patients with inflammatory bowel disease. Cleveland Clin J Med. 1991;58:7–15.

53. Gavaler JS, Delemos B, Belle SH *et al.* Ulcerative colitis disease activity as subjectively assessed by patient-completed questionnaires following orthotopic transplantation for sclerosing cholangitis. Dig Dis Sci. 1991;36:321–8.
54. McLeod RS, Churchill DN, Lock AM *et al.* Quality of life of patients with ulcerative colitis preoperatively and postoperatively. Gastroenterology. 1991;101:1307–13.
55. Kohler LW, Pemberton JH, Zinsmeister AR *et al.* Quality of life after proctocolectomy: a comparison of Brooke ileostomy Kock pouch, and ileal pouch–anal anastomosis. Gastroenterology. 1991;101:679–84.

Section IX
Treatment strategies – reasons and belief

41

New controlled trials for inflammatory bowel diseases: salicylates and others

W. E. FLEIG

Although standard therapy is available for most patients suffering from inflammatory bowel disease, a substantial proportion of patients does not respond well to established modes of treatment. Thus, new controlled trials have been performed using new salicylates and other new therapeutic principles for the following clinical situations:

1. induction of remission in the uncomplicated acute phase of the disease,
2. induction of remission and weaning off steroids in chronic active patients,
3. prevention of recurrence once remission has been achieved,
4. prevention of postoperative recurrence.

The drugs under investigation in such trials are listed in Table 1.

Table 1 'New' drugs under investigation for the treatment of Crohn's disease and ulcerative colitis

Mesalazine and other salicylates
'Splanchnic' steroids: budesonide, tixocortol pivalate, beclomethasone dipropionate
Antibiotics: metronidazole, antimycobacterial agents
Drugs interfering with leukotriene synthesis and action: ω-3 fatty acids, 5-lipoxygenase inhibitors, receptor antagonists
Platelet factor antagonists (e.g triazolodiazepine)
Immunosuppressants: cyclosporin A, methotrexate

MESALAZINE

Mesalazine for Crohn's disease

Mesalazine has been, and still is, investigated for both inflammatory bowel diseases, Crohn's disease and ulcerative colitis. In active Crohn's disease, 2 g mesalazine per day have been shown to be significantly inferior to the standard treatment scheme of 6-methylprednisolone with a starting dose of 48 mg daily as used in the European Cooperative Crohn's Disease Study I[1]. Only 26% of patients were judged as treatment failures with the steroid compared to 79% of those treated with mesalazine. In a large dose-finding trial, Hanauer and co-workers confirmed these results[2]. The outcome of patients treated with 1 g mesalazine per day was identical to, and of those treated with 2 g daily not significantly different from, the untreated control group. It was only in a group of patients treated with 4 g daily that the initial CDAI decreased significantly by 78 points, and 45% of the patients reached clinical remission (compared to 11% of controls and 26% of those receiving 2 g/day). However, these numbers are still far from the efficacy of a standard acute-phase steroid regime as demonstrated in the American[3] and European[4] Crohn's disease studies and the comparative trial of Jenss et al.[1]. Thus, any dose of mesalazine monotherapy for acute phases of Crohn's disease can only be considered in patients refusing to take steroids.

A more promising indication for mesalazine in Crohn's disease could be the prevention of recurrence both after induction of remission by medical management and after resective surgery. The first trial investigating the effect of mesalazine for maintenance of remission was a multinational study published by an International mesalazine study group in 1990[5]. Patients were eligible when disease was clinically inactive for at least 1 month prior to entry (for a mean of 12 months). Recurrence rate was reduced by 1.5 g mesalazine daily from 36% in controls to 24% ($p = 0.04$) almost exclusively by reducing the relapse rate in patients with ileal or ileocolonic disease. Surprisingly, this effect was observed in only three out of the eight participating countries, and the results of this poorly documented report were criticized for several other statistical reasons. Very recently, Prantera et al.[6] reported on 125 patients with inactive Crohn's disease treated for 1 year with either 2.4 g mesalazine or placebo. Relapse rates in the 5-ASA group were significantly reduced from 22% to 12% at 3 months, from 41% to 28% at 6 months and from 55% to 34% at 1 year. The risk of replase was especially reduced in patients with ileal disease, previous resection and prolonged pre-study remission. To date, two other trials have been published in abstract form. Brignola and co-workers reported on 44 patients who were followed for 4 months. Mesalazine patients did no better than controls[7]; however, a tendency in favour of mesalazine was observed in a small subgroup of patients with ileal disease. Furthermore, 4 months of follow-up is not a sufficient observation period to draw any substantial conclusions. Gendre et al.[8] followed 161 patients for 2 years after randomization to receive either placebo or 2 g mesalazine daily. Although the overall number of clinical replases was identical, the recurrence rate was significantly lower in those treated with mesalazine compared to placebo patients who entered the trial less than 3 months after having reached remission. This contrasts the findings of Prantera *et al.*[6], who found reduced relapse rates only in patients with a pre-study remission of more than 9 months.

Studies in postoperative patients have also been published in abstract form. Florent *et al.*[9] randomized a total of 106 patients to receive either 3 g mesalazine or placebo within 15 days after a 'curative' resection of ileal and/or colonic Crohn's disease, and followed them for 12 weeks to detect endoscopic relapse. Slightly more patients had endoscopic relapse after 12 weeks in the placebo group (63%) compared to the mesalazine group (50%), but this difference did not achieve statistic significance. Caprilli and co-workers[10] reported on 70 patients randomized into a placebo or a 2.4 g mesalazine daily group with treatment started 2 weeks after a first resection of diseased ileum or ileocolon. Relapse was defined endoscopically. Statistically significant advantages were observed for mesalazine patients after both 6 and 12 months of follow-up. Data on clinical relapse are lacking. Further trials are clearly needed to clarify this issue.

Mesalazine and other salicylates in ulcerative colitis

Several trials in mild to moderately active left-sided ulcerative colitis indicate that mesalazine, olsalazine and benzalazine are of similar efficacy to equivalent doses of sulphasalazine, but the new salicylates are better tolerated. 5-ASA enemas are effective in distal colitis in doses as low as 1 g daily. Similarly, the equipotency of mesalazine, olsalazine and sulphasalazine for maintenance of remission has been established by several comparative trials; 1 g of mesalazine daily is the appropriate dose (for summary, see ref. 11).

TOPICAL STEROIDS

The long-term use of corticosteroids is associated with chronic systemic side-effects. Thus, much hope has been placed on newly developed corticosteroids, which undergo extensive first-pass metabolism in erythrocytes and the liver resulting in metabolites of minor or no biological activity. Therefore, pharmacological activity is restricted to the area where the drug is administered. Systemic adverse effects are not a problem, and cortisol levels are only partly suppressed, with no effect on the responsiveness of the hypothalamic–pituitary–adrenal system.

Beclomethasone and budesonide retention enemas are both effective in active distal ulcerative colitis[12-14] and budesonide is significantly better than prednisolone without inducing significant suppression of the hypothalamic–pituitary–adrenal axis[12]. Tixocortol pivalate is a non-glucocorticoid, non-mineralocorticoid cortisol derivate with a selectively anti-inflammatory activity when administered topically. Due to extensive metabolism in erythrocytes and the liver it has no systemic effects. Its topical anti-inflammatory effect in active left-sided ulcerative colitis is similar to that of hydrocortisone enemas[15]. Controlled trials of oral or topical budesonide are at present under way for various indications. Since budesonide can be encapsulated in Eudragit for slow release in the distal ileum and colon, it might even be a candidate for the treatment of active Crohn's or ulcerative colitis.

METRONIDAZOLE

The antibiotic agent metronidazole has previously been shown to be effective in suphasalazine-resistant cases of Crohn's disease[16]. Recently, Sutherland and co-workers[17] compared two doses of metronidazole (10 and 20 mg/kg per day) with placebo in a total of 105 patients with active Crohn's disease with a CDAI betwen 180 and 450. After 16 weeks of treatment, both doses of metronidazole were significantly better than placebo. However, a drop-out rate of 47% raises may questions about the validity of the results. Rutgeerts et al.[18] treated 51 operated patients with 20 mg/kg per day of metronidazole or placebo starting 1 week after an ileocaecal resection. While overall endoscopic recurrence within 3 months was not significantly altered by metronidazole compared to placebo (52% endoscopic recurrence versus 75% in placebo patients; $p = 0.09$), the recurrence of severe endoscopic lesions at the ileocolonic anastomosis, which are predictive of subsequent clinical relapse, was significantly reduced (13% versus 43% in placebo patients, $p < 0.02$). Whether or not this result justifies a 3-month postoperative course of metronidazole with a significant risk of severe side-effects remains to be clarified. If mesalazine can be demonstrated to have a similar effect, 5-ASA would probably be the better choice.

DRUGS INTERFERING WITH LEUKOTRIENE SYNTHESIS AND ACTION

Leukotriene synthesis is believed to play an important role in the pathogenesis of inflammation in the bowel wall. Inhibition of the key enzyme 5-lipoxygenase by specific inhibitors such as zileuton would reduce the amount of inflammatory products of the 5-lipoxygenase pathway, especially leukotriene B4. A similar effect results from the administration of large doses of ω-3 fatty acids which compete with the natural substrate of 5-lipoxygenase, arachidonic acid. Furthermore, ω-3 fatty acids have been shown to suppress the synthesis of other inflammatory mediators such as interleukin-1 and tumour necrosis factor in mononuclear cells[19]. While ω-3 fatty acids appear to have some effect in patients with ulcerative colitis[20], they offer no advantage over placebo for the maintenance of remission in patients with Crohn's disease[21].

Zileuton 800 mg b.i.d. inhibits the activity of lipoxygenase by about 80%. In a recent clinical trial in 71 patients with active ulcerative colitis[22], however, the drug was slightly better than placebo with regard to bleeding, stool consistency, symptom score and histology only in patients who were not on sulphasalazine. In those patients who had been on maintenance sulphasalazine and continued to take this dose of SASP during the trial, zileuton offered no advantage over placebo.

IMMUNOSUPPRESSANTS: CYCLOSPORIN A AND METHOTREXATE

About two-thirds of patients with Crohn's disease and ulcerative colitis appeared to respond to cyclosporin A in a series of uncontrolled trials with small numbers of patients. To date, only one countrolled trial of cyclosporin A has been published[23]. Some type of 'response' to the treatment was observed in 59% of patients with chronically active Crohn's disease receiving cyclosporin A in addition to their previous medication of steroids. In contrast, a suprisingly high proportion of 32% of these patients with chronically active Crohn's improved on placebo. Significant improvement was recorded in 31% of the patients receiving cyclosporin A compared to 12% on placebo. Recurrences after stopping cyclosporin were common. The trial was criticized for the definitions of 'response' and 'improvement', because the results could not be validated by harder criteria such as reduction in the CDAI. The results of a recently completed, large randomized European multicentre trial of cyclosporin A in patients with chronically active steroid-resistant and steroid-dependent Crohn's disease will be available in the near future. Results of ongoing controlled trials of methotrexate have only been reported in abstract form[24]. In a small number of prednisone-dependent patients, those treated with methotrexate had less disease flares (46% versus 80% on placebo) than controls, but this is counterbalanced by the occurrence of side-effects necessitating cessation of therapy in 23% of methotrexate-treated patients. Further studies are required to assess adequately the eventual role of this cytotoxic immunosuppressant in Crohn's disease.

CONCLUSIONS

Although fascinating drugs interfering with specific steps or substances involved in the pathogenesis of inflammation in IBD, such as platelet activating factor or 5-lipoxygenase, have been developed, their clinical effect has been disappointing to date. Obviously, drugs with multiple sites of action are more potent; thus mesalazine and other new salicylates, as well as the topical steroids, represent the most promising developments at present. While treatment with mesalazine alone, in whatever dose, is not sufficiently effective in active Crohn's disease, there is evidence that mesalazine at a minimum daily dose of 2.4 g may prevent or delay clinical relapse in subgroups of patients with inactive disease. Whether or not cyclosporin A and methotrexate, as well as antibiotics, will be of value as second-line drugs remains to be evaluated.

References

1. Jenss H, Hartmann F, Schölmerich J. German 5-ASA Study Group. 5-Aminosalicylic acid versus methylprednisolone in the treatment of active Crohn's disease. Gastroenterology. 1989;96:A239 (abstract).

2. Hanauer SB, Belker ME, Gitnick G. *et al.* Multi-center, placebo-controlled, dose-ranging study of oral pentasa (controlled-release mesalamine) for active Crohn's disease: preliminary results. Gastroenterology. 1990;98:A173 (abstract).
3. Summers RW, Switz DM, Sessions JT *et al.* National Cooperative Crohn's Disease Study: results of drug treatment. Gastroenterology. 1979;77:848–69.
4. Malchow H, Ewe K, Brandes JW *et al.* European Cooperative Crohn's Disease Study (ECCDS): results of drug treatment. Gastroenterology. 1984;86:249–66.
5. International Mesalazine Study Group. Coated oral 5-aminosalicylic acid versus placebo in maintaining remission in active Crohn's disease. Aliment Pharmacol Ther. 1990;4:55–64.
6. Prantera C, Pallone F, Brunetti G *et al.* Oral 5-aminosalicylic acid (Asacol) in the maintenance treatment of Crohn's disease. Gastroenterology. 1992;103:363–8.
7. Brignola C, Iannone P, Pasquali S *et al.* Placebo-controlled trial of oral 5-ASA in relapse prevention of Crohn's disease. Dig Dis Sci. 1992;37:29–32.
8. Gendre JP, Mary JY, Florent C *et al.* Does Pentasa prevent relapses in quiescent Crohn's disease? A multicenter placebo-controlled trial (181 patients). Gastroenterology. 1990;98:A171 (abstract).
9. Florent Ch, Cortot A, Quandale P *et al.* Placebo-controlled trial of claversal (C) in the prevention of early endoscopic relapse after 'curative' resection for Crohn's disease (CD). Gastroenterology. 1992;102:A623 (abstract).
10. Caprilli R, Andreoli A, Capurso L *et al.* 5-ASA in the prevention of Crohn's disease postoperative recurrence. An interim report of the Italian Study Group of the Colon. Gastroenterology. 1992;102:A601 (abstract).
11. Peppercorn MA. Advances in drug therapy for inflammatory bowel disease. Ann Intern Med. 1990;112:50–60.
12. Kumana CR, Seaton T, Meghi M, Castelli M, Benson R, Sivakumaran T. Beclomethasone dipropionate enemas for treating inflammatory bowel disease without producing Cushing's syndrome or hypothalamic pituitary adrenal suppression. Lancet. 1982;1:579–83.
13. Van der Heide H, Mulder CJ, Witink EH. Comparison of enema containing beclomethasone dipropionate or prednisone-21-phosphate in the treatment of distal ulcerative colitis [Abstract]. Gastroenterology. 1987;92:1679.
14. Danielsson A, Hellers G, Lyrenas E *et al.* A controlled randomized trial of budesonide versus prednisolone retention enemas in active distal ulcerative colitis. Scand J Gastroenterol. 1987;22:987–92.
15. Hanauer SB, Kirsner JB, Barrett WE. The treatment of left-sided ulcerative colitis with tixocortol pivalate (TP). Gastroenterology. 1986;90:1449 (abstract).
16. Ursing B, Alm T, Bárány F *et al.* A comparative study of metronidazole and sulfasalazine for active Crohn's disease: the cooperative Crohn's disease study in Sweden. II. Result. Gastroenterology. 1982;83:550–62.
17. Sutherland L, Singleton J, Sessions J *et al.* Double blind, placebo controlled trial of metronidazole in Crohn's disease. Gut. 1991;32:1071–75.
18. Rutgeerts P, Peeters M, Hiele M *et al.* A placebo controlled trial of metronidazole for recurrence prevention of Crohn's disease after resection of the terminal ileum. Gastroenterology. 1992;102:A688 (abstract).
19. Endres S, Ghorbani R, Kelley VE *et al.* The effect of dietary supplementation with n-3 polyunsaturated fatty acids on the synthesis of interleukin 1 and tumor necrosis factor by mononuclear cells. N Engl J Med. 1989;320:265–71.
20. Stenson WF, Cort D, Rodgers J *et al.* Dietary supplementation with fish oil in ulcerative colitis. Ann Intern Med. 1992;116:609–14.
21. Lorenz-Meyer H, Purrmann J, Scheurlen C *et al.* Crohnstudie V: Ergebnisse der Studie zur Erhaltung der Remission bei M. Crohn mit Ω-3-FS bzw. einer kohlenhydratarmen Kost. Z Gastroenterol. 1992;30:654 (abstract).
22. Stenson WF, Lauritsen K, Laursen LS *et al.* A clinical trial of Zileuton, a specific inhibitor of 5-lipoxygenase, in ulcerative colitis. Gastroenterology. 1991;100:A253 (abstract).
23. Brynskov J, Freund L, Rasmussen SN *et al.* A placebo-controlled, double-blind, randomized trial of cyclosporine therapy in active Crohn's disease. N Engl J Med. 1989;321:845–50.
24. Anora S, Katkov WN, Cooley J *et al.* A double-blind, randomized, placebo-controlled trial of methotrexate in Crohn's disease. Gastroenterology. 1992;102:A591 (abstract).

42

Use of concomitant drugs – NSAIDs and others

H. SANDBERG-GERTZÉN

This is a summary of reports relating to the influence of drugs on the course and contraction of inflammatory bowel disease (IBD), including reports of drugs causing gut inflammation or gastrointestinal symptoms mimicking IBD.

NSAIDs

NSAIDs often cause dyspeptic symptoms. Although gastric ulcers are frequently found, many patients have normal upper endoscopy. Bjarnason et al. have focused on the adverse effects on the small intestine and found evidence of small intestinal inflammation in as much as 70% of patients on long-term NSAID-medication[1]. Most of these patients remain free of symptoms, but ulcerations and/or strictures of the small intestine have been described. In infants given NSAIDs enterally for closure of ductus Botalli, single or multiple ulcerations of the terminal ileum with haemorrhagic, necrotizing mucosal lesions have been reported[2]. Despite the description of small intestinal damage, reports of colitis or proctitis caused by NSAIDs are mainly anecdotal. One very interesting exception is the prospective study by Tanner and Raghunath[3]. For 18 months they consecutively studied all new patients presenting with bloody or non-bloody diarrhoea in whom there was microscopic evidence of mucosal inflammation. The macroscopic mucosal appearance was either normal or inflamed. The investigation included stool cultures as well as a detailed drug history. In four out of 43 patients there was good evidence that the symptoms were induced by NSAIDs. All resolved after drug withdrawal, although three of them were treated actively with drugs effective for IBD. Two of the four patients were later challenged, with confirming results.

The flaring of a pre-existing colitis has been described after intake of most of the NSAIDs on the market; the relapse tends to occur within a few days of medication. Reports on single patients as well as smaller series exist[4-6]. In two studies the influence of medication during the last 4 weeks preceding clinical attendance was studied. Rampton *et al.*[7] reported that patients who had taken analgesic compounds inclusive of paracetamol significantly more often suffered a relapse. Foster *et al.*[8] found that patients in relapse were more likely to have consumed any analgesic preparation the previous month than were patients in remission, but in this study the difference was not statistically significant. When the use of NSAIDs and paracetamol was analysed separately there was once more a trend but no statistical difference between patients in remission or relapse. Paracetamol is implicated in reports of IBD exacerbation. Further, drugs containing 5-aminosalicylic acid (5-ASA) including sulphasalazine may induce a relapse[9]. This is of special importance as there is a risk of misinterpretation as a non-responding attack of the disease.

The mechanism by which NSAIDs may be noxious to the gut mucosa remains unclear. NSAIDs are potent cyclooxygenase inhibitors, and the ulcerogenic properties of NSAIDs correlate well with their ability to inhibit gastric prostaglandin (PG) production. Whether this is relevant regarding the gut is not known. PGs are supposed to exert a protective effect on the mucosa, and the inhibition of PG synthesis would thus abolish this cytoprotection and compromise intestinal integrity, increase intestinal permeability and allow transmucosal migration of luminal constituents. Despite the theoretical positive effects of PGs, a clinical trial of a synthetic PG analogue for maintenance treatment of ulcerative colitis (UC) failed[10]. Paracetamol is not an inhibitor of gastrointestinal mucosal PG synthesis, giving evidence that if PGs are implicated as a pathogenetic mechanism, they cannot be the only mechanism involved.

During NSAID medication there is a possibility of 'shunting' the arachidonic acid cascade via the 5-lipoxygenase pathway, thus increasing leukotriene production. Leukotrienes appear to be important in the amplification of inflammatory responses, and they are thought to play an important role in IBD. Leukotriene synthesis is elevated in IBD. However, a study of the lipoxygenase inhibitor zileuton in the treatment of UC gave no overwhelming results[11]. In a rat model, NSAID inhibition of cyclooxygenase resulted in a suppression of colonic PGE_2 synthesis and exacerbation of experimental colitis, but this was not accompanied by any significant changes of the leukotriene B_4 synthesis[12]. The problem thus remains as to what is the cause of the disease and what is mere epiphenomenon of the inflammation.

A special entity seems to be the hypersensitivity reactions described for both NSAIDs and 5-ASA-containing drugs[13,14]. Blood and tissue eosinophilia, rash, abnormal liver function tests and eosinophilic colitis have been described, with symptoms resolving rapidly after drug withdrawal.

What should be the practical implications? It is unlikely that the ingestion of NSAIDs is a frequent cause of relapse in IBD, still they should be prescribed with some caution. There is no indication that NSAIDs cause chronic remitting disease. However, a close drug history is always warranted and drug withdrawal should be tried in cases of relevance before a definite diagnosis of IBD is given.

ORAL CONTRACEPTIVES

The development of Crohn's disease (CD), especially of colonic localization, and UC has been associated with the intake of oral contraceptives. The studies reported yield conflicting results[15-18] and have been confounded by the possible simultaneous effects of smoking habits, as women who use the pill tend to be smokers. Smoking is significantly associated with IBD, UC associated with less and CD with an excess of smoking[19-21]. Vascular disease is discussed as one possible cause of Crohn's disease[22], and an association with the pill and with smoking fits well with the theory of an ischaemic element. There are reports of mesenteric vascular ischaemia caused by oral contraceptives inducing gastrointestinal lesions similar to IBD[23-26]. However, if there is an increased risk of contracting IBD due to the pill, the association is probably small. There are no reports of activation of pre-existing disease due to the pill. At the present stage there is not enough substance in this to advise patients to avoid oral contraceptives if they strongly want to use them.

ANTIBIOTICS

Antibiotics may cause pseudomembranous colitis associated with the finding of *Clostridium difficile* and/or its toxin, and an association between *Clostridium difficile* and the exacerbation of UC has been discussed with no convincing results[27-31]. Another form of antibiotic-associated colitis is the acute segmental haemorrhagic colitis reported after amoxicillin or penicillin[32-34]. The risk of these rare complications of antibiotic treatment does not seem to be greater in patients with pre-existing colitis.

COLITIS ASSOCIATED WITH OTHER DRUGS

The colonic mucosa has a limited number of reaction patterns to a variety of noxes. Therefore a number of further drugs and toxins should be considered in the differential diagnosis of IBD: gold salts, parenteral as well as oral preparations, the podophyllotoxin-derived antirheumatic drug prorecid, penicillamine, chemotherapeutic agents, ergot, flucytosine, cimetidine, methyldopa, alcohol and different enema preparations including water-soluble contrast media[35]. All may induce symptoms and findings that mimic those of IBD. These conditions generally resolve on drug withdrawal without further measures and do not induce chronic remitting disease.

CONCLUSION

NSAIDs have the potential of causing a flare of IBD and should be prescribed with caution. There is no evidence that NSAIDs induce remitting IBD. Oral contraceptives may be implicated as a risk factor for the development of IBD. A number of further drugs and toxins may provoke signs and symptoms mimicking IBD that will disappear on discontinuation of medication. Therefore a close history of drug intake is of great importance.

References

1. Bjarnason I, MacPherson A. The changing gastrointestinal side effect profile of non-steroidal anti-inflammatory drugs. Scand J Gastroenterol. 1989;24(suppl 163):56–64.
2. Nagaraj HS, Sandhu AS, Cook LN, Buchino JJ, Groff DB. Gastrointestinal perforation following indomethacin therapy in very low birth weight infants. J Pediatr Surg. 1981;16(6):1003–7.
3. Tanner AR, Raghunath AS. Colonic inflammation and non-steroidal anti-inflammatory drug administration. Digestion. 1988;41:116–20.
4. Rampton DS, Sladen GE. Relapse of ulcerative proctocolitis during treatment with non-steroidal anti-inflammatory drugs. Postgrad Med J. 1981;57:297–9.
5. Schwartz HA. Lower gastrointestinal side effects of non-steroidal anti-inflammatory drugs. J Rheumatol. 1981;8:952–4.
6. Kaufmann HJ, Taubin HL. Nonsteroidal anti-inflammatory drugs activate quiescent inflammatory bowel disease. Ann Intern Med. 1987;107:513–16.
7. Rampton DS, McNeil NI, Sarner M. Analgesic ingestion and other factors preceding relapse in ulcerative colitis. Gut. 1983;24:187–9.
8. Foster PN, Axon ATR, Packman L, Harper A. Non-steroidal anti-inflammatory drugs and the bowel (letter). Lancet. 1989;2:1047–8.
9. Hanauer SB, Stathopoulos G. Risk–benefit assessment of drugs used in the treatment of inflammatory bowel disease. Drug Safety. 1991;6(3):192–219.
10. Goldin E, Rachmilewitz D. Prostanoids cytoprotection for maintaining remission in ulcerative colitis: failure of 15(R),15-methylprostaglandin E_2. Dig Dis Sci. 1983;28:807–11.
11. Stenson W, Lauritsen K, Laursen LS et al. A clinical trial of Zileuton, a specific inhibitor of 5-lipoxygenase, in ulcerative colitis. Gastroenterology. 1991;100(5):253A (abstr.).
12. Wallace JL, Keenan CM, Gale D, Scott Shoupe T. Exacerbation of experimental colitis by nonsteroidal anti-inflammatory drugs is not related to elevated leukotriene B_4 synthesis. Gastroenterology. 1992;102:18–27.
13. Pearson DJ, Stones NA, Bentley SJ, Reid H. Proctocolitis induced by salicylate and associated with asthma and recurrent nasal polyps. Br Med J. 1983;286:1675.
14. Bridges AJ, Marshall JB, Diaz-Ariaz AA. Acute eosinophilic colitis and hypersensitivity reaction associated with naproxen therapy. Am J Med. 1990;89:526–7.
15. Vessey M, Jewell D, Smith A, Yeates D, McPherson K. Chronic inflammatory bowel disease, cigarette smoking, and use of oral contraceptives: findings in a large cohort study of women of childbearing age. Br Med J. 1986;292:1101–3.
16. Logan RFA, Kay CR. Oral contraception, smoking and inflammatory bowel disease. Int J Epidemiol. 1989;18:105–7.
17. Lashner BA, Kane SV, Hanauer SB. Lack of association between oral contraceptive use and Crohn's disease: a community-based matched case-control study. Gastroenterology. 1989;97:1442–7.
18. Lashner BA, Kane SV, Hanauer SB. Lack of association between oral contraceptive use and ulcerative colitis. Gastroenterology. 1990;99:1032–6.
19. Francheschi S, Panza E, La Vecchia C, Parazzini D, Decarli A, Bianchi Porro G. Non-specific inflammatory bowel disease and smoking. Am J Epidemiol. 1987;125:445–52.
20. Tobin MV, Logan RFA, Langman MJS, McConnell RB, Gilmore IT. Cigarette smoking and inflammatory bowel disease. Gastroenterology. 1987;93:316–21.

21. Lindberg E, Tysk C, Andersson K, Järnerot G. Smoking and inflammatory bowel disease: a case control study. Gut. 1988;29:352–7.
22. Wakefield AJ, Dhillon AP, Rowles PM *et al*. Pathogenesis of Crohn's disease: multifocal gastrointestinal infarction. Lancet. 1989;2:1057–62.
23. Hurwitz RL, Martin AJ, Grossman BE, Waddell WR. Oral contraceptives and gastrointestinal disorders. Ann Surg. 1970;172:892–6.
24. Morowitz DA, Epstein BH. Spectrum of bowel disease associated with use of oral contraceptives. Ann Med of District of Columbia. 1973;42:6–10.
25. Camelleri M, Scafler K, Chadwick VS, Hodgson HJ, Weinbren K. Periportal sinusoidal dilatation, inflammatory bowel disease, and the contraceptive pill. Gastroenterology. 1981;80:810–15.
26. Tedesco FJ, Volpicelli NA, Moore FS. Estrogen- and progesterone-associated colitis: a disorder with clinical and endoscopic features mimicking Crohn's colitis. Gastrointest Endosc. 1982;28:247–9.
27. LaMont JT, Trnka YM. Therapeutic implications of *Clostridium difficile* toxin during relapse of chronic inflammatory bowel disease. Lancet. 1980;1:381–3.
28. Bolton RP, Sherriff RJ, Read AE. *Clostridium difficile* associated diarrrhoea: a role in inflammatory bowel disease? Lancet. 1980;1:383–4.
29. Trnka YM, LaMont TJ. Association of *Clostridium difficile* toxin with symptomatic relapse of chronic inflammatory bowel disease. Gastroenterology. 1981;80:693–6.
30. Keighley MRB, Youngs D, Johnson M, Allan RN, Burdon DW. *Clostridium difficile* toxin in acute diarrhoea complicating inflammatory bowel disease. Gut. 1982;23:410–14.
31. Greenfield C, Aguilar Ramirez JR, Pounder RE *et al*. *Clostridium difficile* and inflammatory bowel disease. Gut 1983;24:713–17.
32. Barrison IG, Kane SP. Penicillin-associated colitis. Lancet. 1978;2:843.
33. Heer M, Sulser H, Hany A. Segmentale, hämorrhagische Kolitis nach Amoxicillin-Therapie. Schweiz Med Wochenschr. 1989;119:733–5.
34. Mrowka C, Munch R, Rezzonico M, Greminger P. Akute segmentale hämorrhagische Penicillin-assoziierte Kolitis. Dtsch Med Wochenschr. 1990;115:1750–3.
35. Fortson WC, Tedesco FJ. Drug-induced colitis: a review. Am J Gastroenterol. 1984;79(11):878–83.

43

Monitoring of therapeutic success: empirical or rational?

W. FISCHBACH

As long as the aetiology and the mechanisms of pathogenesis remain unclear, therapy of inflammatory bowel disease (IBD) will continue to be symptomatic. Management efforts concentrate on the treatment of active bowel inflammation, maintenance of remission and prophylaxis of recurrence. Although medical therapy is the usual approach in IBD, there is also a need for well-timed surgery as a consequence of intractable disease and complications or, in some cases, as cancer prophylaxis over the long term. The therapeutic strategy is mainly dependent upon the extent and the localization of bowel involvement. Disease activity, however, represents the decisive criterion to initiate medical therapy and to monitor its effect. Assessment of disease activity must include both inflammatory activity and the patient's perception of disease severity, as they may differ in the individual case. Furthermore, Garrett and Drossman recently postulated also considering psychosocial factors in order to adequately assess the patient's general health status[1]. Table 1 summarizes the various parameters which can be used to estimate disease activity and to monitor the effects of treatment.

Table 1 Parameters indicating disease activity in inflammatory bowel disease

Subjective symptoms
Physical status
Biochemical markers
Faecal markers (e.g. α_1-antitrypsin)
Clinical activity indices (e.g. CDAI, van Hees)
Radiology
Endoscopy
Scintigraphy

Leucocyte scanning using [111]In- or ^{99}Tc-M-HMPAO-labelled autologous granulocytes or, as recently available, monoclonal antibodies against human granulocytes, has been established as a highly sensitive method to detect bowel inflammation[2-4]. By means of a scan-grading, the degree of intestinal inflammation can be estimated semiquantitatively[5].

Measuring the percentage faecal excretion of ^{111}In-labelled neutrophils in a 4-day stool sampling provides an objective assessment of intestinal inflammatory activity[2,6]. As shown by our group and others, this parameter significantly correlates with the inflammatory bowel infiltrate as judged histologically. It is generally accepted as the 'gold standard' for intestinal inflammatory activity.

Conventional radiological methods such as enteroclysis are used to visualize the inflamed small bowel. They can, however, contribute only a little to the assessment of disease activity or to the short-term monitoring of therapy. Computer tomography is mainly reserved for diagnosis of mesenteral or retroperitoneal masses.

The clinical relevance of endoscopy in IBD is mainly based on two aspects. The direct inspection of the mucosa offers the possibility of also detecting small superficial lesions. Thus, IBD and its relapse after surgical resection can be diagnosed at a very early stage. On the other hand, histological examination of endoscopic biopsies allows an exact evaluation of the intestinal inflammation. Ileocolonoscopy is therefore an essential procedure for establishing the diagnosis of IBD. It also seemed highly useful in the monitoring of drug therapy. However, Modigliani and the Groupe d'Etude Therapeutique des Affections Inflammatoires Digestives (GETAID) recently demonstrated, in an outstanding investigation, that there is no correlation between endoscopic findings and clinical severity of Crohn's disease (CD)[7]. In a similar way, Makowiec et al. found an endoscopic relapse rate of 90% within 5 years following bowel resection, whereas only 40% of the patients suffered from clinical symptoms[8]. Therefore, routine endoscopy would be indicated only if clinically asymptomatic patients with endoscopic relapse benefit from early treatment. There has recently been evidence in support of this[9], which needs to be confirmed by further studies.

Due to their invasive nature, and to associated exposure to radiation, the use of scintigraphy, radiology or endoscopy is restricted in the long-term management of IBD patients. Being easily available, various biochemical parameters are used to evaluate the course of disease (Table 2). They generally provide a reliable reflection of systemic inflammation and detect changes rapidly. As non-specific tests they are influenced by extra-intestinal complications and other coexisting diseases. Therefore, estimation of disease activity by biochemical parameters is rarely superior to the clinician's judgement[10]. In a recent investigation we found that various laboratory tests correlate in a very similar way with the faecal excretion of ^{111}In-labelled neutrophils as a specific estimate of bowel inflammation[11]. It seems of little importance, therefore, which one of those commonly used laboratory markers is determined in clinical practice.

Faecal markers represent another approach in assessing the clinical course of disease. Today, faecal excretion of α_1-antitrypsin or calculation of

Table 2 Biochemical markers of inflammation

Acute-phase reactants (CRP, α_1-antitrypsin, acid α_1-glycoprotein)
Serum proteins (albumin, electrophoresis)
ESR
Blood tests (haematocrit, haemoglobin, leucocytosis, thrombocytosis)
Fe
Others

α_1-antitrypsin clearance are the methods of choice for quantitating intestinal protein loss. Furthermore, faecal α_1-antitrypsin correlates well with the activity of CD[12,13]. Using a simplified extraction of native stool and a new immunnephelometric measurement, we also found a significant correlation of faecal α_1-antitrypsin with various biochemical parameters and clinical activity indices[14].

Many clinical activity indices have been devised to quantitatively determine disease activity in an individual patient at a certain stage of the disease. However, to some extent all clinical scales are inadequate to meet this claim fully. In practice they are not widely accepted by clinicians. In this context, the above-mentioned problems of assessing disease activity have to be borne in mind. Measures of systemic inflammation and the patient's experience of illness are very differently represented by the various clinical activity indices. Contrary to indicating the actual patient's status, prognostic scales as developed by Brignola *et al.*[15] deal with the estimation of further clinical course and patient's outcome.

Without question, objective parameters of disease activity are essential in clinical trials. However, what about their use in everyday clinical practice. Do we need them to monitor therapeutic success in the individual case? In this regard we must bear in mind that the various parameters described above are limited with respect to their use and statement, and there is no valid criterion or gold standard for disease activity. A thorough history-taking and physical examination remain the mainstays of evaluation with respect to therapy and monitoring its effects (Fig. 1). They may be complemented by some basic biochemical parameters. Of course it is important to use laboratory tests more often in the severely ill patient, since abnormalities in this case need to be corrected on an ongoing basis. The use of endoscopy,

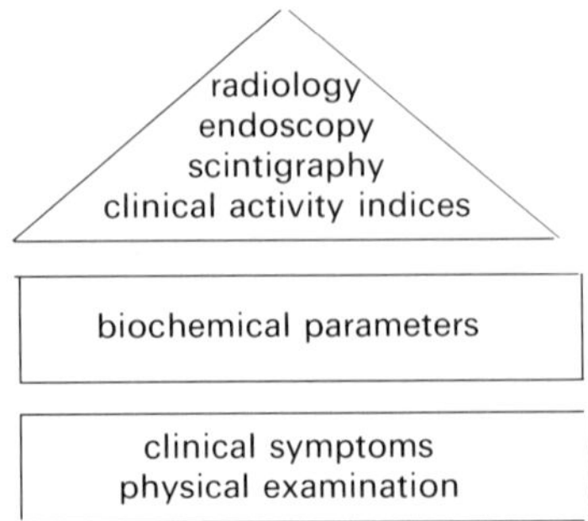

Fig. 1 Parameters to assess disease activity and to monitor therapeutic success

radiology or scintigraphy can be reserved for instances in which specific information is needed to guide management decisions. Summarizing the question, 'Monitoring of therapeutic success: empirical or rational?' can be answered by saying that outside clinical trials monitoring of the efficacy of treatment can be mostly done empirically in the individual case.

References

1. Garrett JW, Drossman DA. Health status in inflammatory bowel disease. Biological and behavioral considerations. Gastroenterology. 1990;99:90–6.
2. Becker W, Fischbach W, Jenett M, Reiners Ch, Börner W. ^{111}In-oxine-labelled white blood cells in the diagnosis and follow-up of Crohn's disease. Klin Wochenschr. 1986;64:141–8.
3. Becker W, Fischbach W, Jenett M, Reiners C, Börner W. In-111-oxin labelled white blood cells in the diagnosis and follow-up of Crohn's disease. Klin Wochenschr. 1986;64:141–8.
4. Saverymuttu SH, Peters AM, Lavender JP, Hodgson JH, Chandwick VS. 111-Indium autologous leucocytes in inflammatory bowel disease. Gut. 1983;26:293–9.
5. Saverymuttu SH, Camilleri M, Rees H, Lavender JP, Hodgson HJF, Chadwick VS. Indium 111-granulocyte scanning in the assessment of disease extent and disease activity in inflammatory bowel disease. Gastroenterology. 1986;90:1121–8.
6. Saverymuttu SH, Peters AM, Lavender JP, Pepys MB, Hodgson HJF, Chadwick VS. Quantitative fecal indium 111-labeled leucocyte excretion in the assessment of disease in Crohn's disease. Gastroenterology. 1983;85:1333–9.
7. Modigliani R, Mary JY, Simon JF, Cortot A, Soule JC, Gendre JP, Rene E and the Groupe d'Etude Therapeutique des Affections Inflammatoires Digestives. Clinical, biological, and endoscopic pictures of attacks of Crohn's disease. Evolution on prednisolone. Gastroenterology. 1990;98:811–18.
8. Makowiec F, Köveker G, Weber P, Jenss H, Starlinger M. Morbus Crohn: Krankheitsaktivität und Rezidiv nach Operation. Dtsch Med Wochenschr. 1990;115:1659–64.
9. Ewe K, Herfarth C, Malchow H, Jesdinsky HJ. Postoperative recurrence of Crohn's disease in relation to radicality of operation and sulfasalazine prophylaxis. A multicenter trial. Digestion. 1989;42:224.
10. Beck IT. Laboratory assessment of inflammatory bowel disease. Dig Dis Sci. 1987;32:26S–41S.
11. Fischbach W, Becker W. Clinical relevance of activity parameters in Crohn's disease estimated by the faecal excretion of 111-In-labeled granulocytes. Digestion. 1991;50:149–52.
12. Meyers S, Wolke A, Field S, Feuer E, Johnson J, Janowitz H. Fecal alpha-1-antitrypsin measurement: An indicator of Crohn's disease activity. Gastroenterology. 1985;89:13–18.
13. Karbach U, Ewe K, Bodenstein H. Alpha-1-antitrypsin, a reliable endogenous marker for intestinal protein loss and its application in patients with Crohn's disease. Gut. 1983;24:718–23.
14. Fischbach W, Deubel M, Boege F, Mössner J. Erste klinische Erfahrungen mit einer vereinfachten Bestimmungsmethode des fäkalen Alpha-1-Antitrypsins. Z Gastroenterol. 1991;29:650–4.
15. Brignola C, Campierieri M, Bazzochi G, Feruggin P, Tragone A, Lanfranchi G. A laboratory index for predicting relapse in asymptomatic patients with Crohn's disease. Gastroenterology. 1986;91:1490–4.

44

Unconventional treatment of ulcerative colitis and Crohn's disease

B. V. KIRKIN and I. L. KHALIF

INTRODUCTION

The use of sulphasalazine, 5-aminosalicylic acid (5-ASA) and corticosteroids enables improvement or remission to be achieved in 80% of colitis patients who suffer from mild or moderate disease. However, unfavourable factors such as hormonal dependence and resistance to certain drugs are often present. In addition, medical treatment does not eliminate the possibility of severe attacks of the disease, with potentially life-threatening complications. For those reasons, colectomy is often considered necessary.

However, this paper puts forward a new approach to the non-surgical treatment of colitis. It is derived from the successful experience of many specialists over a number of years in using extracorporeal detoxification to treat inflammatory bowel disease (IBD). The method has proved its validity in treating not only exogenous and endogenous toxaemia[1-5] but also a range of autoimmune and immune complex conditions[6,7]. As well as detoxification, the new approach encompasses laser therapy[8,9] and hyperbaric oxygenation[10,11] in order to stimulate reparative processes and the epithelialization of the mucosa.

These new, or recently revived, methods have all been implemented clinically. However, it is not a simple matter to evaluate the results achieved unequivocally. Their validity must be determined quantitatively and qualitatively in order to confirm their role in the treatment of ulcerative colitis and Crohn's disease. Nevertheless, although some details remain to be investigated in controlled clinical trials, sufficient experience and clinical data have been amassed for certain conclusions to be drawn about the practical efficacy of these so-called unconventional methods.

Between 1983 and 1991, 1396 patients with ulcerative colitis and 480 patients with Crohn's disease were treated at the hospital of the Institute of Proctology. At various stages of their treatment, for example in order to stop an attack of colitis or at the postoperative stage when complications occurred, many were treated with unconventional methods; 250 underwent haemosorption, 51 plasmapheresis, 186 ultraviolet irradiation of the blood, 54 laser therapy, and 500 hyperbaric oxygenation.

The present study considers cases of exacerbated IBD when unconventional methods were used in addition to medical treatment. The control group consisted of patients who received only conventional medical treatment with corticosteroids, sulphasalazine and 5-ASA. The methods used, their duration and the dosage of drugs were determined exclusively by the severity of the attack.

Techniques used were intended to counter the toxaemia associated with severe attacks of IBD and which reflects a profound disturbance of the ecological equilibrium in the colon. This shift in the microbiological balance leads to the suppression of the strictly glycolitic anaerobes and their elimination from the contact zone of the colon. At the same time, there is a proliferation of potentially harmful anaerobic and aerobic organisms. As a result, the normal trophic and regulatory relationship between microorganisms and their host becomes increasingly disturbed, leading to a reduction in the activity of local T-cell suppressors and therefore to the development of mutual aggression. In turn, this results in the penetration of bacterial metabolites and fragments of bacterial cell membrane into the blood, and endotoxaemia.

Chemically, the toxic products involved are: oligopeptides (usually medium-chain molecules); glycoproteins, which represent the larger fragments of the cellular membranes of certain bacteria; lipopolysaccharides (LPS) from the cell membranes of Gram-negative bacteria such as *E. coli*; and phenols, including the final metabolites of the microflora. Toxins may be present in the blood as either individual molecules or clusters of molecules. The formation of complexes between oligopeptides derived from *E. coli* cell membranes and LPS is to a large extent determined by the interaction between anionic phosphate radicals of lipid A and the cationic radicals of oligopeptide bonds. With regard to phenols, interactions take place between their benzene rings and the chains of fatty acids. It should be noted that bacteraemia is most likely to develop in the later stages of abnormal microflora[12-15].

In the present study, the presence of endotoxaemia was confirmed and its extent estimated by determining the serum concentration of medium-chain molecules, phenol, and proteins of the acute phase of inflammation. Endotoxins originating from the cell membranes of Gram-negative bacteria were detected using mice; mortality was determined 48 h following intraperitoneal injection of 1 ml of the patient's serum.

The clinical and laboratory results showed a correlation between the relapse of ulcerative colitis and Crohn's disease, and an increase in the values of the above markers. In 70–75% of patients tested, there was an increase in all markers and 90% of patients demonstrated an increase in at least one. Values of the markers were, as was expected, higher among patients than among healthy controls. The average concentration of medium-chain molecules among IBD patients was 0.384 ± 0.02 units of optical density and the concentration of phenol was 6.27 ± 0.15 mg/l. Among normal patients the corresponding values were 0.240 ± 0.012 units of optical density, and 2.2 ± 0.9 mg/l, respectively ($p < 0.001$).

As expected, the extent of toxaemia was related to the degree of inflammation, the latter being evaluated by endoscopic examination and the clinical severity of IBD.

Endotoxins derived from Gram-negative bacteria were detected in 70% of the patients tested, among whom 27% showed a strongly positive reaction, 33% a moderately positive reaction, and 10% a mildly positive reaction. It should be stressed that the markers chosen to estimate the extent of toxaemia are of statistical value alone; they should not be considered as accurate means of individual evaluation. In practice, they are of value only for the evaluation of the efficacy of haemosorption and ultraviolet irradiation of the blood.

HAEMOSORPTION

Indications in patients with IBD

Since the end of the 1980s, haemosorption has been more and more widely used in the treatment of patients with IBD. It is technically straightforward and has proved its value in the management of endogenous toxaemia[16]. To date at the Institute of Proctology, haemosorption has been carried out in 211 patients (93 male and 118 female), 159 with ulcerative colitis and 52 with Crohn's disease. Thirty-nine patients with IBD who had undergone haemosorption postoperatively in order to alleviate complications were excluded from the group. Thirty patients were treated for their first attack of ulcerative colitis (acute form) and 129 for the chronic condition; 54 patients had severe and 90 more moderate disease. Of the 52 patients with Crohn's disease, the majority (80%) had the severe or moderate condition (Best's index 452 ± 19). Twenty-six patients with CD had extraintestinal manifestations: 16 had arthritis and arthralgia, five had erythema nodosum and pyoderma gangrenosum, and five had stomatitis aphthosa and eye disorders.

Haemosorption was carried out using Russian-made sorbents at a rate of 80–100 ml/min, exposition was 1.5–2 volumes of circulating blood. The apparatus was joined on a vein-to-vein basis.

Detoxicative effects

Data so far collected indicate that severe attacks of Crohn's disease are accompanied not only by clinical signs of toxicity but also by increased serum concentrations of medium-chain molecules, phenol, and Gram-negative bacterial endotoxin. Changes in these markers which indicate detoxification are shown in Table 1.

After haemosorption, the concentration of medium-chain molecules decreased in 55% of 150 patients, phenol concentrations decreased in 73%, and there was a simultaneous decrease in levels of both in 35% of cases. There was also a dramatic decrease from 26.7% to 3.5% in the number of patients who had Gram-negative bacterial endotoxin in their blood.

Table 1   The change in concentration of toxic metabolites in the blood of patients with IBD under the influence of haemosorption

Groups of patients	Middle-chain molecules (units of optical density)			Phenol (mg/l)		
	Before sorption	After sorption	7 days after sorption	Before sorption	After sorption	7 days after sorption
UC and CD ($n = 150$)	0.339 ± 0.007	0.306 ± 0.006*	0.300 ± 0.009*	5.84 ± 0.20	4.98 ± 0.19*	4.35 ± 0.28*
UC ($n = 121$)	0.354 ± 0.010	0.319 ± 0.009**	0.294 ± 0.012**	6.01 ± 0.22	5.15 ± 0.19***	4.35 ± 0.54***
CD ($n = 29$)	0.279 ± 0.015	0.253 ± 0.010	0.290 ± 0.019	5.02 ± 0.39	4.20 ± 0.40	4.40 ± 0.32

Significance vs original state: *$p < 0.001$;   **$p < 0.05$;   ***$p < 0.01$

Phenol and Gram-negative bacterial endotoxin were the most sensitive to haemosorption of the toxic metabolites discussed here. This was because the adsorbents used (synthetic coals) were non-polar and therefore had a high affinity to lipophilic molecules. LPS has a non-polar fragment, lipid A, and phenol has a non-polar benzene ring. Adsorption of the medium-chain molecules and glycoproteins, which are ionic and polar in nature, was much less successful.

It should be noted that because endotoxin can be present in the adsorbed form on the walls of blood vessels, as well as in the circulating form, the clinical effect of haemosorption is variable. Patients in whom most of the endotoxin is circulating may show better results after the first haemosorption. This factor accounts in part for the variability of laboratory determinations of serum endotoxins.

In recent years, there has been debate about the physiological importance of the post-adsorption period in determining the clinical effect of haemosorption. For example, Yakubovskaya *et al.* showed in 1990 that immediately after haemosorption there is a massive degranulation of neutrophils which leads to a 100–200-fold increase in serum lactopherin concentration[17]. The immunomodulatory and protective effects of lactopherin may therefore be enhanced by haemosorption. In the 24 h immediately after haemosorption, a decrease in the proteins of acute phase inflammation is noted but after 7 days levels return to baseline. Nevertheless, in 16 of 30 patients a verified reduction in the levels of C-reactive protein and seromucoids was detected. This decrease is unlikely to be due to temporary adsorption of these proteins on the column because by day 7 their levels continued to decrease, particularly in patients who had a good clinical response to prednisolone therapy (Table 2).

The clinical effect

The main indications for haemosorption are presented in Fig. 1. Taking into consideration the detoxicative effects of haemosorption, the best results were expected in that group of patients with the most severe disease. It was hoped that the technique might lead to a dramatic improvement and an enhancement of the efficacy of steroid therapy such that colectomy might be avoided.

A total of 72% of patients demonstrated an improvement in general condition as a result of haemosorption, 74% had a reduction in fever, and 50% experienced some relief from abdominal pain. In addition, the stools of some patients were normalized.

The extraintestinal manifestations of disease diminished in 43 of 51 patients as a result of haemosorption. Bacteraemia was eradicated in 16 of 18 cases. Toxic reactions to sulphasalazine were mainly overcome, making it possible to administer the drug at a therapeutic dose (4 g). It should be noted that basic anti-inflammatory therapy was not discontinued; haemosorption was combined with steroid therapy (80–110 mg/d oral prednisolone or 375–500 mg hydrocortisone i.m. or i.v.).

The effect of haemosorption and hence the immediate prognosis was determined by the adequacy of the reaction of patients with the severe form of the disease to steroid therapy.

Table 2 Indicators of anti-inflammatory effect of haemosorption in patients with ulcerative colitis

Indicators	Control	Before haemosorption	After haemosorption	7 days after haemosorption
Properdin (g/l)	30 ± 0.6	40.5 ± 2	38.9 ± 2.8	39.9 ± 2.9
Haptoglobin (g/l)	76 ± 2.6	162.3 ± 12	152.9 ± 11.4	182.4 ± 15.1
Caeruloplasmin (g/l)	27 ± 0.6	38.9 ± 2.5	36.3 ± 2.6	36 ± 2
C-reactive protein (g/l)	0.44 ± 0.02	2.33 ± 0.7	1.7 ± 0.5	1.0 ± 0.6
α_1-Acid glycoprotein (g/l)	80 ± 2	103 ± 7.4	103.3 ± 7.2	114 ± 9
α_1-Antitrypsin (g/l)	155 ± 3	222 ± 15.1	213.6 ± 21.4	229 ± 26
Seromucoid (units of optical density)	0.140 ± 0.019	0.761 ± 0.065	0.701 ± 0.067	0.532 ± 0.062

Post-operative
  patients ($n = 39$):
Peritonitis of various
  aetiology
Perianal abscesses
Hepatic–renal
  insufficiency
Polyvalent allergy
Abscesses in
  abdominal cavity

Patients with
  severe attacks of
  ulcerative colitis
  (54 patients) and
  Crohn's disease
  (29 patients)
  ($n = 83$)
Manifested intoxication
  ($T = 38°$C, pulse rate
  $= 100$ or more,
  leucocytosis with
  elevated neutrophils)
Sepsis, bacteraemia
Toxic dilatation of
  first and second degree
Extraintenstinal
  manifestations: eye
  disorders, skin affection,
  arthritis and arthralgia

Moderate form of the
  disease with moderate
  intoxication ($n = 112$)
Hormonal dependence
Resistant against therapy
Subfebrile temperatures
Bacteraemia
Arthralgia
Toxic and allergic reactions
  to sulphasalazine

Coexisting diseases ($n = 16$):
Bronchial asthma
Rheumatoid arthritis and Bechterew's disease
Psoriasis
Dermatitis

Fig. 1 Indications for haemosorption in patients with IBD ($n = 250$)

Of the group of 54 patients with severe ulcerative colitis who underwent haemosorption, nine (16.7%) subsequently required colectomy. In the control group of 131 patients with severe ulcerative colitis but who did not receive haemosorption 37 (28%) required colectomy almost immediately and a further ten patients (18.5%) were operated on after a delay due to their initial refusal of surgery.

In 29 patients with severe attacks of Crohn's disease, haemosorption led to a decrease in Best's index from 452 ± 19.3 to 365 ± 17. However, the benefits of haemosorption in patients with Crohn's disease have not been confirmed. Of the 29, four (14%) were subsequently treated surgically, compared to 26/288 (9%) in the control group. The analysis did not include surgery conducted because of perianal and abdominal abscesses or intestinal obstruction.

Sixty-eight patients underwent haemosorption because of rapid development of their disease. It was expected that in such cases the technique would overcome drug resistance. However, in only 27 patients (40%) was the expected result achieved; in the remainder no effect was obtained, despite repeated courses of haemosorption. In general, haemosorption was much less successful in severe Crohn's disease than in severe ulcerative colitis.

Plasmapheresis

Plasmapheresis is also an effective means of extracorporeal detoxification[18]. This technique was used in 51 patients with moderate or severe ulcerative colitis. Blood separation was carried out at 200–300 g, blood was delivered at 50–80 ml/min. Erythrocytic mass was withdrawn from the rotor at a rate of up to 100 ml/min and plasmapheresis was conducted taking into account that plasma was to be removed from the patient at a rate of 15–20 mg/kg bodyweight. The results of plasmapheresis are shown in Table 3.

Thus, treatment with haemosorption and plasmapheresis is entirely justified in patients with IBD and leads to a beneficial, though temporary, clinical effect. The temporary reduction in drug resistance obtained can improve the efficacy of steroid therapy and may enable colectomy to be avoided. Nevertheless, the causes of endotoxaemia remain and there is therefore a need to employ further detoxification techniques, for example rapid intestinal lavage plus 5-ASA[19,20].

Table 3 Distribution of patients judging from the indications and efficiency of plasmacytopheresis

Indications	Number of patients	Forms of disease	Direct effect		
			Good	Satisfactory	No effect
Manifested intoxication	29	Moderate	9	6	–
		Severe	7	3	4*
Moderate intoxication	16	Moderate	11	1	4
Subfebrile temperatures	3	Moderate	3	–	–
Extraintestinal manifestations	3	Moderate	3	–	–

*Patients subjected to operation

THE ROLE OF ULTRAVIOLET IRRADIATION OF BLOOD IN THE TREATMENT OF INFLAMMATORY BOWEL DISEASE

A further method of extracorporeal detoxification that is quite popular among Russian specialists is the reinfusion of blood after ultraviolet irradiation. A revival of this method has taken place because of the increasing number of organisms resistant to antibiotics, and because it has been shown to enhance phagocytosis[21,22]. This relatively non-invasive technique was also considered likely to improve the results achieved with haemosorption, the indications for which are the same.

Ultraviolet irradiation (UVI) was performed in 186 patients aged 19 to 57 years; 141 had ulcerative colitis and 45 Crohn's disease. The effectiveness of the treatment was evaluated using the following laboratory markers which indicate the extent of endotoxaemia and inflammation: medium-chain peptide molecules, phenol, and seromucoids. Each was measured on three occasions: before UVI, immediately after it, and 7 days following completion of the treatment. UVI was combined with administration of sulphasalazine or 5-ASA and steroids.

The procedure was conducted using Russian-made apparatus known as ISOLDA. Irradiation was carried out in 10–12 minute sessions, usually at a wavelength of 220–260 nm. The volume of blood irradiated varied from 100 to 180 ml, determined by the weight of the patient (2 mg/kg). Five to ten procedures were conducted, depending on the clinical improvement achieved.

In 18 patients, UVI was used to treat bacteraemia, usually caused by Gram-negative organisms (72%). UVI resulted in sterilization of the blood in 16 of 18 patients, nine of whom did not receive antibiotics. UVI was also beneficial in reducing fever. It was used expressly for this purpose in 38 patients, in 32 of whom temperature was normalized.

It is more difficult to evaluate the efficiency of UVI used to stabilize the effects of haemosorption. Although good results were achieved in 22 of 29 patients treated for this reason, the stabilization effect noted may not have been entirely due to UVI since steroids were also administered.

Seven patients in whom UVI was not able to improve the course of their disease had also failed to respond to hormonal therapy combined with haemosorption.

With regard to Crohn's disease, it should be noted that, judging from Best's index, the level of activity of the disease at the end of the course of treatment did not differ significantly from that in patients treated with combined medical therapy and UVI, or those who received medical treatment alone (Table 4).

Of 30 patients treated with UVI because of the progressive course of their ulcerative colitis, only 10 showed improvement. These benefits included normalization of temperature and improved general condition. However, the procedure seemed to have no effect on intestinal appearance. Extraintestinal symptoms of the disease were treated relatively successfully using UVI; in five patients arthralgia was eliminated and in three there was elimination of erythema nodosum.

However, the clinical effects of detoxification with UVI were much less

Table 4   Changes in index activity in patients with CD in the course of different types of therapy

Groups of patients	Number of patients	Index activity of disease (Best's index)		
		Before sorption	After sorption	After treatment
Haemosorption + UVI + medical treatment (1 group)	11	448 ± 46	351 ± 39	189 ± 49
Haemosorption + medical treatment (2 group)	15	480 ± 43	371 ± 31	261 ± 43
Medical treatment (control group)	35	407 ± 27	–	262 ± 31

obvious than those achieved using haemosorption. There was no clinical effect, but benefits could be seen in terms of changes in laboratory markers (Table 5).

It was thought that UVI plus haemosorption might have an additive effect. However, this was not confirmed clinically; in none of the 29 patients who received the combination was an additive effect detected.

THE ROLE OF HYPERBARIC OXYGENATION IN THE COMPOSITE TREATMENT OF IBD

It has long been recognized that hyperbaric oxygenation (HBO) can lead to the rapid regression of inflammatory processes. The technique is known to have an immunomodulatory action and to stimulate reparation[23,24].

In IBD, disorders in the microcirculation reduce the capacity for regeneration of ulcerative defects of the mucosa, leading to a generally chronic course in both ulcerative colitis and Crohn's disease. Moreover, the administration of glucocorticoids, though having some effect on acute inflammation, slows

Table 5   Influence of various types of detoxicative therapy on levels of toxaemia and inflammatory processes in patients with ulcerative colitis

	Before treatment	After treatment	7 days after treatment
UVI of blood ($n = 76$)			
Middle-chain molecules	0.371 ± 0.020	0.287 ± 0.025***	0.289 ± 0.016**
Phenol	4.17 ± 0.32	4.42 ± 0.34	3.71 ± 0.25
Seromucoid	0.674 ± 0.060	0.517 ± 0.075	0.585 ± 0.070
Haemosorption + UVI ($n = 29$)			
Middle-chain molecules	0.352 ± 0.022	0.276 ± 0.014**	0.261 ± 0.018**
Phenol	5.26 ± 0.46	5.20 ± 0.60	5.06 ± 0.52
Seromucoid	0.720 ± 0.075	0.632 ± 0.079	0.317 ± 0.068*

Significance vs original state: *$p < 0.001$;   **$p < 0.01$;   ***$p < 0.02$

down the reparative process. It should be noted that the leukotriene pathway of arachidonic acid, which is strongly dependent on oxygen, plays an important part in the pathophysiology of ulcerative colitis.

A controlled study involving 500 patients with IBD was conducted in order to evaluate the results of treatment with compressed oxygen. Two hundred and fifty patients with total colitis formed the study group and were divided into subgroups according to the activity of their disease (active or reparative phase), whether or not they were treated with drugs (sulphasalazine, 5-ASA and glucocorticoids), and taking into account the oxygen pressure used (0.13–0.15 MPa or 0.17–0.20 MPa). The control group consisted of 120 patients with total colitis who were not treated with HBO.

Treatment comprised ten sessions of HBO administration of 45–60 min each.

Results of the controlled trial

Evaluation of the direct effects of HBO on the main clinical manifestation of the disease, and on markers, is extremely difficult because of the long duration of treatment involved and, more importantly, the coadministration of medical therapy. For those reasons, it was decided to evaluate only the final outcome of combined therapy on the assumption that HBO would enhance the clinical efficacy of the medical treatment. Results of the controlled trial are shown in Table 6.

HBO administered during the active phase of the disease had a variable effect dependent upon the pressure used and on the drugs coadministered. Administration at a pressure of 0.17–0.20 MPa in combination with sulphasalazine had a deleterious effect; more than 50% of patients experienced acute abdominal pains and increases in bleeding and diarrhoea. These

Table 6 Frequency of remission in the total ulcerative colitis group under the influence of composite therapy consisting of medical treatment and hyperbaric oxygenation

Phase of inflammatory process and medical drug	Controls		Under pressure 0.17–0.20 MPa		Under pressure 0.13–0.15 MPa	
	n	%	n	%	n	%
Active phase:						
Sulphasalazine 3–4 g	47 (28)	59.5	10 (4)	40	14 (9)	64.3
Prednisolone 0.5–1.5 mg/kg of weight of patient per day	50 (30)	60	11 (8)	72.8	33 (16)	48.3
Reparative phase:						
Sulphasalazine 3–4 g	47 (31)	63	15 (14)	93.4	14 (10)	71.5
Prednisolone 0.5–1.5 mg/kg of weight of patient per day	50 (30)	60	13 (13)	100	20 (13)	65

Figures in parentheses show number of patients with remission process

manifestations of the disease may have been provoked by stimulation of colonic motility. A pressure of 0.13–0.15 MPa produced more favourable results, leading to an improvement in general condition and enabling patients to overcome sickness. Nevertheless, HBO administered in the active phase of disease, that is at the beginning of medical treatment, did not significantly affect the final outcome. The proportion of patients achieving remission did not differ significantly between the HBO group and the control group. It was therefore considered more beneficial to prescribe HBO during the reparative phase of the disease. Administration of HBO at the end of treatment led to improved success, including a doubling of the number of remissions. At this phase of the disease, HBO was reasonably well tolerated, even at a pressure of 0.17–0.20 MPa.

The results of the trial thus confirmed the efficacy of HBO at high pressure during the reparative phase, they also indicated that medical treatment was enhanced by this regimen (Table 7). The efficacy of HBO treatment was of the same order as that of steroid therapy.

The administration of 5-ASA, particularly as suppositories and enemas, produced good results even without HBO in patients with left-sided and distal colitis. However, the inclusion of HBO in the regimen for total colitis was advantageous because it enhanced the efficacy of 5-ASA in all patients, even those with severe disease, enabling remission to be attained in 6–8 weeks.

Similar results have been obtained using combined treatment in Crohn's disease. Ninety-six patients who were investigated had no intestinal obstruction or abdominal abscesses. Their primary medical treatment was successful and combined therapy including HBO produced a further reduction in Best's

Table 7 Results of treating patients with IBD in the reparative phase with the help of composite therapy consisting of medical treatment and HBO

		Results of treatment					
		Remission		Improvement		No effect	
Treatment	Number of patients	n	%	n	%	n	%
Sulphasalazine 3–4 g	77	21	27.3	40	51.9	16	20.8
Sulphasalazine + HBO	48	20	41.7	24	50	4	8.3
Sulphasalazine 3–4 g + hydrocortisone 125 mg in enema	76	36	47.4	34	43.4	7	9.8
Sulphasalazine 3–4 g + hydrocortisone 125 mg in enema + HBO	42	21	50	18	42.8	3	7.2
Prednisolone 30–50 mg per day	79	36	45.5	35	44.3	8	10.1
Prednisolone 30–50 mg per day + HBO	48	32	66.7	11	22.9	5	10.4
Prednisolone 60–110 mg per day	175	97	55.4	52	29.7	26	14.9
Prednisolone 60–110 mg per day + HBO	101	67	66.3	26	25.7	8	7.9

index from 387 ± 26.1 to 166 ± 24.5, while in a control group of 35 patients with the same degree of Crohn's disease who were treated medically, a reduction from 407 ± 27 to 262 ± 31 was noted.

Thirty-five patients with IBD who had undergone colectomy received one to three administrations of HBO beginning on the second or third postoperative day. Even a pressure of 0.15 MPa led to the stimulation of intestinal motility accompanied by improvement of emptying of the stomach and its evacuation via a stoma; thus the post-operative complications were overcome.

LASER THERAPY FOR IBD

Copper-vapour lasers are considered to be efficacious in the treatment of erosive and ulcerous disorders of the stomach and duodenum[25]. Irradiation is conducted at two wavelengths, 510.6 nm and 587.2 nm, from the green-yellow band of the spectrum. The laser is operated under a quasi-continuous regimen and has a high frequency of emitting impulses. Irradiation of damaged areas with high intensity pulses can increase the probability of photochemical processes which lead to the decay of complicated biomolecules and hence speed up tissue regeneration.

A study was conducted in order to attempt to achieve therapeutic effects in IBD patients using transendoscopic therapy with a copper-vapour laser. The average emission capacity was 3–5 W and the frequency of repeated impulses was 8–10 kHz. Emission in the lumen was via a 600 mkm quartz-polymer lightdriver inserted into a protective catheter. The catheter included a device for the manual delivery of water using a syringe. Its outer diameter of 2.6 mm would enable it to be inserted through the instrument canals of the majority of endoscopes.

Using this method, laser therapy was administered to 54 patients, 44 had ulcerative colitis and 10 had Crohn's disease. Thirty-four ulcerative colitis patients had the mild condition and ten had the moderate form. Proctosigmoiditis had been diagnosed in 30 patients, 11 had left-sided disorder, and three had total colitis. Thirty-three patients proved on endoscopy to have moderate mucosal inflammation, and 11 showed severe inflammatory processes in the mucosa. Total colitis was diagnosed in seven patients with Crohn's disease and three had left-sided colitis. All patients with Crohn's disease had disorders at the stage of infiltration and the formation of ulcer fissures.

After preparing the colon for endoscopic study, a flexible endoscope was inserted over the damaged area. Laser irradiation was started in the upper proximal areas and was carried out from a distance of 0.5–1 cm. The average emission at the terminal end of the lightdriver was 300–400 mW. The light was continuously transferred from one area to another, each portion being irradiated for about 3–5 s until the entire damaged area had been irradiated.

Irradiation was performed at intervals of 2–3 days. Patients usually received four to seven sessions, depending on the severity of their disease. During the period in which laser therapy was administered, medical treatment was suspended.

After the first session, 40 of 44 patients with ulcerative colitis showed a reduction in bleeding. After two or three sessions, mucosal inflammation diminished and the ulcerative and erosive lesions were free of necrotic stratum; a reduction in contact bleeding was also noted. After four to seven sessions, the number of erosive and ulcerative lesions diminished significantly. However, eight patients with ulcerative colitis (three total, three left-sided and two distal) showed no improvement after the third session and laser treatment was therefore replaced with medical therapy. The remainder of the patients achieved remission, and 14 showed a reduction in acute inflammation of the mucosa.

Seven of ten patients with Crohn's disease showed a reduction in mucosal damage after the first session of laser therapy; they also showed reduced hyperaemia and contact bleeding. After six or seven sessions, eight of the ten patients achieved endoscopically-confirmed remission. No positive effect was seen in the remaining two patients.

At 3 and 6 month follow-up, no relapse was seen. After 12 months relapses were noted in six patients with ulcerative colitis and two with Crohn's disease. Further laser therapy for three to five sessions led to remission in those patients who had relapsed.

The data obtained in the above studies show the promise of laser therapy. It may for example be beneficial in the treatment of patients resistant to pharmacological treatment.

CONCLUSION

The methods of therapy described are not yet substitutes for medical treatment. Thus it is not appropriate to suggest a change from conventional regimens. Indeed, in cases severe enough for the decision to operate to be taken within 24 hours of admission to hospital for ulcerative colitis, extracorporeal detoxification using the techniques described would unnecessarily increase the cost of treatment and, because of the heparinisation of the blood involved, hinder subsequent surgery. However, in cases in which the prognosis is less clear as to the possibility of further severe attacks of colitis, these methods may offer some hope for the patient and the physician. In such cases haemosorption and plasmapheresis can lead to dramatic changes in the course of the disease when combined with parenteral nutrition and steroid treatment. Although the need for urgent colectomy did not diminish as dramatically as expected (from 28% to 16.7%, $p < 0.05$), each patient reported here experienced a beneficial change.

The use of UVI in patients with bacteraemia helps resolve problems over appropriate antibiotic therapy and resistance to it.

HBO has been proven to enhance the effects of medical treatment in the final stages of disease and has become common practice at the authors' clinic for the treatment of IBD.

Laser therapy requires carefully controlled study to confirm its beneficial effects. However, in the meantime it can be of value in treating patients resistant to medication.

ACKNOWLEDGEMENTS

The authors thank those scientists who have developed and put into practice unconventional treatment of IBD: S. A. Fomin, V. G. Rumyantsev, A. F. Ivanov, V. V. Veselov, V. N. Babin and A. V. Dubinin. Many thanks are also due to A. V. Suvurov who translated the manuscript.

References

1. Kirkin BV. Haemosorption in composite treatment of non-specific ulcerative colitis. Sov Med. 1988;8:7–10 (in Russian).
2. Ganichkin AM, Yaitski NA, Dudna VV, Vasiliev SV *et al.* Lymphocytopheresis and lymphosorption as a method of pathogenetic therapy of non-specific ulcerative colitis. Vestnik Chirurgii. 1991;1:28–31 (in Russian).
3. Ganichkin AM, Yaitski NA, Kvasha VI, Grigorian VV *et al.* Plasmacytopheresis in composite therapy of non-specific ulcerative colitis. Vestnik Chirurgii. 1988;2:106–8 (in Russian).
4. Kildushevski AV, Olshanski AY, Ivanenko TV, Fabrikova EA *et al.* Curative plasmapheresis in composite therapy of ulcerative colitis and Crohn's disease. Proceedings of the 1st Conference of Proctologists of Moscow, 'Ways of improving of proctological service'. 1989:90–91 (in Russian).
5. Eroshkina TD, Musin II, Ivanov AF, Fomin SA. Evaluation of methods of detoxication of blood of the patients with IBD. Prob Proctol. 1991;12:191–6 (in Russian).
6. Chuchalin AG, Masuev KA, Shurkalin BK, Evseev NG *et al.* Affection of lungs by immune complex's diseases and the first experience of implementing haemosorption. Ther Arch. 1981;11:15–18 (in Russian).
7. Nasonov EL, Dmitriev AA, Petrova GN, Timofeeva EB *et al.* The influence of haemosorption upon the level of circulating immune complexes by certain diseases of inter organs. Therapeutic Arch. 1982;7:103–7 (in Russian).
8. Lapshin VP, Litvin GD, Nemtsev IZ, Panchenko GA *et al.* Stimulation of the reparation active condition in damage tissues by means of laser radiation. Proceedings of the International Conference: Lasers and Medicine. Collection of theses. Tashkent. 1989; part 1:99.
9. Loginov AS, Sakalova GN, Tkachenko IV, Sakalova SV *et al.* Some aspects of mechanism of stomach ulcer healing with laser therapy. Proceedings of the International Conference: Lasers and Medicine. Collection of theses. Tashkent. 1989:106–7.
10. Polyakova IV, Grigorieva GA, Lukich VL. The possibilities of HBO in treating chronic IBD. Proceedings of the 1st symposium with international participation, 'Hyperbaric oxygenation (New aspects in the practice and theory concerning HBO)'. Moscow, 1989:95 (in Russian).
11. Rumyantsev VG, Kirkin BV, Fomin SA, Ivanov AF. The use of HBO in composite treatment of non-specific ulcerative colitis. Proceedings of the 1st symposium with international participation, 'Hyperbaric oxygenation (New aspects in the practice and theory concerning HBO)'. Moscow, 1989;101–2 (in Russian).
12. Aoki KA. A study of endotoxemia in ulcerative colitis and Crohn's disease. Acta Med Okayama. 1978;32:147–58.
13. Juhlin L, Krause U, Shelley WB. Endotoxin-induced microlots in ulcerative colitis and Crohn's disease. Scand J Gastroenterol. 1980;15:311–14.
14. Colin R, Grancher T, Lemeland J-F, Hecketsweiler P *et al.* Recherche d'une endotoximie dans les entero-colites inflammatories cryptogenetiques. Gastroenterol Clin. 1979;1:15–19.
15. Kruis W, Shussler P, Weinsiorl M. Circulating lipid A antibodies and their relationship to different clinical condition of patients with Crohn's disease. Hepato-gastroenterol. 1987;3:123–6.
16. Lopukchin UM, Molodenkov MN. Haemosorption. Moscow: Medicina; 1985 (in Russian).
17. Yakubovskaya RI, Borisov VI, Nemtsova ER, Kazachkina II *et al.* On the problem of molecular mechanism of agitation of haemosorption. Voprosy Medizin Chim. 1990;4:11–15 (in Russian).
18. Grigorian VV. Plasmacytopheresis in composite therapy of non-specific ulcerative colitis (dissertation). Leningrad: 1st Medical Institute; 1991 (in Russian).

19. Wellman W, Schmidt F. Intestinal lavage in the treatment of Crohn's disease: a pilot study. Klin Wochenschr. 1982;60:371–3.
20. Wellman W. Endotoxaemia in active Crohn's disease. Treatment with whole gut irrigation and 5-aminosalicylic acid. Gut. 1986;7:814–17.
21. Potashov LV, Cheminava RV. Reinfusion of the irradiated blood in surgical patients. Vestnik Chirurg. 1980;10:144–6 (in Russian).
22. Castellanos Y, Owens T, Rudd C. The effect of ultraviolet radiation on early stages of activation of human lymphocytes: inhibitions independent of effect on DNA. Can J Biochem. 1982;60:854–60.
23. Leonov AN. Some metabolitic aspects of hyperbaric oxygenation therapy. In: Metabolitic mechanisms of hyperbaric oxygenation. Voronezsh. 1980:15–18 (in Russian).
24. Efouni SN (ed.). Hyperbaric oxygenation: a manual. Moscow: Medicina; 1986 (in Russian).
25. Loginov AS, Ambartsumian RV, Sakalova GN, Markin EP *et al*. The use of laser of copper vapour in the treatment of longly non-healing stomach ulcers. Proceedings of the International Symposium 'The Use of Laser in Surgery and Medicine'. Samarkand. Moscow: 1988; part 2:125–7 (in Russian).

45
Nutritional therapy

I. H. ROSENBERG and M. E. CAMILO

It is over one half-century since the definitive descriptions of terminal ileitis, now included among related inflammatory diseases of the intestinal tract under the name of Crohn's disease. Over this span of time there has been steady progress in our understanding of some of the complex pathogenetic mechanisms in Crohn's disease and the often-related ulcerative colitis, but in neither condition have we learned the aetiology or the prevention. Thus, while incidence and prevalence have changed over time and place, suggesting the strong involvement of environmental and perhaps dietary factors in the aetiopathogenesis of these diseases, our management continues to depend upon a judicious use of drug therapies directed to the suppression of abnormal inflammation and immune reactivity, and the judicious use of surgical/resective techniques when medical and drug therapy have failed to control obstruction, debilitation or uncontrolled bleeding.

Implicit in the goals of both medical and surgical approaches to management has been the maintenance or restoration of a normal nutritional status with an active and satisfying quality of life and longevity. Indeed, the patient's capacity to eat and maintain weight and nutritional status as an adult, or to achieve normal growth and development in the case of disease onset in childhood, have been major measures of the effectiveness of medical or surgical therapy. One could say that the final pathway of all management in inflammatory bowel diseases, but especially in the case of Crohn's disease, is the ability to maintain a dietary state free of debility and consequences of malnutrition.

During the past quarter-century the place of nutritional management in patients with inflammatory bowel disease received the added impetus of newer approaches to nutritional support in the form of techniques of total parenteral nutrition and enteral nutrition with defined formula diets. With the advent of these new technologies it became possible to maintain full and adequate nutrition support for patients on otherwise highly restricted diets or even on nothing-by-mouth regimens. The concept of primary nutritional therapy for the management of patients with Crohn's disease has been proposed and investigated, as has the possibility that 'total bowel rest' associated with a nothing-by-mouth regimen with intravenous parenteral nutrition would result by that intervention alone in remissions of disease. The capacity to perform total parenteral nutrition for periods of weeks or even months and years, at home in patients with intestinal insufficiency syndromes after surgery, has had a revolutionary impact on the therapeutic armamentarium in these diseases. The ability to use formula diets as supplemental nutritional therapy, or even total nutrition by mouth or by enteral tube, has likewise dramatically expanded management options. The first anecdotal reports of these therapies have given way to retrospective and some prospective studies, and finally to some controlled clinical trials which place these nutritional approaches in the broad perspective of management in inflammatory disease.

Heretofore, we have referred to nutritional management of both Crohn's disease and ulcerative colitis together, but it will be important and necessary to address separately these two main types of inflammatory bowel disease, as we assess our accumulating experience, and that in the literature on nutritional aspects of management.

CROHN'S DISEASE

Crohn's disease is characterized by an unpredictable sequence of remissions and relapses. Nutritional management will differ depending on the clinical setting.

Periods of symptomatic quiescence

The diet must be adequate to meet the individual needs in macro- and micronutrients, to maintain or restore nutritional parameters and growth. Dietary intervention, taking into account the extent and location of disease and/or resection, may involve dietary restrictions or exclusions as well as supplementation.

Patients with a documented lactose intolerance must follow a lactose-free diet, which in the long term may lead to a negative calcium balance. However, most patients will tolerate just a moderate restriction; otherwise or especially in growing children or adolescents, the use of bacterial lactase (LactAid) added at the time of the meal may efficiently reduce symptoms and lactose malabsorption.

Besides dairy products, a variety of foods, mainly cereals (wheat) and vegetables, have been reported to be associated with food intolerance and abdominal symptoms. Personalized food exclusion diets have been reported to induce longer remission periods[1-3]. Whenever under suspicion, three portions of each food were eaten on its test day, and if no symptoms were noted over the next 48 hours the food was subsequently eaten *ad libitum*. If the food induced symptoms, that food was avoided thereafter (though a later challenge might be attempted). Although this approach has not achieved wide acceptance, the concept of food intolerance as a factor in the altered immune response of the intestine in Crohn's continues to have strong adherents.

Fat restriction to 70–80 g/day usually suffices to lessen steatorrhoea and improve calcium, magnesium and zinc balances. Patients with extensive ileal resection or short bowel syndrome may need further reduction, in which case medium-chain triglycerides and/or natural or commercially available carbohydrates are used to augment calorie intake. Dietary fat restriction reduces the absorption of oxalate and decreases the risk of calcium oxalate kidney stones. To further decrease the risk of oxalate renal stones supplemental calcium can be taken along with meals, and the oral intake of fluids should be increased.

Fibre restriction has been widely used, but often without scientific basis. It has been argued that insoluble vegetable fibre may cause further obstruction or encourage bacterial overgrowth proximal to intestinal strictures or narrowing[2], and this may cause exacerbation of symptoms. The individual patient with rigid stenosis may do better with no fibre at all (chemically defined diets), but will almost always need surgery. On the other hand, diets with high fibre and low unrefined carbohydrates have been shown to be of some benefit[4,5]. The majority of asymptomatic patients should be encouraged to eat a normal fibre diet[6]. Long-term restriction of fibre-containing fruits and vegetables may induce marginal deficiencies in folic acid, vitamin C, and other vitamins and minerals. The use of soluble fibre to improve some forms of diarrhoea is under investigation.

Whenever restrictions are needed, the total diet must be naturally or artificially manipulated to provide the proper amount of macro- and micronutrients. Special attention must be paid to patients who are taking drugs that interfere with the absorption or metabolism of nutrients. Corticosteroid therapy interferes with calcium absorption and bone metabolism. Sulphasalazine can induce folate deficiency[7]. Cholestyramine may increase steatorrhoea and the risk of osteomalacia and deficiency of fat-soluble vitamins, folate and B_{12}. Some patients may need specific micronutrient supplementation beyond the standard preventive multivitamin preparation containing one to three times the normal recommended daily allowance (RDA). Higher therapeutic doses (5–10 × RDA) are indicated for an established deficiency and/or a malabsorptive state. Persistent diarrhoea may require supplementation with zinc as zinc sulphate and magnesium as magnesium oxide. Iron deficiency may respond to oral iron supplements, though these are often ill tolerated. We advocate a slower supplementation, preferably in a liquid form, with ferrous salts containing 30–60 mg of elemental iron, along with 500 mg of ascorbic acid for a positive effect on iron absorption. Patients with extensive disease and/or resection of the terminal ileum, or stenosis and bacterial overgrowth, require intramuscular vitamin B_{12} at a dose of 1000 µg with intervals not longer than 3 months. Vitamins B_{12}, A (5000 IU/day p.o.), vitamin D_3 (2500 IU/day p.o.), and eventually K_1 (5 mg/day p.o.) are recommended for patients with extensive ileitis and/or resection or diffuse bowel disease. Prolonged sulphasalazine therapy requires folic acid supplementation (1 mg/day p.o.) and long-term corticosteroids should be accompanied by calcium (after ruling out hypercalciuria) and vitamin D_3 (2500 IU/day p.o.).

Rarely there may be a need for macronutrient supplementation with modular products, either concentrated protein, fat as medium-chain triglycerides or partially digested carbohydrates.

Periods of exacerbation

During flare-ups or complications, management is often based on drug and/or surgical therapy; however, the benefits of nutrition intervention cannot be dismissed. During acute exacerbations, malabsorption, decreased intake, increased nutrient losses or requirements are more conspicuous, increasing the risk of nutritional deficiencies. Nutritional maintenance or repletion by the use of standard diet may be difficult. An *oral low-residue bland diet* enriched with vitamins and minerals is usually prescribed. To achieve a desired high-energy high-nitrogen intake, particularly in malnourished patients, the use of dietary supplements, as a low-residue complete nutritional liquid preparation, has proved to be beneficial both in nutritional and disease activity parameters[8]. The nutritional effect is still observed in more severe cases[9].

Whenever an oral diet is not tolerated, unable to satisfy patients' needs, or its use is precluded (e.g. intestinal obstruction, toxic megacolon, some fistula), a nothing-by-mouth and *parenteral nutrition* (TPN) regimen has been advocated. The rationale is that TPN will provide adequate nutrition for protein synthesis and immune function, while dietary avoidance may decrease intestinal inflammation by decreasing digestive secretions and motility, as well as by reducing the antigenic or trauma chemical response to food and bacterial substances: the 'bowel rest therapy'. Mostly retrospective studies demonstrated that the use of TPN with added drug therapy is associated with a clinical remission in 60–70% of patients, maintenance or improvement of nutritional status and reversal of growth retardation[10]; similar results were later observed with enteral nutrition. The optimal duration of TPN to induce remission is 4–6 weeks. Small intestinal disease is more likely to respond than large bowel disease[10], though there is some benefit in severe acute Crohn's colitis[11]. TPN sometimes allowed a reduction or discontinuation of corticosteroid therapy. Although TPN has proved effective in severe or complicated Crohn's disease, resistant to medical therapy, either in prospective[12,13] or retrospective studies[14], there is no prospective randomized controlled trial comparing TPN alone with standard medical therapy. In addition, the increased risks associated with the permanence of an intravenous access, as well as those derived from the absence of nutrients into the intestinal lumen (enhanced risk of bacterial translocation and systemic infection) has diminished the use of TPN in favour of the more physiological and cost-effective enteral route[1,13]. The evidence indicates that TPN in Crohn's disease should be considered mainly as adjunctive and supportive rather than as primary therapy. However, TPN is associated with a high healing rate in enterocutaneous fistulae without distal obstruction, and in some circumstances is the only therapy available.

It is particularly important in patients with extensive resections, with or without short bowel syndrome, and recurrence of stenosing disease with inflammation. The duration of remission is variable but may be substantial. This finding has led to the use of home TPN for recurrent uncontrolled disease. Home TPN is fundamental in severe short bowel syndrome[15], and may also be used for nutritional repletion prior to surgery, unhealing fistulae or growth retardation[16]. The latter indications presume a previous failure or refusal of the enteral route.

In the past 10 years interest has focused mainly in the provision of *enteral feeding* as primary therapy in acute Crohn's disease. In a number of prospective controlled randomized studies, elemental diets have proved to be as good as, or superior[17,18] to, drug therapy[17,19,20], TPN[1], or polymeric diets[18,21,22]. Polymeric diets have been compared to drug therapy; the remission rate was similar in children[23], but was lower in adults[24,25]. Conflicting results may result from differences in the trial design, as well as in the composition of the chemically defined diets. Lactose-free, fibre-free nutritional liquid formulae are preferred. All of the tested diets provide to a certain extent some degree of 'bowel rest' along with a positive intraluminal nutrient stimulation of mucosal growth. However, elemental diets which are restricted in fat may be more readily absorbed and contain more glutamine (gut-specific) nutrient. In the acute situation the available evidence suggests elemental diets may be superior, and a retrospective study has shown a long-term remission rate similar to that achieved with medical therapy[26]. The poor palatability may be in part overcome by flavouring, cooling or drinking from a straw; failing this, the diet may be administered via a fine-bore nasogastric or nasoenteric tube. Enteral formulas are successful in: reversing nutritional deficits and growth retardation, decreasing subjective and objective signs of disease activity, decreasing fistula drainage and promoting healing. Patients with symptomatic strictures do particularly well, and their remission may be improved by a food exclusion diet[1]. Colonic or perianal diseases have a worse response. At present, enteral nutrition is a valuable tool in the management of the hospitalized or ambulatory patient either as an adjunctive or an alternative to conventional medical treatment, in case of resistance or failure.

ULCERATIVE COLITIS

Nutritional deficiencies are less common and less severe than in Crohn's. Nutritional management has less impact in the patient's outcome.

Quiescent periods

The diet must be adequate to meet the nutritional needs in macro- and micronutrients. Patients with documented lactose intolerance should receive a lactose-restricted diet. There are no objective reasons to reduce fibre as a permanent procedure, yet a low-residue diet is usually prescribed during diarrhoea bouts. Soluble fibres may prove in the future to be helpful, through its positive effect on water reabsorption and production of volatile fatty acids which provide energy to colonocytes. As a consequence of drug maintenance therapy with sulphasalazine, a competitive inhibitor of folic acid absorption, there is a high risk of folic acid deficiency. Folid acid supplementation is advised (1 mg/day) and may have the additional benefit of decreasing the risk of colonic dysplasia[27]. Iron deficiency occurs as a consequence of intermittent or chronic blood loss, a feature of the symptomatic patient. Whenever it occurs, oral supplementation with ferrous salts is usually well tolerated.

Symptomatic colitis

Patients are given a low-residue diet and/or a chemically defined formula. A high-energy, high-nitrogen intake is advocated, and may be better achieved with an enteral formula; this may improve nutrition but not patients' outcome[9]. TPN is regularly used in patients with toxic megacolon. In severe acute colitis a nothing-by-mouth + TPN regimen does not influence outcome when compared with an oral diet[11]. It may still be useful in the individual patient whose intake is not satisfactory[10,11].

References

1. Jones VA. Comparison of total parenteral nutrition and elemental diet in induction of remission of Crohn's disease: long-term maintenance of remission by personalized food exclusion diets. Dig Dis Sci. 1987;32:100S–7S.
2. Raouf AH, Hildray V, Daniel J *et al.* Enteral feeding as sole treatment for Crohn's disease: controlled trial of whole protein v amino acid based feed and a case study of dietary challenge. Gut. 1991;32:702–7.
3. Riordan AM, Hunter JO. Multicentre controlled trial of diet in the treatment of active Crohn's disease (CD). Gastroenterology. 1992;102:A685.
4. Heaton KW, Thorton JR, Emmet PM. Treatment of Crohn's disease with an unrefined-carbohydrate, fibre-rich diet. Br Med J. 1979;2:764–6.
5. Ritchie JK, Wadsworth J, Lennard-Jones JE, Rogers E. Controlled multicentre therapeutic trial of an unrefined carbohydrate, fiber rich diet in Crohn's disease. Br Med J. 1987;295:517–20.
6. Levenstein S, Prantera C, Luzi C, D'Ubaldi A. Low residue or normal diet in Crohn's disease: a prospective controlled study in Italian patients. Gut. 1985;26:989–93.
7. Franklin JL, Rosenberg IH. Impaired folic acid absorption in inflammatory bowel disease: effects of salicylazosulfapyridine (azulfidine). Gastroenterology. 1973;64:517–25.
8. Harries AD, Jones LA, Davis V *et al.* Controlled trial of supplemented oral nutrition in Crohn's disease. Lancet. 1983;1:887–90.
9. Gassull MA, Abad A, Cabre E, Gonzalez-Huiz F, Gine JJ, Dolz C. Enteral nutrition in inflammatory bowel disease. Gut. 1986(Suppl. 1):76–80.
10. Silk DBA, Payne-James J. Inflammatory bowel disease: nutritional implications and treatment. Proc Nutr Soc. 1989;48:355–61.
11. McIntyre PB, Powell-Tuck J, Wood SR *et al.* Controlled trial of bowel rest in the treatment of severe acute colitis. Gut. 1986;27:481–5.
12. Muller JM, Keller HW, Erasmi H, Pichlmaier H. Total parenteral nutrition as the sole therapy in Crohn's disease – a prospective study. Br J Surg. 1983;70:40–3.
13. Greenberg GR, Fleming CR, Jeejeebhoy KN, Rosenberg IH, Sales D, Tremaine WJ. Controlled trial of bowel rest and nutritional support in the management of Crohn's disease. Gut. 1988;29:1309–15.

14. Ostro MJ, Greeberg GR, Jeejebhoy KN. Total parenteral nutrition and complete bowel rest in the management of Crohn's disease. J Parent Ent Nutr. 1985;9:280–7.
15. Purdum PP, Kirby DF. Short-bowel syndrome: a review of the role of nutrition support. J Parent Ent Nutr. 1991;15:93–100.
16. Strobel CT, Byrne WJ, Ament ME. Home parenteral nutrition in children with Crohn's disease: an effective management alternative. Gastroenterology. 1979;77:272–9.
17. Okada M, Yao T, Yamamoto T *et al.* Controlled trial comparing an elemental diet with prednisolone in the treatment of active Crohn's disease. Hepatogastroenterology. 1990;37:72–80.
18. Giaffer MH, North G, Holdsworth CD. Controlled trial of polymeric versus elemental diet in treatment of active Crohn's disease. Lancet. 1990;335:816–19.
19. O'Morain C, Segal AW, Levi AJ. Elemental diets in treatment of acute Crohn's disease: a controlled trial. Br Med J. 1984;2818:1859–62.
20. Saverymuttu S, Hodgson HJF, Chadwick VS. Controlled trial comparing prednisolone with an elemental diet, plus non-absorbable antibiotics in active Crohn's disease. Gut. 1985;26:994–8.
21. Rigaud D, Cosnes J, Le Quintrec Y, Rene E, Gender JP, Mignon M. Controlled trial comparing two types of enteral nutrition in treatment of active Crohn's disease: elemental v polymeric diet. Gut. 1991;32:1492–7.
22. Royall D, Kahan I, Baker YP *et al.* Clinical and nutritional outcome of an elemental vs semi-elemental diet in active Crohn's disease. Gastroenterology. 1992;102:A576.
23. Sanderson IR, Udeen S, Davies PSN, Savage MO, Walker-Smith JA. Remission induced by an elemental diet in small bowel Crohn's disease. Arch Dis Child. 1987;61:123–7.
24. Malchow H, Steinhart HJ, Lorenz-Meyer H *et al.* Feasibility and effectiveness of a defined-formula diet regimen in treating active Crohn's disease. Scand J Gastroenterol. 1990;25:235–44.
25. Lochs H, Steinhardt HJ, Klaus-Wentz B *et al.* Comparison of enteral nutrition and drug treatment in active Crohn's disease. Gastroenterology. 1991;101:881–8.
26. Teahon K, Bjarnason I, Pearson M, Levi AJ. Ten years' experience with an elemental diet in the management of Crohn's disease. Gut. 1990;31:1133–7.
27. Lashner BA, Heidenreich PA, Su GL, Kane SV, Hanauer SB. The effect of folate supplementation on the incidence of dysplasia and cancer in chronic ulcerative colitis: a case–control study. Gastroenterology. 1989;97:255–9.

46

Future treatments: facts, hopes and fantasies

J. E. LENNARD-JONES

INTRODUCTION

Conceptually, it seems likely that the chronic or recurrent inflammation of ulcerative colitis and Crohn's disease begins with an interaction between a factor in the gut lumen and the epithelial barrier between the gut contents and the vulnerable tissues of the mucosa. Chemical compounds or bacteria enter the lamina propria and initiate a complex immunological and inflammatory response. Many types of cytokine and chemical mediator are released which recruit polymorphs, macrophages and lymphocytes to the mucosa. Tissue and vascular damage result which in turn contribute to self-perpetuating or relapsing inflammation.

Factors acting from the lumen may be nutrients, other components of food or drinking water, bacteria, or compounds produced by the action of bacteria on nutrients. A consideration of treatment must therefore begin with food and drink, which may contain an aggravation factor or alternatively be deficient in a substance needed to maintain mucosal integrity or diminish inflammation. Insufficient attention has been given to the role of intestinal bacteria, or viruses, as a trigger or aggravating factor in IBD. Treatments designed to alter the bacterial flora of the gut may therefore be important.

Once initiated, the inflammatory cascade can be reduced by measures which interfere with the synthesis of chemical mediators, which block their action, which reduce the clonal expansion of activated lymphocytes, or which antagonize the effect of toxic inflammatory products such as free oxygen radicals. These mechanisms appear to be the mode of action of the three classes of drug, all shown to have a beneficial effect in IBD, corticosteroids, aminosalicylates and immunosuppressives.

This review will state the facts about each of these modes of treatment, based as far as possible on controlled therapeutic trials, and express hopes about their further development. Where current lines of research and imagination allow I will entertain fantasies about possible new, untested and even undescribed treatments.

NUTRIENTS

Dietary modification could remove an aggravating factor or supply a nutrient which improves the integrity of the epithelium or reduces inflammation.

Facts about removing nutrients from the gut lumen

1. Removal of nutrients from the gut does not reduce the inflammation of acute ulcerative colitis[1,2].
2. There is evidence that surgical diversion of intestinal contents from the intestinal lumen benefits Crohn's disease[3].
3. Removal of nutrients from the gut lumen in Crohn's disease using parenteral nutrition and withholding food by mouth, has been assessed by retrospective comparison with the response of patients to previous treatments. Such comparisons suggest benefit but there has been no direct comparison with an untreated group.
4. There is conflicting evidence as to whether parenteral nutrition and bowel rest gives better or the same results, as parenteral nutrition *and* food by mouth[4,5] or as liquid diets given alone[6].

Facts about altering the consistency or composition of the diet

1. When a blenderized normal diet was compared with a hydrolyzed liquid diet over 2 weeks in patients with ulcerative colitis or Crohn's disease, bowel frequency, and thus a clinical activity index, improved equally in both treatment groups. There was no apparent improvement in laboratory indices of inflammation in either disease or in the appearance of the rectal mucosa in ulcerative colitis[7].
2. Elemental liquid diets have given equivalent results to corticosteroids in a number of small trials, provided that the diet could be tolerated[8,9].
3. A hydrolyzed liquid diet was associated with a slower and reduced remission rate in Crohn's disease as compared with a drug regime of prednisone and sulphasalazine[10].
4. There is dispute as to whether an elemental, hydrolyzed or polymeric diet give the same or different results in active Crohn's disease[11–13].
5. A bran supplement does not prevent relapse in ulcerative colitis[14].
6. A diet low in sugar but high in unrefined carbohydrate does not benefit Crohn's disease[15]; nor does a low-residue diet[16].

Facts about supplying specific additional nutrients

1. A small pilot crossover trial has suggested that sodium butyrate given as a retention enema benefits distal ulcerative colitis[17].
2. Certain polyunsaturated fatty acids, particularly eicosapentanoic acid, can replace arachidonic acid in the cell membrane and affect eicosanoid synthesis with a reduction in the production of leukotriene B4 (LTB4) and other potentially harmful products. So far controlled therapeutic trials have shown the expected changes in the cell membrane but have failed to show clinically significant benefit[18,19].

Hopes

The role of liquid diets in the treatment of Crohn's disease needs clear definition. First, a comparative trial of an elemental, a hydrolyzed and a polymeric diet lasting 4 weeks is required, each of these diets being given by infusion through a nasogastric tube to avoid problems of unpalatability and administration as a liquid bolus. The trial should contain at least 150 patients with proven active Crohn's disease as judged by objective criteria of endoscopy, biopsy and measurement of acute-phase reactants or cytokines in the blood. Patients should be stratified according to the site of their disease. Assessment of the treatments should include both symptoms and the objective criteria to judge whether or not the lesions heal and inflammation is reduced.

If one type of diet proves better than the others, further trials are indicated. First, it should be compared with blenderized normal food to establish the fact that the result is superior to placebo. Second, it should be compared with standard drug therapy. Third, trials should be conducted in which additions are made to the best liquid diet in an effort to establish the basis for its benefit.

If the three types of liquid diet give equivalent results then it will be possible to abandon the unpalatable and expensive elemental diet, and also the hydrolyzed diet, in favour of a more palatable inexpensive (? non-milk-based) polymeric diet.

Fantasies

1. A specific foodstuff or food additive will be discovered as the environmental factor which has caused the increased incidence of Crohn's disease during the past 40 years.
2. A specific dietary supplement, perhaps glutamine or fatty acids will provide a harmless inexpensive treatment for Crohn's disease and/or ulcerative colitis.

BACTERIA

The colon contains a predominance of anaerobic bacteria. During attacks of ulcerative colitis there is an increase in the gut flora of *E. coli* with adhesive properties, and an increase in the proportion of *E. coli* which produce haemolysin and enterotoxin.

Mycobacterium paratuberculosis has been cultured from the mucosa of a few patients with Crohn's disease, and unidentified spheroplasts which have acid-fast properties can be isolated from a larger proportion of patients. An insertion sequence characteristic of *M. paratuberculosis* can be detected by the polymerase chain reaction in the bowel wall of about two-thirds of patients with Crohn's disease, a proportion significantly greater than in tissue removed for ulcerative colitis or other disorders.

Facts

1. A comparative trial in Crohn's disease has shown that metronidazole has approximately the same therapeutic benefit as sulphasalazine[20]. Since sulphasalazine is less effective than corticosteroids (see below) metronidazole is therefore only a moderately effective treatment.
2. Metronidazole in large doses, given over a prolonged period, suppresses inflammation of Crohn's perianal lesions but the lesions tend to give trouble again when the drug is stopped[21].
3. Metronidazole given intravenously to patients with severe acute colitis in one trial did not improve the results of treatment with prednisolone[22].
4. Tobramycin given by mouth to patients with active ulcerative colitis in a controlled trial improved the results of treatment with prednisolone[23].
5. Three controlled trials of antimycobacterial treatment in active Crohn's disease have failed to show benefit[24–27]. A trial of a quadruple-drug regime given to patients with Crohn's disease in remission after corticosteroid treatment reduced the relapse rate over 9 months[28] but this result could have been due to a non-specific effect of the drugs used rather than a specific effect on mycobacteria.

Hopes

It seems possible that relapses of inflammatory bowel disease are due to a change in the gut flora, for example proliferation of an organism with adhesive or toxin-producing capability. If this proves to be the case relapses might be avoided by protecting a patient against such organisms, perhaps by a vaccine or frequent recolonization of the gut with known commensal harmless bacteria to the exclusion of pathogenic strains.

Too little attention has been given to the use of broad-spectrum antibacterial drugs, or those active against aerobic bacteria, in the treatment of acute attacks of ulcerative colitis and Crohn's disease. Further trials of such drugs are needed, preferably supported by microbiological studies. Gut lavage with saline also requires investigation as an early treatment of an acute attack.

Fantasies

In the future, molecular biological techniques may make it possible for rapid and accurate identification of the faecal flora. Organisms at present unrecognized which contribute to worsening of colitis or Crohn's disease may be recognized early and treated specifically.

Crohn's disease is a heterogeneous disorder and some cases may be due to specific infection. Recognition of such cases, and the organism involved, possibly a cell-wall deficient mycobacterium could lead to specific treatment and cure. I dream of a specific treatment for Crohn's disease which changes the whole course of the disease, just as happened with tuberculosis when streptomycin and other drugs were introduced.

AMINOSALICYLATES

The classic experiment of testing sulphasalazine and its two constituent moieties as retention enemas or suppositories in active ulcerative colitis showed that the whole molecule and 5-aminosalicylic acid (mesalazine, 5-ASA), but not sulphapyridine, reduced inflammation. Subsequently 4-aminosalicylic acid (4-ASA), better known as para-aminosalicylic acid (PAS), has been shown to be similarly effective when given by retention enema in ulcerative colitis. Much work has resulted in the development of two compounds with an azo-link (olsalazine and colazide) and various formulations of 5-ASA designed to bring the drug into contact with the whole length of the gut, the distal ileal and colonic mucosa, or the mucosa of the rectum and distal colon. The mode of action of these drugs is not known, though they affect eicosanoid synthesis and also act as scavengers of free oxygen radicals.

Facts

1. Sulphasalazine and 5-ASA compounds or formulations designed to release 5-ASA in the colon, when given by mouth, are effective treatments for moderately active ulcerative colitis, though slower in action than corticosteroids.
2. Sulphasalazine, 5-ASA or 4-ASA when given as a retention enema or foam, are effective treatments for distal colitis, and as suppositories for proctitis.
3. Sulphasalazine and delayed-release 5-ASA preparations reduce the relapse rate in quiescent ulcerative colitis.
4. It has not proved possible to show that sulphasalazine decreases the relapse rate in Crohn's disease but there is increasing evidence that delayed release preparations of 5-ASA, and perhaps 4-ASA, may do so[29,30].

Hopes

It is not known whether the action of aminosalicylates in decreasing relapse in quiescent ulcerative colitis is the same as that which reduces inflammation in active ulcerative colitis. If the mode of action in decreasing relapse could be discovered, more potent but harmless drugs might be introduced which prevent relapse in ulcerative colitis and so greatly affect the natural history of the disease.

4-ASA is a more stable compound than 5-ASA; trials of 4-ASA given by mouth in active ulcerative colitis and Crohn's disease, and as a maintenance treatment in both conditions are warranted.

As in ulcerative colitis, the major problem in Crohn's disease is to prevent relapse, particularly after surgical treatment. The results of trials which include repeated endoscopic observation of anastomoses or previously diseased areas to observe whether the drug leads to healing or prevention of ulceration, are awaited with the hope that the relapse rate can be reduced.

Fantasy

A harmless drug is developed as a result of research on these simple molecules which can be taken long-term to eliminate the relapse rate in inflammatory bowel disease after successful medical or surgical treatment of an acute episode.

CORTICOSTEROIDS

Corticosteroids have multiple actions in reducing the inflammatory cascade. Among other actions they inhibit release of free arachidonic acid from cell membranes, and thus reduce the substrate available for synthesis of eicosanoids, including leukotriene B4, and also reduce lymphoid proliferation. Experimentally, corticosteroids in pharmacological doses reduce immunological reactions most effectively when given just before, or at the time of, exposure to antigen. There has been a long-running controversy as to whether corticosteroids applied locally to the inflamed mucosa of distal colitis act locally or after systemic absorption. The effectiveness of poorly absorbed steroids, or steroids metabolized on first passage through the mucosa or liver, has shown that these steroids have a local effect on inflammation.

Facts

1. Systemic corticosteroids reduce inflammation in a proportion of patients with acute ulcerative colitis; the proportion who improve is inversely related to the severity of the attack.
2. Systemic corticosteroids reduce inflammation in a proportion of patients with active Crohn's disease.
3. Corticosteroids administered topically reduce the inflammation in about two-thirds of patients with active distal ulcerative colitis. This effect is similar whether or not the steroid is absorbed to give potentially therapeutic blood levels.
4. Systemic corticosteroids given in doses low enough to avoid systemic side-effects do not reduce the relapse rate in quiescent ulcerative colitis or Crohn's disease.

Hopes

All clinicians see patients whose ulcerative colitis or Crohn's disease remains under control while they take a corticosteroid in a dose equivalent to prednisolone 10–15 mg daily but in whom disease activity increases if the dose is reduced. Oral administration of a poorly absorbed or rapidly metabolized corticosteroid, perhaps targeted as a delayed-release formulation, requires study in the hope that remission can be achieved by long-term use, yet without side-effects.

Failing this, long-term administration of currently available corticosteroids requires further study, particularly as alternate-day[31] or pulse therapy, and with the simultaneous use of measures to preserve bone density. Research is also needed into why some patients respond to oral or topical corticosteroid treatment and why others do not.

Fantasy

A locally acting corticosteroid drug is developed which is active in every patient and can be continued indefinitely without side-effects. Such a drug leads to healing of the disease and then maintains remission.

IMMUNOSUPPRESSIVE DRUGS

The immunological response in IBD requires activation and clonal amplification of lymphocytes. One mode of action of immunosuppressive agents in treatment of inflammatory bowel disease may be to limit this clonal expansion. In general these drugs are potentially toxic; indications for their use have to be clearly defined and their administration has to be carefully monitored.

Facts

1. Azathioprine and 6-mercaptopurine exert a steroid-sparing effect in chronic active ulcerative colitis and Crohn's disease.
2. 6-Mercaptopurine has an anti-inflammatory effect in chronic active Crohn's disease when given with other drugs. It acts slowly and the mean time to a discernible effect in one trial was 3.2 months[32].
3. Azathioprine, like 6-MP, reduces inflammation in some patients with Crohn's disease and clinical activity tends to recur when the drug is withdrawn, this effect appears independent of the duration of treatment up to 5 years from onset[33].
4. Azathioprine maintains quiescence in some patients with ulcerative colitis shown by the fact that the disease relapses more frequently when the drug is withdrawn than when it is continued[34]. This effect appears to persist for at least 2 years after start of treatment.
5. Cyclosporin benefited a small proportion of patients with chronic active Crohn's disease in one trial[35] while the drug was given, but no significant

effect remained 6 months after discontinuing treatment[36]. Cyclosporin did not prevent relapse in a large series of patients with quiescent Crohn's disease[37].

Hopes

The fact that azathioprine or 6-mercaptopurine reduce inflammation and maintain remission in some cases of chronic active Crohn's disease and ulcerative colitis gives hope that other immunosuppressive drugs may be even more effective. Further trials are needed to define the optimum duration of treatment of these two drugs; does one of them have to be continued indefinitely or can it be stopped after a period of years? In general, the long-term side effects appear few, but the risk of neoplasia requires further assessment and there now appears reasonable hope that it will be low.

Even though early data on the use of cyclosporin in Crohn's disease was encouraging, further study suggests that its use will be restricted to a few patients with complications if special indications for its use can be defined. Anecdotal data now suggest that cyclosporin may have a role in the treatment of severe active ulcerative colitis when given intravenously or chronic active distal colitis when given by retention enema. Hopefully, these reports will be confirmed by controlled trial and a new treatment for steroid-resistant ulcerative colitis will become available.

Methotrexate in an uncontrolled study has given encouraging results in chronic active Crohn's disease and, less so, in ulcerative colitis[38]. The only controlled trial so far reported has suggested that the drug may have a role in reducing the frequency of relapse in chronic active Crohn's disease, but further studies are needed to confirm this hope before the drug is used routinely, especially as its use can be associated with serious side-effects such as interstitial pneumonitis[39].

Fantasies

The steps in the inflammatory cascade are now recognized in some detail. It is apparent that activated lymphocytes, monocytes, and polymorphonuclear leucocytes move into the inflamed area in response to expression by macrophages and lymphocytes of many different cytokines, and the possible presence of chemo-attractants derived from bacteria. Once they have entered the tissue, the activated cells produce a multitude of potentially damaging agents such as antibodies, free oxygen radicals, cytokines, enzymes, kinins and histamine. To check this inflammatory cascade most effectively, the earliest phases of the reaction need to be blocked.

The expansion of CD4+ lymphocytes can be prevented by a monoclonal antibody directed against these cells. Pilot studies have already been undertaken in a few patients with active inflammatory bowel disease with encouraging therapeutic results and no adverse effects[40,41]. Cells with high-affinity receptors to IL2, mainly lymphocytes, can be selectively killed by use of an IL-2 fusion toxin.

Many of the early stages of the inflammatory response are mediated by interleukin-1 (IL-1). There is a natural receptor antagonist, which is available for experimental use and offers a potential treatment. A soluble receptor is also available which can absorb and thus remove this cytokine, so preventing its action.

Leukotriene B4 is a potent cytokine which plays an early role in the inflammatory cascade. Inhibitors of the lipoxygenase enzyme which leads to the synthesis of LTB4 are available and show promise[42,43].

Thus several approaches are already available for depressing specific events in the inflammatory response before the release of multiple potentially damaging compounds by inflammatory cells damage the mucosa. Approaches along these lines in the future may be used to prevent or control inflammation.

FURTHER HOPES AND FANTASIES

Elegant electron microscopic and micro-injection studies have shown that occlusion of blood vessels in the deeper layers of the gut wall is a feature of the pathogenesis of Crohn's disease. It is likely that expression of white cell and vascular endothelial procoagulant activity is the initiating event in fibrin formation. Induction of procoagulant activity is a property of IL-1 and its action is antagonized by prostacyclin synthesis from arachidonic acid by the cyclooxygenase pathway. Prostacyclin inhibits platelet aggregation and is a vasodilator. Measures to reduce vascular thrombosis by blocking the action of IL-1, promoting prostacyclin synthesis, and possibly some form of anticoagulant treatment may decrease tissue damage and prove to be an important treatment. Prostacyclin synthesis is impaired by smoking and may be a reason for advising a reduction in tobacco consumption by patients with Crohn's disease[44].

It is likely that some of the systemic effects of IBD such as anorexia, protein catabolism and growth retardation are mediated by tumour necrosis factor or other cytokines. Monoclonal antibodies directed against them or receptor antagonists may prove to be an important treatment, especially in young people. Whereas current drug treatments have many possible actions in decreasing the inflammatory cascade, specific agents, for example free oxygen radical scavengers, may be developed and prove useful in preventing tissue damage.

CONCLUSION

The role of nutrients and measures to modify the bacterial content of the intestine deserve much greater study, as here may lie the trigger factor for attacks of inflammatory bowel disease. Once the inflammatory cascade begins, established drugs appear to modify it by multiple actions. Drugs and new biological agents are now being developed against specific events in the inflammatory cascade. It remains to be seen whether such treatments prevent, control or modify inflammation sufficiently to give clinical benefit.

References

1. Dickinson RJ, Ashton MG, Axon ATR, Smith RC, Yeung CK, Hill GL. Controlled trial of intravenous hyperalimentation and total bowel rest as an adjunct to the routine therapy of acute colitis. Gastroenterology. 1980;79:1199–204.
2. McIntyre PB, Powell-Tuck J, Wood SR, Lennard-Jones JE, Lerebours E, Hecketsweiler P, Galmiche J-P, Colon R. Controlled trial of bowel rest in the treatment of severe acute colitis. Gut. 1986;27:481–5.
3. Rutgeerts P, Geboes K, Peeters M, Hiele M, Penninckx F, Aerts R, Kerremans R, Vantrappen G. Effect of faecal stream diversion on recurrence of Crohn's Disease in the neoterminal ileum. Lancet. 1991;338:771–4.
4. Greenberg GR, Fleming CR, Jeejeebhoy KN, Rosenberg IH, Sales D, Tremaine WJ. Controlled trial of bowel rest and nutritional support in the management of Crohn's disease. Gut. 1988;29:1309–15.
5. Lochs H, Meryn S, Marosi L, Ferenci P, Hortnagl H. Has total bowel rest a beneficial effect in the treatment of Crohn's disease? Clin Nutr. 1983;2:61–4.
6. Rigaud D, Cerf M, Melchior JC, Sautier C, Rene E, Mignon M. Nutritional assistance (NA) and acute attacks of Crohn's disease (CD): efficacy of total parenteral nutrition (TPN), as compared with elemental (EEN) and polymeric (PEN) enteral nutrition. Gastroenterology. 1989;96:A416.
7. Munkholm Larsen P, Rasmussen D, Ronn D, Munck O, Elmgren J, Binder V. Elemental diet: a therapeutic approach in chronic inflammatory bowel disease. J Intern Med. 1989;225:325–31.
8. O'Morain C, Segal AW, Levi AJ. Elemental diet as primary treatment of acute Crohn's disease; a controlled trial. Br Med J. 1984;288:1859–62.
9. Hunt JB, Payne-James JJ, Palmer KP, Kumar PK, Clark ML, Farthing MJS, Misiewicz JJ, Silk DBA. A randomised controlled trial of elemental diet and prednisolone as primary therapy in acute exacerbations of Crohn's disease. Gastroenterology. 1989;96:A224.
10. Lochs H, Steinhardt HJ, Klaus-Wentz B, Zeitz M, Vogelsang H, Sommer H, Fleig WE, Bauer P, Schirrmeister J, Malchow H. Comparison of enteral nutrition and drug treatment in active Crohn's disease. Gastroenterology. 1991;101:881–8.
11. Rigaud D, Cosnes J, Le Quintrec Y, Rene E, Gendre JP, Mignon M. Controlled trial comparing two types of enteral nutrition in treatment of active Crohn's disease: elemental v polymeric diet. Gut. 1991;32:1492–7.
12. Giaffer MH, North G, Holdsworth CD. Controlled trial of polymeric versus elemental diet in treatment of active Crohn's disease. Lancet. 1990;1:816–18.
13. Raouf AH, Hildrey V, Daniel J, Walker RJ, Krasner N, Elias E, Rhodes JM. Enteral feeding as sole treatment for Crohn's disease: controlled trial of whole protein v amino acid based feed and a case study of dietary challenge. Gut. 1991;32:702–7.
14. Davies PS, Rhodes J. Maintenance of remission in ulcerative colitis with sulphasalazine or a high-fibre diet: a clinical trial. Br Med J. 1978;1:1524–5.
15. Ritchie JK, Wadsworth J, Lennard-Jones JE, Rogers E. Controlled multicentre therapeutic trial of an unrefined carbohydrate, fibre rich diet in Crohn's disease. Br Med J. 1987;295:517–20.
16. Levenstein S, Prantera C, Luzi C, D'Ubaldi A. Low residue or normal diet in Crohn's disease: a prospective controlled study in Italian patients. Gut. 1985;26:989–93.
17. Scheppach W, Sommer H, Kirchner T, Christl SU, Kasper H. Butyrate irrigation for distal ulcerative colitis. Gastroenterology. 1992;102:A691.
18. Hawthorne AB, Daneshmend TK, Hawkey CJ, Belluzi A, Everitt SJ, Holmes GKT, Malkinson C, Shaheen MZ, Willars JE. The treatment of ulcerative colitis with fish oil supplementation: a prospective randomized controlled trial. Gut. 1992;33:922–8.
19. Greenfield SM, Green AT, Teare JP, Punchard NA, Thompson RPH. Final results of a controlled trial of fatty acid supplementation in maintenance treatment of ulcerative colitis. Gastroenterology. 1992;102:A631.
20. Ursing B, Alm T, Barany F, Bergelin I et al. A comparative study of metronidazole and sulfasalazine for active Crohn's Disease: the cooperative Crohn's disease study in Sweden. Gastroenterology. 1982;83:550–62.
21. Brandt LJ, Bernstein LH, Boley SJ, Franks MS. Metronidazole therapy for perineal Crohn's disease: a follow-up study. Gastroenterology. 1982;83:383–7.
22. Chapman RW, Selby WS, Jewell DP. Controlled trial of intravenous metronidazole as an adjunct to corticosteroids in severe ulcerative colitis. Gut. 1986;27:1210–12.

23. Burke DA, Axon ATR, Clayden SA, Dixon MF, Johnston D, Lacey RW. The efficacy of tobramycin in the treatment of ulcerative colitis. Aliment Pharmacol Ther. 1990;4:123–9.
24. Shaffer JL, Hughes S, Linaker BD, Baker RD, Turnberg LA. Controlled trial of rifampicin and ethambutol in Crohn's disease. Gut. 1981;25:203–5.
25. Shaffer JL, Turnberg LA. Does antituberculous chemotherapy for Crohn's disease provide long-term benefit. Gut. 1989;30:A1480.
26. Elliott PR, Burnham WR, Berghouse LM, Lennard-Jones JE, Langman MJS. Sulphadoxine–pyrimethamine therapy in Crohn's disease. Digestion. 1982;23:132–4.
27. Afdhal NH, Long A, Lennon J, Crowe J, O'Donoghue DP. Controlled trial of clofazimine in Crohn's disease. Gut. 1987;28:A1391.
28. Kohn A, Prantera C, Mangiarotti R, Luzi C, Andreoli A. Antimycobacterial therapy and Crohn's disease: a randomized placebo controlled trial. Gastroenterology. 1992;102:A647.
29. International Mesalazine Study Group. Coated oral 5-aminosalacylic acid versus placebo in maintaining remission of inactive Crohn's disease. Aliment Pharmacol Ther. 1990;4:55–64.
30. Prantera C, Pallone F, Brunetti G, Cottone M, Miglioni M and the Italian IBD Study Group. Oral 5-aminosalicylic acid (Asacol) in the maintenance treatment of Crohn's disease. Gastroenterology. 1992;103:363–8.
31. Bello C, Goldstein F, Thornton JJ. Alternate-day prednisone treatment and treatment maintenance in Crohn's disease. Am J Gastroenterol. 1991;86:460–6.
32. Present DH, Korelitz BJ, Wisch N, Glass JL, Sachar DB, Pasternack BS. Treatment of Crohn's disease with 6-mercaptopurine: a long-term, randomized, double-blind study. N Engl J Med. 1980;302:981–1026.
33. O'Donoghue DP, Dawson AM, Powell-Tuck J, Bown RL, Lennard-Jones JE. Double-blind withdrawal trial of azathioprine as maintenance treatment for Crohn's Disease. Lancet. 1978;2:955–7.
34. Hawthorne AB, Logan RFA, Hawkey CJ, Foster PN, Axon ATR, Swarbrick ET, Scott BB, Lennard-Jones JE. Randomised controlled trial of azathioprine withdrawal in ulcerative colitis. Br Med J. 1992;305:20–2.
35. Brynskov J, Freund L, Rasmussen SN et al. A placebo-controlled, double-blind, randomized trial of cyclosporine therapy in active Crohn's disease. N Engl J Med. 1989;321:845–50.
36. Brynskov J, Freund L, Norby Rasmussen S, Lauritsen K, Schaffalitzky de Muckadell O, Williams CN, MacDonald AS, Tanton R, Molina F, Campanini MC, Bianchi P, Ranzi T, Quarto di Palo F, Malchow-Moller A, Ostergaard Thomsen O, Tage-Jensen U, Binder V, Riis P. Final report on a placebo-controlled, double-blind, randomized, multicentre trial of cyclosporin treatment in active chronic Crohn's disease. Scand J Gastroenterol. 1991;26:689–95.
37. Archambault A, Feagan B, Fedorak R, Groll A, Irvine EJ, Kinnear D, Laupacis A, McDonald JWD, Rochon J, Saibil F. The Canadian Crohn's relapse prevention trial (CCRPT). Gastroenterology. 1992;102:A591.
38. Kozarek RA, Patterson DJ, Gelfand MD, Ball TJ, Botoman VA. Long-term use of methotrexate in inflammatory bowel disease: severe disease 3, drug therapy 2. Seventh inning stretch. Gastroenterology. 1992;102:A648.
39. Arora S, Katkov WN, Cooley J, Kemp A, Schapiro RH, Kelsey PB, Podolsky DK. A double-blind, randomized, placebo-controlled trial of methotrexate in Crohn's disease. Gastroenterology. 1992;102:A591.
40. Deusch K, Reiter C, Mauthe B, Riethmuller G, Classen M. Chimeric monoclonal anti-CD4 antibody therapy proves effective for treating inflammatory bowel disease. Gastroenterology. 1992;102:A615.
41. Stronkhorst A, Yong SL, Radema S, ten Berge I, Das PK, Tytgat GN, van Deventer SJH. Phase 1 multiple-dose pilot study of chimeric monoclonal-T412 (anti CD4) antibodies in Crohn's disease. Preliminary data. Gastroenterology. 1992;102:A702.
42. Bukhave K, Laursen LS, Lauritsen K et al. 5-Lipoxygenase inhibition in double-blind trial with zileuton: how much is sufficient in active ulcerative colitis? Gastroenterology. 1991;100:A200.
43. Stenson WF, Lauritsen K, Laursen LS. A clinical trial of zileuton, a specific inhibitor of 5-lipoxygenase, in ulcerative colitis. Gastroenterology. 1991;100:A253.
44. Wakefield AJ, Sawyer AM, Hudson M, Dhillon AP, Pounder RE. Smoking, the oral contraceptive pill, and Crohn's disease. Dig Dis Sci. 1991;36:1147–50.

Section X
Poster presentations

A: Aetiology, animal models

A1

Seasonal appearance of ulcerative colitis

S. KAZIC, B. BRMBOLIC, T. JANKOVIC, S. KOVACEVIC,
B. DAPCEVIC and M. TODOROVIC

According to our experience, more patients with ulcerative colitis are admitted to the hospital during summer months than during other seasons of the year. Therefore, we have retrospectively studied medical records of patients admitted because of ulcerative colitis at Zvezdara Hospital and at the Infectious Disease Hospital in Belgrade in the period 1980–90. Data regarding time of disease onset and intervals of relapses were separately analysed with the chi-square test. There were 74 patients in total, and relapses varied from one to five per patient, making a total of 110 relapses in the whole group.

The first incidence of the disease appeared most frequently in May, June and July. That incidence versus other months of the year was statistically significant ($p < 0.05$). Concerning the intervals between relapses, there was no significant difference between months. We conclude that ulcerative colitis is a disease with prevailing seasonal appearance, and in the May–July period the onset of the disease appears to be more common than in other months of the year.

A2

Experimental studies on dietary aspects of mucosal cell damage: induction of lysosomatic inclusions in macrophages

E. NAGEL, S. SCHATTENFROH, S. BÜHNER and R. PICHLMAYR

Lysosomatic inclusions in mucosal macrophages might be the first stage in the development of granuloma in patients with Crohn's disease (CD). Are these structures inducible by dietary compounds, e.g. heated chemically processed fats (CPF) which are known in pigs to damage the ultrastructure of the mucosal surface similar to CD? We used this model to study deeper mucosal cell layers.

METHODS

Pigs fed either a CPF diet (60% of total energy load; $n = 6$) or normal pig food ($n = 3$) were sacrificed after 3 months. Samples of macroscopically normal ileal mucosa were prepared for transmission electron microscopic analysis.

RESULTS

CPF affected cell structures throughout all mucosal layers. The most striking effects were in the epithelial cell layer: microvilli lesions, mitochondria degeneration, autophagolytic vacuoles, increased number of intraepithelial lymphocytes, goblet cell hyperplasia, widening of intracellular space. Lamina propria: macrophages with big heterogeneous lysosomatic inclusions, infiltration of mast cells, partial axon dilatation.

CONCLUSION

CPF can induce lysosomatic inclusions by mucosal damage. The underlying mechanism could be direct via decomposition of cell membrane structures and/or indirect via accumulation of CPF. It is suggested that these fats can influence immunoresponse in intestinal mucosa.

Supported by the Deutsche Forschungsgemeinschaft grant NA 184/1–2.

A3

Eicosanoids and *Campylobacter* colitis

A. T. COLE, P. EVEREST, P. SIBBONS, R. LEECE, J. KETLEY,
S. KNUTTON, C. J. HAWKEY and P. H. WILLIAMS

The mechanism by which *Campylobacter jejuni* causes colonic inflammation and diarrhoea is unclear. We therefore used a rabbit model to investigate the role of PGE_2, LTB_4 and cAMP in pathogenesis.

Ligated ileal loops were infected with 10^8 viable *C. jejuni* organisms from patients with colitis (four strains) watery diarrhoea (one) or a non-motile mutant strain; $n = 4$ loops each strain. Each rabbit had two test loops, a PBS control and a positive cholera toxin (1 µg) control. Rabbits were sacrificed at 15 h. Tissue and loop fluid were assayed for LTB_4, PGE_2, and cAMP by RIA, and neutrophil infiltrates were scored.

Compared to PBS loops *C. jejuni* isolated from patients with colitis increased mucosal PGE_2 by 14.5 (median, interquartile range 2.6–22.8) ng/g ($n = 16$, $p = 0.088$, Wilcoxon) and cAMP by 0.75 (-1.08 to 4.05) pmol/g and stimulated secretion of 1.5 (median, range 0–18) ml of fluid. This fluid contained 2.16 (median, IQR 1.6–5.22) ng/ml PGE_2 and 0.71 (0.38–4.2) ng/ml LTB_4. Neutrophil infiltration was seen in mucosa from these loops (median grade 2) and correlated with fluid LTB_4 ($p = 0.004$, Pearson) and fluid PGE_2 ($p = 0.02$). Loops with watery diarrhoea or mutant strains showed no neutrophil infiltrate, no fluid production and unchanged PGE_2 ($p = 0.023$, Mann–Whitney, compared to fluid secreting loops) and cAMP production.

In this model *C. jejuni* derived from patients with colitis stimulates an inflammatory response in which PGE_2 is associated with enhanced fluid secretion and LTB_4 and PGE_2 with a neutrophil infiltrate, suggesting these mediators may be important in disease pathophysiology.

A4

Protection in rat colitis models by the sulphydryl modulating compound OR-1364

P. AHO, E. NISSINEN and I.-B. LINDÉN

OR-1364 (3-((3-cyanophenyl)methylene)-2,4-pentanedione) is a cytoprotective compound which forms reversible conjugates with mucosal sulphydryl (SH) groups. Since SH groups are important for maintaining membrane structure and function, we assessed the protective effect of OR-1364 in two models of rat colitis. In the acute model 3.5% acetic acid (AA) was injected into the lumen of the ascending colon. OR-1364 (3–30 mg/kg) was administered intracolonically via rectum 24, 18 and 1 h before and 24 h after AA. In the chronic model 20 mg of trinitrobenzene sulphonic acid (TNB) in 50% ethanol was administered intracolonically and OR-1364 (3–30 mg/kg) was administered 2 h before and 23, 47, 71 and 95 h after TNB. The colonic damage was scored (0–10) and MPO activity was determined 48 h after AA or 96 h after TNB and the release of prostaglandin E_2 (PGE_2) and leukotriene B_4 (LTB_4) from the colons was assayed by RIA.

OR-1364 showed dose-dependent protection in both colitis models decreasing the AA-induced damage score by 53% and MPO activity by 45% at 3 mg/kg and the TNB-damage score by 67% and MPO by 65% at 30 mg/kg. A significant correlation between protection and the initial reaction rate with SH groups was obtained. Although the release of PGE_2 and LTB_4 was increased in the inflamed colons, there was no correlation between damage score and eicosanoid release. Despite a moderate LTB_4 inhibitory activity *in vitro* (IC_{50} 25 μmol/l), OR-1364 did not inhibit eicosanoid production *in vivo*. The findings indicate no crucial role of LTB_4 and PGE_2 in experimental colitis. Instead, the protection by OR-1364 suggests an involvement of mucosal SH groups in the colonic inflammatory process.

A5

Intestinal ischaemia: effects on neuroeffector transmission and neurochemistry of guinea-pig small intestine studied with a pharmacological model

G. M. LEES, P. J. CAMPBELL, S. M. C. CUNNINGHAM, K. N. BROWNING and A. D. CORBETT

Since intermittent ischaemia is thought to play an important role in the aetiology of inflammatory bowel disease, we have examined the effects of anoxia and simulated ischaemia on cholinergic neuroeffector transmission in isolated preparations of guinea-pig small intestine using a new pharmacological model of neuronal ischaemia described by Reiner *et al.* (1990), *Neuroscience Letters*, **119**:175–78.

Sodium cyanide (NaCN; 0.1–3 mmol/l), which blocks oxidative phosphorylation, caused a concentration-dependent, readily reversible inhibition of the electrically evoked contractions of myenteric plexus–longitudinal muscle preparations. These effects were due to both pre- and postjunctional actions. Similar depressions were observed in simple anoxia (95% N_2/5% CO_2) or glucose-free solutions. Blockade of glycolysis by iodoacetic acid (IAA; 0.05–0.5 mmol/l) irreversibly abolished the responses to electrical field stimulation, acetylcholine, histamine and KC1. Interestingly, however, an irreversible blockade of electrically evoked contractions could be induced by a threshold concentration of NaCN in the presence of a subthreshold concentration of IAA.

Incubation (37°C, 45 min) of intestinal segments in either oxygenated Krebs solution containing IAA (0.1 mmol/l) or Krebs solution gassed with 95% N_2/5% CO_2 led to marked enhancement of the immunoreactivity of myenteric and submucous plexus neurones to [Met[5]]enkephalin-Arg[6]-Gly[7]-Leu[8], vasoactive intestinal peptide, and neuropeptide Y.

Supported by the Wellcome Trust.

A6

Bromelin effects on the jejunal mucosa in the heteroimmune and cytostatic enteropathy

F. BARBARINO, E. NEUMANN, C. CRĂCIUM, N. PĂRĂU, P. SZABO and P. LENGYEL

The influence of Bromelin-Merck (EC 3.4.4.24), a proteolytic enzyme obtained from Ananas Comosus, was studied in healthy animals and in two experimental enteropathy models.

In 50 *healthy* guinea pigs Bromelin treatment (50 mg/kg for 3 days intragastrically) enhanced the histochemical activity of some enterocytic enzymes (Lojda–Gossrau–Schiebler methods). It lowered the radioisotope recovery in the isolated duodenojejunal loop (-54.35% [^{3}H]leucine, -57.41% [^{14}C]stearic acid, 30 min after local instillation) and in the 24 h collected faeces plus the colon content (-23.54% [^{131}I]triolein).

'*Heteroimmune*' *enteropathy* was induced in 70 guinea pigs by injecting rabbit antiserum against guinea pig jejunal mucosa and Freund's adjuvant. Bromelin treatment for 4 weeks prevented enterocyte dystrophy and enzyme depression (by 15.22–36.40%), without limiting the mesenchymal cell reaction in the chorion.

In *acute* '*cytostatic*' *enteropathy* (a single intragastric dose of 40 mg methotrexate/kg in 74 rats) Bromelin significantly antagonized the very severe histopathological, infrastructural (EM) and histoenzymatic damage ($LAP = +137.1\%$, $ATPase = +160.5\%$, alkaline phosphatase $= +67.6\%$, $G_6Pase = +100\%$, ANAE-esterase $= +178.4\%$, $NADH_2$-tetrazolium reductase $= +220.5\%$). The decreased radioisotope recovery in the intestinal loop (-28.35% [^{3}H]leucine and -32.13% [^{14}C]stearic acid) and in the faeces (-12.51% [^{131}I]triolein) showed improved digestion and absorption.

It could be postulated that the functional stimulation of enterocytes would influence their reactivity, increasing their resistance to the noxious action of heteroantiserum and methotrexate.

A7

Heterogeneity of IBD empiric risks between Jews and non-Jews

H. YANG, C. McELREE, M. P. ROTH, F. SHANAHAN, S. R. TARGAN and J. I. ROTTER

It has been well established that the Jewish population has an increased frequency of inflammatory bowel disease (IBD) compared to their non-Jewish neighbours. Genetic factors have been implicated in the aetiology of IBD and may have contributed to such ethnic differences. The objectives of this study were to determine the empiric risks for IBD in the first-degree relatives of IBD probands, both for Jews and for non-Jews, for genetic counselling and genetic analysis, as well as to compare these empirical risks for the insight they could contribute to the aetiology of IBD.

A total of 539 IBD patients (300 Jews and 239 non-Jews) were interviewed regarding information on the occurrence of IBD in their 2549 first-degree relatives. In the non-Jewish group we observed crude empirical risk estimates of 1.7% to siblings, 2.3% to parents, and 1.0% to offspring. These estimates are consistently lower than those from the Jewish group, 4.7%, 3.0% and 1.8% respectively. Since IBD has a variable and often late age of onset, crude empirical risk estimates are dependent on the age distribution in relatives. We then utilized age-specific incidence data to estimate the lifetime risks for IBD and to make a valid comparison between different groups. Estimates of lifetime risks for the relatives of non-Jewish patients were 3.9% to siblings, 3.1% to parents, and 4.9% to offspring. These were consistently lower than the corresponding risks for relatives of Jewish patients, 9.3%, 3.8%, and 7.1% respectively ($p < 0.05$). In addition, relatives of CD probands had an increased risk compared to those of UC probands, and this was true for both Jews and non-Jews.

As the familial aggregation of IBD appears largely due to genetic factors, the data showing that there are different empirical risks for relatives of Jewish and non-Jewish probands allow rejection of single Mendelian gene models for susceptibility to IBD. These data are consistent with several other genetic models: multifactorial, multilocus, and especially genetic heterogeneity models. These data suggest that either the genes that predispose to IBD are more common in the Jewish population, or that there is a differential distribution of different genetic factors.

A8

Inflammatory bowel disease (IBD): patients' beliefs about impact of psychosocial factors on the course of their disease

G. MOSER, TH. MAIER-DOBERSBERGER, H. VOGELSANG and H. LOCHS

Patients' beliefs and opinions about their disease are important for their coping style and illness behaviour (compliance). In a half-structured interview we consecutively asked for the opinion of 75 patients with Crohn's disease (CD) and 25 with ulcerative colitis (UC) concerning possible causes for the onset and the course of their illness.

Regarding the onset of disease 59 patients (47 with CD and 12 with UC) said that psychosocial distress was very important. These patients had a significantly ($p < 0.008$) longer disease duration (median 6.9 years vs. 3.9 years). Patients with CD and living in urban areas ($n = 39$) believed more often ($p < 0.008$) that psychological factors were decisive for the onset of the disease (30:9) than patients with CD and living in the country (17:19).

Regarding disease activity 55 patients believed that psychological factors were important. There were no significant correlations between the patients' beliefs and their disease activity at the time of interview.

CONCLUSION

Disease duration influences the beliefs and opinions of patients about their illness. A majority (74%) of the patients felt that psychological factors were important for the course of their disease. From this survey it is not clear if the uncertainty about the cause of the illness and the general stigmatization influenced the assessment of the disease by the patient, or if these causal attributions reflect an actual correlation after many years of illness experience. Our investigation supports earlier data suggesting a correlation between the course of IBD and psychosocial factors. Therefore the data show the need for psychosomatic counselling of patients with IBD.

A9

Additional damage in the pathogenesis of IBD

R. TREUSCH

Because the pathogenesis of IBD is still under discussion, it is necessary first to look at the site of illness.

Undisturbed co-function of gut flora and the intestinal immune system is a guarantee of lasting human health. The mucosa of the intestine is not only attacked by well or badly chewed pieces of food and a lot of different remedies; there are also other things which may damage the epithelium or the gut flora:

1. The abrasives in toothpaste.
2. Surfactants and disinfectants also disturb the gut flora and the lining of mucus with its sIgA. Surfactants loosen the binding of epithelial cells and promote dislocation of bacteria and macromolecules.

Another fact seems to be more dangerous: Hahn *et al.* proved that mercury from amalgam fillings is deposited in the mucosa of the intestine. Here there is a high rate of cell activity: 12–14 g of high quality protein, including immunoglobulins, are produced there. Mercury, with its affinity to sulphur, is also suspect for attaching all –SH groups of proteins, enzymes and metalloenzymes. As Hg^{++} it attaches to the negative molecules of the matrix. Mercury is detoxified by selenium, a component of glutathione peroxidase, which causes a lack of the most efficient scavenger of free radicals.

It is therefore necessary to exclude toothpaste, surfactants, disinfectants and amalgam fillings if the patient has IBD.

A10

Microbiological findings in patients with idiopathic ulcerative colitis

T. HILDEBRAND, D. A. DIOURIA, H. PUZOVA, F. MATEICKA,
F. REMENAR and M. ZAKUCIOVA

Clinical, microbiological and some serologic examinations were carried out in 40 patients with ulcerative colitis. In 30 of them, at the same time, the immunological profile was also examined and HLA typing performed.

In our group of patients the occurrence of HLA-B27 antigen was found in 26.6%. The above occurrence was significantly higher than that of the mentioned antigen in the ordinary population of Slovakia (8.1%).

All HLA-B27 patients frequently had arthritic manifestations and positive evidence of antibodies of *Klebsiella* K_{21}, and particularly K_{23}; this was detected by agglutination reaction. The evidence of specific antibodies IgG K_{23}, when comparing the whole group of patients with healthy individuals, was not statistically significant. The HLA-B27 patients require more intensive monitoring from the standpoint of exacerbations and extraintestinal complications.

B: Immunology

B1

Influence of cumulative doses of prednisone on the mucosal OKT4 and OKT8 T cells and Ig-containing cells in ulcerative colitis

E. A. KONOVICH, I. L. KHALIF and B. V. KIRKIN

The influence of prednisone on the colonic T lymphocytes and Ig-containing cells in patients with severe mucosal inflammation was studied. Nine patients had not received prednisone during the previous month (1); two groups of eight patients each were given oral cumulative doses of prednisone: 600–1200 mg (2) and 1600–6000 mg (3) on the day of investigation. Twelve patients with irritable bowel syndrome were studied as a control group (4).

T cells from the rectal biopsy specimens were studied with monoclonal antibodies (Ortho, USA) in a laser flow cytometry system. Ig cells were investigated with fluorescent antibodies. The results were as follows: OKT4 (%): (1) 38.5 ± 1.8, (2) 41.8 ± 3.1, (3) 38.8 ± 1.8, (4) 44.1 ± 0.7; OKT8: (1) 22.4 ± 1.7, (2) 20.4 ± 1.3, (3) 28.0 ± 1.2 $(p_{2-3} < 0.01)$, (4) 28.4 ± 0.7; OKT4/OKT8: (1) 1.8 ± 0.1, (2) 2.0 ± 0.1, (3) 1.4 ± 0.1 $(p_{2-3} < 0.01)$, (4) 1.56 ± 0.06; IgG cells (%): 13.4 ± 2.1, 11.7 ± 3.3, 12.6 ± 3.2, 4.6 ± 1.5 $(p_{1,2,3-4} < 0.05)$; IgM cells: 7.5 ± 1.6, 8.4 ± 1.1, 7.6 ± 2.4, 0.8 ± 0.3 $(p_{1,2,3-4} < 0.001)$; IgA cells: $6.4 \pm 1.6, 6.8 \pm 1.9, 7.2 \pm 2.0, 6.7 \pm 1.8$, respectively.

Steroids increased the blood OKT8 T cells (*Gut*, 1984, **25**:743) and the Leu-3/Leu-2 ratio *in vitro* (*Z. Gastroenterol.*, 1990;**28**:101).

Cumulative doses of prednisone of more than 1600 mg increase mucosal OKT8 T lymphocytes and have no influence on Ig-containing cells.

B2

Enhanced secretion of TNF-α, IFN-γ, IL-1β and IL-6 by lamina propria mononuclear cells from patients with inflammatory bowel disease

M. STEFFEN, H. C. REINECKER, T. WITTHÖFT, A. VOSS, S. SCHREIBER and A. RAEDLER

Mononuclear cells of the lamina propria (LpMNC), isolated from endoscopically taken biopsies (from the large bowel of patients with ulcerative colitis (UC), of patients with Crohn's disease (CD) or of healthy controls, were analysed for their ability to secrete tumour necrosis factor alpha (TNF-α), interferon-gamma (IFN-γ), interleukin-1β (IL-1β) and interleukin-6 (IL-6).

LpMNC were purified and cultured for 48 h with or without stimulation by pokeweed mitogen. Cytokine concentrations in the culture supernatants were analysed by radioimmunoassay.

All four cytokines were significantly increased in the culture supernatants of LpMNC from patients with inflammatory bowel disease compared to normal controls. Cytokine secretion by LpMNC from inflamed mucosa was higher compared to unaffected mucosa. Interestingly, secretion of IL-6 was found more elevated by LpMNC from UC than from CD.

Our data show that TNF-α, IFN-γ, IL-1β and IL-6 may play a role in the initiation and maintenance of intestinal inflammation. The large amounts of IL-6 observed in UC compared to CD support the concept of a distinct pathogenesis of both diseases.

Quantitative polymerase chain reaction allows the determination of TNF-α mRNA levels in mononuclear cells from mucosal biopsies

T. ANDUS, S. R. TARGAN, R. DEEM and H. TOYODA

Increased numbers of activated mononuclear cells in the mucosa are a characteristic feature in inflamed lesions of patients with inflammatory bowel disease. Activated mononuclear lamina propria cells produce tumour necrosis factor alpha (TNF-α), which has been shown to kill human epithelial targets, such as HT-29. Therefore, we examined the role of TNF-α in the *in situ* inflammatory process using mucosal biopsies. Because only a small number of cells can be obtained from biopsies, we developed a method to measure TNF-α–mRNA by quantitative polymerase chain reaction (PCR).

The TNF-α message was quantitated by co-amplification of cellular RNA (229 bp) with an artificial TNF-α–RNA containing an internal 49 bp deletion after reverse transcription. Because two very similar DNAs were amplified by the same primers, both DNAs were amplified with the same efficiency, as determined by dose–response and time-course experiments.

Using our quantitative PCR method we detected measurable TNFα–RNA in as few as 10^4 lamina propria mononuclear cells. The level of TNF-α message was approximately 8-fold increased in cells from inflammatory lesions of CD patients compared to normal mucosa. OKT-3 stimulated TNF-α–mRNA in isolated lamina propria lymphocytes (LPL) from uninflamed mucosa more than the preactivated LPL from inflamed mucosa.

In conclusion quantitative PCR allows the measurement of *in situ* production of cytokines in mucosal lesions and the study of the regulation of cytokine mRNAs in LPL isolated from mucosal biopsies.

B4

Concentrations of soluble TNF-receptor p55 but not p75 are significantly elevated in plasma of patients with inflammatory bowel disease (IBD)

T. ANDUS, V. GROSS, H. GALLATI, W. GEROK and
J. SCHÖLMERICH

Cytokines such as tumour necrosis factors alpha and beta (TNF) are very powerful inflammatory mediators acting via specific surface receptors. Two distinct soluble inhibitory TNF receptors (TNF-R) with molecular masses of 55 kDa (p55) and 75 kDa (p75) have been found. We examined the plasma concentrations of soluble TNF-R in patients with IBD.

Plasma was obtained from seven patients with active Crohn's disease (CD) (Best index 289 ± 101, mean $\pm$ SD) and from five patients with active ulcerative colitis (UC) (Rachmilewitz index 10.4 ± 4.3). Blood was immediately cooled to $0°C$, centrifuged and plasma was stored at $-20°C$. Concentrations of soluble TNF-R p55 and p75 were measured in duplicate by enzyme linked immunological biological binding assays (ELIBA) (F. Hoffmann La Roche AG, Basle, Switzerland). Normal plasma concentrations for both TNF-R ranged from 0.5 to 1.5 ng/ml. Patients with CD (4.16 ± 2.42 ng/ml) and UC (3.90 ± 1.88 ng/ml) had elevated plasma concentrations of TNF-R p55, whereas TNF-R p75 levels remained normal in most patients with CD or UC (0.79 ± 0.79 ng/ml and 1.46 ± 0.85 ng/ml, respectively).

Systemic treatment with steroids reduced Best and Rachmilewitz indices to 80 ± 71 and 2.6 ± 2.3. Concomitantly plasma concentrations of soluble TNF-R p55 were reduced to 2.62 ± 1.51 ng/ml and 2.23 ± 0.58 ng/ml, respectively. We conclude that plasma concentrations of TNF-R p55 increased in active IBD and reflect disease activity.

Anti-brush border antibodies (ABBA) in inflammatory bowel diseases

O. KOMÁRKOVÁ, B. FIXA and Z. NOŽIČKA

Differential diagnosis between ulcerative colitis and Crohn's disease remains a clinical problem not always solved by usual diagnostic procedures. Therefore a natural tendency exists to prepare new methods that could improve the differential diagnosis of IBD. One of these methods could be testing by ABBA. Our presented results show a significantly higher incidence of ABBA in Crohn's disease in comparison with ulcerative colitis. The diagnostic significance is lowered by the fact that ABBA may be found not only in Crohn's disease, but also in ulcerative colitis and in some other diseases, especially in chronic liver diseases.

B6

Rabbit antibodies to colonic mucosa from patients with ulcerative colitis react with epithelial basal membrane and mucosal vessels

E. A. KONOVICH, I. L. KHALIF and B. V. KIRKIN

Rabbits were inoculated by mucosal supernatants (Sn) from colonic specimens of patients with ulcerative colitis (UC). Anticolon antibodies (Ab) revealed two antigens in immunodiffusion test with Sn of patients with UC. Antigens were not found in 24 human normal organs, including the alimentary tract.

Ab reacted in indirect immunofluorescence on sections with colonic epithelial basal membrane (EBM) and vascular walls in eight of 10 specimens of patients with UC, and in 12 of 14 specimens of uninvolved mucosa of patients with colonic cancer. Ab also reacted with EBM of the colonic specimens in rats and mice. Ab was negative on sections of human aorta and carotid. The involvement of mucosal vessels (T. Halstensen *et al.*, *Gastroenterology*, 1989;**97**:10 and EBM (P. Knoflach *et al.*, *Immunol. Invest.*, 1989;**18**:473) in immunopathogenesis of UC and experimental immune complex disease of intestine are confirmed by these data. We think the targets of immunopathological reactions are interspecies membranous antigens.

Immunization of rabbits by mucosal Sn of patients with UC thus induces Ab to EBM and mucosal vessels.

B7

Autoantibodies against exocrine pancreas (PAB) in acute and chronic pancreatic disorders in Crohn's disease

F. SEIBOLD, A. MÜLLER, G. BÖHMER, C. SCHMIDT-HOLZHÜTER, H. JENSS and P. WEBER

Autoantibodies against exocrine pancreas (PAB) are disease-specific in patients with Crohn's disease (CD). They occur in about one third of these patients (Seibold et al., Gut, 1991;**32**:1192–7). Recently, exocrine pancreatic insufficiency was reported in up to 66% of patients with CD (Hegnhoj et al., Gut, 1990;**31**:1076–9). The association of acute pancreatitis as extraintestinal manifestation of CD was discussed. The role of PAB in CD remains unclear, and therefore we correlated PAB with the incidence of an acute pancreatitis or an exocrine insufficiency in CD.

METHODS

Autoantibodies were detected in indirect immunofluorescence on sections of human pancreas. Sera from 320 patients with CD and 120 controls (pancreatitis, ulcerative colitis, collagen disorders, healthy persons) were tested. Twelve of the patients with CD had an episode of acute pancreatitis, 37 were tested for exocrine insufficiency with the fluorescein-dilaurate test (FDL).

RESULTS

PAB were detected in 102 (32%) patients with CD and in none of the controls. Five of the 12 patients with acute pancreatitis in CD were PAB positive. In the subgroup of patients with CD tested in FDL, 14 out of 37 had PAB. Four of these had a pathological FDL test. None of the patients negative for PAB had a pathological FDL. Occurrence of PAB and of exocrine insufficiency respectively did not correlate with clinical parameters such as disease activity, extent of bowel disease, duration of disease or therapy.

CONCLUSION

PAB occur in a subgroup of patients with CD. There is no evidence that PAB play a role in acute pancreatitis and CD, but preliminary data suggest that PAB could be related to the pathogenesis of an exocrine pancreatic insufficiency in patients with CD.

B8

Lectins applied to intestinal epithelial cells in Crohn's disease

G. BOEHMER, J. PRECHTL, H. MOERK, F. SEIBOLD and P. WEBER

Lectin histochemistry can be used to identify glycoproteins on cell surfaces. The sugar residues are known to be altered in malignant colonic cells compared to normal colon tissue. Recently altered lectin binding by colonic epithelial glycoconjugates was also reported in patients with inflammatory bowel disease. In order to detect the pattern of glycoproteins in different bowel segments we investigated lectin binding on a larger range of tissue samples.

METHODS

Specific binding sites of biopsies and surgical specimens from 19 patients with Crohn's disease (CD) were demonstrated by the direct lectin peroxidase technique. Parallel sections were incubated with labelled lectin alone and with lectin after neuraminidase pretreatment.

RESULTS

Soybean agglutinin (SBA), *Helix pomatia* agglutinin (HPA) and *Dolichus biflorus* agglutinin (DBA) was found in ileum and colon with a high predominance of HPA-binding to N-acetylgalactosamine. Labelling with peanut agglutinin (PNA), *Ulex europaeus* agglutinin (UEA) and *Griffonia simplicifolia* (GS II) was successful only in ileum epithelial cells, whereas in colon no specific epitopes were detected (see Table 1).

CONCLUSION

Carbohydrate residues are involved in adhesion processes of bacteria as well as tumour cells to epithelial cells. The pattern of lectin binding in ileum and colon may be responsible for the pathogenesis of infammation in Crohn's disease.

Table 1

Lectin	Ileum (n = 14)	Colon (n = 14)	Rectosigmoid (n = 16)
SBA α/β-GalNAc	57%	29%	38%
DBA GalNAcal, 3GalNAc	29%	36%	44%
HPA GalNAc	100%	100%	100%
PNA Galβ1, 3GalNAc	57%	7%	6%
UEA I α-L-Fuc	29%	0%	6%
GS II α/β-GlcNAc	21%	0%	0%

B9

Innervation of the intestinal lymphoid follicles

H.-J. KRAMMER and W. STACH

The concept that the immune, nervous and endocrine systems are functionally interconnected is gaining support, although the detailed mechanisms of their intercommunication in healthy and diseased intestine are not yet clear. Two main ways have been suggested through which the nervous system can affect the immune response: an indirect neuroendocrine communication and a direct neural influence on the immune system by the autonomic nervous system (Weihe, E. *Int. J. Neurosci.*, 1991, **59**, 1–23). In the case of the intestine, the enteric nervous system could be involved in the regulation of the immune responses.

Therefore the aim of our study was to investigate contacts between the enteric nervous system and the lymphoid follicles in the human and pig intestine by immunohistochemical techniques. Using antibodies against various nervous-system-specific proteins, an intimate anatomical association between lymphoid nodules and enteric nerves can be demonstrated. The enteric nerves are localized around the follicle in the interfollicular area, the so-called traffic area and in the dome area, which plays an important role in uptake and presentation of antigens. Immunohistochemistry for various neuropeptides provides information on the presence of different neuropeptides in the enteric nerves associated with lymphoid follicles. The presented results of innervation patterns in healthy intestinal lymphoid tissue provide a basis for the investigation of their changes under experimental conditions and in disease.

B10

Influence of therapy and disease activity on perinuclear antineutrophil cytoplasmatic antibodies (p-ANCA) in sera from repeatedly tested patients with ulcerative colitis (UC)

M. ROTH, V. GROSS, J. A. RUMP, H. H. PETER and J. SCHÖLMERICH

Recently Saxon *et al.* (*J. Allergy Clin. Immunol.*, 1990, **86**, 202) suggested that p-ANCA are present in a high percentage of patients with UC. These findings have been confirmed by several other groups including ourselves (Rump *et al.*, *Immunobiology*, 1990, **181**, 406). Since such antibodies may be influenced by treatment or disease activity such as in Wegener's granulomatosis we studied 64 patients with UC of different activity. In addition, 24 patients with positive p-ANCA were followed during treatment under steroids. Our questions were:

1. Is there a correlation to disease activity?
2. Does treatment in particular with steroids or colectomy have an effect on the presence of p-ANCA?

From 37 sera found positive, 31 (84%) were from patients with high activity and only six (16%) had inactive disease. The 27 negative UC sera derived from patients with either long-term steroids ($n = 10$), inactive disease ($n = 7$) or previous colectomy ($n = 2$). The remaining patients ($n = 8$) were active without steroids.

Of the 24 patients with positive p-ANCA (titre 1:100) during follow-up under steroid treatment four patients became negative for p-ANCA and five had only weakly (titre 1:10) positive immunofluorescence. Two patients with complete colectomy after steroid treatment were found negative, in addition.

We conclude that there is an association between p-ANCA positivity and disease activity. Steroid medication influences the disease activity and consecutively the p-ANCA values.

B11

ANCA as a marker of pancolitis or primary sclerosing cholangitis

H. VOGELSANG, S. BAKOS, D. GENSER, H. LOCHS and
E. PENNER

ANCA have been demonstrated in patients with ulcerative colitis (UC) and
primary sclerosing cholangitis (PSC). We investigated 72 patients with
Crohn's disease (CD) (35 male, 37 female; 17 ileal disease, nine colonic
disease, 46 ileocolonic disease), 46 patients with ulcerative colitis (UC) (30
male, 16 female; 24 with disease of the left colon, 22 with pancolitis) and
nine with primary sclerosing cholangitis (PSC) (five male, four female; eight
with UC). ANCA were detected by indirect immunofluorescence.

RESULTS

	MC	*UC*	*PSC*
ANCA (+)	5 (7%)	24 (52%)	9 (100%)

ANCA(+) sera predominantly exhibited a perinuclear pattern (74%). All
five patients with MC and ANCA(+) had colonic involvement. In patients
with UC ANCA were found more often in patients with pancolitis (73%)
than in left-sided colitis (33%) ($p = 0.008$). Patients with ANCA(+) did not
differ from ANCA(−) patients with respect to disease activity (Crohn's
disease activity index, UC activity index, orosomucoid), or alkaline phosphatase.

In conclusion, ANCA are found more frequently in patients with pancolitis
than in left-sided UC, and rarely in patients with CD with exception of
colonic disease. In patients with CD and ANCA(+) the diagnosis of CD
(against UC) has to be discussed. It remains to be investigated whether
ANCA(+) UC patients ultimately develop PSC.

B12

x-ANCA in chronic inflammatory bowel diseases

S. HAUSCHILD, E. CSERNOK, W. H. SCHMITT, A. RAUTMANN and W. L. GROSS

Recently, antineutrophil cytoplasmic antibodies (ANCA) were detected in sera of patients with chronic inflammatory bowel diseases (IBD). However, the frequency and subspecificity of ANCA in IBD are still a matter of discussion.

Therefore, we studied sera from 84 patients suffering from Crohn's disease (CD) and 72 patients with ulcerative colitis (UC). All sera were tested on ethanol and on formaldehyde-fixed granulocytes, and on HEp-2 cells to distinguish perinuclear fluorescence pattern (p-ANCA) from sera with antinuclear antibodies. ELISAs – according to the set-up given by the EC study group – coated with highly purified antigen preparations of proteinase 3 (PR3), myeloperoxidase (MPO), elastase, (HLE), cathepsin G (CG), lactoferrin (LF) and lysozyme (LZ) were employed to detect ANCA directed against these lysosomal proteins.

Forty-five of 72 (62%) UC-sera were ANCA-positive; 17 of 45 showed a perinuclear fluorescence (p-ANCA) and 28 showed a mixture between cytoplasmic and perinuclear fluorescence designated as x-ANCA. From 10 of 84 (12%) ANCA-positive CD sera five had p-ANCA and 5 x-ANCA. There were no c-ANCA found in the sera tested. All sera were negative in PR3 or MPO specific ELISAs. Target antigens of x-ANCA could be detected in only eight out of 33 sera (UC:LZ 5/28, HLE 2/28, CG 1/28 and 20/28 unidentified; CD: 5/5 unidentified). In contrast, p-ANCA in UC sera were directed against HLE (7/17), CG (4/17), LZ (2/17), LF (2/17) and in CD sera against LZ (2/5), CG (1/5) and HLE (1/5).

In conclusion, UC (62%) and CD (12%) proved to be associated with ANCA. We found several autoantibodies against lysosomal proteins causing a p-ANCA fluorescence. The target antigens of the predominantly found x-ANCA could not be identified.

B13

IBD: regulation of T cell cytokine production: is there a defect?

R. L. DEEM and S. R. TARGAN

Reports from other investigators have indicated that mucosal T cells from inflammatory bowel disease (IBD) patients are defective in their ability to produce IL-2 when maximally activated with PMA for 48 h. Such a defect could play a role in IBD by reducing the immune response to potential pathogens, thus maintaining a chronic inflammatory state. Yet others have shown increased IL-2 mRNA expression in active Crohn's disease lesions. Previous results from this laboratory have shown that cytokine production is related to the pathways by which T cells are activated.

This study was designed to examine the ability of T cells from IBD mucosa to produce IL-2 when stimulated with antibodies to the T cell receptor and antigens associated with alternate activation pathways, which might differ from those associated with PMA activation.

Mononuclear cells from the mucosa of normal, ulcerative colitis, and Crohn's disease patients and mononuclear cells from the peripheral blood of normal patients was stimulated with anti-CD3 (OKT3) or anti-CD2 ($T11_2$ and $T11_3$) with and without anti-CD28 (9.3) for 18 h at 37°C. Supernatants were harvested and IL-2 was measured using a CTLL-2 bioassay. Lamina propria lymphocytes (LPL) were more sensitive to stimulation with both anti-CD3 and anti-CD2, and produced greater amounts of IL-2 compared to peripheral blood lymphocytes (PBL). There was no statistically significant difference in IL-2 secretion between LPL isolated from normal, UC, or CD mucosa stimulated with anti-CD3 or anti-CD2.

Co-stimulation of LPL with anti-CD28 markedly increased the secretion of IL-2 from all groups. LPL were stimulated with a wide range of concentrations of antibodies (100 to 0.01 ng/ml anti-CD3 and 1:200 to 1:3200 anti-CD2), suggesting that LPL from IBD mucosa responded identically to LPL from normal mucosa when given either a submaximal or 'maximal' stimulus.

These results demonstrate that T cells from IBD mucosa may not be defective in IL-2 production when stimulated with antibodies to the T-cell receptor or antigens associated with alternate activation pathways. Therefore, any alterations in T cell IL-2 production in active IBD may well be related to the pathway by which these T cells are activated *in vivo*.

B14

IBD: potential role of mucosal T cell cytokine down-regulation

R. L. DEEM, A. NEL and S. R. TARGAN

Previous results from this laboratory have shown that peripheral blood (PBL) and lamina propria (LPL) T cells release TNF-α and IFN-γ when activated through the CD2 or CD3 receptors. These cytokines may be involved in immune-mediated injury of intestinal mucosa. One hypothesis to explain chronic injury in IBD is the relative refractoriness of T cells to important down-regulatory compounds generated during inflammation.

Prostaglandins are one important regulator of immune function that are generated during the inflammatory process in the mucosa of patients with inflammatory bowel disease. This study was designed to examine the relative efficiency of exogenous PGE_2 to down-regulate cytokine production in normal LPL compared to PBL T cells.

Lymphocytes or $CD2^+$ T cells from the lamina propria or peripheral blood were activated with anti-CD2 ($T11_2$ and $T11_3$) or anti-CD3 (OKT3) $\pm$ anti-CD28 (9.3) in the presence or absence of increasing concentrations of PGE_2 and TNF-α and IL-2 production was measured. LPL activated with anti-CD3 were significantly less sensitive to the inhibitory effects of PGE_2 than PBL (ID_{50} of 10^{-8} mol/l, respectively). In addition, activation of CD2+ PBL with PHA for 5 days decreased the ability of PGE_2 to inhibit cytokine production compared to non-activated CD2+ PBL, suggesting that the activation state of the T cell is important in PGE_2-mediated down-regulation. Likewise, the activation pathway seems to play a role in PGE_2 down-regulation, since LPL were more easily inhibited when activated through the CD3 pathway than the CD2 pathway.

Addition of anti-CD28 increased the amount of cytokine produced when LPL or PBL T cells were activated with anti-CD2 or anti-CD3, and decreased the ID_{50} of PGE_2 by 10-fold.

These results suggest: (1) the activation state of the T cell and the pathway by which T cells are activated are important factors in T cell down-regulation by PGE_2; (2) mucosal T cells are in general relatively refractory to down-regulation by PGE_2 compared to PBL, and therefore may be less tightly regulated during inflammation.

B15

Antineutrophil cytoplasmic autoantibodies (ANCA) in sera from patients with ulcerative colitis (UC) after proctocolectomy with ileoanal anastomosis

D. REUMAUX, J. F. COLOMBEL, B. DUCLOS, S. CHAUSSADE,
J. BELAÏCHE, S. JACQUOT, J. L. DUPAS, C. MOLIS and
P. DUTHILLEUL

A distinct subset of ANCA has been described in sera from patients with inflammatory bowel disease and particularly in UC. ANCA in UC may be an epiphenomenon related to colonic inflammation, or may reflect a primitive disturbance of immune regulation. In this regard, study of ANCA status after the whole colorectal mucosa has been removed, could favour one of these two hypotheses.

The aim of the study was therefore to compare the prevalence of ANCA in sera from 70 patients with UC not operated on (37 female, 33 male, mean age 33.6 years) and in sera from 32 patients with UC having had a proctocolectomy with IAA (19 female, 13 male, mean age 38.4) after a follow-up period of an average of 30 months (1–84). Five out of 32 patients had a pouchitis at the time of the study.

METHODS

The detection of ANCA was performed by indirect immunofluorescence assay, according to the guidelines of the first international workshop on ANCA.

RESULTS

Perinuclear ANCA (p-ANCA) were found in 34/70 (49%) patients with UC not operated on, and in 11/32 (34%) patients having had a proctocolectomy with IAA (NS). Two out of five patients with pouchitis had p-ANCA.

CONCLUSION

These preliminary data support the theory that the presence of ANCA in UC reflects an immune disturbance not linked to the presence of the target organ.

Antineutrophil cytoplasmic autoantibodies (ANCA) in patients with ulcerative colitis (UC): influence of disease activity and familial study

D. REUMAUX, J. F. COLOMBEL, L. DELECOURT, L. H. NOËL, A. CORTOT and P. DUTHILLEUL

A distinct subset of ANCA has been described in sera from patients with UC. The relationship between ANCA and disease activity in these patients remains controversial. Recently it has been suggested that ANCA may be a genetic marker of susceptibility to UC.

The aim of the study was to assess further these two points: (1) the influence of disease activity on presence of ANCA in sera from 25 repeatedly tested patients with UC at $T0$ and after a mean 3.6 months (0.5–10) follow-up period; (2) the prevalence of ANCA in 91 first-degree and nine second-degree relatives of 30 patients with UC.

METHODS

The detection of ANCA was performed by indirect immunofluorescence assay in a blinded fashion by two investigators, according to the guidelines of the first international workshop on ANCA. The control group included 60 healthy blood donors and 10 spouses of patients with UC.

RESULTS

p-ANCA were present respectively in 13/25 (52%) of patients with UC at $T0$ and in 15/30 (50%) patients with UC of familial study and in 0/70 controls. No change in p-ANCA status in serum occurred at follow-up in 17/25 patients with UC (68%); in six patients, improvement of UC was associated with the appearance of p-ANCA. None of the 100 relatives of patients with UC had ANCA.

CONCLUSIONS

In our series: (1) the presence of p-ANCA may reflect an underlying immunological disturbance, not linked to the disease activity in patients with UC; (2) ANCA did not appear as being potentially a genetic marker of susceptibility to UC.

B17

Clinical significance of ulcerative colitis (UC) linked anti-neutrophil cytoplasmic antibody (p-ANCA) and Crohn's disease (CD) linked antibody to the kD-45/48 mycobacterial antigen in patients with inflammatory bowel disease (IBD)

M. OUDKERK POOL, B. M. E. VON BLOMBERG,
R. GOLDSCHMEDING, G. BOUMA, B. U. RIDWAN, H. BRIL,
P. K. DAS, R. VAN ES, A. KROMHOUT, A. S. PEÑA and
S. G. M. MEUWISSEN

Antibodies (Ab) against neutrophils (p-ANCA) have been demonstrated in 68% of UC patients (*J. Allergy Clin. Immunol.*, 1990, **86**, 202–10). A specific IgG Ab against a kd-45/48 mycobacterial antigen (M.Ab) was shown in 75% of CD patients by immunoblotting (*Gastroenterology*, 1989, **96**, A111). Sera from 196 IBD patients were examined for M.Ab using a solid-phase kD 45/48 enzyme-linked immunoadsorbent assay (ELISA). Sera from 214 IBD patients were tested for p-ANCA in an immunofluorescence assay.

Sensitivity of p-ANCA detection for the diagnosis of ulcerative colitis in IBD was 0.70 (77/100 patients, specificity 0.87 (90/104 patients, positive predictive value of 0.85 (77/91 patients). In 117 p-ANCA negative IBD patients, M.Ab detection had a positive predictive value of 0.86 (60/70 patients) for the diagnosis of Crohn's disease. No correlation was found between the presence of antibody and disease activity, duration or localization of disease, previous surgery or steroids.

In conclusion, detection of Ab against kD 45/48 M.Ab in p-ANCA negative patients may support the diagnosis of Crohn's disease. In addition, both serological tests may be of value in unravelling the heterogeneity of IBD within its different clinical subgroups.

Table 1

	M.Ab		p-ANCA		p-ANCA	M.Ab	UC	CD
	+	−	+	−	+	−	28	4
CD	72	30	14	90	−	+	10	60
UC	45	49	77	33	+	+	35	12
		$p < 0.002$		$p < 0.0001$	−	−	21	26

C: Pathophysiology

C1

Fatty acid profile of inflamed mucosa

S. BÜHNER, E. NAGEL, H. STOCKHORST, J. KÖRBER and
R. PICHLMAYR

The physiology of the intestinal mucosa substantially depends on its fatty acid profile, being the dynamic result of diet and absorption, endogenic consumption and synthesis.

We assessed the fatty acid profile (C14:0–C22:6) of ileal and colonic mucosal biopsies from patients with active Crohn's disease (CD; $n = 12$, 6 female, 6 male) and controls ($n = 12$, 6 female, 6 male). In CD biopsies were excised from macroscopically inflamed areas. Fatty acids of whole lipid fraction were analysed by capillary column gas chromatography (GC) using C17:0 as internal standard.

Comparing CD and controls the most striking differences were seen in the n-6 series: there was a lower amount of linoleic acid (18:2) and a higher amount of arachidonic acid (20:4) in CD than in controls. This was true for the ileum as well as the colon. Data from ileum and colon showed only small variations. The lower level of 18:2 could indicate a higher consumption for the synthesis of 20:4. Since 20:4 is a precursor of pro-inflammatory mediators, the question arises why there is an increase and not a reduction in this fatty acid? Probably the level of 20:4 varies with the development of the inflammation. This is supported by previous experimental findings in pigs where histological and ultrastructural lesions of ileal mucosa were accompanied by low 18:2 but an almost normal level of 20:4. The mucosal changes were found to be similar to those seen in macroscopically normal mucosal areas of patients with active CD.

Supported by the Deutsche Forschungsgemeinschaft grant NA 184/1-2.

C2

Intraluminal concentration of prostaglandin E (PGE), a marker of ulcerative colitis (UC) activity

M. LUKÁŠ, K. LUKÁŠ, M. JÁCHYMOVÁ and R. JIROUŠEK

AIMS OF THE STUDY

(1) To establish the relationship between a change of PGE concentration and UC activity, evaluated by clinical, endoscopic and histological criteria; (2) to establish the relationship, if there is any, between PGE production and the course and development of the disease.

METHODS

In 53 patients with UC in different stages of disease activity assessed by clinical, endoscopic and histological criteria, PGE concentration was determined, using radioimmunoassay, from the rectal dialysate obtained *in vivo*.

RESULTS

In 16 volunteers, mean PGE concentration was 0.364 ng/ml, in 11 patients with inactive UC, PGE concentration was 0.498 ($p > 0.1$); it was 1.67 ng/ml in patients with mild activity of the disease, and 2.97 ng/ml in those with high activity of the disease ($p < 0.05$). PGE correlated best with histological activity of the disease (mean PGE concentration values were 0.45, 1.62 and 3.14 ng/ml in inactive UC, mildly and highly active UC, respectively ($p < 0.01$); a significant correlation was also demonstrated between endoscopic activity and PGE concentration (0.60, 2.23 and 2.83 ng/ml in inactive UC, mildly and highly active UC, respectively) ($p < 0.05$). The loosest correlation existed between PGE concentration and clinical signs of activity (1.11, 2.55 and 2.40 ng/ml in inactive UC, mildly and highly active UC, respectively) ($p < 0.1$).

Patients with a high PGE value (over 2.0 ng/ml) showed a protracted or remitting course of the disease and progressive development of the disease.

CONCLUSIONS

(1) Changes in the intraluminal concentration of PGE significantly correlate with UC activity assessed using clinical, endoscopic and histological criteria; (2) a high PGE concentration occurs in the unfavourable form of the disease.

C3

Intraluminal concentrations of leukotriene B4 (LTB4) and activity of ulcerative colitis (UC)

K. LUKÁŠ, M. LUKÁŠ and M. JÁCHYMOVÁ

AIM OF THE STUDY

To establish the relationship, if there is any, between intraluminal concentrations of LTB4 and UC activity evaluated by clinical, endoscopic and histological criteria.

METHODOLOGY

Overall, 35 patients with UC in various stages of disease activity were assessed by our own clinical, endoscopic and histological criteria; their rectal dialysate was obtained and LTB4 concentrations were determined by radioimmunoassay.

RESULTS

Mean LTB4 concentration in patients in complete remission was 0.28 ng/ml, it was 2.37 ng/ml in those in the stage of mild activity, and 2.11 ng/ml in patients with severe activity of the disease; mean LTB4 value was 1.38 ng/ml in a control group of healthy volunteers. No statistically significant differences were found between the groups. No difference was seen between LTB4 concentrations and histological severity (mean LTB4 concentrations were 0.895, 2.826, and 1.92 ng/ml in remission, and in the stages of mild and severe activity, respectively); significant differences were noted between LTB4 concentrations and the endoscopic severity of the disease (0.91, 3.35 and 1.48 ng/ml in remission, and in patients with mild and severe activity, respectively); LTB4 concentrations correlated only with clinically expressed severity of the disease ($p < 0.05$) (1.42, 2.38 and 3.42 ng/ml in remission, and in the stage of mild and severe activity, respectively.

CONCLUSIONS

(1) UC activity is associated with an increase in the intraluminal concentrations of LTB4 correlating with the clinically expressed activity of the disease. (2) No correlation was demonstrated between the endoscopic and histological criteria of the disease and LTB4 concentration.

C4

Mucosal histamine secretion and tissue histamine content in Crohn's disease

M. RAITHEL, H. W. BAENKLER and E. G. HAHN

Increased numbers of mucosal mast cells that contain histamine have been found in lesions of Crohn's disease (CD; active = a, not active = na). This study investigated the mucosal histamine content (HC; medians (range), pg/mg dry weight) and its secretion pattern from colorectal mucosa specimens, both with and without inhibition of the two main histamine catabolizing enzymes (DAO diamine oxidase and HNMT histamine N-methyltransferase) of the gut.

The histamine release of 309 biopsies (10 patients control group (CG), 19 CD) was measured at 5 min intervals for 30 min in an air-bubbled incubation medium (37°C) that prevented the occurrence of cold or warm ischaemia for the mucosal particles. The HC was obtained by addition of the released amounts of histamine and the remaining tissue histamine detected after heat inactivation of the samples. Histamine amounts were measured using a radioimmunoassay.

The secretion pattern of histamine in CD was significantly different from that of the CG. Similar mucosal HCs (without inhibition of the histamine catabolism) were obtained in CDna (19.1 (102) pg/mg) and in the CG (23.6 (87.8) pg/mg), but both were significantly lower than in CDa (54.6 (273) pg/mg). All inhibition experiments confirmed higher histamine levels in CDa than in CDna.

Furthermore, the specific inhibition of the histamine-degrading enzymes (DAO + HNMT) caused clearly different increasing rates of the tissue histamine (CG 76.6%; CDna 34%; CDa 20.6%) suggesting that also alterations of the histamine catabolism may occur in the gut mucosa of CD.

In conclusion, these results demonstrate significant elevations of the mucosal histamine in actively inflamed areas of CD, and indicate that changes of the mucosal histamine involved in the inflammatory process may thus cause, modify or at least accompany the transition of the inactive disease stage to the active one.

C5

Reduced neutrophil neutral endopeptidase 24:11 in ulcerative colitis

A. T. COLE, C. SMITH, L. KURLAK and C. J. HAWKEY

Neutral endopeptidase 24.11 (NEP) is expressed by neutrophils and can down-regulate neutrophil chemotaxis and activation by degrading substance P, endorphins and FMLP. We have therefore compared peripheral blood neutrophil NEP activity in patients with active ulcerative colitis with that in normal volunteers.

Peripheral blood was obtained concurrently from six ulcerative colitis patients age 41 (median range 22–62) and six normal volunteers, age 21 (20–33). Patients had symptom scores of 5 (2 to 10 – modified Powell Tuck) and sigmoidoscopy scores 3 (1 to 3), two were receiving steroids, three steroid enemas, five oral salicylates and four azathioprine. Neutrophils were separated from heparinized venous blood and stored frozen at $-20°C$. The degradation of succinyl-alanyl-alanylphenylalanyl (4-amido-4-methyl)-coumarin was used to measure NEP activity with thiorphan 10^{-3} mol/l as a specific NEP inhibitor. Log transformed data were compared using the unpaired t-test.

The coefficient of variation of NEP activity in three separate samples from one volunteer was 2.8%. Normal volunteers showed NEP activity of 2.24 (geometric mean 95% CI 1.27 to 3.95) $\times 10^{-6}$ mol/l per 30 min per 10^5 neutrophils. Ulcerative colitis patients showed lower NEP activity of 1.07 (geometric mean, 95% CI 0.58 to 1.98). Differrence from normal patients $p = 0.048$ (confidence interval for ratio of means 0.23 to 0.98).

These data show reduced peripheral blood NEP activity in a group of patients with active ulcerative colitis compared to a group of normal volunteers. Impaired down-regulation of neutrophil activation as a consequence of reduced NEP activity could be a characteristic of subjects with ulcerative colitis.

C6

Some features of electromechanical activity of severely affected human small intestine

P. PLEVOKAS, S. PLEVOKAS and A. MIKALIŪKŠTIENE

We studied 36 patients with a small intestinal obstruction caused by inflammatory illness of the gut or abdominal cavity: destructive appendicitis, 16; perforated peritonitis, 10; gynaecological diseases, 6; Crohn's disease, 3; and Meckel's diverticulum, 1. All these patients were treated by operative closed enterodecompression and postoperative enterodrainage using tubes of our design. To record electromechanical activity (EMA) of the affected small intestine EMA probes of our design were attached to enterodrainage tubes. EMA probes keep stable electrical contact between their electrodes and mucosa even if the probes are moved by intestinal contraction. EMA probes are soft and do not injure the mucosa. The duration of the studies was 3–4 h every day. EMA of the small intestine returned within 3 days in 21 patients and within 6 days in the rest. The latter group suffered from inflammatory delayed obstruction of the small intestine. Among them we observed tonic intestinal contractions without myoelectrical spike activity, significant electrical neural activity in the mucosa, hyperintensive single spikes, and electrical activity of unusual form without intestinal contractions.

The data show that unusual EMA of inflamed affected small intestine would be an alarm sign suggesting the need for more intensive therapeutic treatment.

C7

Assessment of ileum function in inflammatory bowel disease and in short bowel syndrome

J. RYZKO, M. WROBLEWSKA, J. SOCHA, L. TOMASZEWSKI and M. WOYNAROWSKI

The aim of the study was to assess the usefulness of the following tests in determining ileal function: (1) fat in faeces; (2) α_1-antitrypsin in faeces (α_1-AT); (3) postprandial bile acids in serum; (4) SeHCAT test.

The study was carried out in five patients with Crohn's disease in remission, in 34 patients with ulcerative colitis, and in five patients after partial resection of ileum (0.5–10 years before the study). The function of ileum was determined by measurement of fat content in 3 days stool collection, α_1-AT content in stool sample, postprandial serum level of total bile acids and cholyglycyl bile acid, retention of SeHCAT in the body 7 days after exposure.

RESULTS

Steatorrhoea was found only in patients with short bowel syndrome. The increase of α_1-AT in stools (more than 2 mg/g stool weight) was found in patients with steatorrhoea and hypoalbuminaemia. Patients with Crohn's disease and after ileal resection had flat bile acid curves (particularly with respect to cholyglycyl bile acid). The lowest values of SeHCAT retention were found in patients after ileal resection (0–6%) and Crohn's diseases (10–16%).

CONCLUSIONS

Complex investigations are required for assessment of ileal function: α_1-AT in stools and SeHCAT test were of particular importance.

C8

Bone demineralization in Crohn's disease

J. KOCIÁN and J. KOCIÁNOVÁ

In a group of 43 patients in different stages of Crohn's disease bone mineralization was studied by measuring clavicular corticodiaphyseal indices, and intestinal Ca absorption was measured with 47-Ca using a whole-body counter.

A linear correlation between degree of bone mineralization and Ca intake in the organism was found; the Ca intake was calculated from dietary Ca intake and the degree of its intestinal absorption.

In an acute attack of the disease Ca absorption was abnormally decreased; during rest periods there was a lower decrease of Ca absorption and successful resection of the afflicted intestinal segments leads to normalization of Ca absorption in spite of the decreased intestinal absorption area. Bone demineralization is due also to reduced dietary Ca intake (lactose intolerance) and impaired conversion of vitamin D in the liver, and is negatively affected by corticosteroid treatment.

C9

Prolonged indocyanine-green half-life in active Crohn's disease

A. TROMM, D. HÜPPE, H. D. KUNTZ and B. MAY

In inflammatory bowel disease involvement of the liver has been previously described as fibrosis, pericholangitis, primary sclerosing cholangitis, hepatic abscesses, fatty liver or changes in standard laboratory tests (AST, ALT). There is little current information concerning indocyanine-green half-life as a test for the flow-dependent elimination performance of the liver, particularly with respect to disease activity (Kuntz, 1988).

PATIENTS AND METHODS

We determined the indocyanine-green (ICG) half-life in relation to disease activity in 38 examinations of 25 patients with Crohn's disease = CD (14 female, 11 male; mean age 33.04 ± 11.2 years) and 20 healthy controls. Twenty tests were performed in patients with active Crohn's disease, whereas 18 tests were performed in remission by clinical and endoscopical criteria. ICG half-life was determined using a photometric assay after injection of 0.8 mg/kg ICG (Paumgartner, 1975).

RESULTS

The results indicate a significant increase of ICG half-life in patients with active CD (4.63 ± 1.1 min) compared to patients in remission (3.71 ± 0.9 min; $p < 0.05$) and healthy controls (2.6 ± 0.4 min; $p < 0.01$). A total of 94.1% of patients with active CD showed pathologically elevated levels of the ICG half-life (> 3.0 min; range: 3.68–6.8 min), whereas only 10% showed elevated standard liver tests (AST, ALT). Regarding the localization of the disease the increase of ICG half-life was most evident ($p < 0.05$) in patients with total colonic involvement (5.28 ± 1.0 min; $n = 6$) compared to patients with limited ileitis (3.83 ± 0.5 min; $n = 5$). No influence of treatment by steroids or oral contraceptives and no correlation to the commonly used liver function tests (AST, ALT) could be demonstrated. Moreover short-term follow ups as an intraindividual comparison ($n = 9$) after treatment with steroids and 5-ASA for 22 days did not show any significant changes (4.33 ± 0.62 vs 4.42 ± 1.1 min). In contrast follow-ups ($n = 4$) after more than

3 months in clinical remission led to a significant decrease of ICG half-life
(5.67 ± 0.99 vs 3.22 ± 0.59 min).

DISCUSSION

The results indicate a temporary increase of ICG half-life in active CD. We
suggest the influence of inflammatory mediators (cytokines, endotoxins) in
the enterohepatic circulation. Further investigations should focus more
attention on the gut–liver axis in inflammatory bowel disease.

C10

Intestinal protein loss in diabetes mellitus

Z. SAJEWICZ

Gastrointestinal disturbances in patients with diabetes mellitus are not uncommon, and are described as diabetic enteropathy. The aim of this study was to evaluate intestinal protein loss in diabetes mellitus by means of $[^{131}I]$polyvinylopyrrolidone.

The author examined 20 healthy volunteers (control group), 30 patients without vascular complications of diabetes, 25 patients with diabetic microangiopathy and 14 patients with diabetic enteropathy.

RESULTS

Intestinal protein loss in the control group was $0.32 \pm 0.183\%$, in uncomplicated diabetes mellitus it was $0.39 \pm 0.200\%$ (n.s.), in diabetic microangiopathy it was $0.45 \pm 0.203\%$ (n.s.) and in diabetic enteropathy it was $1.52 \pm 0.807\%$ ($p < 0.001$).

CONCLUSIONS

1. Increased intestinal protein loss was demonstrated in patients with diabetic enteropathy.
2. In diabetes mellitus without vascular complications and with microangiopathy the protein loss into intestinal lumen was normal.

C11

Increased permeability through paracellular pathways (^{51}Cr-EDTA) in Crohn's disease is due to extent of disease

M. PEETERS, P. RUTGEERTS, Y. GHOOS, M. HIELE, K. GEBOES and G. VANTRAPPEN

Intestinal permeability for water-soluble macromolecules is increased in Crohn's disease. It is not known whether the increased permeation is a secondary phenomenon or is of primary importance. To investigate the permeability of macroscopically normal mucosa in IBD, we studied the permeation of two probes, i.e. PEG-400 and ^{51}Cr-EDTA. After an overnight fast a 100 cm segment of normal upper intestine of patients with Crohn's disease, ulcerative colitis and normal controls was isolated with a distal water-filled balloon and perfused with a standard liquid meal (250 ml Nutrison®) containing the two probes. This 2 h perfusion was followed by a perfusion of 500 ml water to stimulate diuresis. Distally of the balloon all contents were aspirated. Urines were collected for 3 h. ^{51}Cr-EDTA was measured by scintillation counting and PEG-400 by gas chromatography.

RESULTS

	^{51}Cr-EDTA	PEG-400	PEG/Cr
Controls ($n = 10$)	0.32% ± 0.024	20.06% ± 1.28	65.73 ± 6.12
Crohn ileitis ($n = 12$)	0.92% ± 0.24	17.63% ± 0.71	33.04 ± 6.26
	0.023 (S)	0.052 (S)	0.0041 (S)
Crohn colitis ($n = 7$)	0.28% ± 0.12	24.63% ± 3.49	395.30 ± 203.29
	0.241 (NS)	0.107 (NS)	0.107 (NS)
Colitis ulcerosa ($n = 3$)	0.11% ± 0.034	10.49% ± 0.77	106.96 ± 18.38

The results show a significant increased permeability through paracellular pathways (Cr-EDTA) in Crohn's ileitis. In patients with colitis there is no significant increased permeability. This suggests a diffuse nature of ileal disease affecting the paracellular transport route. Increased permeability is probably not of primary importance.

C12

Effect of mucosal inflammation on colonic smooth muscle contraction

Y. N. XIE, W. T. GERTHOFFER, V. E. EYSSELEIN and W. J. SNAPE, Jr

Previous studies showed that colonic smooth muscle develops less contractile force to neurohumoral stimulation when associated with mucosal inflammation. This study evaluated (1) bethanechol-induced inositol 1,4,5-triphosphate [Ins(1,4,5)P$_3$) production; (2) the calcium dependence for colonic smooth muscle contraction; (3) the maximum velocity of muscle shortening (V_{max}); (4) changes in 20 kDa myosin light chain (MLC) phosphorylation; and (5) content of actomyosin in distal colonic muscle from healthy rabbits and from rabbits with experimental colitis, induced by formalin and immune complexes.

The isometric tension of intact muscle stimulated with bethanechol or KCl was ($p < 0.05$) less in animals with colitis compared to the control group. Ins(1,4,5)P$_3$ increased about 2-fold over basal after bethanechol stimulation in both groups ($p < 0.05$). But this increase was not significantly different between both groups ($p > 0.05$). In saponin-skinned muscle the amplitude of the maximal tension at $[Ca^{2+}]$ of 3×10^{-7} mol/l was decreased ($p < 0.05$) in colitis animals ($4.3 \pm 0.9 \times 10^4$ N/m^2, $n = 7$) compared to healthy animals ($10.5 \pm 2.4 \times 10^4$ N/m^2, $n = 6$). However, the EC$_{50}$ for Ca^{2+} stimulation was similar ($p > 0.05$) in both groups.

When MLC was thiophosphorylated with ATPγS, the tension development was decreased ($p < 0.01$) in colitis ($2.1 \pm 0.3 \times 10^4$ N/m^2, $n = 5$) compared to normals ($5.0 \pm 1.4 \times 10^4$ N/m^2, $n = 5$). In healthy animals phosphorylation of 20 kDa MLC increased rapidly to $51.2 \pm 3.1\%$ within 15 s after stimulation, and subsequently declined to $19.0 \pm 2.1\%$ at 5 min. V_{max} was maximal ($0.14 L_o$/s) 13 s after stimulation and declined prior to maximal active isometric stress. In colitis animals the 20 kDa MLC phosphorylation ($p < 0.05$) and the V_{max} ($p < 0.01$) were decreased. Myosin content decreased in each colitis sample including those with mild mucosal inflammation. In severe colitis the actin content was also decreased compared to control ($p < 0.05$). These studies suggest that: (1) isometric tension development is decreased in colitis muscle; (2) the Ins(1,4,5)P$_3$ production and the Ca^{2+} sensitivity for contraction is not decreased in colitis; (3) 20 kDa MLC phosphorylation and V_{max} are decreased in colitis. Decreased shortening velocity may be secondary to lower myosin phosphorylation levels. (4) Decreased isometric force may result from decreased actin and myosin content. This decreased content of actomyosin or a possible change in isoform of contractile proteins may contribute to the abnormal actin myosin cross-bridge formation in colitis.

C13

Regulation of substance P gene expression in experimental colitis

M. REINSHAGEN, A. PATEL, M. SOTTILI, W. DAVIS and
V. E. EYSSELEIN

We have previously shown (*Gastroenterology*, 1991, **101**, 1211–19) that substance P (SP) decreases early in the colon muscle layer in a rabbit colitis model. Since the SP content in the colonic muscle layer was unchanged by sensory denervation with capsaicin (data not shown) we assume that SP is located in intrinsic neurones of the colon, and that the decrease of SP during inflammation reflects changes in intrinsic SP content. However, damage of SP neurones by inflammation is another explanation for the SP decrease.

The aim of this study was to determine SP gene expression in intrinsic (colonic muscle layer) and extrinsic sensory (dorsal root ganglia) neurones to prove that SP transcription and therefore neuronal function is intact.

METHODS

Colitis was induced in adult white New Zealand rabbits by a formalin enema (4 ml of 0.4% formalin) followed by 0.85 ml immune complex i.v. 2 h later. The animals were sacrificed 48 h after induction of colitis. The colon and the dorsal root ganglia were dissected and processed for radioimmunoassay (SP-AB kindly provided by C. Sternini) and Northern blot analysis. 10 µg of total RNA was electrophoresed, blotted to nitrocellulose filters and hybridized with ^{32}P βppT-cRNA (β-preprotachykinin, kind gift of J. Krause). Results were quantitated by densitometry.

RESULTS

	Control	Colitis 48 h
Colon muscle layer		
mRNA βppT		
OD units	1.78 ± 0.24	2.16 ± 0.44
SP-IR	6.15 ± 0.4	3.82 ± 0.8*
nmol/g protein		
Dorsal root ganglia (S4-L4)		
mRNA βppT		
OD units	4.52 ± 0.89	4.71 ± 0.57
SP-IR	13.4 ± 3.3	5.3 ± 1.1*
pmol/ml		

*$p < 0.05$ compared to control.

CONCLUSION

The marked decrease of SP in the colitis muscle layer is not accompanied by decreased SP message suggesting that (a) the intrinsic SP neurones are intact and (b) that SP is released during inflammation. The decrease of SP-IR in the DRG with unchanged SP message suggests additional release of SP from extrinsic nerve fibres during inflammation.

C14

Dual effects of TGE-β_1 on epithelial chloride secretion

C. M. GELBMANN, L. ECKMANN, M. VAJANAPHANICH,
M. F. KAGNOFF and K. E. BARRETT

Several proinflammatory and immunoregulatory cytokines are increased during intestinal inflammation. To examine whether they modulate the secretory function of the epithelium and perhaps predispose to secretory diarrhoea, we studied whether various cytokines (IL-1β, IL-2, IL-6, TNF-α, GM-CSF and TGF-β_1) alter chloride secretion by T_{84} cells. After incubation of cell monolayers for 20–24 h with the cytokine to be examined, chloride secretion was measured in modified Ussing chambers as changes in short circuit current (I_{SO}) induced by carbachol, VIP and a cell-permeant analogue of cAMP, Bt_2cAMP/AM. Under these conditions, only TGF-β_1 had significant effects on cell responses. While it had no effect on carbachol-induced Cl^- secretion, two independent effects could be observed on the response to VIP. One effect was a dose-dependent enhancement of the secretory response. 0.1, 1 and 10 ng/ml TGF-β_1 enhanced VIP-induced Cl^- secretion by $24.9 \pm 24.7\%$, $64.5 \pm 11.6\%$ ($p < 0.01$), and $70.8 \pm 10.0\%$ ($p < 0.01$), respectively. In other experiments TGF-β_1 dose-dependently inhibited the response to VIP ($5.2 \pm 12.8\%$, $47.5 \pm 7.3\%$ ($p < 0.05$) and $32.3 \pm 3.9\%$ ($p < 0.05$) at 0.1, 1 and 10 ng/ml, respectively). Stimulatory or inhibitory effects of TGF-β_1 on VIP-induced secretion were consistent within a given experiment. However, when secretion was induced by Bt_2cAMP/AM only the inhibitory effect could be observed. Thus the stimulatory effect of TGF-β_1 may reflect changes in second messenger production, whereas the inhibitory effect presumably occurs downstream of cAMP synthesis. None of the cytokines tested affected tight junction integrity. In summary, we found that physiological doses of TGF-β_1 modulate epithelial sensitivity and, under some circumstances, might predispose the intestine to secretory diarrhoea.

D: Therapy

D1

The effect of interferon alpha-2a on clinical and endoscopic findings in chronic active ulcerative colitis

N. SÜMER, A. R. BEYLER, M. PALABIYIKOĞLU, A. ERTEN, K. BAHAR, A. ÖZDEN and Ö. UZUNALIMOĞLU

It has been accepted that immunological factors have a place in the pathogenesis of IBD. In this study the effect of interferon alpha-2a (IFN), which has immunomodulatory properties, has been sought in chronic active ulcerative colitis (UC) while being used by the parenteral route (s.c.). The patients were all unresponsive to classical therapy and had bloody diarrhoea, pain and weight loss for 8–12 months, as well as a bloody defaecation rate of 12–25 per day. Out of 12 patients, four were female and the mean age was 32.2. In five patients the whole colon, in six patients only the left descending colon and in one patient the left colon up to the middle of the transverse colon were affected, having a fragile mucosa with many bleeding foci. There were disseminated grape-bunch-like pseudopolyps in four individuals while others had less.

No amoebiasis was detected among patients whose biopsies revealed UC. Hypoalbuminaemia, hypokalaemia, iron-deficiency anaemia and haematochezia were important laboratory findings.

After they had been hospitalized for 10 days without any therapy, the patients were started on IFN at a dose of $3 \times 9 \times 10^6$ IU in the first week, $3 \times 6 \times 10^6$ IU in the second week, $3 \times 3 \times 10^6$ IU in the third week and then $3 \times 3 \times 10^6$ IU in every week for 5 months. At the end of the first week, 83% of the patients began responding to therapy, and after 3 or 4 weeks clinical and endoscopically full remission was observed; anaemia and electrolyte imbalance also improved. Pseudopolyps lessened in number and became smaller. No recurrence was determined during 5 months of therapy. In addition, the patients gained physical activity and weight, suffering only from short-period fever and fatigue as side-effects of IFN at the beginning of the course. Seventeen per cent of patients were unresponsive to IFN therapy.

It is accepted that the therapeutic effect of IFN probably results from its immunomodulatory properties.

D2

Treatment of inflammatory bowel disease with monoclonal antibody

J. EMMRICH, M. SEYFARTH, W. E. FLEIG and F. EMMRICH

Recent experimental and clinical data demonstrate that the T helper lymphocyte subset plays a central role in the pathogenesis of inflammatory bowel disease. We have used a monoclonal antibody (mAb) to CD4 in a pilot study for the treatment of Crohn's disease and ulcerative colitis.

PATIENTS AND METHODS

One patient with Crohn's disease (patient 1) and four patients with ulcerative colitis resistant to conventional therapy were treated for 7 days with an anti-CD4 mAb (MAX 16H5) at a daily dose of 0.3 mg/kg body weight mAb.

RESULTS

Immunological monitoring revealed a transient, selective depletion of CD4 T cells after each infusion. The proliferative response of peripheral blood mononuclear cells to mitogens was significantly diminished after cessation of antibody treatment. Human anti-mouse antibodies could be detected after 14 days. Patients 1, 2 and 5 responded to anti-CD4 treatment clinically, but relapsed after 1 month. Laboratory findings (ESR, CRP, orosomucoids) also revealed remission of the inflammatory process throughout this month. Patient 3, however, reached a complete clinical, endoscopic and biochemical remission, lasting now for more than 10 months. Patient 4 was unresponsive to mAb treatment.

CONCLUSION

Anti-CD4 mAb may be of value as a second-line treatment of inflammatory bowel disease when conventional therapy has failed. Optimal dosage and timing of this treatment are still to be defined. There were no side-effects.

D3

Decreased responsiveness of platelets to iloprost in patients with Crohn's disease. Reversal by n-3 polyunsaturated fatty acids (n-3 PUFA)

M. SCHEURLEN, K. JASCHONEK and M. R. CLEMENS

n-3 PUFA can reduce inflammatory responses by inhibition of leukotriene B_4 biosynthesis and by decreasing the formation of cytokines. Additionally, an interference of these fatty acids with platelet function has been observed.

We monitored the responsiveness of platelets to the stable prostacyclin analogue iloprost, and the specific iloprost binding sites in six patients with active Crohn's disease during the application of eicosapentaenoic acid (EPA) and docosahexaenoic acid (DHA) for 6 months.

During the study the concentration of iloprost required for half-maximum inhibition of ADP-induced primary platelet aggregation was measured. Additionally, the binding of 5 nmol/l $[^3H]$iloprost was determined in the presence and absence of 20 μmol/l of the unlabelled ligand to determine specific binding. Resorption and incorporation of the n-3 PUFA into membrane lipids were monitored in red blood cell ghosts by gas chromatography after methylation of the fatty acids.

Before therapy the patients' platelet responsiveness to iloprost and $[^3H]$iloprost binding were reduced by 79% and 40%, respectively, as compared with normal controls. During supplementation with n-3 PUFA over 6 months, a continuous normalization of platelet function was observed.

The enchancement of platelet PGI_2-receptor surface expression observed in this study could be due to changes of the receptor lipid microenvironment. This effect of n-3 PUFA can be expected to reduce the risk of vascular complications in Crohn's disease, and to modulate inflammatory reactions by the reduction of local platelet accumulations that may give rise to formation of specific platelet-derived proinflammatory eicosanoids.

D4

Butyrate: a new therapeutic principle in distal ulcerative colitis

W. SCHEPPACH, H. SOMMER, T. KIRCHNER, P. BARTRAM,
F. RICHTER, S. U. CHRISTL and H. KASPER

Short-chain fatty acid irrigation of the colonic mucosa has been shown to ameliorate inflammation in diversion colitis. As this type of colitis is endoscopically and histologically similar to ulcerative colitis (UC), the effect of rectal butyrate irrigation was tested in patients with distal UC.

Twelve patients who had been unresponsive or intolerant to standard therapy for 8 weeks were treated with sodium butyrate (100 mmol/l) or sodium chloride enemas for two 2-week periods in random order (placebo-controlled, single-blind trial with crossover design). Before and after treatments, clinical symptoms were noted and the endoscopic appearance of the mucosa was evaluated (endoscopic score, range 0–10). In biopsies the overall inflammatory change was graded histologically (grade 0–3) and cell proliferation was assessed by autoradiography (*in vitro* incorporation of tritium-labelled thymidine).

After butyrate irrigation, stool frequency (n/day) decreased from 4.5 ± 0.4 to 2.2 ± 0.5 ($p < 0.004$, Wilcoxon test) and discharge of blood ceased in 11 of 12 patients. The endoscopic score fell from 6.8 ± 0.4 to 3.8 ± 0.6 ($p < 0.004$). The histological degree of inflammation decreased from 2.4 ± 0.2 to 1.4 ± 0.2 ($p < 0.008$). Overall crypt proliferation was unchanged, but the upper crypt labelling index fell from 0.086 ± 0.019 to 0.032 ± 0.003 ($p < 0.03$). On placebo, all these parameters were unchanged.

Unlike anti-inflammatory drugs, intestinal nutrients (e.g. butyrate) may help to suppress disease activity by raising energy availability to colonocytes. This new therapeutic concept has been shown to be efficient in diversion colitis but may also prove valuable in distal UC.

D5

Treatment of bone demineralization in Crohn's disease

J. KOCIÁNOVA, K. AXMANN and J. KOCIÁN

Bone demineralization found mainly in a group of patients with active form of Crohn's disease is worsened by therapeutic use of corticoids.

During 20 years we have measured the bone indices in a group of 98 patients with Crohn's disease.

In the treatment of demineralization we used a high-calcium diet. This condition could not be fulfilled in patients who suffered from lactose intolerance and Ca had to be supplemented by medication. Small doses of vitamin D increase Ca intestinal absorption. Moderate doses of Naf are tolerated well, and with the exception of acute stages of Crohn's disease all other patients have to load their bones with regular exercises. This combined treatment can restore bone mineralization to normal rates, but it must be complex, continuous and over a sufficiently long period of time.

D6

Our experience with conservative therapy of complications of Crohn's disease

K. AXMANN, V. KOS, M. SKVARILOVÁ, J. KAMLER and J. HRBEK

The surgical score of patients with Crohn's disease ranged from 2.4 to 20. Repeated resections lead to reduction of the functional part of the intestine. The aim of surgery, and mainly of conservative therapy, is to retain a large resorption area of the intestine.

The authors report on their experience with the therapy of stenoses and fistulae in 20 patients with Crohn's disease. In the period 1989–92, 10 men and 10 women were given a complete parenteral or enteral infusion for 4–8 weeks. At the same time, six patients were subjected to endoscopic dilatations of stenoses in anastomoses, four patients with fistulae were administered continual infusions with somatostatin, and two men were treated with a local Salofalk enema. The closure of fistulae, diameter of the intestine, laboratory results, subjective complaints and clinical findings were evaluated.

On the basis of the results, the following conclusions were drawn:

1. Surgery is indicated in 20% of patients.
2. Prerequisite to successful therapy of fistulae in patients with Crohn's disease is a complete parenteral infusion + corticotherapy.
3. Continual infusions with somatostatin do not affect the rate of fistular closure.
4. Endoscopic pneumatic dilatation of stenoses in anastomoses is a therapeutic modality of choice.
5. Local application of Salofalk enema reduces the number of endoscopic dilatations.
6. Conservative therapeutic modalities applied to patients are evaluated in detail and if necessary.

D7

Natural history of perianal fistulae in Crohn's disease – 2-year results of a prospective study

M. STARLINGER, F. MAKOWIEC, M. WEINLICH and H. D. BECKER

Perianal fistulae occur in more than half of patients with Crohn's disease. The natural course of the fistulae is thought to be benign; however, prospective data to substantiate this theory are lacking. The aim of the study was to evaluate the course of perianal disease, the inactivation and healing of fistulae and recurrence of fistula activity.

METHODS

Eighty-nine consecutive patients with perianal fistulae seen in a specialized Crohn's disease clinic were followed prospectively (clinically, rectoscopy, endosonography, nuclear magnetic resonance, NMR) at regular intervals. Fistula activity was defined as presence of purulent discharge and/or pain. Rectal disease activity was assessed by rectoscopy. Deep perianal abscesses were identified by endosonography and NMR. Active fistulae and abscesses were treated by seton or catheter drainage. Healing of fistulae was defined as closure of the fistula for more than 1 month duration. Median observation time was 14 months. Results were calculated by life-table analysis.

RESULTS

Fifty-five patients had active fistulae, 34 patients inactive fistulae at study entrance. Drainage of active disease resulted in inactivation in 50% of the patients within 6 weeks and in 80% within 12 weeks. The probability of fistula healing was 20% after 1 year. One year after inactivation, the probability of recurrent fistula activity was 52%. Recurrence rate depended on the type of fistula (subcutaneous 20%, trans-sphincteric 50% and complex fistulae 65%), but not on rectal disease activity or the presence of a stool-deviating ostomy.

DISCUSSION

Whereas conservative treatment (drainage) of perianal fistulae in patients with Crohn's disease results in a relatively rapid resolution of symptoms, the chance of healing is small. Half of the patients have a symptomatic recurrence within 1 year, irrespective of a disease activity in the rectum or the presence of a diverting ostomy. Whether a more aggressive treatment is able to change this natural course remains to be determined.

D8

Crohn's disease of gastroduodenum

Z. BENEŠ, V. KRTEK, I. LÍBALOVÁ and M. DUBOVSKÁ

Crohn's disease can affect practically the whole gastrointestinal tract, but there are localities which are affected very rarely; they include the gastroduodenal area. It is stated that effects in the stomach occur in 1–5% of all cases.

Clinical difficulties rely mainly on the extent of affliction. They can be quite inconspicuous or significant; sometimes symptoms are similar to ulcerous disease of the stomach. The affliction of Crohn's disease is also connected with other localities. It can occur in stomach as primary affliction of Crohn's disease or the involvement can be secondary, such as the consequence of continuous disease of small bowel. Stomach changes occur most often in the pylorobulbar area. In the macroscopic picture we can see aphthae or ulcerations of various sizes. Sometimes it is possible to observe a polypoid mucosa.

Various intensified infiltrative stomach changes leading to stenosis can be seen. They can also imitate malignant changes, especially by X-ray examination. Gastroscopy with biopsy is the decisive examination. The final diagnosis can sometimes be confirmed only by surgery, mainly in patients with long-term non-healing ulcers or infiltrative inflammation of stomach mucosa with obscure biopsy findings.

We present here our own experiences with diagnostic Crohn's disease of stomach; the data are from three patients (two women and one man). The stomach locality of Crohn's disease with affliction of small bowel was found in two patients, and one isolated form of stomach of Crohn's disease was found.

D9

Ulcerative colitis in the elderly

J. HOCH, F. ANTOS, Z. JECH and P. SLAUF

While the frequency of ulcerative colitis (UC) in older patients is high in western countries, this entity is rare in Czechoslovakia until now. The severity of the disease, its location, symptoms and prognosis are different in young people and in the old. Older patients with UC may be more likely to suffer from a severe initial attack, expressed also with higher mortality. Grave complications such as toxic megacolon or perforation occur in the elderly more frequently than in younger patients. Contrary to that the response to medical therapy after OMGE survey is better in the elderly.

From the surgical point of view we describe our own experience. We treated nine patients with UC in both our departments in 1991. They all were over 70, the oldest was 79. The initial attack of UC was discovered in six patients. Inflammatory bowel disease (IBD) history occurred in three patients, but they had been treated irregularly or not at all during the past 10 years. Typical signs of colitis were noted in eight patients. One patient suffered from stubborn constipation. Due to the seriousness of their condition they were admitted and intensive conservative treatment by surgery was necessary in six patients, in five for toxic megacolon, and in one for bowel perforation. No surgery was performed electively. Subtotal colectomies and ileostomies were done. The rectal stump was blindly closed and in two patients pulled out in the form of a mucous fistula. The death of a 79-year-old man from pulmonary embolism was the only serious complication; the others healed without problems.

The whole large bowel was involved in all operated patients. In three patients successfully treated in a conservative way only the distal segment was involved.

Mesalazine, both peroraly and rectally, has been administered to such patients until now. Only Salofalk suppository administration is sufficient in patients who underwent surgery.

The key point of UC in the elderly is influenced by early diagnosis and treatment. Risk of surgery is influenced more by age and presence of concomitant disease than by UC alone. We consider the vital prognosis of the older patient with UC to be favourable if we succeed with conservative or surgical treatment of the initial attack of the illness.

The presence of an intestinal stenosis in Crohn's disease does not predict perforating complications

F. MAKOWIEC, M. STARLINGER and H. D. BECKER

Perforating complications leading to surgery in Crohn's disease are associated with higher morbidity and mortality than non-perforating complications. According to a current hypothesis perforating complications (abscess, fistula, free perforation) are facilitated by the presence of an intestinal stenosis. To test this hypothesis we evaluated the occurrence of perforating (P) and obstructing (ileus/subileus; O) complications and the predictive value of an intestinal stenosis on the appearance of both types of complications in 384 patients.

METHODS

The charts of 492 patients with Crohn's disease (mean follow-up 5.2 years) were reviewed. To assess the prognostic value of a stenosis (endoscopically/radiologically proven) at time of diagnosis for the development of a subsequent complication, patients with surgery within 3 months after diagnosis were excluded ($n = 108$). The probabilities for the occurrence of complications were calculated using survival analysis.

RESULTS

One hundred and thirty patients (34%) had intestinal surgery. Of these 62 (48%) had an O-, 18 (14%) a P-, and 12 (9%) both O- and P-complication. Forty per cent of the patients with P-complications had simultaneous O-complications, but only 17% with O-complications had experienced a P-complication. At the time of diagnosis 143 patients (37%) showed stenosing lesions. The 5-year probabilities for complications requiring surgery (all), for O- and for P-complications are given in Table 1.

Patients with stenosis at time of diagnosis had a higher risk for surgery (overall) and for an obstruction, but not for a perforating complication. Only one of six obstructions was associated with a P-complication. Patients with P-complications do not more often have an obstruction than all patients operated on. The presence of an intestinal stenosis early in the disease course does not favour the development of a perforating complication.

Table 1

Stenosing lesion	Type of complication		
	All	*O*	*P*
Yes	43%	42%	20%
No	32%	29%	18%
p	<0.01	<0.01	n.s.

CONCLUSIONS

Stenotic lesions promote perforating complications in some but not all patients with Crohn's disease. A treatment policy aimed at the prophylactic operation of a stenosis to prevent a perforation does not seem justified.

D11

Perforating and non-perforating complications in Crohn's disease – no difference in postoperative course

F. MAKOWIEC, H. D. BECKER and M. STARLINGER

Perforating Crohn's disease was reported to represent an aggressive form of the disease with a short preoperative disease duration, higher postoperative recurrence rate and repeated perforating complications as indication for reoperation. To test this hypothesis we evaluated the disease course of primary perforating or non-perforating Crohn's disease in 492 patients with a mean follow-up of 5.2 years.

METHODS

A total of 238 patients had primary surgery during the study period. Indications for surgery were classified as perforating (abscess, fistula, free perforation; P) or non-perforating (NP). Symptomatic postoperative recurrence was defined as need for therapy because of an acute flare-up of the disease, reoperation as need for a second operation because of recurrent Crohn's disease. Reoperation rate was analysed by actuarial methods.

RESULTS

Seventy-three patients (30.7%) had a P-complication and 165 patients (69.3%) a NP-complication at primary surgery. Both groups were comparable for age and disease location. Patients with a P-complication had a shorter preoperative disease duration than patients with a NP-complication (median 3.6 vs 10.9 months; $p < 0.05$). A symptomatic recurrence occurred in 7/73 patients (9.6%) with P-complication and in 30/165 patients (18.2%) with NP-complication (n.s.). The 5-year reoperation rate was 19.8% (P) and 21.3% (NP; n.s.). Thirty-nine patients were reoperated (14 with P and 25 with NP at primary surgery). The indication for reoperation (P or NP) showed no significant correlation to the indication for primary surgery in these patients.

CONCLUSION

The presence of a perforating complication may characterize an initial aggressive form of Crohn's disease but has no prognostic relevance for the later course of the disease.

D12

Lactase activity in duodenal mucosa in Crohn's disease after right hemicolectomy with milk intolerance syndrome

J. KOCIÁNOVÁ and Z. LOJDA

In a group of 67 patients with Crohn's disease hemicolectomy and resection of terminal ileum was performed.

In 27 patients (40%) after this operation lactose intolerance on milk products appeared.

In 11 patients of this group gastroduodenojejunoscopy (JFB_4) was performed and bioptic specimens were taken from the third part of the duodenum and from the jejunum. The specimens were processed by histochemical methods.

By this method we have found various degrees of lactase deficiency in the mucosa of duodenum and jejunum.

D13

Preoperative diagnosis of perianal fistulae in Crohn's disease: nuclear magnetic resonance versus clinical examination

M. WEINLICH, F. MAKOWIEC and M. STARLINGER

Perianal fistulae in Crohn's disease are frequently characterized by complex fistula tracts and deep abscess formation which are often difficult to identify by simple clinical examination. In this prospective study we examined the value of nuclear magnetic resonance (NMR) imaging in the preoperative diagnosis of complex perianal Crohn's disease.

METHODS

In 36 patients with active perianal Crohn's disease (abscess, purulent discharge), clinical examination including rectoscopy was compared with the results of an NMR examination. To assess their diagnostic value, both were then compared with the intraoperative findings.

RESULTS

Fistulae

Clinical examination and NMR showed identical findings in 10 patients. Subcutaneous fistulae could not be identified by NMR in three patients. With NMR, deep, complex fistulae could be identified in 18 patients. They were missed by clinical examination in five of these patients (28%).

Abscesses

All abscesses found intraoperatively were diagnosed preoperatively by NMR ($n = 20$). They were not identified by clinical examination in seven patients (35%).

DISCUSSION

NMR imaging plays an important role in preoperative diagnosis of complex fistulae and deep abscess formation in patients with perianal Crohn's disease. The NMR offers exact localization of fistulae and abscesses without irradiation or contrast medium. As a non-invasive diagnostic mean NMR allows detection of deep perianal abscesses and complex fistulae which cannot be identified by clinical and rectoscopic examination in one-third of the patients.

D14

Quality of life in Crohn's disease: patient experience and satisfaction after drug or surgical treatment

S. SHIVANANDA

Despite advances in the past 20 years in diagnosis and management, Crohn's disease remains one of the major challenges in clinical medicine today. Much attention has been given to the assessment of laboratory parameters consequent to these advances, but few reports have examined the quality of life of patients with this disease in comparison to those without the disease. We investigated this question in a retrospective case–control epidemiological study at the University Hospital Rotterdam 'Dijkzigt' in the Netherlands.

The study population in the survey consisted of 120 cases with established Crohn's disease and 75 neighbourhood controls with similar age, sex and social class and no prior history of chronic gastrointestinal complaints. They were interviewed by trained interviewers using a structured questionnaire. The questionnaire was designed in consultation with the patients' association for colitis and Crohn's disease in the Netherlands and using measures of quality of life discussed at an international workshop in Uppsala.

Of the 120 patients, 73% had some complaints even when the disease was in remission, this figure rising to 97% during reactivation. Most complaints were related to difficulties in the social domain such as coping with work, friends and family, and this was reflected in a significantly higher divorce rate ($p < 0.03$) among cases than controls. Seventy-seven per cent of the patients felt the disease had influenced the quality of their lives and this was independent of the extent, duration or disease severity. Patients' evaluation of the benefits of surgery on quality of life declined rapidly with reoperation and inversely their estimation of drug treatment improved. Surgery clearly improved levels of activity but patients had significantly greater problems with employment than controls. Persistence of abdominal pain, chronic tiredness without underlying cause and a cluster of other problems such as anxiety and depression interfered with the personal, domestic and occupational life of the patient. Patient satisfaction after drug or surgery treatment reported in this study suggests a need for reassessment of the relative benefits of these therapeutic measures in the long-term management of Crohn's disease.

Acknowledgement

The authors wish to thank the National Institute of Public Health of the Government of the Netherlands for financial support of this investigation.

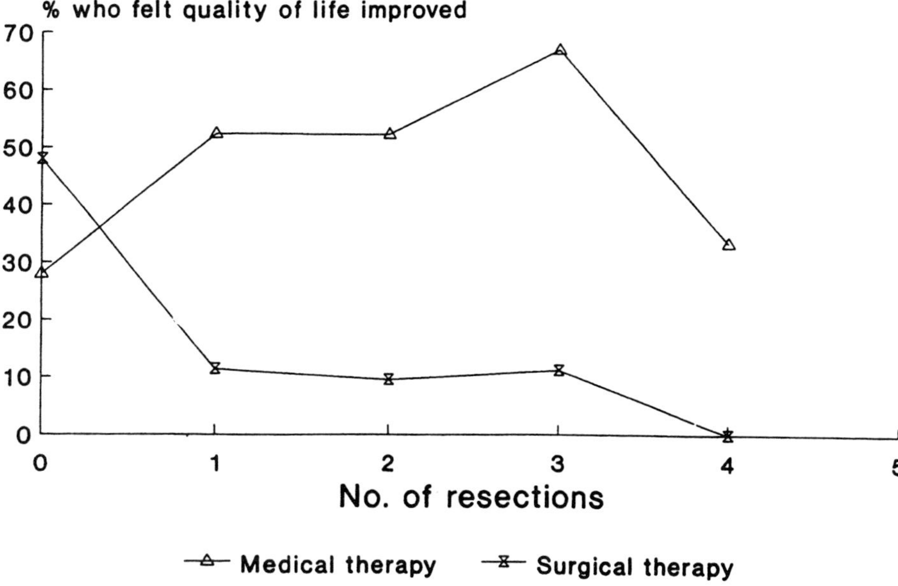

Fig. 1 Patients' perception of the value of medication or surgery on quality of life. Patients' evaluation of the benefits of surgery declined rapidly after the first resection and subsequently remained uniformly low; however, their estimation of drug treatment improved and remained significantly better ($\chi^2 = 34$, $p < 0.001$)

D15

Small intestinal transit of oral mesalazine (5-ASA) from a microsphere preparation in humans

J. KELLER, P. LAYER, U. KLOTZ and H. GOEBELL

Delivery of mesalazine (5-aminosalicylic acid, 5-ASA) from an enteric coated microsphere preparation (Pentasa®) to different small intestinal sites following oral administration was studied in six healthy volunteers who were intubated with an 11-lumen oro-ileal tube for marker perfusion and aspiration from the duodenal, mid-jejunal and terminal ileal lumen.

Subjects swallowed two capsules of Pentasa® (total 5-ASA dose 500 mg) together with a semi-liquid test meal. Intraluminal concentrations of 5-ASA and its main metabolite acetyl-5-ASA (ac-5-ASA) were measured by high-performance liquid chromatography at each intestinal site, in plasma and in urine for 400 min, and deliveries to intestinal sites were calculated using recovery marker techniques.

RESULTS

5-ASA was delivered to the duodenum, together with the meal marker, suggesting approximately parallel gastric emptying. Urinary excretion was 17.6 ± 2.2 mg in 7 h (98% acetylated).

	Duodenum	Jejunum	Ileum	Plasma
Plateau concentration $\pm$ SE				
5-ASA (µg/ml)	52 ± 5	59 ± 17	64 ± 13	0.06 ± 0.03
ac-5-ASA (µg/ml)	38 ± 13	82 ± 4	104 ± 8	0.34 ± 0.04
Plateau duration $\pm$ SE (min)	170 ± 27	180 ± 28	203 ± 27	>300
Amount in solution				
5-ASA (% of dose)	10.7	9.2	8.1	
ac-5-ASA (% of dose)	6.4	13.3	12.1	

SUMMARY

Gastric emptying of a 5-ASA microsphere preparation occurred together with the meal. Intraluminal 5-ASA concentration increased from proximal to distal intestinal sites, while substantial 5-ASA release occurred in the duodenal lumen. Fifty per cent of liberated luminal 5-ASA was as the acetylated metabolite. The intraluminal kinetics, the small proportion of urinary excretion and the low plasma levels suggest that the major part of the dose remained unabsorbed by the small intestine and reached the large bowel.

CONCLUSION

The relatively high intraluminal 5-ASA concentration throughout the small bowel following oral administration of this prepartion may be of importance in the treatment of small intestinal Crohn's disease.

D16

Strictureplasty in the treatment of Crohn's disease

F. ANTOŠ, J. HOCH and P. ŠLAUF

Strictureplasty is one of the surgical alternative methods for resection of the diseased bowel. The indications for strictureplasty are not very broad, and this operative method still is seldom used in Czechoslovakia.

According to our experience with structureplasty performed in 13 cases (altogether 24 strictureplasties) we can conclude that this operative method, when used in the right circumstances, is very useful, and gives the patient the chance of further conservative treatment – e.g. Salofalk.

Modulatory effects of anti-inflammatory drugs on cytokine release by monocytes from patients with inflammatory bowel disease

H.-G. LESER, V. GROSS, T. ANDUS, H. FENNER and
J. SCHÖLMERICH

Mononuclear phagocytes seem to play a pivotal role in the pathophysiology of inflammatory bowel disease (IBD). We have recently shown (*Gastroenterology*, 1991, **100**, A593) that the release of inflammatory mediators such as IL-1, IL-6, and TNF from monocytes of patients with IBD can be modulated by a new IL-1 response modifier (Ro 31-3948). In this study we performed a comparative analysis on the effects of anti-inflammatory drugs such as 5-aminosalicylic acid (5-ASA, 630 µg/ml), sulphasalazine (SAS, 1.2 mg/ml), Ro 31-3948 (100 µg/ml), and beclomethasone (BM, 10^{-6} and 10^{-9} mol/l) on the cytokine release from monocytes of patients with IBD ($n = 7$) and healthy controls ($n = 10$).

Isolated monocytes were cultured for 24 h *in vitro* with or without endotoxin (LPS 10 pg–100 ng/ml) to stimulate monokine release. Spontaneous and LPS-induced cytokine production was measured in monocyte supernatants by enzyme-linked immunoadsorbent assay (IL-1, TNF) and B9 cell assay (IL-6), respectively. LPS induced the expected dose-dependent increase of IL-1, IL-6, and TNF production in monocytes from healthy controls. In comparison, LPS induced production of IL-1 and TNF was even more pronounced in monocytes of IBD patients. Addition of Ro 31-3948, BM 10^{-6} and 10^{-9} mol/l did not lead to significant inhibition of LPS induced IL-6 production by monocytes either from healthy persons or from IBD patients, whereas 5-ASA and SAS led to inhibition of IL-6 production in both groups. In contrast, all tested drugs inhibited spontaneous and LPS-induced IL-1 production in monocytes of patients with IBD, but only 5-ASA, SAS and BM 10^{-6} mol/l did so in healthy controls. In addition, spontaneous and LPS-induced TNF production was inhibited by all tested drugs in monocytes from IBD patients, but only by 5-ASA, SAS and BM 10^{-6} mol/l in monocytes of healthy controls.

In conclusion, our data suggest that anti-inflammatory drugs already used in the treatment of IBD have different inhibitory effects on the cytokine release of activated monocytes of patients with IBD, in contrast to control persons.

D18

Oral slow-release budesonide induces remission in active Crohn's disease with little effect on adrenal function

M. ROTH, B. UEBERSCHAER, K. EWE, V. GROSS and
J. SCHÖLMERICH

Corticosteroids are the cornerstone of treatment for active Crohn's disease (CD). However, they induce significant side-effects due to their systemic action. Furthermore, they suppress the hypothalamic–pituitary–adrenal axis (HPA). Budesonide, due to a very high first-pass effect in the liver has low systemic bioavailability. It has been used successfully as enema in active distal ulcerative colitis.

In order to test its potential in active CD we studied the effect of 9 mg oral budesonide daily in a slow-release preparation in nine patients. All patients responded with a decrease of the Crohn's disease activity index (CDAI) from initially 278 ± 63 to 114 ± 109 after 2 weeks and 96 ± 94 after 4 weeks. Three patients (one with interenteric fistulae and abscess, one with a rectovaginal fistula and interenteric conglomerate tumour and one with systemic extraintestinal manifestations) presented with an increase of the CDAI during continued therapy, requiring surgery and/or treatment with methylprednisolone. In one patient a slight increase of the CDAI (up to 90) occurred after week 4; upper endoscopy revealed stomach involvement.

In six patients a cortisol-releasing factor (CRF) test was done before and after 6 weeks. Basal cortisol was decreased after treatment in five of six patients (initial: 160 ± 41 ng/ml; 6 weeks 33 ± 43 ng/ml). The increase of plasma cortisol after CRF test was preserved in all patients except in one who had a rather high basal value (271 ng/ml) after treatment.

We conclude that budesonide shows a comparable effect as conventional steroids with regard to treatment. It somewhat suppresses basal cortisol at the dose used, but the HPA is still functioning. This drug requires further intensive study in controlled trials.

D19

Selective decontamination of digestive tract as treatment of cholestasis in patients on long-term parenteral nutrition

Th. MAIER-DOBERSBERGER, M. RUDAS, H. VOGELSANG and H. LOCHS

Cholestasis is a common complication in total parenteral nutrition (TPN) of patients with very short bowel syndrome (VSBS). It may be caused by bacterial translocation from the digestive tract.

We report on three female patients (ages 31, 32 and 37 years) who had VSBS because of multiple resections due to Crohn's disease. After approximately 1 year of home parenteral nutrition all three patients developed increasing cholestasis (serum alkaline phosphatase 510, 290 and 876 U/l and serum bilirubin 2.09, 1.03 and 3.0 mg/dl, respectively). Furthermore signs of infection (fever, leucocytosis) and positive blood cultures (*Candida albicans, Enterococcus faecalis* and *Enterobacter cloacae*) could be found. All patients were treated with selective decontamination of digestive tract (2 × 80 mg gentamicin and 4 × 6 ml amphotericin orally per day).

Laboratory tests and clinical symptoms were normalized without intravenous chemotherapy by selective decontamination of digestive tract (SDD) in all three patients.

In patient 1 SDD was discontinued after 6 months and the condition of the patient deteriorated; she eventually died of sepsis. Histology showed cholestatic fibrosis and infectious infiltration of the liver. In the other two patients SDD is still given, and both have normal liver function tests. Our data indicate that cholestasis in VSBS patients on long-term TPN can be caused by bacterial translocation from the digestive tract. We therefore recommend long-term SDD as concomitant therapy in these patients.

D20

Specific increase of colonic Na^+ pump activities after short-term treatment with topical steroids in inflammatory bowel disease (IBD)

C. SCHEURLEN, H. ALLGAYER, W. KRUIS and R. GUGLER

Topical administration of steroids quickly improves diarrhoeal symptoms in patients with left-sided IBD. To study these therapeutic actions in more detail we measured colonic Na^+ pump activities i.e. $(Na^+ + K^+)$-ATPase and specific $[^3H]$ouabain binding (sp^3H) (representing the number of enzyme molecules) in IBD patients before and after treatment (3 days) with topical steroids.

Sigmoidoscopy with biopsy sampling was performed in 19 patients (six with Crohn's disease, five with ulcerative colitis, eight with normal mucosa) before and after treatment with hydrocortisone acetate enemas (100 mg b.i.d.). Inflammation was assessed macroscopically and histologically. $(Na^+ + K^+)$-ATPase was defined as the ouabain inhibitable (1 mmol/l) portion of the total ATPase. Mg^{2+} was calculated from the difference between the two activities. sp^3H was measured with the rapid filtration technique.

Topical steroid treatment increased colonic $(Na^+ + K^+)$-ATPase both in controls (from $5.07 \pm 0.85\,\mu$mol Pi/mg per hour to 11.37 ± 0.04; $x \pm$ SEM) and in diseased patients (from 3.16 ± 0.38 to 6.40 ± 1.43; $p < 0.05$). sp^3H was increased by 160% from 0.18 ± 0.01 pmol/mg to 0.24 ± 0.04 in controls and from 0.11 ± 0.02 to 0.21 ± 0.04 in IBD ($p < 0.05$). In contrast, Mg^{2+}-ATPase remained unchanged, as well as macroscopic and histological signs of inflammation.

Our study shows that one of the early treatment effects of topical steroids in IBD is the specific increase of colonic Na^+-pump activities partially due to an increased number of pump sites as sp^3H was enhanced. These observations support the view that topical steroids may have therapeutic effects on mucosal function even before they lead to a decrease of local inflammation.

Renal–tubular damage in patients with inflammatory bowel disease treated with 5-aminosalicylic acid and sulphasalazine

E. ZEHNTER, H. DÖRHÖFER, D. J. ZIEGENHAGEN, C. SCHEURLEN,
C. A. BALDAMUS and W. KRUIS

There are some case reports on renal dysfunction in patients with IBD under either 5-aminosalicylic acid (5-ASA) or sulphasalazine (SASP). To answer the question whether medical treatment of IBD may cause impairment of renal function we examined 48 consecutive patients (20 male, 28 female, age 18–55 years, 34 Crohn's disease (CD), 14 ulcerative colitis (UC)) who either received 5-ASA ($n = 20$), or SASP ($n = 11$), or steroids ($n = 7$) or none ($n = 10$).

MEASUREMENTS

We measured blood creatinine, blood urea, the excretion of protein, albumin, gamma-glutamyl-transpeptidase (γGT), alkaline phosphatase (AP), β-N-acetyl-glucosaminidase (NAG), α_1-microglobulin (α_1-M) in the urine. We also made urine stix and performed a SDS-PAGE of the urine aliquots.

RESULTS

All patients had normal values for blood creatinine, urea and a normal urine stix. None of the parameters determined showed any significant differences between CD and UC, active or inactive patients or with respect to disease duration. Different therapeutic modalities did not influence the excretion of protein, albumen, α_1-M and NAG. The excretion of the tubular enzyme AP was significantly higher in the patients who received either 5-ASA or SASP, γ-GT showed a trend to higher values. The patients treated with these drugs had a higher number of pathological SDS-PAGEs, demonstrating a pattern indicative for tubular alterations (Table 1).

Pathology findings	5-ASA/SASP	others
γ-GT (U/mmol creatinine)	3.08 ± 1.69	2.20 ± 1.11
NAG (U/mmol creatinine)	0.38 ± 0.30	0.18 ± 0.13
AP (U/mmol creatinine)	1.44 ± 1.33*	0.49 ± 0.31* $p < 0.01$

SDS-PAGE

Seventeen patients showed a pathological SDS-PAGE, 15 of the 5-ASA/SASP group. All patients with a tubular proteinuria belonged to the 5-ASA/SASP group.

CONCLUSIONS

Despite normal values of creatinine, urea and a normal urine stix, more sensitive tests showed evidence for tubular damage in a considerable number of patients with IBD. Renal dysfunction showed a relationship to treatment with 5-ASA and SASP.

Therefore in patients with IBD treated with 5-ASA or SASP control of renal function should include not only standard tests but also additional investigations such as SDS-PAGE or enzyme excretion.

Crohn Study V: Results of a trial with n-3 PUFAs or carbohydrate-reduced diet for maintenance of remission in Crohn's disease

H. LORENZ-MEYER, J. PURRMANN, C. SCHEURLEN,
M. SCHEURLEN, W. B. FLEIG, P. BAUER, C. MASCHLER,
B. SCHULZ and L. CARR

There is no established therapy for maintaining remission in patients with Crohn's disease. n-3 PUFAs have been shown to possess anti-inflammatory effects in patients suffering from ulcerative colitis. Additionally epidemiological studies suggest that patients' eating habits may play a causative role in Crohn's disease. Thus both potential interventions for maintaining remission were tested using either 5 g/day of a highly concentrated n-3 PUFA compound or a carbohydrate-reduced diet (72 g/day).

A total of 204 patients were recruited in 23 participating centres. Patients were included after an acute relapse of their disease in which remission (CDAI < 150) was attained under steroid therapy. Patients were randomized to receive either 3 PUFAs ($n = 70$), placebo ($n = 65$) or diet ($n = 69$). Low-dose prednisolone was given to all patients for the first 8 weeks of intervention and then discontinued. Follow-up visits were initially at monthly intervals, followed by 3-month intervals for 1 year. CDAI and CRP were used as test criteria. Patients were asked to document their eating habits for 3 days prior to each follow-up visit.

Patient visits, mailings and telephone contacts by a diet specialist served to monitor patient compliance. Intention-to-treat analysis of the data was performed using Kaplan–Meier life tables.

RESULTS

Intention-to-treat analysis and analysis of only those patients adhering to the protocol, did not reveal a significant effect of n-3 PUFAs on extending remission in Crohn's disease. Patients able to maintain a carbohydrate-reduced diet, however, did gain benefit from the diet taken in the framework of a trial and patient care provided ($p < 0.05$). The diet group, however, contained the highest numbers of drop-outs (20 of 69). Intention-to-treat analysis of the diet group showed no significant difference from placebo. The question still remains as to whether these patients dropped out early because they sensed a relapse approaching, or whether their condition deteriorated because they failed to comply with the dietary guidelines.

D23

Morbus Crohn – ergebnisse aus 20 Jahren chirurgischer Therapie

H. KESSLER and F. P. GALL

Die Analyse von 505 Patienten der Chirurgischen Universitätsklinik Erlangen, bei denen zwischen dem 1.1.1970 und dem 1.1.1990 insgesamt 567 Darmresektionen wegen eines Morbus Crohn durchgeführt wurden, läßt Wandel in Indikationsstellung und Operationsverfahren erkennen. Bei einer Unterteilung des Gesamtzeitraums in drei gleiche Abschnitte fällt unter den Komplikationen vor Operation eine Zunahme der Patienten mit Mangelernährung von 13% im Zeitabschnitt 1970 bis 77 auf 33% während der Jahre 1984 bis 1990 auf. Ebenso waren Patienten mit einer Stenose als führendem Symptom im letzten Zeitraum mit 53% gegenüber 2% im Abschnitt 1970 bis 77 stark gehäuft. Dies spiegelt den Trend zu längerer konservativer Therapie wieder. Gleichzeitig findet sich ein Trend zur begrenzten Darmresektion. Wurde in den Jahren 1970 bis 77 noch in 28.7% eine Rektumexstirpation mit evtl. Colektomie durchgeführt, so sank diese Rate im Zeitraum 1984 bis 90 auf 7.1%. Insgesamt verminderte sich die Rate ausgedehnter Resektionen während beider oben genannter Zeiträume von 70% auf 31%, während gleichzeitig die Häufigkeit limitierter Resektionen von 11% auf 37% anstieg. Die durchschnittliche resezierte Länge des Dünndarms sank von 50.6 cm auf 35.6 cm, des Dickdarms von 46.9 cm auf 24.9 cm. Gleichzeitig ging die Rate postoperativer Komplikationen wie Anastomoseninsuffizienz von 2.7% auf 0.9% zurück, die Häufigkeit letaler Komplikationen von 7.1% auf 0.5%. Dennoch sollte das Vorhandensein deutlicher aktiver Crohnläsionen am Resektionsrand vermieden werden. In einer Follow-up-Untersuchung (medianer Nachbeobachtungszeitraum 7.2 Jahre) waren Spätrezidive mit 37.8% bei aktivem Crohn am Resektionsrand bei der primären Resektion deutlich häufiger, als wenn der Resektionsrand keine (21.3%) oder nur minimale Crohnläsionen (22.7%) aufwies. Die Strikturoplastik (n = 43) konnte ohne postoperative Komplikationen und Letalität erfolgreich in das Therapiekonzept aufgenommen werden; im Follow-up traten keine Rezidive am Ort der primären Strikturoplastik auf, langfristig waren 83% der Patienten beschwerdefrei.

D24

Bioavailability of hydrocortisone after rectal administration in healthy volunteers

J. BARTH, T. WAGNER, S. TUNN, A. TROMM, H. DERENDORF, M. KRIEG, H. MÖLLMANN and G. HOCHHAUS

The topical treatment of distal ulcerative colitis with corticosteroids is based on the concept that a high activity of the steroid can be produced at the site of administration. In addition the degree of systemic side-effects can be minimized because of a low absorption of the steroid.

Retention enemas and a foam preparation of hydrocortisone acetate (HC-A) are frequently used steroids for this purpose. As yet, however, there is only little information about the absorption rate of hydrocortisone (HC) from the rectum; even more, only a few studies have been published to address the absolute bioavailability (BA) of HC after systemic administration. To have information on this parameter is a prerequisite to calculate and compare bioavailabilities after different modes of drug application.

METHODS

The pharmacokinetics and BA of HC were determined after intravenous injection (20 mg HC), oral administration (20 mg HC tablets), and single rectal administration (100 mg HC-A as foam preparation) given to healthy volunteers ($n = 8$ each group, intraindividual study design). Endogenous cortisol was suppressed totally by dexamethasone; plasma levels of HC were determined with a sensitive RIA, the data were subjected to compartmental and non-compartmental pharmacokinetic analysis.

RESULTS

After i.v. administration HC was eliminated with a total body clearance of 18 l/h. Oral BA averaged 96%. After rectal administration the absolute BA was only about 2% and maximal HC levels – reached after 2 h – were extremely low (24–35 ng HC/ml compared to 300 mg after oral application).

CONCLUSIONS

From the data it can be concluded that in healthy subjects, and after single administration of HC foam, only a very small part of the rectal dose was absorbed. The determined plasma levels were 10-fold lower than those obtained after oral administration of a 5-fold lower dose. The induction of systemic side-effects by those low levels seems unlikely.

D25

Systemic absorption from hydrocortisone acetate rectal foam after single and multiple administration in healthy volunteers

Th. WAGNER, J. BARTH, A. TROMM, S. TUNN, M. KRIEG, H. DERENDORF and H. MÖLLMANN

The rationale for administration of a corticosteroid by the topical route is that the side-effects associated with the systemic administration may be decreased or avoided because the drug is administered directly to the target organ in total amounts smaller than used systemically. Recently published studies demonstrate clinical efficacy of rectal applied hydrocortisone acetate foam (HCA) in the treatment of chronic inflammatory bowel diseases. Only a little is known about the degree of systemic absorption of HCA after single and multiple administration.

METHODS

The degree of hydrocortisone absorption after rectal application of a hydrocortisone acetate foam was determined after single, twice and four times a day administration of 100 mg hydrocortisone acetate in 5 ml foam in eight to 10 healthy volunteers. Endogenous cortisol secretion was suppressed during the study to < 10 ng/ml by oral administration of 4 mg dexamethasone at 10 p.m. the day before. Plasma hydrocortisone concentrations were measured by radioimmunoassay and corrected to the individual pre-dose levels (mean pre-dose level $= 8.3 \pm 1.3$ ng/ml). The area under the plasma–time curve (AUC) was calculated using the trapezoidal rule.

RESULTS

The single rectal administration of hydrocortisone acetate leads to very low systemic steroid levels. The AUC was 109 ± 45 ng/h per ml. Maximum hydrocortisone levels of 35 ± 24 ng/ml were observed after 2.1 ± 0.9 h. For the twice a day treatment no accumulation could be observed, since almost all of the drug was eliminated before the second dose was applied. With the four times daily administration a slow increase of plasma steroid levels is produced. The maximum concentrations were after the first 20 ± 9 ng/ml, second 30 ± 10 ng/ml, third 39 ± 14 ng/ml and fourth application 42 ± 12 ng/ml, respectively.

CONCLUSIONS

From the data it can be concluded that rectal administration of hydrocortisone acetate foam in healthy volunteers leads only to a low systemic absorption. The biological bioavailability was nearly 2%. This kind of therapy is a safe application mode with respect to potential systemic side-effects, even if it is used manifold and at short time intervals.

D26

Pharmacokinetics and bioavailability of hydrocortisone after single and multiple rectal administration of hydrocortisone acetate foam in patients with distal chronic and inflammatory bowel diseases in comparison to healthy volunteers

H. W. MÖLLMANN, J. BARTH, A. TROMM, Ch. BIGALKE,
T. WAGNER, U. SCHWEGLER, S. TUNN, H. DERENDORF, M. KRIEG,
B. MAY and G. HOCHAUS

Local corticoid therapy of distal proctocolitis has been shown to be effective. Many patients prefer the foam to a liquid steroid enema because it is easier to handle and to retain, and causes less interference with social and occupational activities.

However, there is little information on the degree of systemic absorption of hydrocortisone acetate (HCA), after rectal administration. We have recently reported the pharmacokinetics of hydrocortisone (HC) after single and multiple administration of hydrocortisone acetate foam. The measured HC levels were 10-fold lower than those obtained after oral administration of a 5-fold lower dose (20 mg) of hydrocortisone in the same subjects.

METHODS

The pharmacokinetics of hydrocortisone after rectal administration of 100 mg hydrocortisone acetate (Colifoam®, Trommsdorf, Germany) in 26 patients were investigated and compared with data obtained after i.v. administration of a 20 mg dose (Hydrocortisone Hoechs®) and data obtained from healthy volunteers. For the multiple-dose studies the drug was administered in two different schedules: for the twice-a-day administration (b.i.d.) at 8 a.m. and 4 p.m. and for the four-times-a-day administration (q.i.d.) at 8 a.m., 11 a.m., 2 p.m. and 5 p.m. Hydrocortisone concentrations were measured by radioimmunoassay in serum and corrected for the individual pre-dose levels. The data were subjected to non-compartmental pharmacokinetic analysis.

RESULTS

Only a very small part of the rectal dose (100 mg) was absorbed. The mean absolute bioavailability was about 2%. There was substantial intersubject variability. Maximum hydrocortisone levels after single or multiple dose every 8 h were reached 2 h after dosing and ranged from 24 to 35 ng/ml. After multiple dosing every 3 h maximum concentrations were found 1.7 h after dosing and reached 42 ng/ml.

Pharmacokinetics after single and multiple rectal administration of hydrocortisone acetate in patients were nearly consistent with those obtained in healthy volunteers. Hydrocortisone levels after single rectal administration were very low. The AUC was 267.5 ng/h per ml and the average bioavailability 2.9%. For the b.i.d. treatment every 8 h no accumulation could be observed, since almost all of the drug was eliminated before the second dose. The mean maximum concentration after the first dose (64 ± 7 ng/ml) was not essentially different from that after the second dose (61 ± 12 ng/ml), and they both occurred after 3–4 h. The average area under the curve was 665.7 ng.h/ml. This corresponds to an average bioavailability of 3.7%.

For the q.i.d. treatment every 3 h plasma levels increased slowly. The maximum concentration for the 4-h doses were 45 ± 9, 55 ± 10, 63 ± 14, and 78 ± 12 ng/ml. These occurred after a t_{max} of 2.5, 2.5, 1.5 and 1.6 h, respectively. The area under the curve was 827.4 ng.h/ml. This corresponds to an average bioavailability of 2.3% (Table 1).

Table 1

Treatment	AUC (ng.h/ml), healthy volunteers	AUC (ng.h/ml), patients	Bioavailability (%), healthy volunteers	Bioavailability (%), patients
1 × 100 mg HCA	159.9	167.5	1.8	2.9
2 × 100 mg HCA	506.1	665.7	2.8	3.7
3 × 100 mg HCA	528.4	827.4	1.5	2.3

CONCLUSIONS

The plasma concentrations observed after single and multiple dosing in patients was slightly higher than in healthy volunteers. Due to the short half-life of hydrocortisone only a very low systemic accumulation can be expected, which is insignificant for side-effects. The extremely low bioavailability of $\sim 3\%$ in combination with positive clinical reports on the therapeutic effectiveness makes hydrocortisone acetate foam a very safe and suitable dosage form for local treatment of chronic inflammatory bowel diseases.

D27

Circa (semi) annual rhythms of ulcerative colitis and drug treatment

I. DURIS, M. HUORKA, J. PAYER, M. MIKULECKY and
I. TISCHLEROVA

A semiannual and annual history of attacks in ulcerative colitis was noted before sulphasalazine and corticosteroids were used in treatment (Ransaude *et al.*, 1939; Maratka, 1948). We were interested to see whether this periodicity would be present also under long-term therapy with these drugs. A total of 274 attacks of ulcerative colitis between 1974 and 1990 were processed by Fischer's periodogram and Halberg's cosinor analysis. The presence of 6- and 12-month periodicity and highly significant ($p < 0.001$) linearly increasing trend over 17 years was revealed. The fitted yearly plexogram (Fig. 1) displays two peaks in the monthly numbers of attacks: a higher one in March and a lower one in September.

Times of decreased resistance have been identified. Different results from various authors in evaluation of drug efficacy could be dependent on the period of the year at which they are used.

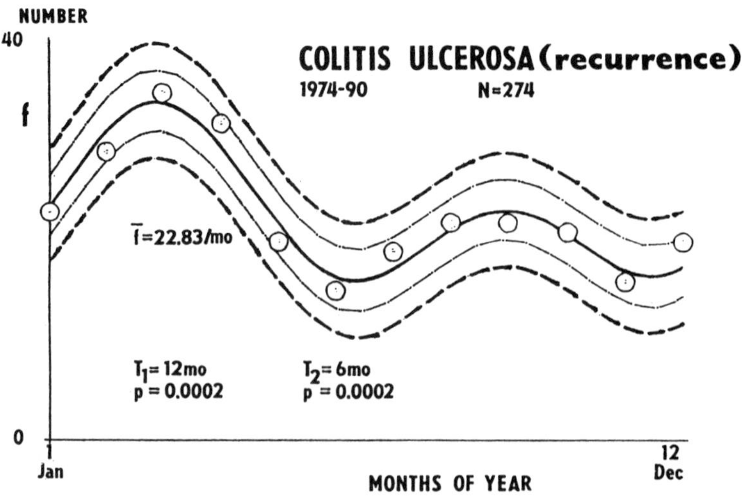

Fig. 1 Fitted annual plexogram with observed numbers of attacks (circles), 95% confidence (narrower) and 95% tolerance corridor.

Index